Essentials of Peritoneal Dialysis

Essentials of Peritoneal Dialysis

Edited by Abigail Lloyd

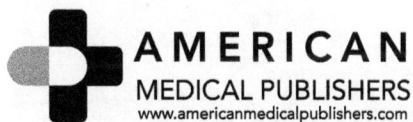

AMERICAN
MEDICAL PUBLISHERS
www.americanmedicalpublishers.com

American Medical Publishers,
41 Flatbush Avenue,
1st Floor, New York,
NY 11217, USA

Visit us on the World Wide Web at:
www.americanmedicalpublishers.com

ISBN: 978-1-63927-269-3

Cataloging-in-Publication Data

Essentials of peritoneal dialysis / edited by Abigail Lloyd.
     p. cm.
Includes bibliographical references and index.
ISBN 978-1-63927-269-3
1. Peritoneal dialysis. 2. Hemodialysis. 3. Dialysis. 4. Blood--Filtration. I. Lloyd, Abigail.
RC901.7.P48 E77 2022
617.461 059--dc23

Table of Contents

Preface...IX

Chapter 1 **Fluid Status in Peritoneal Dialysis Patients: The European Body Composition Monitoring (EuroBCM) Study Cohort** 1
Wim Van Biesen, John D. Williams, Adrian C. Covic, Stanley Fan, Kathleen Claes, Monika Lichodziejewska-Niemierko, Christian Verger, Jurg Steiger, Volker Schoder, Peter Wabel, Adelheid Gauly, Rainer Himmele

Chapter 2 **The Potential Role of HMGB1 Release in Peritoneal Dialysis-Related Peritonitis** 10
Shirong Cao, Shu Li, Huiyang Li, Liping Xiong, Yi Zhou, Jinjin Fan, Xueqing Yu, Haiping Mao

Chapter 3 **Aliskiren Prevents the Toxic Effects of Peritoneal Dialysis Fluids during Chronic Dialysis in Rats** 22
Juan Pérez-Martínez, Francisco C. Pérez-Martínez, Blanca Carrión, Jesús Masiá, Agustín Ortega, Esther Simarro, Syong H. Nam-Cha, Valentín Ceña

Chapter 4 **NFκB in the Development of Endothelial Activation and Damage in Uremia: An In Vitro Approach** 32
Carolina Caballo, Marta Palomo, Aleix Cases, Ana M. Galán, Patricia Molina, Manel Vera, Xavier Bosch, Gines Escolar, Maribel Diaz-Ricart

Chapter 5 **Prevalence and Risk Factors of Fluid Overload in Southern Chinese Continuous Ambulatory Peritoneal Dialysis Patients** 41
Qunying Guo, Chunyan Yi., Jianying Li, Xiaofeng Wu, Xiao Yang, Xueqing Yu

Chapter 6 **Good Glycemic Control is Associated with Better Survival in Diabetic Patients on Peritoneal Dialysis** 51
Dong Eun Yoo, Jung Tak Park, Hyung Jung Oh, Seung Jun Kim, Mi Jung Lee, Dong Ho Shin, Seung Hyeok Han, Tae-Hyun Yoo, Kyu Hun Choi, Shin-Wook Kang

Chapter 7 **Lean Body Mass Predicts Long-Term Survival in Chinese Patients on Peritoneal Dialysis** 59
Jenq-Wen Huang, Yu-Chung Lien, Hon-Yen Wu, Chung-Jen Yen, Chun-Chun Pan, Tsai-Wei Hung, Chi-Ting Su, Chih-Kang Chiang, Hui-Teng Cheng, Kuan-Yu Hung

Chapter 8 **Impact of Individual and Environmental Socioeconomic Status on Peritoneal Dialysis Outcomes** 65
Rong Xu, Qing-Feng Han, Tong-Ying Zhu, Ye-Ping Ren, Jiang-Hua Chen, Hui-Ping Zhao, Meng- Hua Chen, Jie Dong, Yue Wang, Chuan-Ming Hao, Rui Zhang, Xiao-Hui Zhang, Mei Wang, Na Tian, Hai-Yan Wang

Chapter 9 **Higher Peritoneal Protein Clearance as a Risk Factor for Cardiovascular Disease in Peritoneal Dialysis Patient** 73
Tae Ik Chang, Ea Wha Kang, Yong Kyu Lee, Sug Kyun Shin

Chapter 10   **Back to Basics: Pitting Edema and the Optimization of Hypertension Treatment in Incident Peritoneal Dialysis Patients (BRAZPD)**.. 80
Sebastião R. Ferreira-Filho, Gilberto R. Machado, Valéria C. Ferreira,
Carlos F. M. A. Rodrigues, Thyago Proença de Moraes, José C. Divino-Filho,
Marcia Olandoski, Christopher McIntyre, Roberto Pecoits-Filho

Chapter 11   **Seeking Clarity within Cloudy Effluents: Differentiating Fungal from Bacterial Peritonitis in Peritoneal Dialysis Patients**.. 86
Ruchir Chavada, Jen Kok, Sebastiaan van Hal, Sharon C-A. Chen

Chapter 12   **Laparoscopic versus Open Peritoneal Dialysis Catheter Insertion**.. 91
Sander M. Hagen, Jeffrey A. Lafranca, Ewout W. Steyerberg, Jan N. M. IJzermans,
Frank J. M. F. Dor

Chapter 13   **Predictors and Prevalence of Latent Tuberculosis Infection in Patients Receiving Long-Term Hemodialysis and Peritoneal Dialysis**.. 102
Chin-Chung Shu, Vin-Cent Wu, Feng-Jung Yang, Sung-Ching Pan, Tai-Shuan Lai,
Jann-Yuan Wang, Jann-Tay Wang, Li-Na Lee

Chapter 14   **Safety Issues of Long-Term Glucose Load in Patients on Peritoneal Dialysis**.. 108
Hon-Yen Wu, Kuan-Yu Hung, Tao-Min Huang, Fu-Chang Hu, Yu-Sen Peng,
Jenq-Wen Huang, Shuei-Liong Lin, Yung-Ming Chen, Tzong-Shinn Chu,
Tun-Jun Tsai, Kwan-Dun Wu

Chapter 15   **The Spectrum of Podoplanin Expression in Encapsulating Peritoneal Sclerosis**.. 115
Niko Braun, M. Dominik Alscher, Peter Fritz, Joerg Latus, Ilka Edenhofer,
Fabian Reimold, Seth L. Alper, Martin Kimmel, Dagmar Biegger,
Maja Lindenmeyer, Clemens D. Cohen, Rudolf P. Wüthrich, Stephan Segerer

Chapter 16   **Peritoneal Dialysis-Related Peritonitis due to *Staphylococcus aureus*: A Single-Center Experience over 15 Years**.. 125
Pasqual Barretti, Taíse M. C. Moraes, Carlos H. Camargo, Jacqueline C. T. Caramori,
Alessandro L. Mondelli, Augusto C. Montelli, Maria de Lourdes R. S. da Cunha

Chapter 17   **Transcriptional Patterns in Peritoneal Tissue of Encapsulating Peritoneal Sclerosis, a Complication of Chronic Peritoneal Dialysis**.. 132
Fabian R. Reimold, Niko Braun, Zsuzsanna K. Zsengellér, Isaac E. Stillman,
S. Ananth Karumanchi, Hakan R. Toka, Joerg Latus, Peter Fritz, Dagmar Biegger,
Stephan Segerer, M. Dominik Alscher, Manoj K. Bhasin, Seth L. Alper

Chapter 18   **The Associations between the Family Education and Mortality of Patients on Peritoneal Dialysis**.. 147
Zhi-Kai Yang, Qing-Feng Han, Tong-Ying Zhu, Ye-Ping Ren, Jiang-Hua Chen,
Hui-Ping Zhao, Meng-Hua Chen, Jie Dong, Yue Wang, Chuan- Ming Hao,
Rui Zhang, Xiao-Hui Zhang, Mei Wang, Na Tian, Hai-Yan Wang

Chapter 19   **Pneumonia and Mortality Risk in Continuous Ambulatory Peritoneal Dialysis Patients with Diabetic Nephropathy**.. 154
Feng He, Xianfeng Wu, Xi Xia, Fenfen Peng, Fengxian Huang, Xueqing Yu

Chapter 20   **The Associations of Uric Acid, Cardiovascular and All-Cause Mortality in Peritoneal Dialysis Patients**.. 161
Jie Dong, Qing-Feng Han, Tong-Ying Zhu, Ye-Ping Ren, Jiang-Hua Chen, Hui-Ping Zhao, Meng-Hua Chen, Rong Xu, Yue Wang, Chuan-Ming Hao, Rui Zhang, Xiao-Hui Zhang, Mei Wang, Na Tian, Hai-Yan Wang

Chapter 21   **High-Sensitivity C-Reactive Protein Predicts Mortality and Technique Failure in Peritoneal Dialysis Patients**.. 168
Shou-Hsuan Liu, Yi-Jung Li, Hsin-Hsu Wu, Cheng-Chia Lee, Chan-Yu Lin, Cheng-Hao Weng, Yung-Chang Chen, Ming-Yang Chang, Hsiang-Hao Hsu, Ji-Tseng Fang, Cheng-Chieh Hung, Chih-Wei Yang, Ya-Chung Tian

Chapter 22   **Glycosylated Hemoglobin and Albumin-Correcte Fructosamine are Good Indicators for Glycemic Control in Peritoneal Dialysis Patients**... 178
Szu-Ying Lee, Yin-Cheng Chen, I-Chieh Tsai, Chung-Jen Yen, Shu-Neng Chueh, Hsueh-Fang Chuang, Hon-Yen Wu, Chih-Kang Chiang, Hui-Teng Cheng, Kuan-Yu Hung, Jenq-Wen Huang

Chapter 23   **Histological and Clinical Findings in Patients with Post-Transplantation and Classical Encapsulating Peritoneal Sclerosis**... 187
Joerg Latus, Sayed M. Habib, Daniel Kitterer, Mario R. Korte, Christoph Ulmer, Peter Fritz, Simon Davies, Mark Lambie, M. Dominik Alscher, Michiel G. H. Betjes, Stephan Segerer, Niko Braun

Chapter 24   **Serum Potassium Levels and its Variability in Incident Peritoneal Dialysis Patients: Associations with Mortality** 196
Qingdong Xu, Fenghua Xu, Li Fan, Liping Xiong, Huiyan Li, Shirong Cao, Xiaoyan Lin, Zhihua Zheng, Xueqing Yu, Haiping Mao

Permissions

List of Contributors

Index

Preface

Peritoneal dialysis (PD) is a dialysis technique in which the peritoneum is used as the membrane for the exchange of fluid and dissolved substances with blood. It is performed in individuals with kidney failure, to sustain the continued removal of excess fluid and toxins. It affords better tolerability and greater flexibility in people with heart disease. In peritoneal dialysis, a solution made of hydrogen carbonate, sodium chloride and an osmotic agent is introduced through a tube in the lower abdomen, until it is removed later. This can happen at regular intervals throughout the day, or at night. A person on PD should be monitored to ensure adequate dialysis, and evaluated for complications. Since infections commonly occur with dialysis, an appropriate medical regimen should be established to ensure its prevention. This book outlines the techniques and applications of peritoneal dialysis in detail. Also included in this book is a detailed explanation of the modern practices of performing peritoneal dialysis. This book, with its detailed analyses and data, will prove immensely beneficial to professionals and students involved in nephrology at various levels.

The information contained in this book is the result of intensive hard work done by researchers in this field. All due efforts have been made to make this book serve as a complete guiding source for students and researchers. The topics in this book have been comprehensively explained to help readers understand the growing trends in the field.

I would like to thank the entire group of writers who made sincere efforts in this book and my family who supported me in my efforts of working on this book. I take this opportunity to thank all those who have been a guiding force throughout my life.

Editor

Fluid Status in Peritoneal Dialysis Patients: The European Body Composition Monitoring (EuroBCM) Study Cohort

Wim Van Biesen[1]*, **John D. Williams**[2], **Adrian C. Covic**[3], **Stanley Fan**[4], **Kathleen Claes**[5], **Monika Lichodziejewska-Niemierko**[6], **Christian Verger**[7], **Jurg Steiger**[8], **Volker Schoder**[9], **Peter Wabel**[9], **Adelheid Gauly**[9], **Rainer Himmele**[9], on behalf of the EuroBCM study group

1 University Hospital Ghent, Ghent, Belgium, 2 University Hospital of Wales College of Medicine, Cardiff, United Kingdom, 3 University "Gr T Popa" and University Hospital "C I Pharon", Iasi, Romania, 4 The Royal London Hospital, London, United Kingdom, 5 University Hospital Leuven, Leuven, Belgium, 6 Dialysis Center NephroCare, Gdansk University, Gdansk, Poland, 7 University Hospital René Dubos, Pontoise, France, 8 University Hospital Basel, Basel, Switzerland, 9 Fresenius Medical Care Deutschland GmbH, Bad Homburg, Germany

Abstract

Background: Euvolemia is an important adequacy parameter in peritoneal dialysis (PD) patients. However, accurate tools to evaluate volume status in clinical practice and data on volume status in PD patients as compared to healthy population, and the associated factors, have not been available so far.

Methods: We used a bio-impedance spectroscopy device, the Body Composition Monitor (BCM) to assess volume status in a cross-sectional cohort of prevalent PD patients in different European countries. The results were compared to an age and gender matched healthy population.

Results: Only 40% out of 639 patients from 28 centres in 6 countries were normovolemic. Severe fluid overload was present in 25.2%. There was a wide scatter in the relation between blood pressure and volume status. In a multivariate analysis in the subgroup of patients from countries with unrestricted availability of all PD modalities and fluid types, older age, male gender, lower serum albumin, lower BMI, diabetes, higher systolic blood pressure, and use of at least one exchange per day with the highest hypertonic glucose were associated with higher relative tissue hydration. Neither urinary output nor ultrafiltration, PD fluid type or PD modality were retained in the model (total R^2 of the model = 0.57).

Conclusions: The EuroBCM study demonstrates some interesting issues regarding volume status in PD. As in HD patients, hypervolemia is a frequent condition in PD patients and blood pressure can be a misleading clinical tool to evaluate volume status. To monitor fluid balance, not only fluid output but also dietary input should be considered. Close monitoring of volume status, a correct dialysis prescription adapted to the needs of the patient and dietary measures seem to be warranted to avoid hypervolemia.

Editor: Carmine Zoccali, L' Istituto di Biomedicina ed Immunologia Molecolare, Consiglio Nazionale delle Ricerche, Italy

Funding: Fresenius Medical Care (Bad Homburg, Germany) provided the BCM device and the equipment necessary for the trial to the participating centres. Adelheid Gauly, Rainer Himmele, Volker Schoder and Peter Wabel are employees of Fresenius Medical Care, and helped the other authors with the data collection, analysis and preparation of the manuscript.

Competing Interests: Adelheid Gauly, Rainer Himmele, Volker Schoder and Peter Wabel are employees of Fresenius Medical Care. Wim Van Biesen received speaker's fees from Fresenius Medical Care, Baxter and Gambro on different occasions, however none related to the current study. Stanley Fan received speaker's fees from Fresenius Medical Care and Baxter on different occasions, however none related to the current paper. His department received educational and research support grants from Baxter and Fresenius, but none related to the current study. Adrian Covic and John Williams have worked as consultants for Fresenius Medical Care. There are no patents, products in development or marketed products to declare. This does not alter the authors' adherence to all the PLoS ONE policies on sharing data and materials, as detailed online in the guide for authors.

* E-mail: wim.vanbiesen@ugent.be

Introduction

Euvolemia is a predictor of outcome in peritoneal dialysis (PD) patients, as [1,2]volume overload is related to cardiac dysfunction [3,4,5], inflammation [6] and mortality [7]. Euvolemia is probably a more important adequacy parameter than small solute clearance, as fluid status [7] but not small solute clearance [8] predicts outcome. Guidance on how to achieve and maintain euvolemia in individual PD patients is hampered by the absence of a convenient device to measure volume status, and by the lack of

insight in the prevalence of and factors associated with volume overload.

In clinical practice, the assessment of volume status is relatively crude. Volume status is often assessed indirectly by measuring fluid removal, failing to take into account fluid balance by omission of dietary fluid intake. Ultrasonic evaluation of inferior vena cava diameter (IVC) only assesses intravascular volume, and is also influenced by diastolic dysfunction [9] [10], and is thus a reflection of preload, and not of tissue hydration[11]. Parameters, such as Brain Natriuretic Peptide (BNP) or NT-proBNP can reflect changes in hydration status [12], but are also influenced both by preload and ventricular abnormalities, and in patients with renal failure, accumulation can occur [13]. Direct measurement of extracellular (ECW) and total body water (TBW) by dilution methods is considered as the golden standard, but these techniques are laborious and expensive [14].

Bio-impedance spectroscopy (BIS) represents a different approach to the assessment of fluid status [11,15,16]. By measuring the flow of electrical current through the body, resistance and reactance can be measured, and in BIS, this is performed at different frequencies [17]. The Body Composition Monitor (BCM, Fresenius Medical Care, Germany) is a bio-impedance spectroscopy device for clinical use, validated by isotope dilution methods [18], and reference body composition methods [19], and has been used in hemodialysis (HD) [20,21,22,23] and PD [24].

The fluid status in PD patients has so far not been characterized by a method that allows comparison to the normal healthy populations. Some studies have evaluated the volume status of PD patients in relation to modality (APD vs. CAPD) [25,26] transport status, residual renal function [27], or inflammation [28]. However, whereas these studies contribute information on relative volume status in different groups of PD, they were hampered to express the degree of true fluid overload due to the lack of a reference population. In contrast, Wieskotten et al [29] evaluated a large cohort of 688 healthy persons using the BCM to derive reference ranges, allowing to compare fluid overload as measured by BCM to age and gender matched values of the normal healthy population. In addition, expressing extracellular and intracellular water as absolute values induces the problem of scaling to body size. In previous studies using bio-impedance, ratios of extracellular water to height, weight, body surface area, intracellular water or total body water [30] have been used to express "fluid overload", but the ideal scaling parameter remains a matter of debate [14]. The use of relative Δtissue hydrationdiminishes the problem of scaling nearly completely, and allows comparison to the healthy population [29]. In HD patients [20] relative Δtissue hydration is associated with mortality, indicating the clinical relevance of this parameter.

The European Body Composition study (EuroBCM study) in PD was designed to measure hydration status in a large, multicentric cohort of PD patients using the BCM device, as compared to a healthy reference population, and to establish associations between clinical and practice related parameters and volume status.

Methods

Study objectives

The EuroBCM study in PD was a cross sectional, observational, multi center trial in 28 centers in 6 European countries. The primary objective was to analyze hydration status in a representative sample of prevalent PD patients as compared to the healthy population, and to identify associations between hydration status and patient characteristics (age, gender, diabetes, peritoneal transport characteristics, residual renal function, and daily ultrafiltration) and treatment practice (type of PD solution, use of APD vs CAPD) to find out which conditions should alert the clinician to potential fluid overload.

Centers

Patients were recruited from 6 different European countries (Belgium, France, Poland, Romania, United Kingdom, and Switzerland). Centers were selected to reflect the distribution of

PD in that country, aiming to an overall inclusion of ±10% of the total number of PD patients of that country.

Patients

In each center, all prevalent patients on PD were assessed for eligibility for inclusion (prevalent cross-sectional cohort approach) if they were older than 18 years of age and wanted to sign informed consent. Patients were excluded if they had a cardiac pacemaker or metallic implants, were amputees or were pregnant. Patients were evaluated during a routine clinical visit. All patients signed informed consent, and ethical advice was obtained from the individual ethics committees as per country protocol. This trial has been registered at the Cochrane Renal Group trials registry (http://www.cochrane-renal.org) under the number CRG110800153.

Measurements of hydration and body composition

BCM measurements were in each center performed by one reference PD physician or nurse, using a portable whole body bio-impedance spectroscopy device, the BCM (Fresenius Medical Care). The BCM measures the impedance spectroscopy at 50 different frequencies between 5 kHz and 1 MHz. The BCM was validated intensively against all available gold-standard methods [19]. Clinically relevant parameters were registered in the case report form (CRF).

Electrodes were attached to one hand and one foot at the ipsilateral side, after the patient had been in recumbent position for at least 5 minutes. Due to bio-physical reasons, bio-impedance spectroscopy does not measure sequestered fluid in the trunk [25,31,32,33]. Therefore, presence or absence of PD fluid in the abdomen does not influence the readings of hydration status. For determination of weight, we used the weight adjusted for empty abdomen.

Extracellular water (ECW), intracellular water (ICW) and total body water (TBW) were determined from the measured impedance data following the model of Moissl et al [18]. Reproducibility of BCM derived parameters is high, with a coefficient of variation for the interobserver variability ECW and TBW around 1.2% [34]. Therefore, only one BCM measurement was performed in each individual patient.

Absolute ΔTissue Hydration (AΔTH) was derived from the impedance data based on a physiologic tissue model [35,36]. Absolute ΔTissue Hydration represents the difference between the amount of ECW in the tissue as actually detected by the BCM and the amount of water present in tissue, as predicted by physiological models under normal physiological (normohydrated) conditions [36]. Of note, AΔTH has no direct relation to circulating volume.

All values of AΔTH were compared with and categorized according to the 10th (corresponding to −1.1l) and 90th (corresponding to +1.1l) percentiles of a population of the same gender distribution and with a comparable age band out of a healthy reference cohort, where hydration status was measured with the identical technology [29,37].

AΔTH is further normalized to extracellular water, and expressed as a ratio called Relative ΔTissue Hydration (RΔTH = AΔTH/ECW). In the normal reference population, the 90th percentile of RΔTH is 7%. Accordingly, when RΔTH was greater than 7%, this was classified as "fluid overload". As a RΔTH ratio >15% is related to mortality [20], this cut off was used to define "severe fluid overload".

Blood pressure was recorded as the mean of two consecutive measurements with 5 minutes interval, using one single calibrated device in each center. Height and weight were measured using one single calibrated device in each center.

Patient characteristics

Diabetes was assumed to be present in patients using glucose lowering drugs or insulin.

Congestive heart failure was defined according to the New York Heart Association (NYHA) classification. Ultrafiltration was calculated from the patient's charts as a daily mean of ultrafiltration (in ml) obtained during the last month preceding the measurement. Due to the daily variation, residual diuresis was assessed in a categorical way (<100 ml, between 100 and 500 ml/day, between 500 and 1000 ml/day, or >1000 ml/day) based on the reported current urine production. Total fluid output was estimated as the sum of urinary, taken as the halfway value of the cohort, and ultrafiltered volume per 24 hour. In this way, a patient with zero ultrafiltration and a reported urinary output in the 500–1000 ml/day has a total output of 750 ml, the cut off value in the EAPOS study [38].

The following biochemical parameters were determined in the local laboratories from blood collected during the routine visit: hemoglobin, hematocrit, albumin, CRP, urea, creatinine.

Peritoneal membrane characteristics were determined based on results of the last available PET test preceding the BCM measurement, according to Twardowski [39]. If no PET test was available the last four months, transport status was noted as "unknown"

Statistical analysis

Continuous data are expressed as mean ± standard deviation. Categorical variables are expressed as percentage of total. For univariate comparisons, student's t-test, Mann Whitney U-test and Fisher's exact test were used. One-way ANOVA was used to compare multiple categories, with post hoc testing.

Multivariate linear regression analysis was performed with relative Δtissue hydration as the target variable, to find factors which were independenly associated with overhydration, and should thus alert the physician for this condition. Switzerland was excluded from the multivariate analysis as the low patient number made the models unstable. Since the implementation of APD and polyglucose was very low in Romania and Poland, it was decided to analyse only patients from UK, Belgium and France in the multivariate analysis.

Variables were selected for entry in the model selection procedure either because of univariate $p<0.1$ or for biological plausibility. Regression diagnostics was performed to detect and eliminate outliers and highly influential observations.

All analyses were done with SAS V9.2 (SAS Institute inc, Cary, North Carolina).

Results

Of the prevalent patients in the study centers, 734 were eligible for the study, 73 of whom were excluded because of predefined contra-indications for BCM measurement: metal implants or artificial joints: n = 48, pacemakers or implanted pumps: n = 15, amputations: n = 10. From the remaining 661 patients, 22 patients had incomplete data.

Patients were recruited from Belgium (5 centers, n = 98), France (5 centers, n = 65), Poland (5 centers, n = 82), Romania (9 centers, n = 218), United Kingdom (2 centers, n = 167) and Switzerland (1 center, n = 9).

The baseline demographic, clinical, relevant laboratory data and hydration parameters of the population are provided in table 1. In this population, 24.4% were diabetic, and 32.1% had signs of heart failure (9.7, 12.2, 8.1 and 2.0% NYHA class 1, 2, 3 or 4 respectively). Some patients had previously been treated by HD (18.3%), or had a failed transplant (4.9%). Average time on PD was 32.6±31.0 months. At least one type of antihypertensive

drug was taken by 85.4% of the patients (44.9% diuretics, 46.8% Beta blocking agents, 41.5% calcium antagonists, 51.2% inhibitors of the renin- angiotensin system, 9% central acting drugs).

Underhydration (AΔTH<10th percentile), normohydration and overhydration (AΔTH>90th percentile), as defined by the 10th and 90th percentile of values obtained in the normal population [29], were present in 6.7, 39.9 and 53.4% of the EuroBCM cohort. Fluid overload and severe fluid overload, as defined by a relative Δtissue hydration (AΔTH/ECW) above 7% or above 15% were present in 53.4 and 25.2% of the study population.

Univariate analysis

There was a substantial scatter on the linear relationship between AΔTH and systolic blood pressure, diastolic blood pressure or pulse pressure (correlation coefficients 0.23, 0.02 and 0.29 respectively). As described elsewhere for HD patients [22,37], different zones (figure 1) can be identified in the plot of systolic blood pressure (Y-axis) versus AΔTH (X-axis), of patients who are both normohydrated and normotensive (26.8%, zone A), who are both fluid overloaded and hypertensive (25.8%, zone B), who are hypertensive despite being normo- or underhydrated (13.3%, zone C), who are normo- and hypotensive despite being fluid overloaded (27.5%, zone D) and patients who are hypotensive and normohydrated or normotensive and underhydrated (6.6%, zone E)

Males (vs females, 2.19±2.57 vs 1.03±1.82 l, p<0.001) and diabetics (vs non diabetics, 1.92±2.12 vs 1.52±2.38 l, p = 0.06) had a higher AΔTH. The prevalence of PD patients with a AΔTH>90th percentile of the normal healthy reference population was also higher in males as compared to females (65.0 vs 39.3%). There was no impact of "vintage on PD" on AΔTH (time on PD of patients with an AΔTH >1.1 liter vs euvolaemic patients 32.5±28.0 vs 33.4±34.4 months, p = 0.66).

There was a correlation between transport status and AΔTH (figure 2), with a declining trend from fast (2.04±2.75 l) to fast average (1.63±2.34 l), slow average (1.23±1.97 l) and slow (0.76±1.71 l) transport status (ANOVA: p<0.001). However the interquartile range in each group was substantial, and there is considerable overlap in AΔTH between the groups. AΔTH was most increased in those patients where transport status had not routinely been measured in the last four months (2.48±2.42 l, post-hoc p-value vs. slow transport status p<0.0001). There was a trend for declining AΔTH with increasing urinary output from <100 ml/day (1.99±2.38 l), over 100–500 ml/day (1.84±2.77 l) and 500–1000 ml/day (1.55±2.12 l) to those with a urinary output greater than 1000 ml/day (1.28±1.99 l) (one way ANOVA: p<0.001), but with large interquartile range and overlap. There was no correlation between AΔTH and daily ultrafiltration (R = 0.10), and only a weak correlation between AΔTH and estimated daily total fluid output (residual diuresis + peritoneal ultrafiltration) (R = 0.17).

There was a negative relation between AΔTH and serum albumin (R = −0.42), hemoglobin (R = −0.34) and hematocrit (R = −0.31). There was no correlation between AΔTH and glomerular filtration rate or CRP-level.

There was a difference in AΔTH in the univariate analysis between patients using or not using polyglucose (0.9±2 vs 1.4±2 l resp, p = 0.04) in the countries without logistical impediment to the use of polyglucose. The relation between hydration status and use of polyglucose was complex, with more patients being overhydrated in the group using polyglucose in Belgium, whereas in UK and France, patients using polyglucose were less overhydrated (table 2). In countries where the use of polyglucose was restricted (Romania and Poland), the few patients using polyglucose tended

Table 1. Demographic, clinical and fluid status data of the EuroBCM study cohort (N = 639).

	mean or percentage	Standard deviation
Gender Male	55%	
Age (years)	58.8	14.8
Height (cm)	165.7	9.6
Weight (kg)	72.2	15.4
Body Mass Index (kg/m^2)	26.3	5.1
Blood pressure (mmHg)		
Systolic	136.9	25.6
Diastolic	79.9	14.3
Residual GFR (ml/min)	6.6	7.2
Ultrafiltration (ml/day)	940	580
Residual urine output		
<100 ml/day	19.1%	
100–500 ml/day	21.9%	
500–1000 ml/day	23.5%	
>1000 ml/day	32.6%	
Missing data	3.0%	
Treatment modality Automated PD§	53.1%	
Use of polyglucose§	63.7%	
Transport status		
Fast	16.6%	
Fast average	33.3%	
Slow average	28.3%	
Slow	5.9%	
Not known	15.9%	
Serum levels		
Albumin (g/l)	36.3	6.0
Creatinine (mg/dl)	8.1	3.0
Urea (mg/dl)	117.0	39.7
C-reactiveprotein (mg/l)	11.6	23.5
Hemoglobin (g/dl)	11.3	1.6
Hematocrit (%)	34.3	5.1
HbA1C (%)	6.5	1.7
Absolute ΔTissue Hydration (AΔTH) (l)	1.7	2.3
	Q25: 0.2; Median 1.3; Q75: 2.9	
Relative ΔTissue Hydration (%) (Ratio AΔTH/ECW)	8.6	11.5
	Q25: 1.1; Median 7.8; Q75: 15.1	
Total Body Water (l)	35.8	7.7
Extracellular Water (l)	17.2	3.8
Intracellular water (l)	18.5	4.5
Extracellular/Intracellular water	0.95	0.15
Intracellular resistance Ri (Ohm/m)	569.6	117.5
Extracellular resistance Re (Ohm/m)	1611.6	479.5
Phase angle at 50 kHz	4.9	1.2

§after exclusion of patients from countries where polyglucose and APD are not liberally available due to logistical reasons.

to be more overhydrated (table 2), potentially indicating a bias by indication.

There was a small difference in AΔTH in univariate analysis between patients on CAPD vs APD (1.3 ± 2.0 vs 0.9 ± 1.9 l resp, p = 0.06) in these countries without logistical impediment to the use of APD (Belgium, France, UK).

Multivariate analysis of tissue hydration

Because of the strong interaction, the multivariate analysis included only patients from countries with unrestricted access to APD and alternative PD solutions.

In this multivariable linear regression analysis adjusted for country effects (table 3), older age, male gender, lower serum albumin, lower BMI, diabetes, higher systolic blood pressure, and use of at least once per day highest hypertonic glucose were associated with higher relative tissue hydration. Neither urinary output nor ultrafiltration was retained in the model. The use of alternative dialysis solutions (including polyglucose) did not contribute to the model (total R^2 of the model = 0.57).

Discussion

The EuroBCM study is the first large multi-centre study of hydration status and its associated factors in PD patients in Europe allowing comparison to a healthy reference population. Fluid overload was a frequent finding in PD patients as compared to a

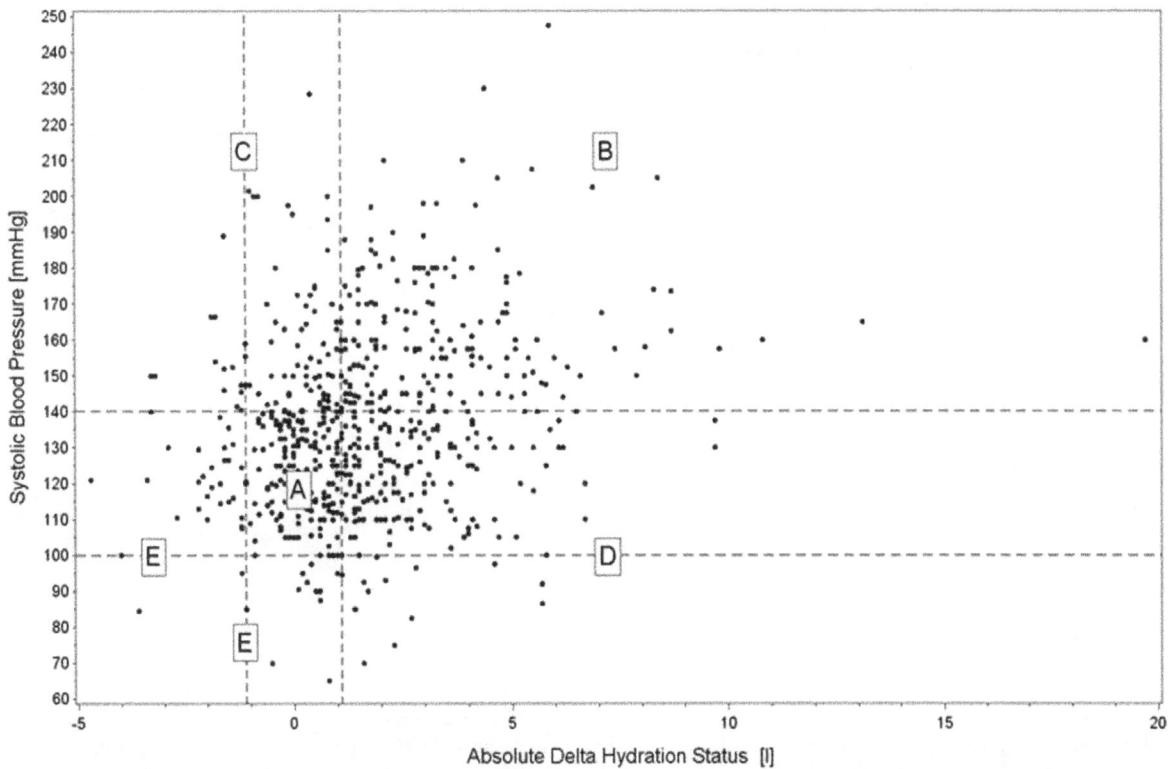

Figure 1. Scatter plot of the relation between absolute Δtissue hydration (litres) in the X-axis and systolic blood pressure (mmHg) in the Y-axis in the individual patients of the EuroBCM study cohort. Dotted vertical lines indicate the 10th and 90th percentile of absolute Δtissue hydration in the healthy population (−1.1 and +1.1 liter respectively), representing thus the limits of "normohydration". Dotted horizontal lines indicate the "normotensive range" for systolic blood pressure.

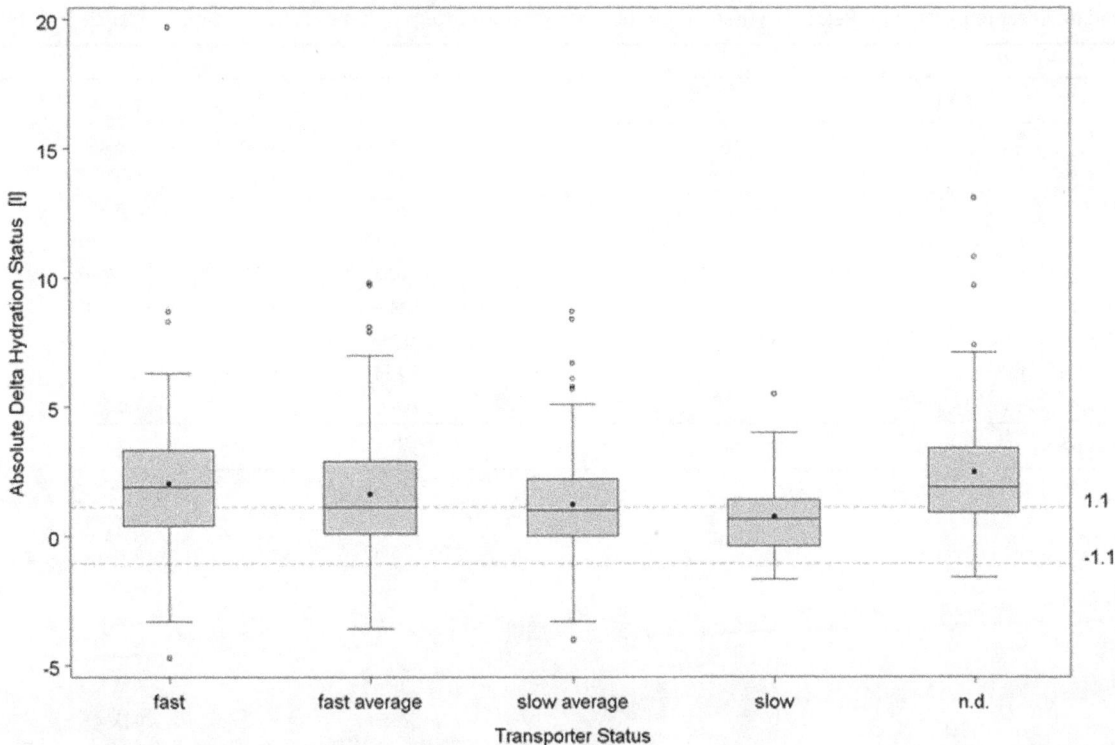

Figure 2. Box and whisker plots (median, 25th and 75th quartile, outliers) of Absolute ΔTissue Hydration (in liters) in the different transport categories. n.d.: no peritoneal transport characteristics available in the 4 months before the BCM measurement.

Table 2. Tissue hydration related to percentiles of the normal reference population stratified for the use of polyglucose or not.

	% <10th percentile of normal population	% between 10th and 90th percentile of normal population	% >90th percentile of normal population
Belgium			
Polyglucose (n = 59)	6.8	42.4	50.8
No polyglucose (n = 39)	5.1	56.4	38.5
France			
Polyglucose (n = 44)	9.1	54.5	36.4
No polyglucose (n = 21)	4.8	33.3	61.9
United Kingdom			
Polyglucose (n = 113)	16.8	47.8	35.4
No polyglucose (n = 54)	9.3	38.9	51.8
Switzerland			
Polyglucose (n = 7)	0.0	0.0	100.0
No polyglucose (n = 2)	0.0	50.0	50.0
Romania			
Polyglucose (n = 17)	1.0	33.0	66.0
No polyglucose (n = 203)	2.8	35.3	60.0
Poland			
Polyglucose(n = 9)	4.1	35.6	60.3
No polyglucose (n = 73)	11.1	44.4	44.4

healthy reference population [29], but comparable to that reported in HD patients [20,22,23]. The deviation from the relation between blood pressure and tissue hydration was substantial, pointing out that blood pressure is not a good tool to evaluate hydration status in PD patients. Overhydration was associated with higher age, male gender, diabetes, lower BMI, higher systolic blood pressure, and use of hypertonic solutions, and

in these conditions, physicians should have enhanced awareness for volume status. Use of polyglucose or biocompatible glucose solutions or the type of PD modality was not independently associated with hydration status.

In the large cohort of the EuroBCM in PD study, a substantial portion of patients were fluid overloaded by more than 1.1 litre, the 90th percentile of absolute Δtissue hydration in the normal

Table 3. Multivariate linear regression for Relative ΔTissue Hydration from the subgroup of patients from Belgium, France and UK.

Parameter	Coefficient	95% CI		p-value
Intercept	**30.27**	20.65	39.88	<0.0001
Age (per year)	**0.10**	0.05	0,16	0.0002
Sex (female vs male)	**−3.04**	−4.55	−1.52	0.0001
Albumin per g/l	**−0.75**	−0.91	−0.59	<0.0001
BMI per kg/m^2	**−0.66**	−0.83	−0.50	<0.0001
Diabetes (vs no diabetes)	**4.86**	3.14	6.59	<0.0001
Systolic BP (per mmHg)	**0.09**	0.05	0.12	<0.0001
Glucose at least once 2.5% vs. 1.5% only	**−0.73**	−2.56	1.11	0.80
Glucose at least once 3.86/4.25% vs. 1.5% only	**5.18**	2.62	7.74	<0.0001
Not included due to p>0.1				
Ultrafiltration				0.86
Urine output				0.66
Hypertension stage				0.41
NYHA Stage				0.39
Liver disease				0.56
Time on PD per month				0.25
Transport status				0.83
Type of PD solution				0.12
PD modality				0.27

Model adjusted for country effects (Belgium, France and UK), total R^2 of the model = 0.57, n = 299.
NYHA = New York Heart Association classification of heart failure.

reference population [29], and 25% of patients had a relativeΔ tissue hydration/extracellular water ratio above 15%, a value associated with increased mortality in HD patients [20]. Substantial fluid overload is therefore indeed a prevalent problem in PD patients, and more attention should be given to its assessment and correction. Nevertheless, it is important to note that comparable numbers of severe fluid overload have been reported in HD patients [20,22,23,24], and already in early stages of renal impairment, patients tend to be more fluid overloaded [40,41].

Many physicians estimate hydration status by using clinical parameters, such as edema, weight gain or blood pressure[42]. Although there was a direct correlation between systolic blood pressure and tissue hydration, a substantial proportion of patients did not comply with this paradigm. A number of patients had systolic hypertension, despite normohydration or even tissue underhydration. These are probably patients who suffer from vascular stiffness [2]. Further dehydration of these patients in an attempt to normalize blood pressure might be dangerous, as it might abruptly compromise coronary perfusion [43]. A number of patients had a low or normal blood pressure, despite being fluid overloaded. It is conceivable that many of these patients suffer congestive heart failure. Normotension in these patients should not be seen as equivalent to euvolemia, as also reported in HD patients [22].

In many studies on fluid overload, attention is focused on fluid output (ultrafiltration and/or diuresis), neglecting that fluid status is a balance of fluid output and input. In the EuroBCM study, there was a very weak association between fluid overload and diuresis, but this association disappeared in the multivariate analysis. Davison et al [25] found a small influence of residual GFR, but not of peritoneal ultrafiltration or daily urine output, on volume status. Wiggins et al [44] demonstrated that total fluid output one month after the initiation of PD was not associated with patient survival. All these point out that in studies on fluid status, both fluid input and output should be considered. In addition, and maybe even more of importance, clinicians should be aware that patients can be overhydrated because of dietary incompliance, despite having substantial residual diuresis. Dietary intake of fluid and salt should thus be conisdered when managing fluid overloaded patients.

In our BCM cohort, the use of high hypertonic bags was associated with fluid overload. It is tempting to attribute this observation to bias by indication. However, an alternative potential hypothesis could be that the strategy of using hypertonic bags is not effective in returning patients back to euvolemia for a sustained period of time, as it can lead to dysregulation of glycemic control, and thus to hyperosmolarity and thirst. Sustained exposure to hypertonic exchanges can also negatively impact on the peritoneal membrane function [45], leading to further detrimental consequences on fluid balance. Further studies in this regard are warranted. This is compatible with the negative impact of high initial peritoneal fluid removal [44]: it is likely that those with a high fluid output achieved this at the expense of increased use of hypertonic bags, thus damaging the peritoneal membrane in the long term.

There was an association between peritoneal membrane transport characteristics and tissue hydration, as already demonstrated by others [27]. Nevertheless, there was a substantial overlap between groups, and the effect was rather small and disappeared in the multivariate analysis. In the study by Davison et al [25], transport status explained only 1.6% of the variation in volume status. It can be hypothesized that fluid overload is induced by not adapting the dwell time appropriately to the transport status of the patient [46]. Although it has been stated that removal of salt can be impaired in patients on APD [47], hydration status in patients on APD and CAPD was comparable in the multivariate analysis in the EuroBCM cohort, just as in previous observations [25,26]. Of note, in one of these studies [25], the number of cycles per night was limited, so the dwell time was probably long enough to allow diffusive sodium transport. To maintain fluid balance, fast transporters need short dwells, to avoid negative ultrafiltration, and implementing APD might be of value in this patient category. On the other hand, slow transporters need long dwells to avoid sodium sieving, and APD with short cycles might be detrimental in this patient group. Johnson et al [48] recently reported that APD was associated with better survival in fast, but with worse survival in low transporters, an observation that is compatible with this paradigm.

As Davison et al (23), we found a negative association between serum albumin and overhydration. As this is a cross-sectional cohort, it is however impossible to determine whether low albumin is a consequence or a cause of overhydration.

In the EuroBCM study cohort, polyglucose use was associated with less overhydration and more underhydration in some countries, whereas the opposite was true in other countries, pointing to potential underlying differences in practice related to the use of polyglucose (table 2). In a subcohort of the EuroBCM trial, excluding countries were alternative PD solutions and APD are not liberally available due to logistical reasons, we observed a neutral impact both of the solution type and the PD modality on fluid overload, just as it was found in the cohort of Davison et al [25].

This study is a cross sectional study, and as such, no causal relations can be drawn. However, our observations can generate some interesting hypotheses on the association between practices and hydration status. It would be interesting e.g. to study the impact on hydration status and residual renal function using a prospective protocol where implementation of polyglucose, dwell length and use of APD vs CAPD is guided by BCM based assessment of fluid overload. Another limitation is the rather crude evaluation of fluid output using patient charts as a reference, which might induce inaccuracies. However, this is the way fluid output is measured in real life. Of special interest for a future prospective study in this regard is the potential impact of bag overfill on the overestimation of ultrafiltration and fluid overload [49]. It can be that the overestimation of real ultrafiltration by neglecting overfill can lead to overhydration, as it gives the patient and the physician the false feeling of adequate ultrafiltration.

In conclusion, the EuroBCM study demonstrates some interesting issues on volume status in PD patients: fluid overload is a frequent problem, and relying only on clinical parameters for its assessment might be misleading. Fluid overload is related to prescription practices, gender and diabetes. Despite good ultrafiltration and residual diuresis, patients still can be fluid overloaded, stressing the important role of dietary restriction of salt and fluid intake. Although indication bias cannot be excluded, attempts to increase ultrafiltration by the long term use of hypertonic bags [46] seem to be no guarantee for achieving sustained euvolemia. Objective measurement of fluid status as a basis for an integrated approach to fluid balance is warranted. As fluid overload has been linked to mortality [7,20], further studies evaluating whether awareness of hydration status can improve volume management and patient outcome are warranted.

Acknowledgments

We thank all the nurses and the patients in the participating centres for their contribution.

EuroBCM Study group:

Romania: Christian Klein, Dialysis Center NephroCare Devila, Bucharest; Olimpia Cretu, County Hospital Alexandria, Alexandria; Mihai Voiculescu, Fundeni Institute Bucharest, Bucharest; Adrian Covic, Nephrocare Dialysis Center Iasi, Iasi; Viorica Butnaru, County Hospital Ploiesti, Ploiesti; Dorin Ionescu, Emergency University Hospital Bucharest, Bucharest; Cezarina Bejan, City Hospital Barlad, Barlad; Cristian Serafinceanu, Institute for Metabolic Disease, Bucharest; Marcel Pravat, County Hospital Slobozia, Slobozia;

Poland: Monika Lichodziejewska-Niemierko, Fresenius Nephrocare Gdansk, Gdansk; Magdalena Krajewska, Akademickie Centrum Kliniczne, Wroclaw; Andrzej Kaczmarek, Fresenius Nephrocare Pleszew, Pleszew; Bernadeta Marcykiewicz, Fresenius Nephrocare Krakow, Krakow; Mirosław Kroczak, Fresenius Nephrocare Sieradz, Sieradz;

Switzerland: Jürg Steiger, Universitätsspital Basel, Basel;

France: Agnès Caillette-Beaudoin, Calydial Vienne, Vienne; Christian Verger, CHU Dubos, Pontoise;

Karine Moreau, CHU Pellegrin, Bordeaux; Marie-Christine Mavel, Centre Hospitalier André Grégoire, Montreuil;

Nasredine Ghali, Centre Hospitalier Marc Jacquet, Melun;

Belgium: Wim van Biesen, UZ Ghent, Ghent; Kathleen Claes, UZ Leuven, Leuven; Serge Treille, CHU - Hôpital Civil de Charleroi, Charleroi; Christophe Bovy, CHU de Liège, Liège; Dierik Verbeelen, UZ Brussels, Brussel;

UK: Steve Riley, John Williams, Cardiff University, Cardiff; Stanley Fan, Royal London Hospital, London.

All authors declare that the results presented in this paper have not been published previously in whole or part, except in abstract format.

Author Contributions

Conceived and designed the experiments: WVB RH AG VS PW. Performed the experiments: WVB JDW ACC SF KC ML-N CV JS. Analyzed the data: WVB VS AH RH PW SF. Wrote the manuscript: WVB JDW ACC SF KC ML-N CV JS AG RH PW VS.

References

1. Lo WK, Bargman JM, Burkart J, Krediet RT, Pollock C, et al. (2006) Guideline on targets for solute and fluid removal in adult patients on chronic peritoneal dialysis. Perit Dial Int 26: 520–522.
2. Van Biesen W, Verbeke F, Devolder I, Vanholder R (2008) The relation between salt, volume, and hypertension: clinical evidence for forgotten but still valid basic physiology. Perit Dial Int 28: 596–600.
3. Wang AY, Lam CW, Wang M, Chan IH, Goggins WB, et al. (2007) Prognostic value of cardiac troponin T is independent of inflammation, residual renal function, and cardiac hypertrophy and dysfunction in peritoneal dialysis patients. Clin Chem 53: 882–889.
4. Konings CJ, Kooman JP, Schonck M, Dammers R, Cheriex E, et al. (2002) Fluid status, blood pressure, and cardiovascular abnormalities in patients on peritoneal dialysis. Perit Dial Int 22: 477–487.
5. Enia G, Mallamaci F, Benedetto FA, Panuccio V, Parlongo S, et al. (2001) Long-term CAPD patients are volume expanded and display more severe left ventricular hypertrophy than haemodialysis patients. Nephrol Dial Transplant 16: 1459–1464.
6. Demirci MS, Demirci C, Ozdogan O, Kircelli F, Akcicek F, et al. Relations between malnutrition-inflammation-atherosclerosis and volume status. The usefulness of bioimpedance analysis in peritoneal dialysis patients. Nephrol Dial Transplant.
7. Paniagua R, Ventura MD, Avila-Diaz M, Hinojosa-Heredia H, Mendez-Duran A, et al. (2010) NT-proBNP, Fluid volume overload and dialysis modality are independent predictors of mortality in ESRD patients. Nephrol Dial Transplant 15.
8. Paniagua R, Amato D, Correa-Rotter R, Ramos A, Vonesh EF, et al. (2000) Correlation between peritoneal equilibration test and dialysis adequacy and transport test, for peritoneal transport type characterization. Mexican Nephrology Collaborative Study Group. Perit Dial Int 20: 53–59.
9. Leunissen KM, Kouw P, Kooman JP, Cheriex EC, deVries PM, et al. (1993) New techniques to determine fluid status in hemodialyzed patients. Kidney Int Suppl 41: S50–56.
10. Aurigemma GP, Gaasch WH (2004) Clinical practice. Diastolic heart failure. N Engl J Med 351: 1097–1105.
11. Kraemer M, Rode C, Wizemann V (2006) Detection limit of methods to assess fluid status changes in dialysis patients. Kidney Int 69: 1609–1620.
12. Jacobs LH, van de Kerkhof JJ, Mingels AM, Passos VL, Kleijnen VW, et al. (2009) Inflammation, overhydration and cardiac biomarkers in haemodialysis patients: a longitudinal study. Nephrol Dial Transplant.
13. Sommerer C, Heckele S, Schwenger V, Katus HA, Giannitsis E, et al. (2007) Cardiac biomarkers are influenced by dialysis characteristics. Clin Nephrol 68: 392–400.
14. Woodrow G (2007) Body composition analysis techniques in adult and pediatric patients: how reliable are they? How useful are they clinically? Perit Dial Int 27(Suppl 2): S245–249.
15. Matthie JR (2008) Bioimpedance measurements of human body composition: critical analysis and outlook. Expert Rev Med Devices 5: 239–261.
16. Jaffrin MY, Morel H (2008) Body fluid volumes measurements by impedance: A review of bioimpedance spectroscopy (BIS) and bioimpedance analysis (BIA) methods. Med Eng Phys 30: 1257–1269.
17. Kotanko P, Levin NW, Zhu F (2008) Current state of bioimpedance technologies in dialysis. Nephrol Dial Transplant 23: 808–812.
18. Moissl UM, Wabel P, Chamney PW, Bosaeus I, Levin NW, et al. (2006) Body fluid volume determination via body composition spectroscopy in health and disease. Physiol Meas 27: 921–933.
19. Wabel P, Chamney P, Moissl U, Jirka T (2009) Importance of whole-body bioimpedance spectroscopy for the management of fluid balance. Blood Purif 27: 75–80.
20. Wizemann V, Wabel P, Chamney P, Zaluska W, Moissl U, et al. (2009) The mortality risk of overhydration in haemodialysis patients. Nephrol Dial Transplant 24.
21. Wizemann V, Rode C, Wabel P (2008) Whole-body spectroscopy (BCM) in the assessment of normovolemia in hemodialysis patients. Contrib Nephrol 161: 115–118.
22. Passauer J, Petrov H, Schleser A, Leicht J, Pucalka K. Evaluation of clinical dry weight assessment in haemodialysis patients using bioimpedance spectroscopy: a cross-sectional study. Nephrol Dial Transplant 25: 545–551.
23. Machek P, Jirka T, Moissl U, Chamney P, Wabel P. Guided optimization of fluid status in haemodialysis patients. Nephrol Dial Transplant 25: 538–544.
24. Devolder I, Verleysen A, Vijt D, Vanholder R, Van Biesen W. Body composition, hydration, and related parameters in hemodialysis versus peritoneal dialysis patients. Perit Dial Int 30: 208–214.
25. Davison SN, Jhangri GS, Jindal K, Pannu N (2009) Comparison of volume overload with cycler-assisted versus continuous ambulatory peritoneal dialysis. Clin J Am Soc Nephrol 4: 1044–1050.
26. Davenport A, Willicombe M (2009) Comparison of fluid status in patients treated by different modalities of peritoneal dialysis using multi-frequency bioimpedance. Int J Artif Organs 32: 779–786.
27. Konings CJ, Kooman JP, Schonck M, Struijk DG, Gladziwa U, et al. (2003) Fluid status in CAPD patients is related to peritoneal transport and residual renal function: evidence from a longitudinal study. Nephrol Dial Transplant 18: 797–803.
28. Gangji AS, Brimble KS, Margetts PJ (2009) Association between markers of inflammation, fibrosis and hypervolemia in peritoneal dialysis patients. Blood Purif 28: 354–358.
29. Wieskotten S, Heinke S, Wabel P, Moissl U, Becker J, et al. (2008) Bioimpedance-based identification of malnutrition using fuzzy logic. Physiol Meas 29: 639–654.
30. Engel B, Davies SJ (2007) Achieving euvolemia in peritoneal dialysis. Perit Dial Int 27: 514–517.
31. Foster KR, Lukaski HC (1996) Whole-body impedance–what does it measure? Am J Clin Nutr 64: 388S–396S.
32. Cooper BA, Aslani A, Ryan M, Zhu F, Ibels LS, et al. (2000) Comparing different methods of assessing body composition in end stage renal failure. Kidney Int 58.
33. Passauer J, Schewe J, Parmentier S, Palm C, Herbrig K (2009) Influence of peritoneal fluid on measurements of fluid overload by bio-impedance spectroscopy in peritoneal dialysis patients. World Congres of Nephrology 2009: SU450.
34. Wabel P, Chamney P, Moissl U (2007) Reproducibility of bioimpedance spectroscopy for the assessment of body composition and dry weight. J Am Soc Nephrol 18: A255.
35. Chamney PW, Wabel P, Moissl UM, Muller MJ, Bosy-Westphal A, et al. (2007) A whole-body model to distinguish excess fluid from the hydration of major body tissues. Am J Clin Nutr 85: 80–89.
36. Wang J, Pierson R (1976) Disparate hydration of adipose and lean tissue require a new model for body water distribution in man. J Nutr 106: 6.
37. Wabel P, Moissl U, Chamney P, Jirka T, Machek P, et al. (2008) Towards improved cardiovascular management: the necessity of combining blood pressure and fluid overload. Nephrol Dial Transplant 23: 2965–2971.
38. Brown EA, Davies SJ, Rutherford P, Meeus F, Borras M, et al. (2003) Survival of functionally anuric patients on automated peritoneal dialysis: the European APD Outcome Study. J Am Soc Nephrol 14: 2948–2957.
39. Twardowski Z, Nolph K, Khanna R (1987) Peritoneal equilibration test. Perit Dial Bull 7.
40. Bellizzi V, Scalfi L, Terracciano V, De Nicola L, Minutolo R, et al. (2006) Early changes in bioelectrical estimates of body composition in chronic kidney disease. J Am Soc Nephrol 17: 1481–1487.
41. Essig M, Escoubet B, de Zuttere D, Blanchet F, Arnoult F, et al. (2008) Cardiovascular remodelling and extracellular fluid excess in early stages of chronic kidney disease. Nephrol Dial Transplant 23: 239–248.

42. Cocchi R, Degli Esposti E, Fabbri A, Lucatello A, Sturani A, et al. (1999) Prevalence of hypertension in patients on peritoneal dialysis: results of an Italian multicentre study. Nephrol Dial Transplant 14: 1536–1540.

43. Covic A, Haydar AA, Bhamra-Ariza P, Gusbeth-Tatomir P, Goldsmith DJ (2005) Aortic pulse wave velocity and arterial wave reflections predict the extent and severity of coronary artery disease in chronic kidney disease patients. J Nephrol 18: 388–396.

44. Wiggins KJ, Rumpsfeld M, Hawley CM, O'Shea A, Isbel NM, et al. (2007) Baseline and time-averaged fluid removal affect technique survival in peritoneal dialysis in a non-linear fashion. Nephrology (Carlton) 12: 218–223.

45. Davies SJ, Brown EA, Reigel W, Clutterbuck E, Heimburger O, et al. (2006) What is the link between poor ultrafiltration and increased mortality in anuric patients on automated peritoneal dialysis? Analysis of data from EAPOS. Perit Dial Int 26: 458–465.

46. van Biesen W, Heimburger O, Krediet R, Rippe B, Lamilia V, et al. (2010) Evaluation of peritoneal membrane characteristics: a clinical advice for prescription management by the ERBP working group. Nephrol Dial Transplant 25: 2052–2062.

47. Rodriguez-Carmona A, Fontan MP (2002) Sodium removal in patients undergoing CAPD and automated peritoneal dialysis. Perit Dial Int 22: 705–713.

48. Johnson DW, Hawley CM, McDonald SP, Brown FG, Rosman JB, et al. (2010) Superior survival of high transporters treated with automated versus continuous ambulatory peritoneal dialysis. Nephrol Dial Transplant, 25: 1973–1979.

49. Davies SJ (2006) Overfill or ultrafiltration? We need to be clear. Perit Dial Int 26: 449–451.

2

The Potential Role of HMGB1 Release in Peritoneal Dialysis-Related Peritonitis

Shirong Cao[1⑨], Shu Li[1,2⑨], Huiyang Li[1], Liping Xiong[1], Yi Zhou[1], Jinjin Fan[1], Xueqing Yu[1], Haiping Mao[1]*

1 Department of Nephrology, The First Affiliated Hospital, Sun Yat-sen University, Key Laboratory of Nephrology, Ministry of Health, Guangzhou, China, 2 Department of Rheumatology, The Second Xiangya Hospital, Central South University, Changsha, Hunan, China

Abstract

High mobility group box 1 (HMGB1), a DNA-binding nuclear protein, has been implicated as an endogenous danger signal in the pathogenesis of infection diseases. However, the potential role and source of HMGB1 in the peritoneal dialysis (PD) effluence of patients with peritonitis are unknown. First, to evaluate HMDB1 levels in peritoneal dialysis effluence (PDE), a total of 61 PD patients were enrolled in this study, including 42 patients with peritonitis and 19 without peritonitis. Demographic characteristics, symptoms, physical examination findings and laboratory parameters were recorded. HMGB1 levels in PDE were determined by Western blot and ELISA. The concentrations of TNF-α and IL-6 in PDE were quantified by ELISA. By animal model, inhibition of HMGB1 with glycyrrhizin was performed to determine the effects of HMGB1 in LPS-induced mice peritonitis. In vitro, a human peritoneal mesothelial cell line (HMrSV5) was stimulated with lipopolysaccharide (LPS), HMGB1 extracellular content in the culture media and intracellular distribution in various cellular fractions were analyzed by Western blot or immunofluorescence. The results showed that the levels of HMGB1 in PDE were higher in patients with peritonitis than those in controls, and gradually declined during the period of effective antibiotic treatments. Furthermore, the levels of HMGB1 in PDE were positively correlated with white blood cells (WBCs) count, TNF-α and IL-6 levels. However, pretreatment with glycyrrhizin attenuated LPS-induced acute peritoneal inflammation and dysfunction in mice. In cultured HMrSV5 cells, LPS actively induced HMGB1 nuclear-cytoplasmic translocation and release in a time and dose-dependent fashion. Moreover, cytosolic HMGB1 was located in lysosomes and secreted via a lysosome-mediated secretory pathway following LPS stimulation. Our study demonstrates that elevated HMGB1 levels in PDE during PD-related peritonitis, at least partially, from peritoneal mesothelial cells, which may be involved in the process of PD-related peritonitis and play a critical role in acute peritoneal dysfunction.

Editor: Cordula M. Stover, University of Leicester, United Kingdom

Funding: This work was supported by grants from the National Natural Science Foundation of China (81070553, 81270783). The funders had no role in study design, data collection and analysis, decision to publish, or preparation of the manuscript.

Competing Interests: The authors have declared that no competing interests exist.

* E-mail: haipingmao@126.com

⑨ These authors contributed equally to this work.

Introduction

Peritoneal dialysis (PD) is the most important home dialysis therapy for patients with end-stage renal disease. Although the rate of peritoneal dialysis-related peritonitis has been significantly reduced, it remains a major complication of PD [1]. The repeated or severe peritonitis may cause peritoneal membrane dysfunction and eventually leads to dropout of PD.

The peritoneum is composed of an extensive monolayer of mesothelial cells resting upon a thin basement membrane. During peritonitis, mesothelial cells are activated by proinflammatory cytokines, such as tumor necrosis factor α (TNF-α) and interleukin-6 (IL-6) derived from peritoneal macrophages, and play critical roles in amplification of peritoneal inflammation though release of many proinflammatory cytokines and mediators [2].

High mobility group box protein 1 (HMGB1), a ubiquitous nonhistone nuclear protein, can be released actively by innate immune cells (macrophages, monocytes) or other cell types as well as passively by injured and necrotic cells [3,4]. During systemic inflammation, TNF-α and IL-6 regulate HMGB1 release from various cells. Once released, HMGB1 may serve as a mediator of delayed endotoxin lethality and systemic inflammation, contributing to disease pathogenesis by upregulation of endothelial adhesion molecules, stimulation of epithelial cell barrier failure and enhancing the synthesis of proinflammatory cytokines [5,6]. HMGB1 is not detectable in serum of normal subjects, but it is significantly increased in clinical inflammatory conditions such as sepsis, rheumatoid arthritis, and chronic kidney disease [7,8,9,10]. Administration of HMGB1 via intracerebroventricular, intratracheal, intraperitoneal and intraarticular routes induces marked inflammatory responses, and activates various innate immune cells [6]. At the same time, targeting HMGB1 with either antibodies or specific antagonists has been demonstrated to blunt inflammatory response and confer protective effects in animal models, including lethal endotoxemia or sepsis, collagen-induced arthritis, and ischemia-reperfusion induced tissue injury [5,11,12,13]. However, the potential role of HMGB1 in PD-related peritonitis has not been investigated.

In this study, we hypothesized that HMGB1 levels would be elevated in PDE and associated with peritonitis in PD patients. We also explored the effect of HMGB1 on peritoneal function in LPS-induced peritonitis in mice and further examined the source and the process of HMGB1 release using human peritoneal mesothelial cell line (HMrSV5) *in vitro*.

Results

Patient Characteristics

The baseline clinical characteristics of continuous ambulatory peritoneal dialysis (CAPD) patients with and without peritonitis were presented in Table 1. There were no significant differences in mean age, gender, the percentage of patients with diabetes, dialysis duration, hemoglobin (Hb), Kt/V_{urea}, and residual glomerular filtration rate (GFR) between patients with or without peritonitis. However, patients with peritonitis had a higher high-sensitivity C-reactive protein (hsCRP) and lower levels of serum albumin (Alb) as compared with the control patients ($P<0.05$). The above results were similar in patients with Gram-positive or Gram-negative peritonitis.

Levels of HMGB1 in PDE during Peritonitis

To determine whether HMGB1 levels are elevated in PD-related peritonitis, intraperitoneal HMGB1 concentrations were first determined by immunoblot analysis. As shown in Figure 1A and B, the levels of HMGB1 were significantly elevated in PDE samples of patients with peritonitis as compared with the controls. Moreover, levels of HMGB1 were significantly higher in patients with Gram-negative than those with Gram-positive peritonitis (Fig. 1C and D). HMGB1 levels in PDE samples were further confirmed by specific ELISA kits. Consistent with results obtained by immunoblot analysis, HMGB1 levels in PD patients with peritonitis were significantly increased compared to the controls (12.73 *versus* 5.93 ng/ml, $P<0.01$) (Fig. 1E), and also significantly higher in patients with Gram-negative peritonitis than those with Gram-positive peritonitis (17.14 ng/ml *versus* 10.79 ng/ml, $P<0.01$) (Fig. 1F). Importantly, dynamic observation of HMGB1 levels in peritonitis patients showed that high levels of HMGB1

were evident at the onset of peritonitis, gradually diminished and barely captured on day 7 after effective antibiotic treatment (Fig. 2A and B). Taken together, these findings suggest that increased PDE HMGB1 levels are associated with the severity of PD related-peritonitis, and LPS, endotoxin from Gram-negative bacteria may play additional direct role in stimulating HMGB1 secretion.

Levels of TNF-α and IL-6 and their Correlation with HMGB1 in PDE

In parallel analyses, we examined both TNF-α and IL-6 levels in PDE of the first day of peritonitis by ELISA. As shown in Figure 3A and B, levels of TNF-α and IL-6 in PDE of controls were almost undetectable, whereas levels of both cytokines markedly elevated in peritonitis patients. Similarly, PDE levels of TNF-α and IL-6 were higher in patients with Gram-negative as compared to Gram-positive peritonitis ($P<0.01$, Fig. 3C and D). Further, there was a significant positive correlation between HMGB1 levels and WBC counts (r = 0.86, $P<0.01$, Fig. 4A), TNF-α level (r = 0.75, $P<0.01$, Fig. 4B) as well as IL-6 level (r = 0.81, $P<0.01$, Fig. 4C) in PDE of patients with peritonitis.

Inhibition of HMGB1 Expression Attenuated LPS-induced Peritoneal Dysfunction

Since elevated expression of HMGB1 in PDE was associated with the presence of PD-related peritonitis, we further evaluated whether HMGB1 could play a role in peritoneal function during peritonitis. To this end, acute peritonitis in mice was generated by intraperitoneal injection of LPS as previously described [14]. Compared with the control group, LPS administration significantly enhanced the peritoneal edema, recruitment of inflammatory cells in both the parietal and visceral peritoneum in mice (Fig. 5A). Further, the total number of WBC in dialysate was elevated (Fig. 5B) and the percentage of neutrophils increased (7.50±1.24% *versus* 25.00±5.85%, $P<0.05$) in parallel with a decrease in lymphocytes (72.70±7.90% *versus* 55.50±6.20%,

Table 1. Patients Characteristics.

Characteristic	No peritonitis (n = 19)	Peritonitis (n = 42)	G⁺ peritonitis (n = 27)	G⁻ peritonitis (n = 15)
Age (years)	48.43±18.67	55.23±15.25	56.70±15.30	52.75±15.33
Gender (%, male)	57.9	61.9	66.7	53.3
Cause of ESRD (%)				
Diabetes mellitus	26.3	23.8	25.9	20.0
Glomerulonephritis	52.6	64.3	55.6	60
Other	21.1	11.9	11.1	20.0
PD duration(month)	22(6, 25)	11(4,17)	9(3,16)	12(9,24)
BMI (kg/m²)	22.51±2.31	22.71±2.72	23.43±2.22	21.51±3.11[b]
Hb (g/L)	100.75±23.93	95.4±21.25	93.21±23.31	99.10±22.12
Serum albumin (g/L)	35.67±3.57	31.55±5.26[a]	31.66±4.71[a]	31.35±6.24[a]
hs-CRP (mg/dL)	2.52(0.74,7.17)	9.28(3.88,12.21)[a]	8.00(4.07,11.82)	10.74(3.56,12.90)[a]
Total Kt/V	2.12(1.95,2.48)	2.20(1.97,2.73)	2.15(1.95,2.61)	2.23(2.20,2.73)
rGFR (ml/min/1.73 m²)	2.18(0.77,2.37)	2.06(1.43,3.47)	3.01(1.67,3.68)	2.1(0.96,2.69)

Note: ESRD, end-stage renal disease; PD, peritoneal dialysis; BMI, body mass index; Hb, haemoglobin; hsCRP, high-sensitivity C-reactive protein; Kt/V, solute clearance as a dialysis adequacy index; rGFR, residual glomerular filtration rate calculated by mean of creatinine and urea clearance.
Characteristics are presented as the mean ± SE or as median (interquartile range) for continuous variables and percentages for categorical variables.
[a]$p<0.05$, vs no peritonitis group.
[b]$p<0.05$,vs Gram-positive peritonitis group.

A

B

C

D

E

F

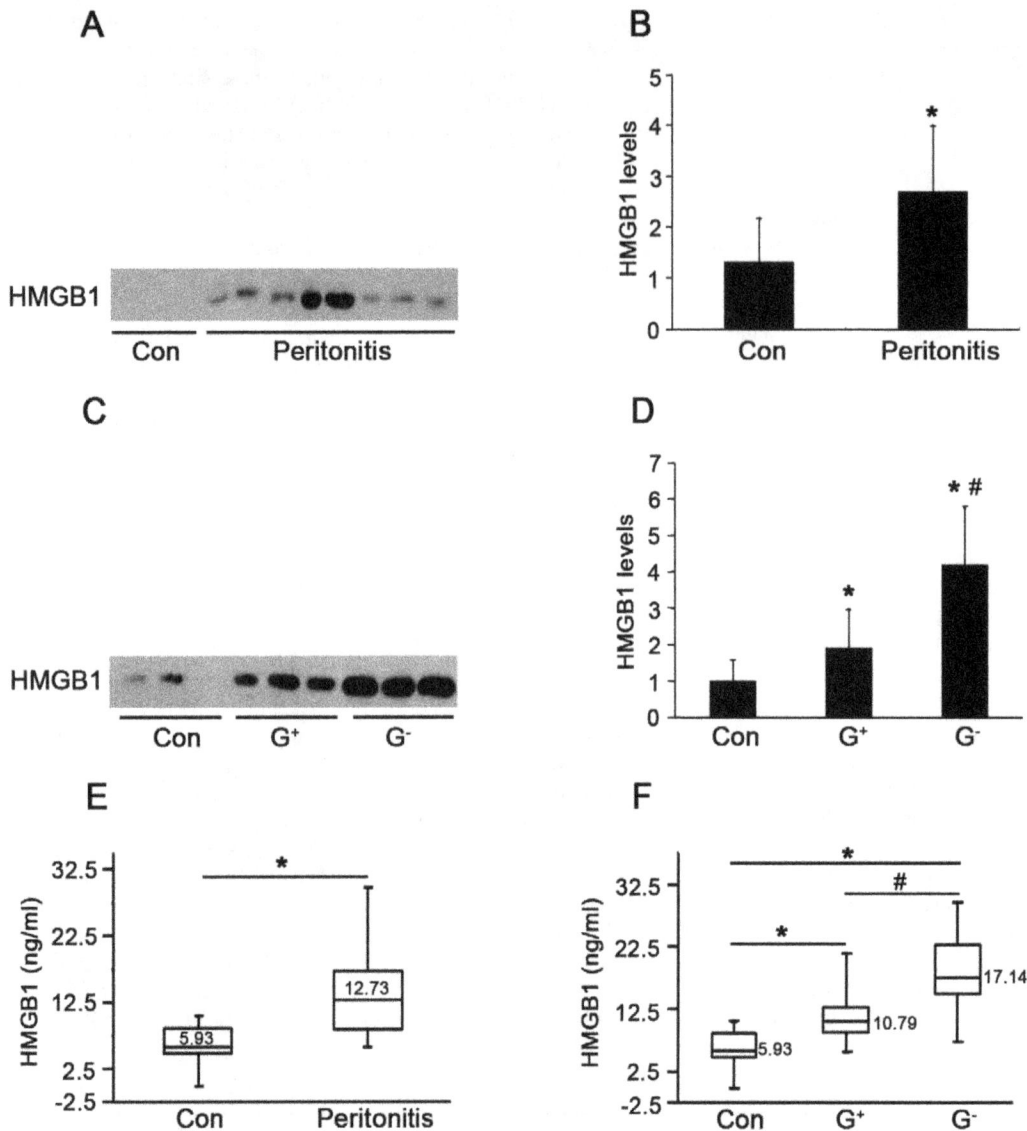

Figure 1. HMGB1 levels in peritoneal dialysis effluents (PDE). (A) Levels of HMGB1 in PDE of patients with or without peritonitis were detected by western blotting. PD patients without peritonitis served as controls (Con). (B) Densitometry of HMGB1 in immunoblots. Data are means ± SE ($n = 3$), *$P<0.05$ *versus* control subjects. (C) Representative immunoblot for HMGB1 in PDE among patient subgroups, including patients without peritonitis, with Gram-positive (G^+) and Gram-negative (G^-) peritonitis. (D) Quantitative determination of the relative abundance of HMGB1 protein among different groups. Data are means ± SE ($n = 3$), *$P<0.05$ *versus* control subjects. (E) Levels of HMGB1 in PDE of patients with or without peritonitis were quantified by ELISA. (F) Levels of HMGB1 in PDE among patient subgroups were assayed by ELISA. The box plot in E and F represents (from the top) values of the maximum, the third quartile, the median, the first quartile and the minimum, respectively ($n = 4$). *$P<0.05$ *versus* no peritonitis, #$P<0.05$ *versus* Gram-positive peritonitis.

$P<0.05$). Mice with acute LPS-associated peritonitis were accompanied by loss ultrafiltration (Fig. 5C), a progressive increase in the dialysate to plasma ratio for urea (Fig. 5D) and a progressive reabsorption of glucose from the dialysate (Fig. 5E). Pretreatment with glycyrrhizin, a known HMGB1 inhibitor [15], significantly attenuated these alterations, although glycyrrhizin did not affect LPS-induced increase in the percentage of neutrophils (data not shown). These findings suggest that inhibition of HMGB1 may provide protection against LPS-induced acute peritoneal inflammation and dysfunction. Of note, glycyrrhizin per se did not cause obvious cell toxicity in mice (data not shown).

LPS Induced HMGB1 Release and Cytoplasmic Translocation in HMrSV5 Cells

Given that HMGB1 is released by a variety of activated immune and non-immune cells [16,17,18] and peritonitis can cause injury to mesothelial cells, it would be of interest to know whether the elevated HMGB1 in PDE of patients with peritonitis can be directly released from damaged peritoneal mesothelial cells. Because of the significantly higher release of HMGB1, TNF-α and IL-6 in Gram-negative peritonitis, LPS was used to examine HMGB1 release in peritoneal mesothelial cells. We found that LPS stimulation for 48 hr caused a dose-dependent active HMGB1 release in culture media from HMrSV5 cells (Fig. 6A and B). Notably, the release of HMGB1 was independent on cell

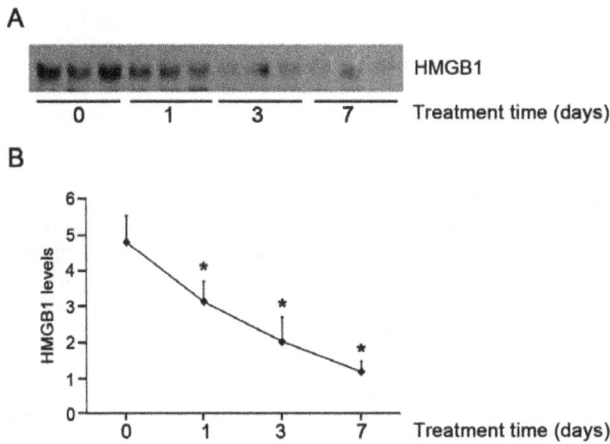

Figure 2. Serial changes in HMGB1 levels in PDE during peritonitis. (A) Representative HMGB1 immunoblot on PDE samples after antibiotic treatment. (B) Quantitative determination of relative HMGB1 levels in PDE after treatment. Data are expressed as mean ± SE from 3 independent experiments, *$P<0.05$ *versus* HMGB1 levels before treatment.

death at the dose of LPS from 0.5 to 2 µg/ml, because it did not significantly affect cell viability (Fig. 6C). However, a high dosage of LPS (5 µg/ml) exhibited cytotoxicity and consequently triggered a more pronounced, robust HMGB1 release, possibly as a result of both active and passive HMGB1 release (Fig. 6A, B and C). In addition, exposure of cells to LPS (2 µg/ml) induced active HMGB1 release in a time-dependent fashion within 48 hr, since it showed a cytotoxic effect on cells at 72 hr after LPS treatment (Fig. 6D, E and F).

Because HMGB1 resides primarily in the nucleus, we further speculated the relocation of HMGB1 from the nucleus to the cytoplasm after LPS treatment. As shown by immunofluorescence, HMGB1 was noted predominantly in the nucleus in the absence of LPS stimulation, but it appeared to move from the nucleus to the cytoplasm by displaying a punctuate staining in both nucleus and cytoplasm in the presence of LPS treatment for 24 hr (Fig. 7A). To further confirm those findings, cytoplasm and nuclear fractions were isolated and subjected to immunoblot analysis with antibodies specific for HMGB1, fibrillarin (a marker of nuclear protein) and tubulin (a marker of cytoplasm protein), respectively. Consistent with immunofluorescence results, HMGB1 was located primarily in the nucleus under the baseline condition. LPS treatment resulted in HMGB1 increase in the cytoplasm and

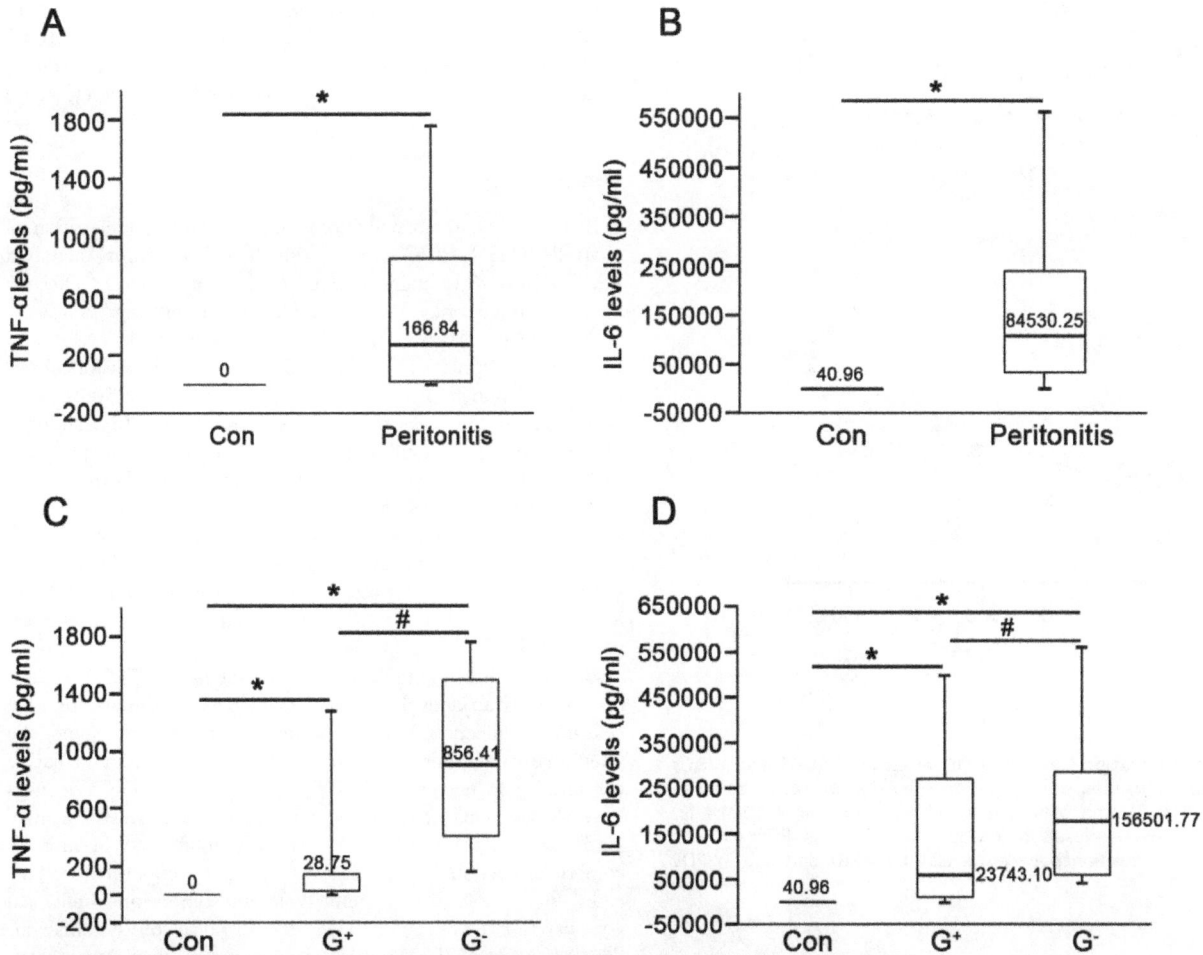

Figure 3. Levels of TNF-α and IL-6 in PDE during peritonitis. TNF-α levels (A) and IL-6 levels (B) in PDE were measured by ELISA from PD patients with or without peritonitis. The concentrations of TNF-α (C) and IL-6 (D) in PDE among subgroups of patients were determined by ELISA. The values represented the maximum, the third quartile, the median, the first quartile and the minimum, respectively (n = 4). *$P<0.05$ *versus* no peritonitis, #$P<0.05$ *versus* Gram-positive peritonitis.

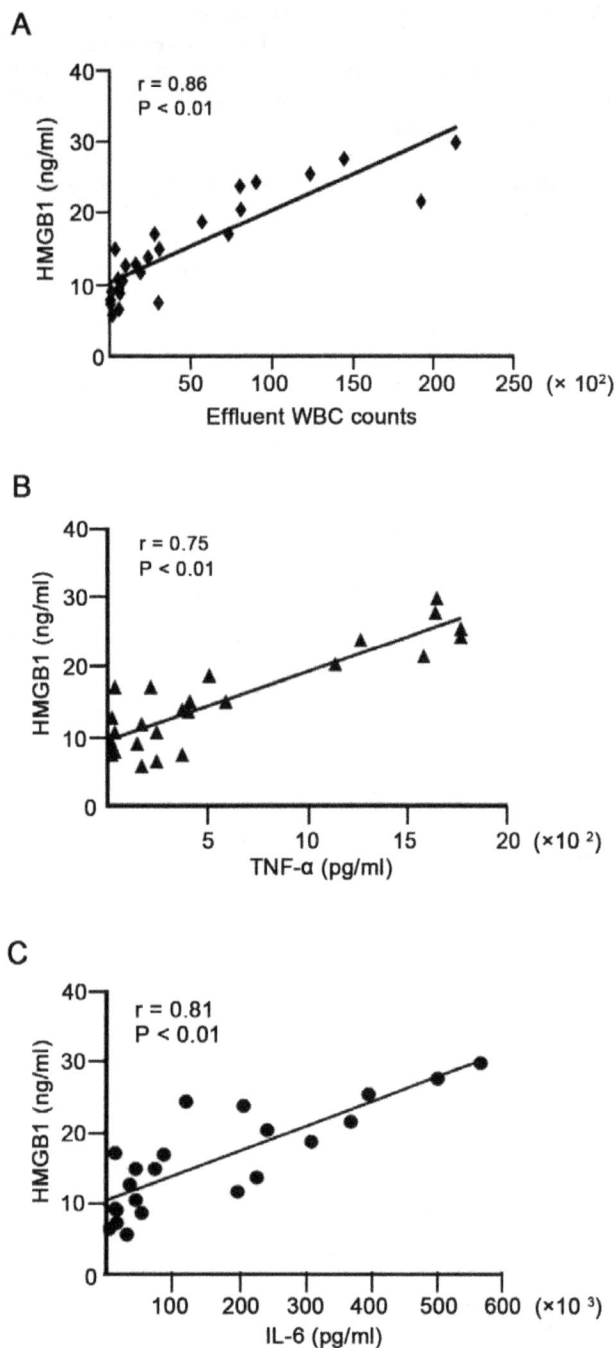

Figure 4. Correlation between PDE levels of HMGB1 and WBCs as well as cytokines during peritonitis. (A) Correlation between levels of HMGB1 and WBC counts in PDE ($r = 0.86$, $P < 0.01$). (B) Correlation between levels of HMGB1 and TNF-α in PDE ($r = 0.75$, $P < 0.01$). (C) Correlation between levels of HMGB1 and IL-6 in PDE ($r = 0.81$, $P < 0.01$).

corresponding decrease in the nucleus (Fig. 7B and C). Both immunofluorescence staining and immunoblot analysis indicate that LPS treatment causes HMGB1 nuclear-cytoplasmic translocation before releasing it into the extracellular milieu in peritoneal mesothelial cells.

HMGB1 was Secreted via Secretory Lysosome by HMrSV5 Cells

HMGB1 shuttles continually from the nucleus to the cytoplasm in quiescent cells [19]. However, HMGB1 lacks a leader peptide and thus not secreted via the Golgi/ER pathway. It has been reported that HMGB1 secretion was mediated by secretory lysosomes in innate immune cells, such as macrophages/monocytes [20]. To test whether peritoneal mesothelial cells share the same secretory pathway with macrophages, LPS-activated HMrSV5 cells were homogenized. Lysosome fractions were collected by a Lysosome Enrichment Kit and subjected to immunoblot analysis. Cathepsin D was used as a marker for the purity of lysosome fraction. As shown in Figure 8A and B, a few amount of HMGB1 was present in lysosome extracts under a baseline condition and showed a marked increase after LPS treatment (lane 1 and 2). In contrast, HMGB1 was not detectable in the presence of Triton X-100 (lane 3 and 4). The distribution of HMGB1, as revealed by the immunofluorescent staining, further confirmed an extensive colocalization of HMGB1 with the lysosome marker LAMP2a (Fig. 8C).

We showed that LPS stimulated a time-dependent release of HMGB1. To explore whether the increase of extracellular HMGB1 levels was associated with a reduction of lysosomal levels, the lysosomes were isolated and examined for HMGB1. After LPS exposure for 48 hr, lysosomal HMGB1 levels significantly decreased (Fig. 7D and E), suggesting that HMGB1 nuclear-cytoplasmic translocation induced by LPS may locate in a dense vesicular compartment of lysosome and secrete upon exocytosis of these organelles.

Discussion

In this study, we first demonstrated a significant elevation of HMGB1 in PDE of PD patients with clinical peritonitis. Increased HMGB1 levels gradually declined during the period of effective antibiotic treatments. Moreover, HMGB1 levels were markedly and positively correlated with WBC counts and with TNF-α and IL-6 levels. Inhibition of HMGB1 augmented peritoneal inflammation and improved peritoneal function in LPS-associated peritonitis in mice. *In vitro* studies showed that LPS induced HMGB1 nuclear-cytoplasmic translocation in peritoneal mesothelial cells. Upon low doses of LPS stimulation, HMGB1 was released actively into extracellular media and cytosolic HMGB1 secreted via a lysosome-mediated secretory pathway. These findings provide significant insights that HMGB1 is involved in PD-related peritonitis process and elevated HMGB1 in PDE are actively secreted, at least in part, from activated peritoneal mesothelial cells.

HMGB1 has been implicated as a key mediator of inflammatory disease. It is an actively secreted cytokine from innate immune cells during infection. HMGB1 triggers, amplifies and extends the inflammatory response by inducing cytokine release and mediating cell injury and necrosis [16,21,22]. A large number of evidences have shown that pharmacologic inhibition of HMGB1 activity (antibodies, antagonist proteins, release inhibitors) in animals confers protection against various infectious inflammatory diseases, suggesting a pathogenic role and important biological activities for extracellular HMGB1 in local or systemic inflammation [16,23]. However, it has never been investigated whether HMGB1 levels are elevated in PDE of patients with peritonitis. Our study showed that PDE HMGB1 levels in patients with peritonitis were significantly higher than those in control subjects and correspondingly elevated levels decreased gradually after effective antibiotic treatment. Analysis of a subgroup of

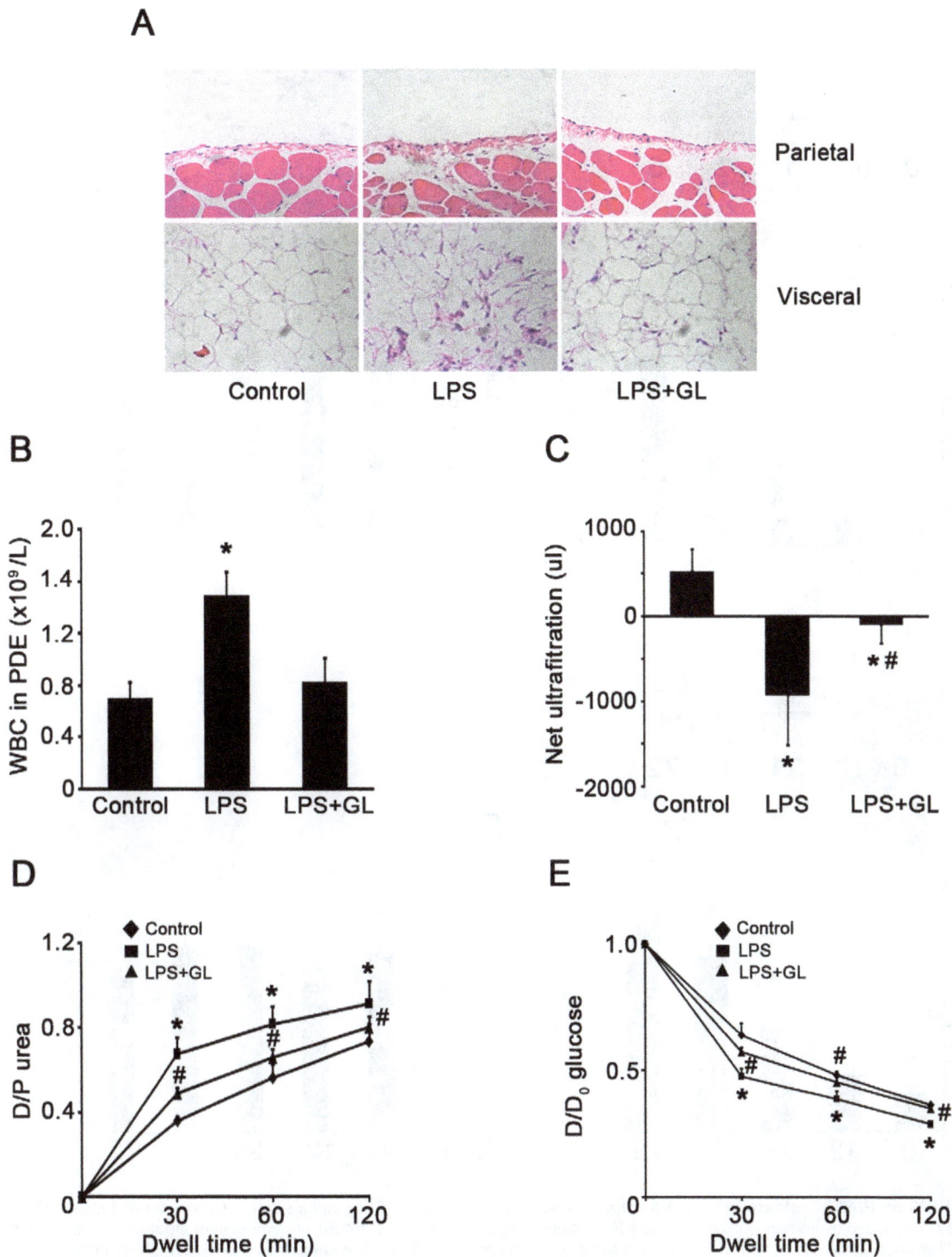

Figure 5. Effects of HMGB1 inhibitor on peritoneal inflammation and function. (A) Representative HE staining showed morphological changes and inflammatory infiltrate in both parietal and visceral peritoneum in each condition. Original magnification×200. (B) The total number of WBCs and the percentage of leukocytes in PDE among different group. (C–E) PD transport parameters to ultrafiltration, urea and glucose among different groups. Values are expressed as net ultrafiltration, D/P urea or D/D_0 glucose. Data in C, D and E are mean $\pm$ SE ($n=6$), *P<0.05 *versus* control, # P<0.05 *versus* LPS-treated without glycyrrhizin (GL) administration.

patients revealed that patients with Gram-negative peritonitis had greater HMGB1 levels in PDE compared with Gram-positive peritonitis, which underlying cause(s) has not been fully understood. Consistent with other previous reports, our data showed

that PDE levels of TNF-α and IL-6 were markedly elevated on the first day of peritonitis. Importantly, there was a significant positive correlation between PDE levels of HMGB1 and TNF-α, IL-6, as well as WBCs counts during peritonitis. In line with previous

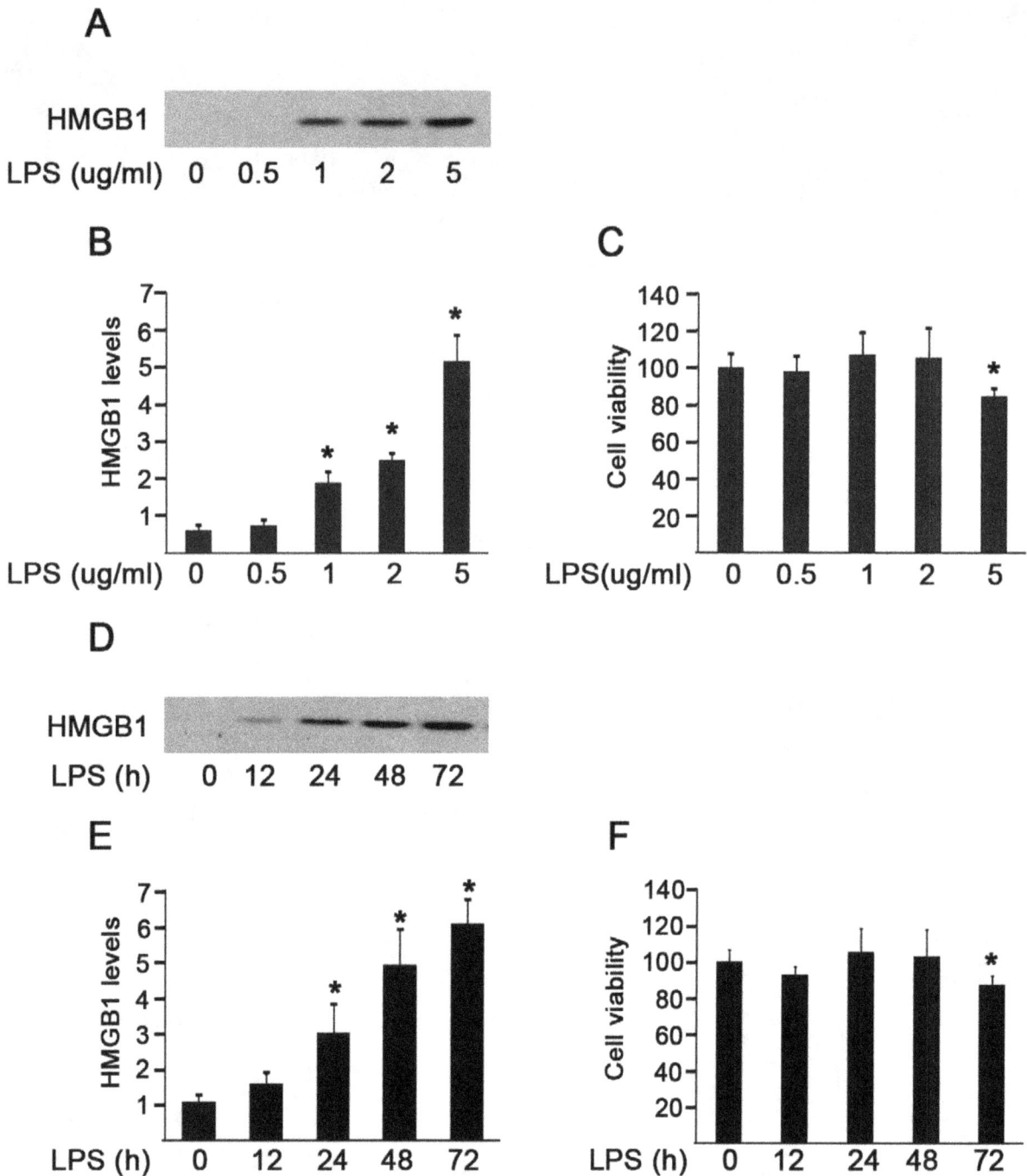

Figure 6. Effects of LPS on HMGB1 release in HMrSV5 cells. (A) Cells were treated with LPS at various concentrations for 48 hr. Cell culture media were collected and analyzed by immunoblotting with HMGB1 antibody. (B) Densitometry of HMGB1 proteins in immunoblots. (C) Cell viability was evaluated by MTT assay after treatment with LPS at the indicated concentrations for 48 hr. (D) Immunoblot analysis of HMGB1 in cell culture supernatants following 2 µg/ml LPS stimulation for the indicated time. (E) Quantitative determination of the relative abundance of HMGB1 proteins among different groups. (F) Cell viability was assayed by MTT at different time following LPS incubation. Data in B, C, E and F are expressed as mean ± SE ($n = 6$). *$P < 0.05$ *versus* control group.

studies [11,24,25,26], our results also showed that inhibition of HMGB1 by glycyrrhizin significantly attenuated LPS-induced peritoneal inflammatory cells infiltration and improved peritoneal function in mice, supporting the potential pathogenic role of HMGB1 in LPS-associated peritonitis. Taken together, these findings indicate that the HMGB1 levels in the PDE may be related to the process and severity of PD-related peritonitis.

The peritoneal macrophages in peritoneal cavity form the first line of defense against invading microorganisms. These cells are activated by microbial components resulting in complement activation and the release of proinflammatory mediators. It has been reported that both immune and non-immune cells actively release HMGB1 [5,16,19,23]. There is also evidence suggesting that the peritoneal mesothelial cells play a pivotal role in the local

A

LPS (h)   0   12   24   48

B

HMGB1

Tubulin

Fibliarian

LPS (h)   0   12   24   48   0   12   24   48

Cytosolic extract   Nuclear extract

C

LPS (h)   0   12   24   48   0   12   24   48

Cytosolic extract   Nuclear extract

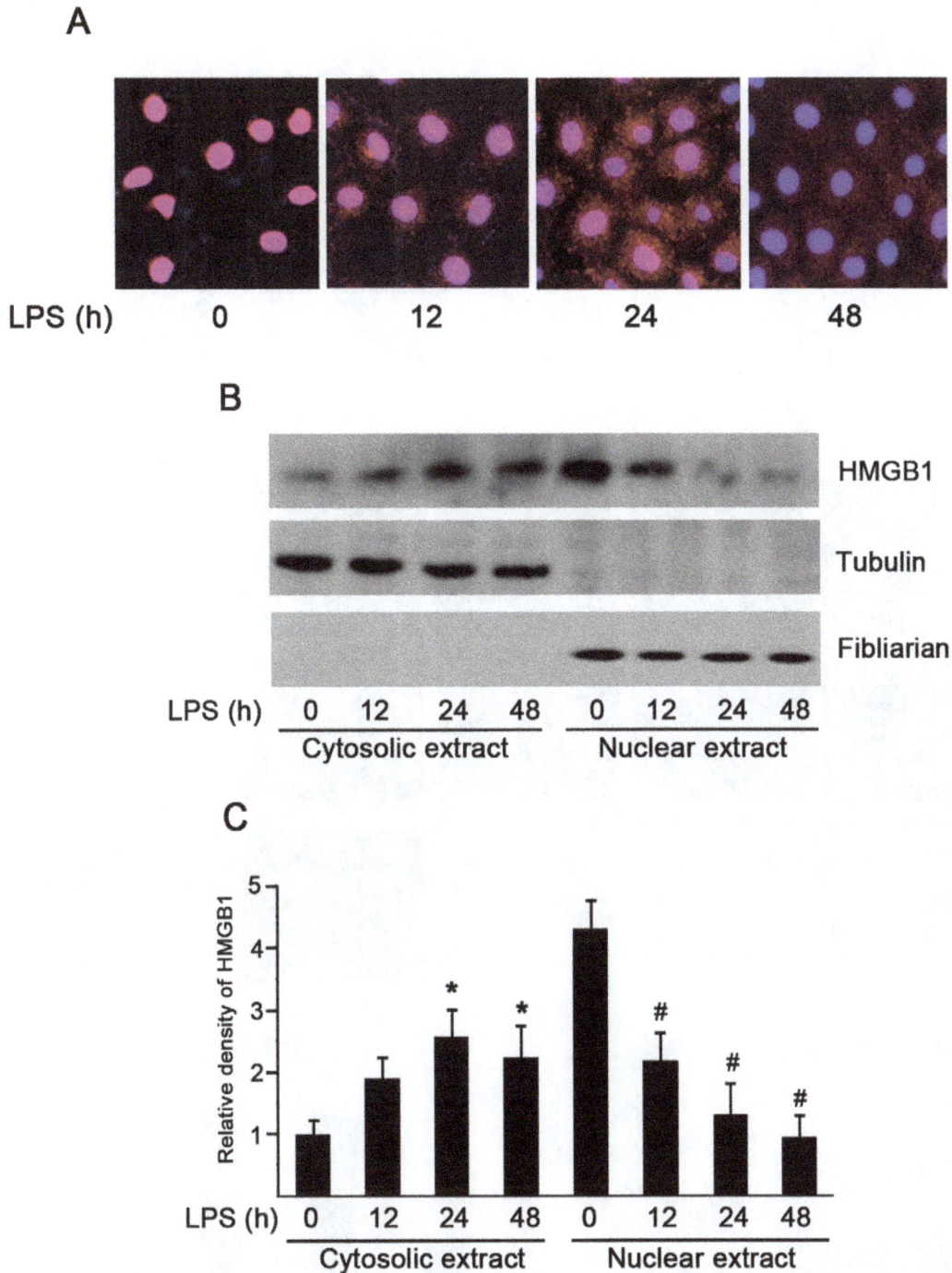

Figure 7. HMGB1 nuclear-cytoplasmic translocation in LPS-induced HMrSV5 cells. Cells were treated with 2 µg/ml LPS for the indicated time period. (A) Representative confocal microscopic images showed the cellular localization of HMGB1 (red) and nuclear staining (blue) by indirect immunofluorescence staining in cells. Original magnification ×400. (B) HMGB1 content in cytoplasm and nuclear fractions after LPS stimulation were assessed by Western blot analysis. (C) Quantitative determination of the relative abundance of HMGB1 in the cytoplasm and the nucleus among different groups. Data are expressed as mean±SE of three experiments. *$P<0.01$ *versus* negative control in the cytoplasm; #$P<0.01$ *versus* negative control in the nucleus.

defense by their ability to produce various cytokines [27,28]. However, it is unclear whether HMGB1 can be expressed and released by mesothelial cells during peritonitis. Our studies showed that at nontoxic concentrations of LPS exposure, the release of HMGB1 in HMrSV5 cells was not dependent on cell death, suggesting that the active release of HMGB1 occurred in peritoneal mesothelial cells following a sublethal dose of LPS stimulation. However, at slight cytotoxic dosages, LPS (5 µg/ml) might also cause passive HMGB1 leakage from peritoneal mesothelial cells. These findings support the notion that peritoneal mesothelial cells might be a source or additional source for extracellular HMGB1.

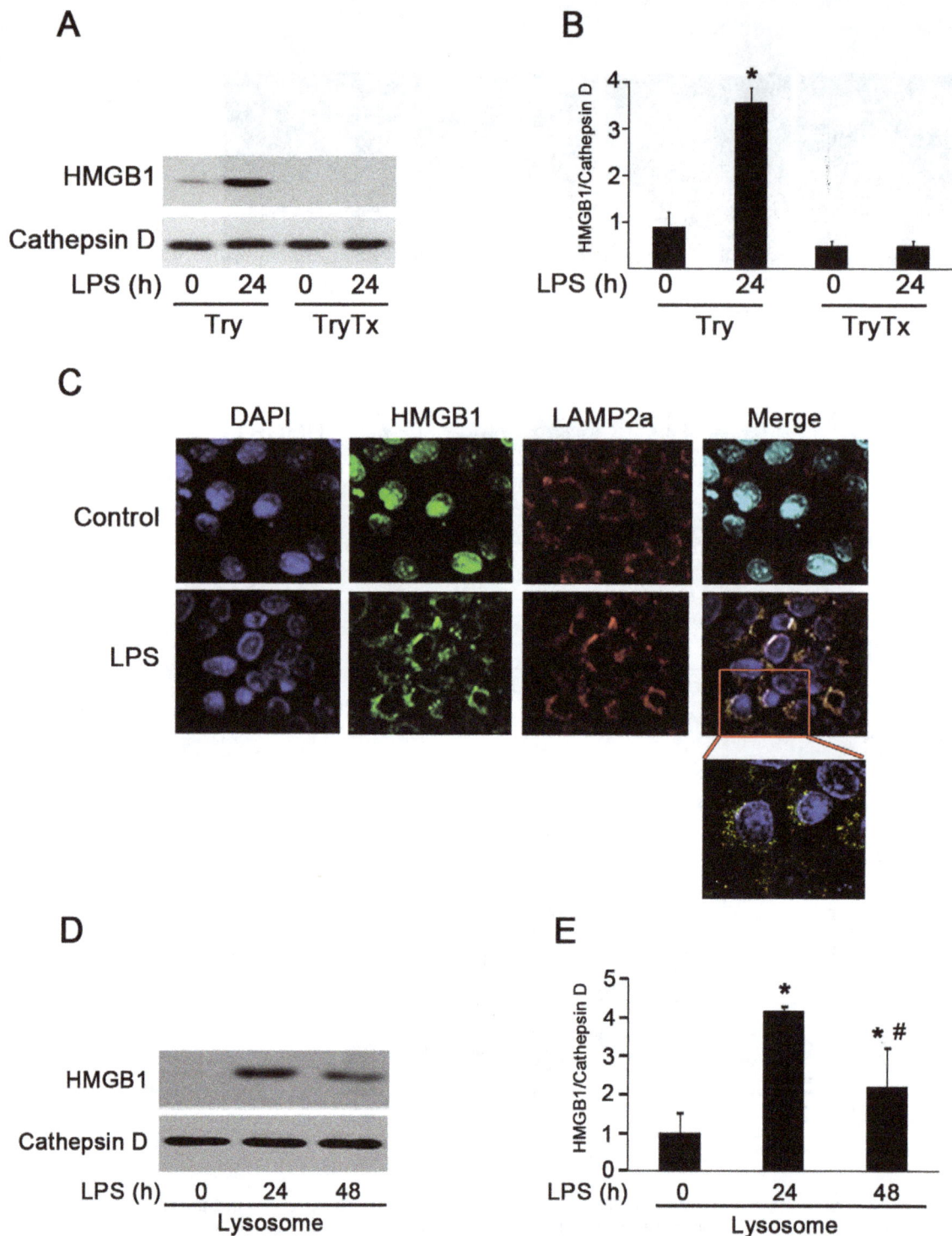

Figure 8. HMGB1 was secreted via lysosome-mediated secretory pathway in response to LPS stimulation. (A). HMGB1 was present in vesicles cofractionating with lysosomes after LPS administration. Lysosome fractions were untreated (lanes 1 and 2, Try) or solubilized (lanes 3 and 4, TyrTx) with Triton X-100 (TX) before trypsin (Try) digestion and subjected to Western blot analysis with anti-Cathepsin D and anti-HMGB1 antibodies. (B) Densitometry of HMGB1 content in different groups. Data are expressed as mean ± SE, $n = 3$ per treatment, *$P < 0.05$ versus Try treated only group. (C) Cells were treated with LPS (2 ug/ml) for 24 hr. Representative immunofluorescence analysis of cellular localization of HMGB1 (green) and LAMP2a (red), a maker of lysosome in cells. Original magnification×400. (D) HMGB1 protein contents in lysosome fractions following LPS treatment were determined by Western blotting. (E) Quantitative determination of the relative abundance of HMGB1 among different groups. Data are expressed as mean ± SE, $n = 3$ per treatment, *$P < 0.05$ versus control group, # $P < 0.05$ versus LPS treated for 24 hr.

As a non-histone chromosomal protein, HMGB1 localizes mainly in the nucleus of most cells under basal condition. It has been reported that HMGB1 secretion from monocytes/macrophages depends on relocalization from the nucleus to special cytoplasmic organelles, the secretory lysosomes [20]. In agreement with previous studies, we also observed that LPS induced HMGB1 nuclear-cytoplasmic translocation and once moving in the cytoplasm of peritoneal mesothelial cells, HMGB1 was loaded into secretory lysosomes. More importantly, these alterations were associated with the corresponding increased HMGB1 levels in extracellular milieu, supporting a lysosome-mediated HMGB1 export from LPS-stimulated human mesothelial cells.

In conclusion, our study reveals that HMGB1 levels in PDE are elevated and may play a critical role in peritoneal dysfunction during PD-related peritonitis. Activated or damaged peritoneal mesothelial cells may contribute to the increased HMGB1 in PDE. Thus, we propose that blockage of HMGB1 might represent a potential therapeutic strategy in PD-related peritonitis.

Materials and Methods

Ethics Statement

The study protocol was approved by the Ethics Committee of the First Affiliated Hospital, Sun Yat-sen University (Guangzhou, China). All participants provided written informed consent.

Patients

This was a longitudinal observational study. 42 PD patients within 24 hr of the onset of the first clinical signs and symptoms of peritonitis during the period from August 2008 to May 2009 in our PD center were recruited in the study. 19 PD patients without peritonitis were randomly selected during the study period and served as controls. The two groups were comparable in age, sex, primary renal disease, duration of dialysis, and co-morbidities. Peritonitis was defined as the presence of two of the following criteria: abdominal pain, cloudy effluent with ≥ 100 white blood cells (WBC)/μl and $\geq 50\%$ polymorphonuclear cells, or positive dialysate microbiological culture [29]. Episodes of peritonitis were initially treated with intraperitoneal ceftazidine, 1.0 g/2 L, and cefazolin, 1.0 g/2 L for one exchange daily for 14 days. The antibiotic regimen was modified on the basis of organism identification and drug sensitivity. Patients with PD-associated peritonitis were divided into two groups (Gram-positive and Gram-negative) based on the results of the Gram stain and the microbiological culture. Subjects with polymicrobial, fungal peritonitis, other organisms or culture negative were excluded.

All samples were taken when the patients were entered into this study. WBCs in PDE and serum haemoglobin were analyzed by standard techniques. Serum urea, creatinine, total cholesterol, triglycerides and albumin were measured by an autoanalyser (COBAS INTEGRA 400 plus, Roche). Serum hs-CRP was measured by using a latex enhanced immunoturbidimetric method with detection limit 0.07 mg/L (Roche Diagnostic, Mannheim, Germany). Residual GFR was defined as the average of 24-hr urinary urea and creatinine clearances. Total Kt/V was calculated using the PD Adequest 2.0 computer program for Windows (Baxter Healthcare Corp, Deerfield, IL).

Collection of PDE

The serial PDE samples were collected before the initiation of antibiotic treatment and after 1, 3, 7 and 14 days of treatment. All PDE samples were overnight dialysate effluent (1.36 g/dL glucose concentration) and examined by routine microbiology laboratory analysis and microbiological culture. The remaining dialysate was centrifuged at 4000×g for 15 min. The supernatants were collected and stored at −80°C until analysis.

Reagents and Antibodies

Reagents were obtained from the following sources: LPS (*Escherichia coli serotype 0111:B4*) and Glycyrrhizin were from Sigma-Aldrich (St. Louis, MO, USA). Anti-HMGB1 and anti-fibrillarin antibodies were purchased from Abcam (Cambridge, MA, USA). Anti-Cathepsin D was from Calbiochem (Merck, Darmstadt, Germany). Anti-β-tubulin was from Boster Biological Technology (Wuhan, China). Horseradish peroxidase (HRP) - conjugated anti-mouse IgG, HRP-conjugated anti-rabbit IgG and Alexa Fluor 546-conjugated anti-rabbit IgG were purchased from Cell Signal Technology (Beverly, MA, USA).

Enzyme-linked Immunosorbent Assay (ELISA)

The concentrations of HMGB1 (HMGB1 ELISA Kit II, Shino-Test Corporation, Tokyo, Japan), TNF-α and IL-6 (R&D Systems, Inc., Minneapolis, MN, USA) in PDE of patients were measured by using commercially available ELISA kits according to the manufacturer's instructions. The sensitivity of the HMGB1, TNF-α and IL-6 was 1 ng/mL, 0.70 pg/mL and 1.6 pg/mL, respectively. Each sample was run in triplicate and compared with a standard curve. The mean concentration was determined for each sample.

Animal Studies

Adult male C57 BL/6J mice (20–25 g) were obtained from Guangdong Medical Experimental Animal Center (Guangzhou, China). The animal experimental protocols were approved by Animal Care and Use Committee of the Sun Yat-sen University. Acute peritonitis was generated in mice by intraperitoneal injection of a single dose of LPS (10 mg/kg) in 1 ml sterile saline, as previously described [14,30]. 10 mg/mouse glycyrrhizin was administrated intraperitoneally 1 hr before LPS treatment. Glycyrrhizin was diluted in 50 mM NaOH at 37°C and pH was adjusted to pH 7.0–7.5 by the addition of 1 M Tris-HCl [15]. Control mice received the same volume sterile saline. Peritoneal function was evaluated by a 2-hr peritoneal equilibration test (PET) at 48 hr after LPS injection, as previously described [14]. The dialysate and blood samples were collected during PET. Dialysate WBCs and the differential count were counted by an automatic hematology analyzer. Concentrations of urea nitrogen and glucose in serum and dialysate were measured using an autoanalyser (COBAS INTEGRA 400 plus, Roche). Peritoneal solute transport was calculated from the dialysate concentration at 2 hr relative to its concentration in the initial infused dialysis solution (D/P creatinine) for urea nitrogen, and the dialysate-to-plasma concentration ratio (D/D$_0$ glucose) at 2 hr for glucose. Peritoneal tissues were collected and subjected to immunohisto-chemical analysis using hematoxylin-eosin (HE) staining.

Cell Culture and Viability

The in *vitro* studies were performed in human peritoneal mesothelial cell line (HMrSV5) as previously reported [14]. Cells were cultured in DMEM Nutrient Mix F12 media (Invitrogen Life Technologies, Carlsbad, CA, USA) supplemented with 10% fetal bovine serum. Cells were grown to approximately 70–80% confluence and subjected to serum-deprivation for 24 hr before LPS exposure. Cell viability was determined by the MTT [3-(4, 5-dimethylthiazol-2-yl)-2, 5-diphenyl tetrazolium bromide] test.

Preparation of the Cell Culture Media and Cellular Extracts

After exposure to the indicated experimental conditions, cell media were collected and filtered through Millex-GP (Millipore, Bedford, MA) to remove cell debris and macromolecular complexes. Superntants were then concentrated with Amicon Ultra-4 -10000 NMWL (Millipore, Bedford, MA) according to the manufacturer's instructions.

Cells were harvested and washed twice with cold PBS. Nuclear and cytoplasmic extracts were isolated as in our previous study using NE-PER Nuclear and Cytoplasmic Extraction Reagents (Pierce, Rockford, IL, USA) [31].

Lysosome-enriched fractions were enriched by using the Lysosomes Extract Kit following the manufacturer's instruction (Pierce, Rockford, IL, USA). In brief, cells with or without LPS treatment were harvested and cell pellets were incubated with Lysosome Enrichment Reagent A and B, then centrifuged at $500 \times g$ for 10 min at 4°C to remove nuclei and cell debris. Post-nuclear supernatants were mixed with the OptiPrep™ Cell Separation Media (Pierce, Rockford, IL, USA) to make a final concentration of 15% OptiPrep™ Media and subjected to gradient centrifugation. Lysosome lysis was collected from the top of the gradient, treated with 100 µg/ml trypsin for 30 min on ice, in the absence or presence of 1% Triton X-100, and subjected to immunoblot analysis.

Western Blot Analysis

Proteins were isolated from PDE samples, cell culture media or cell extracts. The protein concentration was measured by the Bradford protein assay (Bio-Rad, Hercules, CA). Equal volume (40 µl) of the concentrated PDE sample or cell culture media and equal amounts of proteins from cellular extracts were loaded and separated by 10% SDS-PAGE and transferred onto nitrocellulose membrane. The blots were probed overnight at 4°C with specific antibodies, and detected using the ECL system as previously described [31]. Densitometric analysis was performed with the image analysis program (FluorChem 8900; Alpha Innotech Corp, San Leandro, CA).

Immunouorescence and Immunohistochemical Analysis

Indirect immunofluorescence staining was performed following conventional procedures as described in our previous study [31]. Briefly, cells were cultured on glass coverslips and stimulated with 2 µg/ml LPS for the indicated time. Subsequently, cells were fixed in 4% formaldehyde, permeabilized with 0.1% Triton-X-100 in PBS and sequentially incubated with the indicated primary antibodies, washed 3 times in PBS and incubated for 1 hr with each of the corresponding secondary antibodies. All images were collected by a laser scanning confocal microscopy (Zeiss LSM 510 META, Carl Zeiss, Germany).

Both parietal and visceral peritoneum were fixed in 10% phosphate buffer formalin, dehydrated through graded alcohol and xylene, embedded in paraffin, sectioned at 2-µm thickness, and then stained with hematoxylin and eosin. Histological examinations were observed by light microscopy and evaluated in a blinded manner.

Statistical Analysis

Continuous data were expressed as mean ± standard deviation (SD) or median (interquartile range IQR) and categorical data were expressed as frequencies and percentage. Differences among groups were analyzed by one way-ANOVA analysis. Significant variation in the data within groups was investigated using a Kruskal Wallis test. Frequency data (e.g., gender) were analyzed by the Chi-square test. The Spearman or Pearson correlation coefficient test was used to evaluate associations between two quantitative variables. P values <0.05 were considered significant. All statistical analyses were conducted using SPSS 15.0 statistics software (version 15.0, SPSS Inc, Chicago, IL).

Author Contributions

Conceived and designed the experiments: HPM XQY SRC SL. Performed the experiments: SRC SL HYL LPX JJF YZ. Analyzed the data: SRC SL HPM. Contributed reagents/materials/analysis tools: SRC SL XQY. Wrote the paper: SL HPM.

References

1. Nessim SJ (2011) Prevention of peritoneal dialysis-related infections. Semin Nephrol 31: 199–212.
2. Yung S, Li FK, Chan TM (2006) Peritoneal mesothelial cell culture and biology. Perit Dial Int 26: 162–173.
3. Lotze MT, Tracey KJ (2005) High-mobility group box 1 protein (HMGB1): nuclear weapon in the immune arsenal. Nat Rev Immunol 5: 331–342.
4. Scaffidi P, Misteli T, Bianchi ME (2002) Release of chromatin protein HMGB1 by necrotic cells triggers inflammation. Nature 418: 191–195.
5. Wang H, Bloom O, Zhang M, Vishnubhakat JM, Ombrellino M, et al. (1999) HMG-1 as a late mediator of endotoxin lethality in mice. Science 285: 248–251.
6. Wang H, Yang H, Tracey KJ (2004) Extracellular role of HMGB1 in inflammation and sepsis. J Intern Med 255: 320–331.
7. Goldstein RS, Bruchfeld A, Yang L, Qureshi AR, Gallowitsch-Puerta M, et al. (2007) Cholinergic anti-inflammatory pathway activity and High Mobility Group Box-1 (HMGB1) serum levels in patients with rheumatoid arthritis. Mol Med 13: 210–215.
8. Bruchfeld A, Qureshi AR, Lindholm B, Barany P, Yang L, et al. (2008) High Mobility Group Box Protein-1 correlates with renal function in chronic kidney disease (CKD). Mol Med 14: 109–115.
9. Sunden-Cullberg J, Norrby-Teglund A, Rouhiainen A, Rauvala H, Herman G, et al. (2005) Persistent elevation of high mobility group box-1 protein (HMGB1) in patients with severe sepsis and septic shock. Crit Care Med 33: 564–573.
10. Borde C, Barnay-Verdier S, Gaillard C, Hocini H, Marechal V, et al. (2011) Stepwise release of biologically active HMGB1 during HSV-2 infection. PLoS One 6: e16145.
11. Yang H, Ochani M, Li J, Qiang X, Tanovic M, et al. (2004) Reversing established sepsis with antagonists of endogenous high-mobility group box 1. Proc Natl Acad Sci U S A 101: 296–301.
12. Dehbi M, Uzzaman T, Baturcam E, Eldali A, Ventura W, et al. (2012) Toll-like receptor 4 and high-mobility group box 1 are critical mediators of tissue injury and survival in a mouse model for heat stroke. PLoS One 7: e44100.
13. Andrassy M, Volz HC, Igwe JC, Funke B, Eichberger SN, et al. (2008) High-mobility group box-1 in ischemia-reperfusion injury of the heart. Circulation 117: 3216–3226.
14. Li S, Zhou Y, Fan J, Cao S, Cao T, et al. (2011) Heat shock protein 72 enhances autophagy as a protective mechanism in lipopolysaccharide-induced peritonitis in rats. Am J Pathol 179: 2822–2834.
15. Sitia G, Iannacone M, Muller S, Bianchi ME, Guidotti LG (2007) Treatment with HMGB1 inhibitors diminishes CTL-induced liver disease in HBV transgenic mice. J Leukoc Biol 81: 100–107.
16. Andersson U, Tracey KJ (2011) HMGB1 is a therapeutic target for sterile inflammation and infection. Annu Rev Immunol 29: 139–162.
17. Rendon-Mitchell B, Ochani M, Li J, Han J, Wang H, et al. (2003) IFN-gamma induces high mobility group box 1 protein release partly through a TNF-dependent mechanism. J Immunol 170: 3890–3897.
18. Maugeri N, Franchini S, Campana L, Baldini M, Ramirez GA, et al. (2012) Circulating platelets as a source of the damage-associated molecular pattern HMGB1 in patients with systemic sclerosis. Autoimmunity 45: 584–587.
19. Wang H, Yang H, Czura CJ, Sama AE, Tracey KJ (2001) HMGB1 as a late mediator of lethal systemic inflammation. Am J Respir Crit Care Med 164: 1768–1773.
20. Gardella S, Andrei C, Ferrera D, Lotti LV, Torrisi MR, et al. (2002) The nuclear protein HMGB1 is secreted by monocytes via a non-classical, vesicle-mediated secretory pathway. EMBO Rep 3: 995–1001.
21. Bogdanovich S, Krag TO, Barton ER, Morris LD, Whittemore LA, et al. (2002) Functional improvement of dystrophic muscle by myostatin blockade. Nature 420: 418–421.

22. Wang H, Vishnubhakat JM, Bloom O, Zhang M, Ombrellino M, et al. (1999) Proinflammatory cytokines (tumor necrosis factor and interleukin 1) stimulate release of high mobility group protein-1 by pituicytes. Surgery 126: 389–392.

23. Liu S, Stolz DB, Sappington PL, Macias CA, Killeen ME, et al. (2006) HMGB1 is secreted by immunostimulated enterocytes and contributes to cytomix-induced hyperpermeability of Caco-2 monolayers. Am J Physiol Cell Physiol 290: C990–999.

24. Sitia G, Iannacone M, Aiolfi R, Isogawa M, van Rooijen N, et al. (2011) Kupffer cells hasten resolution of liver immunopathology in mouse models of viral hepatitis. PLoS Pathog 7: e1002061.

25. Orlova VV, Choi EY, Xie C, Chavakis E, Bierhaus A, et al. (2007) A novel pathway of HMGB1-mediated inflammatory cell recruitment that requires Mac-1-integrin. Embo J 26: 1129–1139.

26. Andersson U, Harris HE (2010) The role of HMGB1 in the pathogenesis of rheumatic disease. Biochim Biophys Acta 1799: 141–148.

27. Topley N (1995) The host's initial response to peritoneal infection: the pivotal role of the mesothelial cell. Perit Dial Int 15: 116–117.

28. Yung S, Davies M (1998) Response of the human peritoneal mesothelial cell to injury: an in vitro model of peritoneal wound healing. Kidney Int 54: 2160–2169.

29. Li PK, Szeto CC, Piraino B, Bernardini J, Figueiredo AE, et al. (2011) Peritoneal dialysis-related infections recommendations: 2010 update. Perit Dial Int 30: 393–423.

30. Ni J, McLoughlin RM, Brodovitch A, Moulin P, Brouckaert P, et al. (2010) Nitric oxide synthase isoforms play distinct roles during acute peritonitis. Nephrol Dial Transplant 25: 86–96.

31. Zhou Y, Mao H, Li S, Cao S, Li Z, et al. (2010) HSP72 inhibits Smad3 activation and nuclear translocation in renal epithelial-to-mesenchymal transition. J Am Soc Nephrol 21: 598–609.

3

Aliskiren Prevents the Toxic Effects of Peritoneal Dialysis Fluids during Chronic Dialysis in Rats

Juan Pérez-Martínez³, Francisco C. Pérez-Martínez⁴, Blanca Carrión⁴, Jesús Masiá³, Agustín Ortega³, Esther Simarro⁵, Syong H. Nam-Cha⁶, Valentín Ceña¹,²*

1 Unidad Asociada Neurodeath, Departamento de Ciencias Médicas, CSIC-Universidad de Castilla-La Mancha, Albacete, Spain, 2 CIBERNED, Instituto de Salud Carlos III, Madrid, Spain, 3 Department of Nephrology, Complejo Hospitalario Universitario, Albacete, Spain, 4 Department of Research and Development, NanoDrugs, S.L., Parque Científico y Tecnológico, Albacete, Spain, 5 Department of Clinical Chemistry, Complejo Hospitalario Universitario, Albacete, Spain, 6 Department of Pathology, Complejo Hospitalario Universitario, Albacete, Spain

Abstract

The benefits of long-term peritoneal dialysis (PD) in patients with end-stage renal failure are short-lived due to structural and functional changes in the peritoneal membrane. In this report, we provide evidence for the *in vitro* and *in vivo* participation of the renin-angiotensin-aldosterone system (RAAS) in the signaling pathway leading to peritoneal fibrosis during PD. Exposure to high-glucose PD fluids (PDFs) increases damage and fibrosis markers in both isolated rat peritoneal mesothelial cells and in the peritoneum of rats after chronic dialysis. In both cases, the addition of the RAAS inhibitor aliskiren markedly improved damage and fibrosis markers, and prevented functional modifications in the peritoneal transport, as measured by the peritoneal equilibrium test. These data suggest that inhibition of the RAAS may be a novel way to improve the efficacy of PD by preventing inflammation and fibrosis following peritoneal exposure to high-glucose PDFs.

Editor: Rajesh Mohanraj, UAE University, Faculty of Medicine & Health Sciences, United Arab Emirates

Funding: This work has been supported, in part, by grants PI081434 from Fondo de Investigaciones Sanitarias, BFU2011-30161-C02-01 from Ministerio de Ciencia e Innovación and PII1I09-0163-4002 and POII10-0274-3182 from Consejería de Educación, JCCM to V.C.; and PI10/01420 from the Fondo de Investigaciones Sanitarias, Ministerio de Ciencia e Innovación; and PI-2009/32 from Consejería de Salud y Bienestar Social, JCCM, to J.P.-M. The funders had no role in study design, data collection and analysis, decision to publish, or preparation of the manuscript. No additional external funding was received for this study.

Competing Interests: The authors have read the journal's policy and have the following conflicts: - The corresponding author, VC, is an Academic Editor for the journal. - FCP-M and BC are employed by NanoDrugs, S.L. This does not alter the authors' adherence to all the PLoS ONE policies on sharing data and materials.

* E-mail: valentin.cena@gmail.com

Introduction

Chronic kidney disease is a worldwide public health problem with increasing incidence and prevalence, poor outcomes and high costs [1] Long-term peritoneal dialysis (PD) is a suitable and effective therapy option for patients with end-stage renal failure, and has been widely used for more than 20 years [2]. Nevertheless, the benefits of PD are short-lived, mainly due to structural and functional changes in the peritoneal membrane caused by the use of conventional PD fluids (PDFs) [3,4], which contain high concentrations of glucose as the osmotic agent [5,6]. However, a loss of peritoneal mesothelial cells (PMCs), progressive peritoneal fibrosis (PF), membrane hyperpermeability and ultrafiltration failure develop when using glucose-based solutions [7–9], although the physiopathological mechanisms underlying these changes are not fully understood.

Angiotensin II, a component of the renin–angiotensin–aldosterone system (RAAS), is constitutively expressed within PMCs [10,11]. Noxious stimuli induce activation of the local peritoneal angiotensin II, which initiates production of transforming growth factor-β1 (TGF-β1), thus contributing to extracellular matrix accumulation and inducing PF [12,13]. Functionally, these changes translate into reduced ultrafiltration capacity of the peritoneal membrane, which is a significant cause of the failure of the technique among patients on long-term PD [11]. Aliskiren

decreases angiotensin II production [14] and it is therefore effective in lowering blood pressure and holds considerable potential for organ protection beyond blood pressure reduction [14,15].

We studied the protective effects of aliskiren on PMCs exposed to glucose-enriched solutions *in vitro* as well as on the peritoneal membrane in rats dialyzed with PDFs for four weeks. We found that, at concentrations achievable in humans, aliskiren prevents high glucose-mediated PDF-induced thickening and fibrosis of the peritoneum, decreases cellular damage markers and, by decreasing fibrosis, preserves the efficacy of PDFs. These results strongly suggest that a RAAS blockade may increase the effective time of PDF therapy, paving the way for the development of new, less toxic PD solutions.

Results

Aliskiren Protects PMCs From PDF Toxicity *In Vitro*

In cultured rat PMCs, PDFs containing high levels of glucose induced increases in free-radical production that amounted to approximately $162.5 \pm 8.5\%$ of control levels at 8 h of exposure (Fig. 1a). Phosphorylation of p38 mitogen-activated protein kinase (MAPK) is a generally accepted index of toxicity for PMCs [16]. Exposure to a high-glucose PDF for 48 h caused a marked increase in the phospho-p38 (p-p38) MAPK/p38 MAPK protein ratio compared to control cells (Fig. 1b). This toxicity may activate the cell death cascade, as indicated by the increase in caspase-3 activity observed in rat PMCs following exposure to a high-glucose PDF for 18 h (Fig. 1c). Aliskiren, at concentrations equal to or higher than 50 μmol/L, significantly prevented the observed increase in the studied toxicity markers for PMCs *in vitro* (Fig. 1). Moreover, exposure to a high-glucose PDF for 24 h caused a marked increase in mRNA levels of the pro-apoptotic markers p53 (Fig. 2a) and Bax (Fig. 2b), and a decrease in the mRNA level of the anti-apoptotic marker Bcl-2 (Fig. 2c) in rat-cultured PMCs. On the other hand, exposure to a high-glucose PDF for 24 h increased mRNA levels of fibrosis markers such as collagen III (Fig. 2d) and fibronectin (Fig. 2e). RAAS inhibition using aliskiren markedly decreased the production of these fibrosis and pro-apoptotic markers, as well and increased Bcl-2 mRNA expression (Fig. 2).

Aliskiren Prevents Damage Induced *In Vivo* by High-Glucose PDFs

To explore PDF-mediated toxicity *in vivo*, we dialyzed rats daily using commercial PDFs containing three different glucose

concentrations (1.5%, 2.3% and 4.5%) for four weeks. At the end of the study, the peritoneum was removed and analyzed for levels of mRNA encoding for proteins involved in the death/survival pathway. The p53 mRNA levels increased in PMCs collected from the peritoneum of rats dialyzed with 4.5% PDF as compared to the vehicle group (Fig. 3a). The addition of aliskiren (100 mg/l) to the PD solution prevented the PDF-mediated increase in p53 mRNA levels (Fig. 3a). Moreover, Bax mRNA levels were significantly higher in the rat peritoneum after chronic dialysis than in the vehicle-dialyzed group. The increase in Bax mRNA levels following dialysis was much smaller when aliskiren was added to the PDF (Fig. 3b), with a concentration-dependent effect from aliskiren. The above data indicate that aliskiren prevents the PDF-induced increase in pro-apoptotic gene expression. In addition, chronic dialysis using 2.3% and 4.5% PDFs decreased mRNA levels of the anti-apoptotic protein Bcl-2 in the peritoneum (Fig. 3c). The addition of aliskiren to the PD solution markedly increased Bcl-2 mRNA levels well above basal levels (between 2- and 5-fold) (Fig. 3c). Surprisingly, this effect was not observed in vehicle-dialyzed rats and was only evident

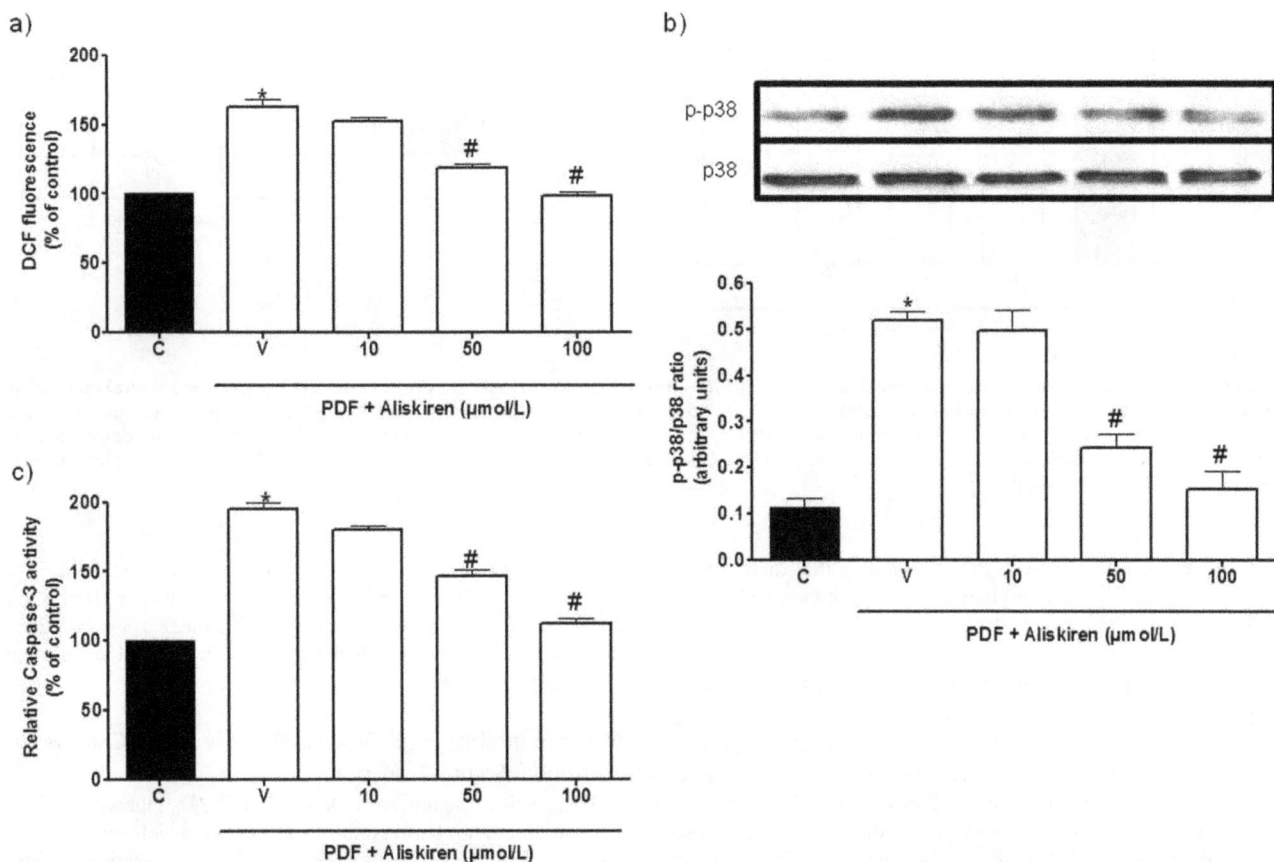

Figure 1. Aliskiren decreases toxicity induced by peritoneal dialysis fluids (PDFs) in rat peritoneal mesothelial cells (PMCs). a) Effect of aliskiren on PDF-mediated reactive oxygen species (ROS) production in PMCs. Cells were treated for 8 h with a 1.5%-glucose PDF diluted 1:1 in culture medium in the absence (V) or the presence of aliskiren. ROS production was measured using dichlorodihydrofluorescein (DCF) as described in Methods. Results represent mean ± s.e.m. of 4 experiments. *p<0.05 as compared to untreated control cells (C). #p<0.05 as compared to cells treated with vehicle and high-glucose PDF (V). b) Effect of aliskiren on phospho-p38 (p-p38) mitogen-activated protein kinase (MAPK)/p38 MAPK ratio in rat PMCs exposed to a high-glucose PDF for 24 h. PMCs were treated as above, in the absence (V) or presence of aliskiren and then both p-p38 MAPK and p38 MAPK protein levels were determined by western blot. The histograms represent a densitometric analysis of the p-p38 MAPK/p38 MAPK ratio. Data represent mean ± s.e.m. of 4 experiments.*p<0.05 as compared to C. #p<0.01 as compared to V. c) Effect of aliskiren on caspase-3 activity in rat PMCs exposed to a high-glucose PDF for 18 h. PMCs were treated as above, in the absence (V) or presence of aliskiren and then caspase-3 activity was determined (see Methods). Data represent mean ± s.e.m. of 4 experiments. *p<0.05 as compared to C. #p<0.05 as compared to V.

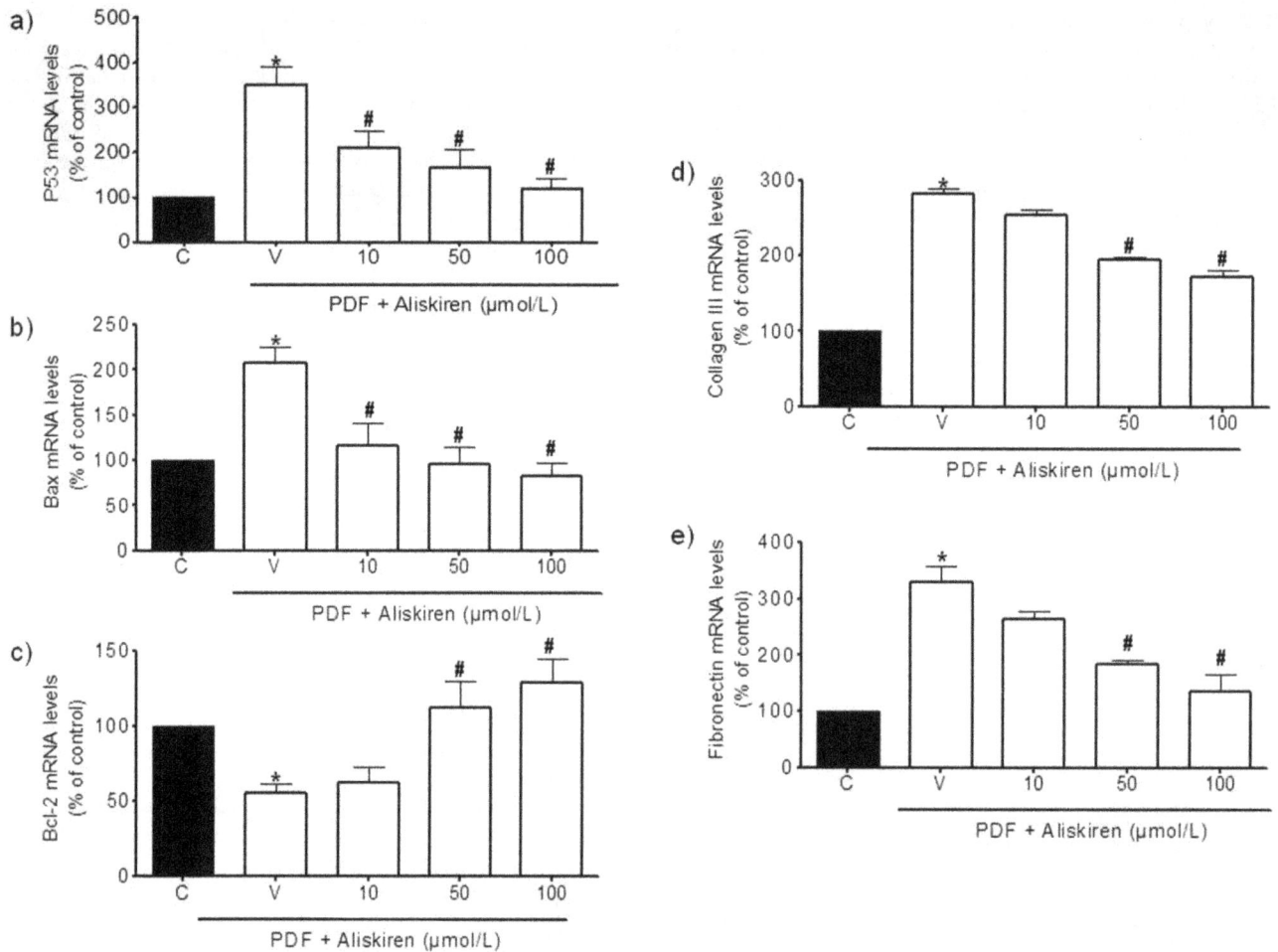

Figure 2. Aliskiren decreases fibrosis markers and inhibits changes in apoptosis markers induced by peritoneal dialysis fluids (PDFs) in rat peritoneal mesothelial cells (PMCs). Cells were treated for 24 h with a 1.5%-glucose PDF diluted 1:1 in culture medium in the absence (V) or the presence of aliskiren, and the levels of mRNA for p53 (a), Bax (b), Bcl-2 (c), collagen III (d) and fibronectin (e) were determined by real-time RT-PCR. Data represent mean ± s.e.m. of 4 experiments. *p<0.05 as compared to untreated control cells (C). #p<0.01 as compared to cells treated with vehicle and PDF (V).

following chronic dialysis with PDF, suggesting that dialysis with bio-incompatible PD solutions may sensitize peritoneal cells to the actions of aliskiren.

Aliskiren Reduces Inflammation and Fibrosis Produced by High-Glucose PDFs

After four weeks of daily PD, a Peritoneal Equilibrium Test (PET) adjusted for rats was performed using 2.3% PDF. The C reactive protein (CRP) and amyloid-P protein level inflammation markers were increased in both serum and dialysate when the rats were dialyzed using 4.25% PDF in the absence of aliskiren (Figs. 4a and 4b). Moreover, amyloid-P protein levels were also significantly increased in the group dialyzed with 2.3% PDF. The addition of aliskiren (100 mg/l) to the PDFs prevented the increase observed in the levels of inflammation markers CRP and amyloid-P protein in both serum and dialysate (Figs. 4c and 4d).

Consistent with well-known PD complications, fibrosis markers such as fibronectin and collagen III mRNA levels were markedly elevated in PMCs collected from the 2.3% and 4.25% PDF groups when compared to the vehicle group (Figs. 5a and 5b). These changes in fibronectin and collagen III gene expression after PDF exposure correlated with an increase in the thickness of the

peritoneal membrane (Fig. 5c). The inclusion of aliskiren in the PD solution markedly reduced fibronectin and collagen III mRNA levels in response to chronic dialysis with the 2.3% and 4.25% PDFs and decreased the thickness of the peritoneal membrane after chronic dialysis (Fig. 5).

Aliskiren Inhibits High-Glucose PDF-Mediated Changes in Peritoneal Solute Transport

There was no significant difference in D_2/D_0 glucose and D_2/P_2 creatinine ratios between the groups dialyzed with vehicle in the absence or presence of aliskiren (Fig. 6). The peritoneal solute transport in the group dialyzed with 1.5% PDF for four weeks was no different from that observed in the group dialyzed with saline alone (vehicle group), and the presence of different doses of aliskiren in the 1.5% PDF did not have any effect. On the other hand, D_2/D_0 glucose ratios were significantly lower, and D_2/P_2 creatinine ratios were significantly higher in the 2.3% and the 4.25% PDF groups as compared to the vehicle group (Fig. 6) indicating a high transporter status that is consistent with the observed inflammatory changes. The groups dialyzed with both 2.3% and 4.25% PDFs supplemented with aliskiren showed higher D_2/D_0 glucose and lower D_2/P_2 creatinine ratios than their

a)

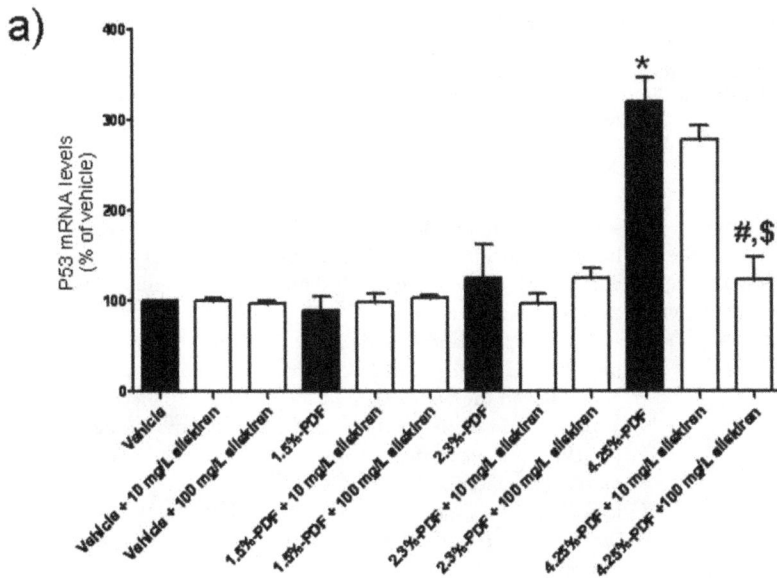

b)

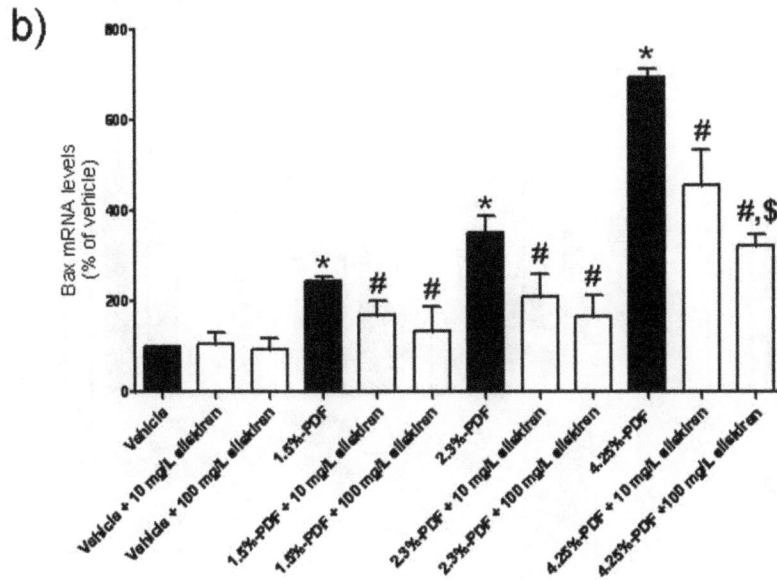

c)

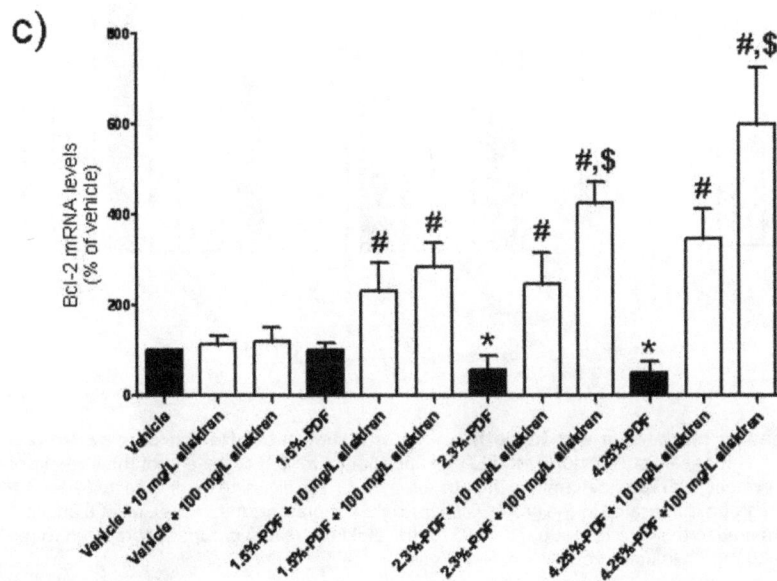

Figure 3. *In vivo* effect of aliskiren on p53, Bax and Bcl-2 mRNA levels in the peritoneum after daily peritoneal dialysis for 4 weeks. Twelve groups of 6 rats each one were dialyzed daily as described in Methods for 4 weeks in the absence (black histograms) and in the presence of aliskiren (10 and 100 mg/L). At the end of this period, peritoneal mesothelial cells (PMCs) were isolated and the mRNA levels for p53 (a), Bax (b), and Bcl-2 (c) quantified and normalized to the the β-actin mRNA levels. The dialysis fluid and the treatment for each group is indicated in the graph. Each histogram represents mean ± s.e.m. of 6 animals. *p<0.05 as compared to the vehicle group. #p<0.05 for the aliskiren-treated groups as compared to the same PDF in absence of aliskiren. $p<0.05 as compared to 10 mg/L aliskiren groups.

respective groups dialyzed with high-glucose PDFs in the absence of aliskiren indicating a lower transporter status. Moreover, the effect of aliskiren was dose-dependent, with a significantly higher D_2/D_0 glucose ratio and a significantly lower D_2/P_2 creatinine ratio in the group dialyzed with 4.25% PDF supplemented with 100 mg/l aliskiren than the group dialyzed with 4.25% PDF supplemented with 10 mg/l aliskiren (Fig. 6).

Discussion

PD is an effective therapy for patients with end-stage renal failure [8]. Nevertheless, the benefits of PD are short-lived, due mainly to structural and functional changes in the peritoneal membrane caused by the use of conventional high-glucose PDFs. These changes can cause deterioration of the peritoneal membrane, thereby inducing a failure in peritoneal transport of solutes and ultrafiltration [17]. This failure results in patients having to turn to hemodialysis therapy for end-stage renal failure, and enduring the medical, social and economic limitations related to this type of treatment.

There is substantial evidence to support a pathogenic role of high-glucose PDFs in the development of structural and functional alterations in the peritoneum of long-term PD patients, including an increase in oxidative stress, p38 MAPK activity and apoptosis [18,19]. Previous studies have shown that all these PMC damage markers are increased in PMCs exposed to high-glucose solutions in a dose- and time-dependent manner [19,20]. We observed in our study that rat PMCs exposed *in vitro* to a high-glucose PDF showed increases in damage markers, such as reactive oxygen species (ROS) production, p38 MAPK phosphorylation, caspase-3 activity and mRNA expression of p53 and Bax. The addition of

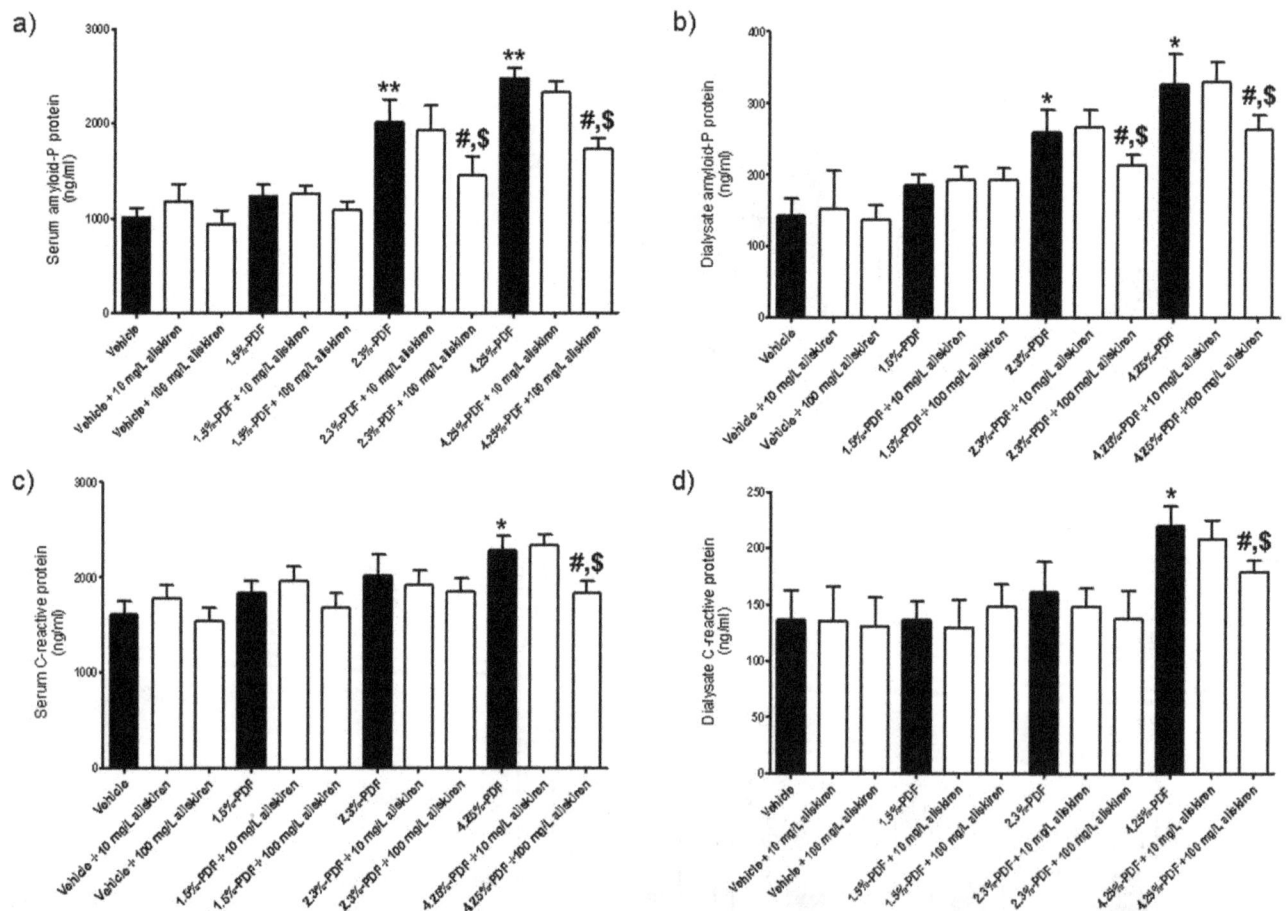

Figure 4. Aliskiren decreases the levels of inflammatory markers *in vivo* in both serum and dialysate after chronic peritoneal dialysis. The groups of animals were the same as in Fig. 3. A Peritoneal Equilibration Test (PET) was performed for 2 h at the end of the 4 weeks of dialysis. The levels of amyloid-P protein (a, b) and C-reactive protein (c, d) were determined in both serum (a, c) and dialysate (b, d) collected after 2 h dwell time. The dialysis fluid used and the treatment for each group is indicated in the graph. Each histogram represents mean ± s.e.m. of 6 animals. *p<0.05 as compared to the vehicle group. **p<0.01 as compared to the vehicle group. #p<0.05 for the aliskiren-treated groups as compared to the same PDF in absence of aliskiren. $p<0.05 as compared to 10 mg/L aliskiren groups.

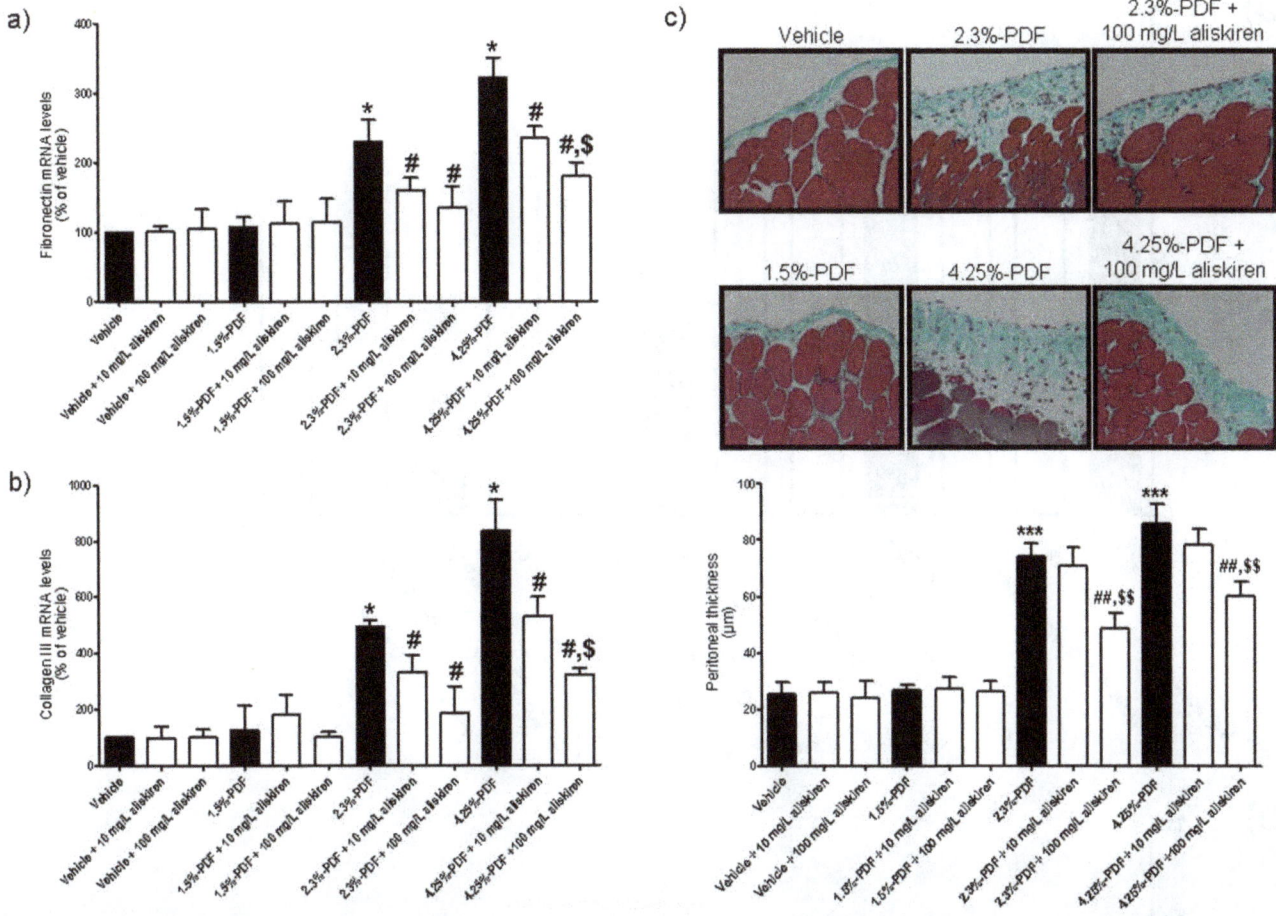

Figure 5. Aliskiren reduces the peritoneal fibrosis *in vivo* after chronic peritoneal dialysis. The groups of animals were the same as in Fig. 3. At the end of the 4 week-dialysis period, peritoneal mesothelial cells (PMCs) were isolated and the fibronectin (a) and collagen III (b) mRNA levels were determined in PMCs and normalized to the β-actin mRNA levels. The dialysis fluid used and the treatment for each group is indicated in the graph. Each histogram represents mean ± s.e.m. of 6 animals. *$p < 0.05$ as compared to the vehicle group. #$p < 0.05$ for the aliskiren-treated groups as compared to the same PDF in absence of aliskiren. $p < 0.05$ as compared to 10 mg/L aliskiren groups. c) Masson's trichrome staining of parietal peritoneum. <u>Top panel</u>. Histological sections from the vehicle, 1.5%-PDF, 2.3%-PDF, 4.25%-PDF, 2.3%-PDF plus aliskiren (100 mg/L) and 4.25%-PDF plus aliskiren (100 mg/L) groups at 200× magnification. Bottom panel. Quantification of the peritoneal thickness. The dialysis fluid used and the treatment for each group is indicated in the graph. Each histogram represents mean ± s.e.m. of 6 animals. ***$p < 0.001$ as compared to the vehicle group. ##$p < 0.01$ for the aliskiren-treated groups as compared to the same PDF in absence of aliskiren. $$p < 0.01$ as compared to 10 mg/L aliskiren groups.

aliskiren to the culture medium markedly reduced damage to PMCs in culture suggesting that a blockade of angiotensin synthesis may be beneficial during PD by protecting PMCs from high-glucose PDF-mediated damage. These protective actions of aliskiren may be explained by the known growth factor properties of angiotensin II, which when over-produced may cause PF [12]. Moreover, angiotensin receptor blockers and angiotensin converting-enzyme inhibitors ameliorate chlorhexidine gluconate-induced PF in rats [21]. On the other hand, high-glucose-induced angiotensin II synthesis has been observed in cardiac fibroblasts [22], vascular smooth muscle cells [23] and renal mesangial cells [24], among others. Furthermore, angiotensin II produced by PMCs mediates high-glucose PDF-induced up-regulation of TGF-β1 and fibronectin expression and this up-regulation is mediated by ROS [10]. Aliskiren inhibits angiotensin I generation from angiotensinogen by inhibiting renin leading to decreased angiotensin II production [14]. *In vitro* studies have shown that local RAAS is physiologically active in many cell types, including

PMCs. An RAAS inhibitor could therefore be a powerful tool for preserving peritoneal function during PD.

As with our results, previous studies have shown that the deleterious effect of chronic PD using PDFs with elevated glucose levels is characterized by the activation of apoptotic processes, accumulation and deposition of excess matrix proteins within the interstitial area, neoangiogenesis and vasculopathy of the peritoneal microvasculature [25,26]. In our study, we analyzed the effect of aliskiren addition to PD solutions during chronic (28 days) dialysis of rats. We found that PMCs isolated from the peritoneum of rats dialyzed daily for four weeks showed increased mRNA levels of fibrosis (collagen III and fibronectin) and pro-apoptotic (p53 and BAX) markers, as well as decreased Bcl-2 mRNA (an anti-apoptotic marker), similar to that observed in acutely isolated cultured PMCs *in vitro*, indicating that the response to high-glucose PDFs is similar *in vitro* and *in vivo*. This expression pattern suggests that, during chronic PD, PMCs suffer damage that activates death-signaling pathways. However, in rats treated with aliskiren-containing PDFs, changes in those cell damage markers were

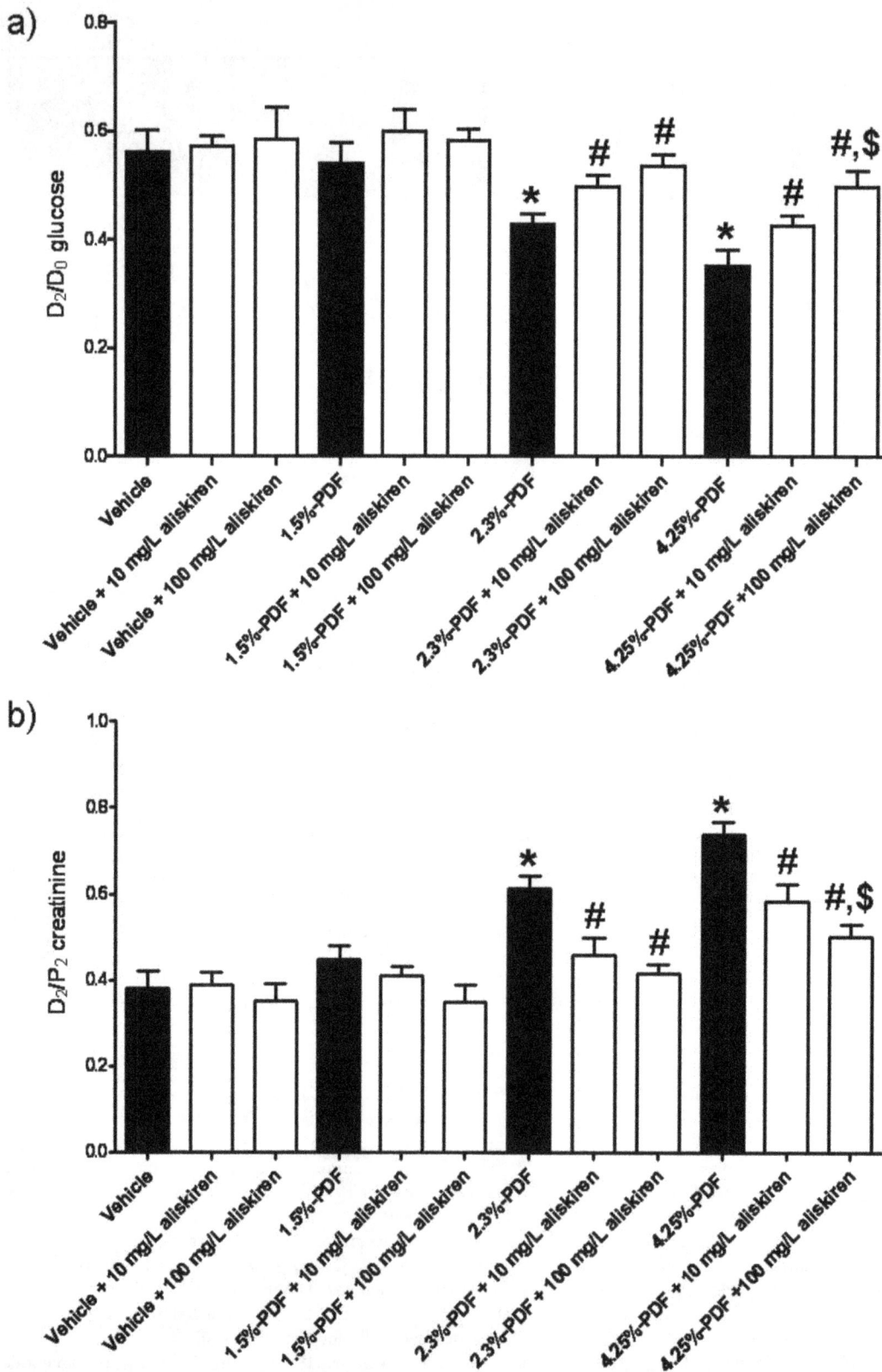

Figure 6. Aliskiren reduces changes in solute transport through the peritoneal membrane during chronic dialysis using high-glucose peritoneal dialysis fluids. The groups of animals were the same as in Fig. 3. A Peritoneal Equilibration Test (PET) was performed for 2 hours at the end of the 4 weeks of dialysis and the ratios D_2/D_0 glucose level (a) and D_2/P_2 creatinine level (b) were determined. The dialysis fluid used and the treatment for each group is indicated in the graph. Each histogram represents mean $\pm$ s.e.m. of 6 animals. *$p<0.05$ as compared to the vehicle group. #$p<0.05$ for the aliskiren-treated groups as compared to the same PDF in absence of aliskiren. $$p<0.05 as compared to 10 mg/L aliskiren groups.

significantly reduced, which is consistent with recent studies showing that aliskiren suppressed *in vivo* gene expression of pro-apoptotic factors inhibiting degeneration [27,28]. Taken as a whole, these data indicate that aliskiren may protect PMCs *in vivo*, which would be useful to extending the period during which PD may be used without peritoneal damage and thus delaying the initiation of hemodialysis.

After peritoneal membrane injury (especially to the mesothelial cell layer), a process of tissue repair begins. This process can be described as an inflammatory response that is characterized by remesothelialization of the wounded area, neovascularization and fibrosis of the submesothelial cell extracellular matrix [29]. We observed that levels of fibrosis markers fibronectin and collagen III mRNAs were significantly lower in PMCs collected from animals dialyzed with PDFs containing aliskiren than in control animals dialyzed with PDFs lacking aliskiren. Accordingly, high-glucose PDFs also increased the thickness of the peritoneum, as well as serum and dialysate CRP (one of the acute phase proteins whose levels increase during systemic inflammation) and amyloid-P protein (an acute phase protein during inflammation that can bind to apoptotic and necrotic cells) levels. All these changes were at least partially reversed by the addition of aliskiren to the PDFs. This result supports the idea that aliskiren protects PMCs from PDF-induced damage, thus decreasing the inflammation and fibrosis associated with peritoneal PMC damage.

One important issue is whether these protective actions of aliskiren are correlated with improved peritoneal membrane function during PD. To explore this issue, we performed a PET, which reflects the rates of glucose and creatinine transfer through the peritoneal membrane, after four weeks of PD using high-glucose PD solutions. Chronic dialysis using high-glucose PDFs produced a glucose-dependent decrease in the D_2/D_0 glucose ratio and an increase in the creatinine D_2/P_2 ratio, indicating a high transporter status. This type of transport is generally associated with less efficient ultrafiltration due to the more rapid absorption of glucose and an earlier loss of the osmotic driving force for fluid transport across the peritoneal membrane [5], which leads to an early transfer to hemodialysis due to failure of the PD [30]. In addition, a high transporter status is also associated with reduced survival of patients receiving PD [31]. The addition of aliskiren to the PDFs during chronic dialysis markedly increased the D_2/D_0 glucose ratio while decreasing the creatinine D_2/P_2 ratio, thus slowing the transport rate to values obtained in rats dialyzed with vehicle, which was due to the protective action on PMCs against PDF-induced damage. This indicates that the addition of aliskiren markedly improves the efficacy of PD, probably by preventing PMC damage and subsequent inflammation and fibrosis following peritoneal exposure to high-glucose PDFs.

We therefore propose that inhibition of the RAAS by aliskiren protects against high-glucose PDF-induced oxidative stress, apoptosis, inflammation, and fibrosis *in vitro* and *in vivo*. Moreover, the addition of aliskiren to PDFs prevents alterations in peritoneal transport as measured by the PET. These data suggest that inhibition of the RAAS may be a novel solution for preventing long-term PD-related modifications in the peritoneal membrane, thereby improving the efficacy of PD.

Materials and Methods

Materials

All chemicals, unless otherwise stated, were obtained from Sigma-Aldrich Chemical Company (St. Louis, MO, USA), and all tissue culture plastics were purchased from TPP (Trasadingen, Switzerland).

Animals

Seventy-two female Sprague–Dawley rats weighing 200 g to 220 g (Charles River Breeding Laboratories) were used for *in vivo* experiments. The animals were housed at a constant room temperature, with 12-hour light and dark cycles. Food and water were given *ad libitum*. All experimental protocols were carried out in accordance with the European Community Council Directive 2003/65/CE and with the experimental protocols approved by the CHU Albacete Institutional Animal Care and Use Committee.

Dialysis Experimental Design

Rats were randomly divided into 12 groups of 6 animals each. Four different dialysates were used: Vehicle (saline), 1.5% glucose PDF (1.5% PDF; CAPD/DPCA 2, Fresenius Medical Care, St. Wendel, Germany), 2.3% glucose PDF (2.3% PDF; CAPD/DPCA 4, Fresenius Medical Care) and 4.25% glucose PDF (4.25% PDF; CAPD/DPCA 3, Fresenius Medical Care). Each dialysate was administrated to three different groups incorporating aliskiren at 0 mg/l, 10 mg/l (low-dose) or 100 mg/l (high-dose) in the dialysate. The animals received 20 ml dialysate via a 30-gauge needle daily for four weeks. Furthermore, a group of animals was not dialyzed and the data obtained were not significantly different from animals dialyzed with vehicle (data not shown). Body weight was monitored at the beginning and the end of the experimental period. No rats were lost and all animals appeared to be healthy during the study, which involved repeated infusions of PDF.

Peritoneal Equilibration Test (PET)

After four weeks of treatment with the dialysates, a PET was performed during a 2-hour dwell with a 2.3% glucose PD solution. PETs were also performed on rats from the control group. During each PET, rats were given 30 ml of conventional 2.3% PDF (Fresenius Medical Care) via a 30-gauge needle to the peritoneal cavity. Dialysate samples (1 ml) were taken at time 0 (immediately after infusion) and 120 minutes after infusion. Blood samples were taken from the tail vein at the start and end of the PET. During the PET, animals were awake and had free access to water and food.

The dialysate and blood samples were centrifuged and stored at $-20°C$ until assayed. Concentrations of creatinine and glucose in serum and dialysate were measured using enzymatic methods on a DSX automated analyzer (DYNEX Technologies Inc., Chantilly, VA, USA). Amyloid-P protein and CRP quantification in serum and dialysate were measured using ELISA kits (GenWay Biotech Inc., San Diego, CA, USA). Peritoneal solute transport was calculated from the dialysate concentration at 2 h relative to its concentration in the initial infused dialysis solution (D_2/D_0 glucose) for glucose, and the dialysate-to-plasma concentration ratio (D_2/P_2 creatinine) at 2 h for creatinine.

At the end of the PET, animals were euthanized and biopsies of the parietal peritoneum were taken for light microscopy. Rat PMCs were also isolated from the parietal peritoneum and cultured as described below. Similar samples were taken from rats not exposed to PD solution. Peritoneal thickness was determined in Masson's trichrome stained tissue specimens by measurement of the combined thickness of the mesothelium and submesothelial interstitium using a 200× objective lens via a computer imaging analysis system (Image-Pro Plus, Media Cybernetics, Bethesda, MD, USA) as described previously [32]. The thickness of the parietal peritoneum was measured at a minimum of 10 points in each sample.

Rat Peritoneal Mesothelial Cells (PMCs) Culture

Rat PMCs were isolated from the peritoneum of rats by enzymatic digestion as previously described [33]. To identify PMCs, the cells were examined for specific markers and morphology as described elsewhere [33]. Cells between passages 3 and 6 were used for experiments. Experimental procedures were carried out according to the guidelines of the European Community on Welfare of Research Animals (Directive 2003/65/CE) and the CHU Albacete Institutional Animal Care and Use Committee.

To determine the effect of high-glucose solutions, subconfluent PMCs were incubated with serum-free media for 24 h to arrest and synchronize cell growth as previously described [34]. The PMCs were then treated for 48 h with serum-free media containing aliskiren (10 µmol/l to 100 µmol/l) or vehicle (distilled water), before stimulation with a 1.5% glucose PDF diluted to twice the volume with serum-free M199 medium in the presence or absence of aliskiren.

Reactive Oxygen Species (ROS) Determination

Intracellular formation of ROS was detected using 5-(and-6)-chloromethyl-2,7-dichlorodihydrofluorescein diacetate (DCF [CM-H2DCFDA: Invitrogen, Barcelona, Spain]), as previously described [35]. DCF was added at a final concentration of 10 µmol/l, and the cells were incubated for 60 minutes at 37°C in the dark. Cells were then washed, resuspended in PBS, and kept on ice for immediate detection by flow cytometry (BD-LSR, BD Biosciences, San Jose, CA, USA). Data were acquired and analyzed using the CellQuest program (BD Biosciences).

Western Blot Analysis

Proteins (20 µg/lane) were separated on 10% polyacrylamide-SDS gels in reducing conditions [36]. After electrophoresis, samples were transferred onto nitrocellulose membranes (Bio-Rad Laboratories, Hercules, CA, USA), blocked with 5% nonfat milk in blocking TTBS buffer (50 mmol/l Tris HCl, 150 mmol/l NaCl, and 0.05% Tween 20; pH 7.5), and incubated overnight at 4°C with a mouse monoclonal anti-p-p38 MAPK antibody (1:1.000, Cell Signaling, Beverly, MA, USA) or a rabbit polyclonal anti-p38 MAPK antibody (1:1000, Santa Cruz Biotechnology, Santa Cruz, CA, USA). Afterwards, blots were washed and incubated at room temperature for 1 h with a secondary antibody and developed using an enhanced chemiluminescence system (Millipore, Bedford, MA, USA). Densitometric analysis of immunoreactive bands was performed using Quantity One Software (Bio-Rad Laboratories).

Caspase-3 Activity

Caspase-3 activity was determined as previously described [37]. Cell extracts (40 µg of protein) were incubated in reaction buffer (25 mmol/l HEPES, 10% sucrose, 0.1% CHAPS buffer, and 10 mmol/l DTT) containing 50 µmol/l fluorescence substrate Asp-Glu-Val-Asp-7-amino-4 trifluoromethyl-coumaryl (Z-DEVD-AFC) at 37°C for 1 h. Cleavage of the AFC fluorophore was determined at 37°C on an Infinite 200 microplate reader (Tecan Group, Salzburg, Austria) at an excitation wavelength of 400 nm and a fluorescence emission wavelength of 505 nm.

Real-time RT-PCR Analysis

RNA expression was evaluated by real-time RT-PCR in cultured PMCs isolated from rats used for *in vivo* experiments. cDNA was synthesized from the purified total RNA using a High Capacity cDNA Reverse Transcription Kit (Applied Biosystems, Foster City, CA, USA) according to the manufacturer's instructions. For real-time RT-PCR, cDNA was amplified using SYBR Green PCR Master mix with the StepOne Real-Time PCR System and StepOne v2.0 software (Applied Biosystems). The following primer sets were used to amplify: fibronectin, 5′-GCA-CAG-GGG-AAG-AAA-AGG-AG-3′ (sense) and 5′-TTG-AGT-GGA-TGG-GAG-GAG-AG-3′ (antisense); collagen III, 5′-ATA-TCA-AAC-ACG-CAA-GGC-3′ (sense) and 5′-GAT-TAA-AGC-AAG-AGG-AAC-AC-3′ (antisense); p53, 5′-CCT-CCT-CAG-CAT-CTT-ATC-CG-3′ (sense) and 5′-CAC-AAA-CAC-GCA-CCT-CAA-A-3′ (antisense); Bax, 5′-GAT-GCG-TCC-ACC-AAG-AA-3′ (sense) and 5′-AGT-AGA-AGA-GGG-CAA-CCA-C-3′ (antisense); and Bcl-2, 5′-CCC-AAG-GGA-AGA-CGA-TG-3′ (sense) and 5′-GAG-CGG-GTA-GGG-AAA-GA-3′ (antisense). The real-time RT-PCR reaction was maintained at 95°C for 10 minutes, followed by 40 cycles of 95°C for 15 seconds and 60°C for 1 minute. The dissociation curves were analyzed to ensure amplification of a single PCR product. In order to ensure reliability of the results, all samples were processed in triplicate. Quantification was performed by the comparative cycle threshold (Ct) method [38]. To normalize the data, the β-actin RNA expression level was used as a housekeeping gene.

Statistical Analysis

Statistical significance was evaluated by nonparametric variance analysis (Kruskal-Wallis) followed by Dunn's test, with $p < 0.05$ considered statistically significant. The SPSS software application (version 13.0: SPSS, Chicago, IL) was used for all statistical analyses.

Acknowledgments

We thank Ana B. García for her technical assistance.

Author Contributions

Conceived and designed the experiments: JP-M FP-M VC. Performed the experiments: JP-M BC JM AO ES SN. Analyzed the data: JP-M FP-M. Contributed reagents/materials/analysis tools: VC. Wrote the paper: JP-M FP-M VC.

References

1. Bailie GR, Uhlig K, Levey AS (2005) Clinical practice guidelines in nephrology: evaluation, classification, and stratification of chronic kidney disease. Pharmacotherapy 25: 491–502.

2. Lameire N, Van BW (2010) Epidemiology of peritoneal dialysis: a story of believers and nonbelievers. Nat Rev Nephrol 6: 75–82.

3. Nagy JA (1996) Peritoneal membrane morphology and function. Kidney Int Suppl 56: S2–11.

4. Krediet RT (1999) The peritoneal membrane in chronic peritoneal dialysis. Kidney Int 55: 341–356.

5. Davies SJ (2004) Longitudinal relationship between solute transport and ultrafiltration capacity in peritoneal dialysis patients. Kidney Int 66: 2437–2445.

6. Holmes C, Mujais S (2006) Glucose sparing in peritoneal dialysis: implications and metrics. Kidney Int Suppl. pp S104–S109.

7. Heimburger O, Waniewski J, Werynski A, Tranaeus A, Lindholm B (1990) Peritoneal transport in CAPD patients with permanent loss of ultrafiltration capacity. Kidney Int 38: 495–506.

8. Davies SJ, Phillips L, Naish PF, Russell GI (2001) Peritoneal glucose exposure and changes in membrane solute transport with time on peritoneal dialysis. J Am Soc Nephrol 12: 1046–1051.

9. Mortier S, De Vriese AS, Lameire N (2003) Recent concepts in the molecular biology of the peritoneal membrane - implications for more biocompatible dialysis solutions. Blood Purif 21: 14–23.

10. Noh H, Ha H, Yu MR, Kim YO, Kim JH, et al. (2005) Angiotensin II mediates high glucose-induced TGF-beta1 and fibronectin upregulation in HPMC through reactive oxygen species. Perit Dial Int 25: 38–47.

11. Nessim SJ, Perl J, Bargman JM (2010) The renin-angiotensin-aldosterone system in peritoneal dialysis: is what is good for the kidney also good for the peritoneum?. Kidney Int 78: 23–28.

12. Weber KT, Swamynathan SK, Guntaka RV, Sun Y (1999) Angiotensin II and extracellular matrix homeostasis. Int J Biochem Cell Biol 31: 395–403.

13. Margetts PJ, Bonniaud P, Liu L, Hoff CM, Holmes CJ, et al. (2005) Transient overexpression of TGF-{beta}1 induces epithelial mesenchymal transition in the rodent peritoneum. J Am Soc Nephrol 16: 425–436.

14. Jensen C, Herold P, Brunner HR (2008) Aliskiren: the first renin inhibitor for clinical treatment. Nat Rev Drug Discov 7: 399–410.

15. Muller DN, Luft FC (2006) Direct renin inhibition with aliskiren in hypertension and target organ damage. Clin J Am Soc Nephrol 1: 221–228.

16. Nakagami H, Morishita R, Yamamoto K, Yoshimura SI, Taniyama Y, et al. (2001) Phosphorylation of p38 mitogen-activated protein kinase downstream of bax-caspase-3 pathway leads to cell death induced by high D-glucose in human endothelial cells. Diabetes 50: 1472–1481.

17. Aroeira LS, Aguilera A, Sanchez-Tomero JA, Bajo MA, del Peso G, et al. (2007) Epithelial to mesenchymal transition and peritoneal membrane failure in peritoneal dialysis patients: pathologic significance and potential therapeutic interventions. J Am Soc Nephrol 18: 2004–2013.

18. Jiang N, Qian J, Lin A, Lindholm B, Axelsson J, et al. (2008) Initiation of glucose-based peritoneal dialysis is associated with increased prevalence of metabolic syndrome in non-diabetic patients with end-stage renal disease. Blood Purif 26: 423–428.

19. Gotloib L (2009) Mechanisms of cell death during peritoneal dialysis. A role for osmotic and oxidative stress. Contrib Nephrol 163: 35–44.

20. Xu ZG, Kim KS, Park HC, Choi KH, Lee HY, et al. (2003) High glucose activates the p38 MAPK pathway in cultured human peritoneal mesothelial cells. Kidney Int 63: 958–968.

21. Bozkurt D, Cetin P, Sipahi S, Hur E, Nar H, et al. (2008) The effects of renin-angiotensin system inhibition on regression of encapsulating peritoneal sclerosis. Perit Dial Int 28 Suppl 5: S38–S42.

22. Singh VP, Baker KM, Kumar R (2008) Activation of the intracellular renin-angiotensin system in cardiac fibroblasts by high glucose: role in extracellular matrix production. Am J Physiol Heart Circ Physiol 294: H1675–H1684.

23. Lavrentyev EN, Malik KU (2009) High glucose-induced Nox1-derived superoxides downregulate PKC-betaII, which subsequently decreases ACE2 expression and ANG(1–7) formation in rat VSMCs. Am J Physiol Heart Circ Physiol 296: H106–H118.

24. Singh R, Singh AK, Alavi N, Leehey DJ (2003) Mechanism of increased angiotensin II levels in glomerular mesangial cells cultured in high glucose. J Am Soc Nephrol 14: 873–880.

25. Fusshoeller A (2008) Histomorphological and functional changes of the peritoneal membrane during long-term peritoneal dialysis. Pediatr Nephrol 23: 19–25.

26. Chaudhary K, Khanna R (2010) Biocompatible peritoneal dialysis solutions: do we have one? Clin J Am Soc Nephrol 5: 723–732.

27. Westermann D, Riad A, Lettau O, Roks A, Savvatis K, et al. (2008) Renin inhibition improves cardiac function and remodeling after myocardial infarction independent of blood pressure. Hypertension 52: 1068–1075.

28. Singh VP, Le B, Khode R, Baker KM, Kumar R (2008) Intracellular angiotensin II production in diabetic rats is correlated with cardiomyocyte apoptosis, oxidative stress, and cardiac fibrosis. Diabetes 57: 3297–3306.

29. Yung S, Thomas GJ, Davies M (2000) Induction of hyaluronan metabolism after mechanical injury of human peritoneal mesothelial cells in vitro. Kidney Int 58: 1953–1962.

30. Churchill DN, Thorpe KE, Nolph KD, Keshaviah PR, Oreopoulos DG, et al. (1998) Increased peritoneal membrane transport is associated with decreased patient and technique survival for continuous peritoneal dialysis patients. The Canada-USA (CANUSA) Peritoneal Dialysis Study Group. J Am Soc Nephrol 9: 1285–1292.

31. Chung SH, Heimburger O, Lindholm B, Lee HB (2005) Peritoneal dialysis patient survival: a comparison between a Swedish and a Korean centre. Nephrol Dial Transplant 20: 1207–1213.

32. Ke CY, Lee CC, Lee CJ, Subeq YM, Lee RP, et al. (2010) Aliskiren ameliorates chlorhexidine digluconate-induced peritoneal fibrosis in rats. Eur J Clin Invest 40: 301–309.

33. Carrión B, Pérez-Martínez FC, Monteagudo S, Pérez-Carrión MD, Gómez-Roldán C, et al. (2011) Atorvastatin reduces high glucose toxicity in rat peritoneal mesothelial cells. Perit Dial Int 31: 325–331.

34. Ha H, Yu MR, Choi HN, Cha MK, Kang HS, et al. (2000) Effects of conventional and new peritoneal dialysis solutions on human peritoneal mesothelial cell viability and proliferation. Perit Dial Int 20 Suppl 5: S10–S18.

35. Simoncini S, Sapet C, Camoin-Jau L, Bardin N, Harle JR, et al. (2005) Role of reactive oxygen species and p38 MAPK in the induction of the pro-adhesive endothelial state mediated by IgG from patients with anti-phospholipid syndrome. Int Immunol 17: 489–500.

36. Jordan J, Galindo MF, Calvo S, Gonzalez-Garcia C, Ceña V (2000) Veratridine induces apoptotic death in bovine chromaffin cells through superoxide production. Br J Pharmacol 130: 1496–1504.

37. Posadas I, Vellecco V, Santos P, Prieto-Lloret J, Ceña V (2007) Acetaminophen potentiates staurosporine-induced death in a human neuroblastoma cell line. Br J Pharmacol 150: 577–585.

38. Livak KJ, Schmittgen TD (2001) Analysis of relative gene expression data using real-time quantitative PCR and the 2(-Delta Delta C(T)) Method. Methods 25: 402–408.

NFκB in the Development of Endothelial Activation and Damage in Uremia: An In Vitro Approach

Carolina Caballo[1], Marta Palomo[1], Aleix Cases[2], Ana M. Galán[1], Patricia Molina[1], Manel Vera[2], Xavier Bosch[3], Gines Escolar[1], Maribel Diaz-Ricart[1]*

1 Hemotherapy-Hemostasis Department, Centre de Diagnòstic Biomèdic, Institut d'Investigacions Biomèdiques August Pi i Sunyer, Hospital Clinic, Universitat de Barcelona, Barcelona, Spain, 2 Nephrology Department, Institut d'Investigacions Biomèdiques August Pi i Sunyer, Hospital Clinic, Universitat de Barcelona, Barcelona, Spain, 3 Cardiology Department, Institut d'Investigacions Biomèdiques August Pi i Sunyer, Hospital Clinic, Universitat de Barcelona, Barcelona, Spain

Abstract

Impaired hemostasis coexists with accelerated atherosclerosis in patients with chronic kidney disease (CKD). The elevated frequency of atherothrombotic events has been associated with endothelial dysfunction. The relative contribution of the uremic state and the impact of the renal replacement therapies have been often disregarded. Plasma markers of endothelial activation and damage were evaluated in three groups of patients with CKD: under conservative treatment (predialysis), on hemodialysis, and on peritoneal dialysis. Activation of p38 MAPK and the transcription factor NFκB was assessed in endothelial cell (EC) cultures exposed to pooled sera from each group of patients. Most of the markers evaluated (VCAM-1, ICAM-1, VWF, circulating endothelial cells) were significantly higher in CDK patients than in controls, being significantly more increased in the group of peritoneal dialysis patients. These results correlated with the activation of both p38 MAPK and NFκB in EC cells exposed to the same sera samples, and also to the peritoneal dialysis fluids. Hemodialysis did not further contribute to the endothelial damage induced by the uremic state observed in predialysis patients, probably due to the improved biocompatibility of the hemodialysis technique in recent years, resulting in lower cellular activation. However, peritoneal dialysis seemed to exert a significant proinflammatory effect on the endothelium that could be related to the high glucose concentrations and glucose degradation products present in the dialysis fluid. Although peritoneal dialysis has been traditionally considered a more physiological technique, our results raise some doubts with respect to inflammation and EC damage.

Editor: Aernout Luttun, Katholieke Universiteit Leuven, Belgium

Funding: This work has been partially supported by grants: SAF2011-28214, SAF 2009-10365 (Ministerio de Economía y Competitividad); PI08/0156, CP04-00112, PS09/00664 (Fondo de Investigaciones de la Seguridad Social); German José Carreras Leukaemia Foundation (R 07/41v); and RD06/0009/1003 (Red HERACLES, Instituto de Salud Carlos III). The funders had no role in study design, data collection and analysis, decision to publish, or preparation of the manuscript.

Competing Interests: The authors have declared that no competing interests exist.

* E-mail: mdiaz@clinic.ub.es

Introduction

Patients with chronic kidney disease (CKD) suffer from complex hemostasis disorders. Both a bleeding tendency and an increased risk of accelerated atherosclerosis, with a high incidence of cardiovascular death, have been described to coexist [1]. Moreover, these patients are known to be exposed to a chronic proinflammatory state and oxidative stress, leading to endothelial cell dysfunction. In hemodialyzed patients, humoral factors such as uremic toxics accumulated in plasma and cytokines released by cellular activation are involved in the development of these pathological processes [2,3,4,5].

The vascular endothelium has been recognized as a complex endocrine organ that regulates many physiological functions such as vascular tone, vascular smooth muscle cell growth and migration, vascular permeability to solutes and blood cells, and regulation of hemostasis, among others [6]. The endothelium is able to adapt to pathophysiological challenges. However, depending on the nature and intensity of the stimuli, the endothelium may become dysfunctional. In this regard, there is clinical [7,8,9] and experimental evidence of endothelial activation and damage in uremia [10,11,12,13]. In patients

with CKD, the progression of atherothrombosis is accelerated [14], causing early cardiovascular complications [15]. In this regard, mortality from cardiovascular disease is nearly tenfold higher in patients with end-stage renal disease (ESRD) on dialysis than in the general population (US Renal Data System, USRDS 2009 Annual Data Report). This clinical situation cannot be fully explained by an increased prevalence of traditional cardiovascular risk factors such as hypertension, diabetes, hyperlipidemia or smoking, in ESRD [16]. Similarly, an enhanced cardiovascular risk has been reported in patients with CKD not on dialysis [17].

Using endothelial cells in culture, our group has previously characterized the endothelial activation and damage occurring in association with CKD. When exposed to growth media containing sera from patients on hemodialysis, cells showed morphological alterations [13], increased proliferation [13], signs of inflammation with no evidence of apoptosis [12,13], and an increased thrombogenicity of the generated extracellular matrix [18,11]. A more recent proteomic approach revealed that there are changes in the expression of some molecules related to inflammation, such as HMGB1 and aldose reductase, and to oxidative stress, such as superoxide dismutase and glutathione peroxidase. These changes were correlated with the activation of the transcription factor NFκB [19].

Most of the studies on the endothelial damage in CKD patients have been conducted in patients undergoing hemodialysis treatment. In the present study, we have investigated the relative contribution of uremia and renal replacement therapies (RRT), hemodialysis and peritoneal dialysis, to the development of endothelial damage in patients with CKD. We applied two different approaches: *ex vivo* analysis of plasma markers of endothelial activation and damage, and *in vitro* evaluation of the signaling mechanisms involved.

Results

Main demographic characteristics and biochemical parameters of the patients included in the study

The present studies were carried out in four different groups: i) 15 healthy donors (control group), ii) 11 patients under conservative treatment (PreD group), iii) 15 patients undergoing hemodialysis (HD group), and iv) 9 patients under peritoneal dialysis (PD group). Patients with diabetes and/or dyslipidemia, and smokers were excluded. The main demographic characteristics and biochemical parameters are detailed in Table 1.

Levels of endothelial damage markers are increased in dialyzed patients, specially in those under peritoneal dialysis

Plasma sVCAM-1, sICAM-1, and VWF increased significantly in the three groups of patients (p<0.01, p<0.05, and p<0.01 vs. control). Values of sPECAM-1, sE-SELECTIN, and sP-SELECTIN were higher in PreD and PD groups. However, ADAMTS-13 activity was within the normal range (table 2).

Circulating EC, identified as CD45−/CD146+/CD31+/CD133+ by flow cytometry, were above the control values (<100 CEC/mL) in all CKD groups, being significantly higher in the PD group with respect to the rest of groups (see table 2).

Uremic media promotes activation of the p38 MAPK and NFκB p65/RelA signaling pathways

Changes in the activation state of both p38 MAPK and NFκB, expressed as the relative extent of the phosphorylated target protein, are shown in figure 1 and 2, respectively. Two different techniques were applied: a phosphospecific antibody cell-based ELISA, which is faster but probably less sensitive, and immunoblotting as a reference method.

In relation to p38 MAPK, a statistically significant increase in the levels of the phosphorylated protein was observed in cells exposed to sera from the PD group, after 1 and 15 min (increases of 71.4±2.5% and 28.4±1.9% vs. control, respectively, both

Table 1. Main demographic characteristics and biochemical parameters.

	Control (n = 15)	PreD (n = 11)	HD (n = 15)	PD (n = 9)
Age, yr, mean±SD	42.3±10.0	62.4±11.2	51.2±14.5	61.4±20.4
Gender male/female	7/8	10/1	8/7	5/4
Mean glomerular filtration rate (ml/min/1.73 m²±SD)	–	19.0±7.8	–	–
Residual renal function (ml/min) mean±SD	–	–	0	5.3±4.8
Mean time on dialysis, months±SD	–	–	55.9±70.5	16.1±6.2
Serum Albumin (g/dl) mean±SD	4.2±0.3	4.5±0.2	4.1±0.3	3.7±0.2
Hemoglobin (g/dl) mean±SD	12.2±1.1	12.8±1.8	11.8±1.3	12.1±1.1
Leukocytes (10⁹/l) mean±SD	7.5±1.2	7.6±1.1	6.21±1.96	7.0±1.6
Causes of CKD n (%)				
glomerulonephritis		3 (27.3%)	4 (26.7%)	0
interstitial nephropathy		2 (18.2%)	0	0
renal hypoplasia		1 (0.9%)	0	0
polycystic kidney disease		0	3 (20.0%	2 (22.2%)
systemic lupus erythematosus		0	1 (0.7%)	0
hemolytic uremic syndrome		0	1 (0.7%)	0
bilateral nephrectomy		0	1 (0.7%)	0
obstructive kidney disease		0	1 (0.7%)	0
nephrosclerosis		0	0	2 (22.2%)
unknown		4 (36.4%)	4 (26.7%)	5 (55.6%)
Hypertension n (%)	0	9 (81.8%)	15 (100%)	4 (44.4%)
Use of statins n (%)	0	7 (63.6%)	5 (33.3%)	8 (88.9%)
Use of vitamin D n (%)	0	8 (72.7%)	5 (33.3%)	9 (100%)
Use of erythropoietin n (%)	0	3 (27.3%)	12 (80.0%)	8 (88.9%)
Use of inhibitors of the Renin-Angiotensin System	0	5 (45.5%)	1 (6.7%)	4 (44.4%)

Table 2. Levels of soluble biomarkers of endothelial activation and damage measured in plasma.

	Control (n = 15)	Predialysis (n = 11)	Hemodialysis (n = 15)	Peritoneal dialysis (n = 9)
sVCAM-1 (ng/ml)	816.9±64.2	1496.0±190.4**	1427.5±191.0**	1781.4±254.1**
sICAM-1 (ng/ml)	130.8±14.0	281.7±15.6*	296.6±20.4*	376.2±35.3*
sPECAM-1(ng/ml)	145.3±21.0	226.7±40.0	155.1±15.3	251.1±40.1*
sE-selectin (ng/ml)	88.8±10.3	109.5±15.8	70.7±7.7	86.1±11.0
sP-selectin (ng/ml)	244.1±22.2	347.6±37.3*	225.3±23.6	331.8±35.4*
VWF (%)	83.6±11.3	153.4±11.4**	210.8±31.9**	173.2±15.7**
CEC/ml	<100	263.3±75.3	155.6±52.2	471.0±119.2*
ADAMTS-13 (%)	103.0±20.0	104.7±6.3	100.1±6.6	93.2±5.1

Data are means±S.E.M.
*$p < 0.05$ and
**$p < 0.01$ vs. the control group.

$p < 0.05$, n = 6). Levels of p38 MAPK activation in the PreD and HD groups were similar to those observed in the control group. Increases of 7.4±0.3% and 4.2±0.01% in response to PreD and HD sera, respectively, were detected after 1 min of activation, and no significant variations were detected after 15 min. Activation of p38 MAPK in cells exposed to the conditions under study was confirmed by immunoblotting (see figure 1). Although activation of p38 MAPK was observed in the C, PreD and HD groups, specially at 15 min, it was mild. Phosphorylation of p38 MAPK increased progressively when cells were exposed to sera from the PD group from 15 to 60 min, being really significant at 60 min (increase of the mean intensity from 0 to 60%, $p < 0.001$).

Additionally, NFκB p65/ReIA showed a higher ratio of phosphorylation when EC were exposed to the sera of the three groups of uremic patients when compared to the control group. The most notable changes were observed when EC were incubated with the sera from PD patients at 1 and 15 min of exposure (increases of NFκB activation of 65±2.9% and 85±2.6% vs. control, respectively, both $p < 0.05$, n = 6). Although not statistically significant, there was also an activating effect of the HD sera (increases of 19±4.5% and 27±3.8% at 1 and 15 min of exposure, n = 6). Sera from PreD patients also caused a significant activation of NFκB at 15 min (46±2.1%, $p < 0.05$ vs. control, n = 6).

Western-blot analysis of phospho-IκB showed that this transcription factor was equally activated in cells exposed to the sera from the three groups of patients and it was not detected in cells exposed to control sera (see figure 2). Mean intensity of phosphorylation in cells exposed to sera from the three different groups of uremic patients was maximal at 15 min of exposure ($p < 0.001$) and was sustained till 30 min in the HD group ($p < 0.001$).

Effect of the glucose and its degradation products on endothelial damage and inflammation

The results obtained throughout the present study led us to explore the potential causes of endothelial activation in the group of peritoneal dialysis patients. Glucose degradation products (GDP) present in heat-sterilized dialysis solutions are thought to contribute to cellular dysfunction and membrane damage during peritoneal dialysis. Therefore, we examined the impact of conventional and low GDP peritoneal dialysis solutions with different concentrations of glucose (1.5%, 2.3%, and 4.25%), and

Icodextrin, on the activating state of the signaling molecules explored.

Phosphorylation of both p38 MAPK and NFκB p65/ReIA, expressed as the phosphorylation signal measured at 450 nm and corrected by the relative number of cells measured at 595 nm, was really significant in cells exposed to all the solutions tested for 15 min (see figure 3).

When compared to the basal condition, phosphorylation levels of p38 MAPK increased 85±2.5% ($p < 0.01$) in response to the PD sera, and 44±2.8% ($p < 0.05$) in response to icodextrin. When cells were exposed to the 1.5%, 2.3% and 4.25% c-PDS, phosphorylation of p38 MAPK was more notable and occurred in a concentration-dependent manner, increasing in 76±2.3%, 87±3.4% and 127±5.6% (all $p < 0.01$). The activating effect of the low GDP-PDS, although significant vs. the basal state and in a concentration dependent manner, was always below that induced by the PD pool of sera (increases of phosphorylation of 9±1.9%, 13±0.9% and 28±2.5%, $p < 0.05$, in response to the 1.5%, 2.3% and 4.25% GDP-PDS vs. the basal state).

In relation to the the NFκB, results were similar to those observed for p38 MAPK. Activation vs. the basal state increased to 114±3.0% with PD sera, 53±3.2%, 125±3.1% and 134±4.0% in response to the 1.5%, 2.3% and 4.25% c-PDS, and 35±1.8%, 54±1.7% and 34±0.9% in response to the 1.5%, 2.3% and 4.25% GDP-PDS. The effect of Icodextrin was much more intense on the phosphorylation of the transcription factor NFκB, even above all the conditions studied (increase of 178±4.9% vs. the basal state).

Discussion

The present study was focused to discern the contribution of uremia and the RRT to the development of endothelial activation and damage. The *ex vivo* and *in vitro* approaches applied revealed that uremia *per se* causes a proinflammatory state on the endothelium, as derived from results in pre-dialysis patients. The hemodialysis technique with the current advances (generalized use of biocompatible membranes and ultrapure water, among others) did not exhibit a damaging effect on the endothelium additionally to that observed in patients with advanced CKD managed conservatively. Interestingly, peritoneal dialysis was the most proinflammatory condition, as demonstrated by a higher presence of soluble markers of endothelial activation and damage in plasma, and a more intense activation of both p38 MAPK and NFκB signaling pathways in cultured endothelial cells. These effects

A

B

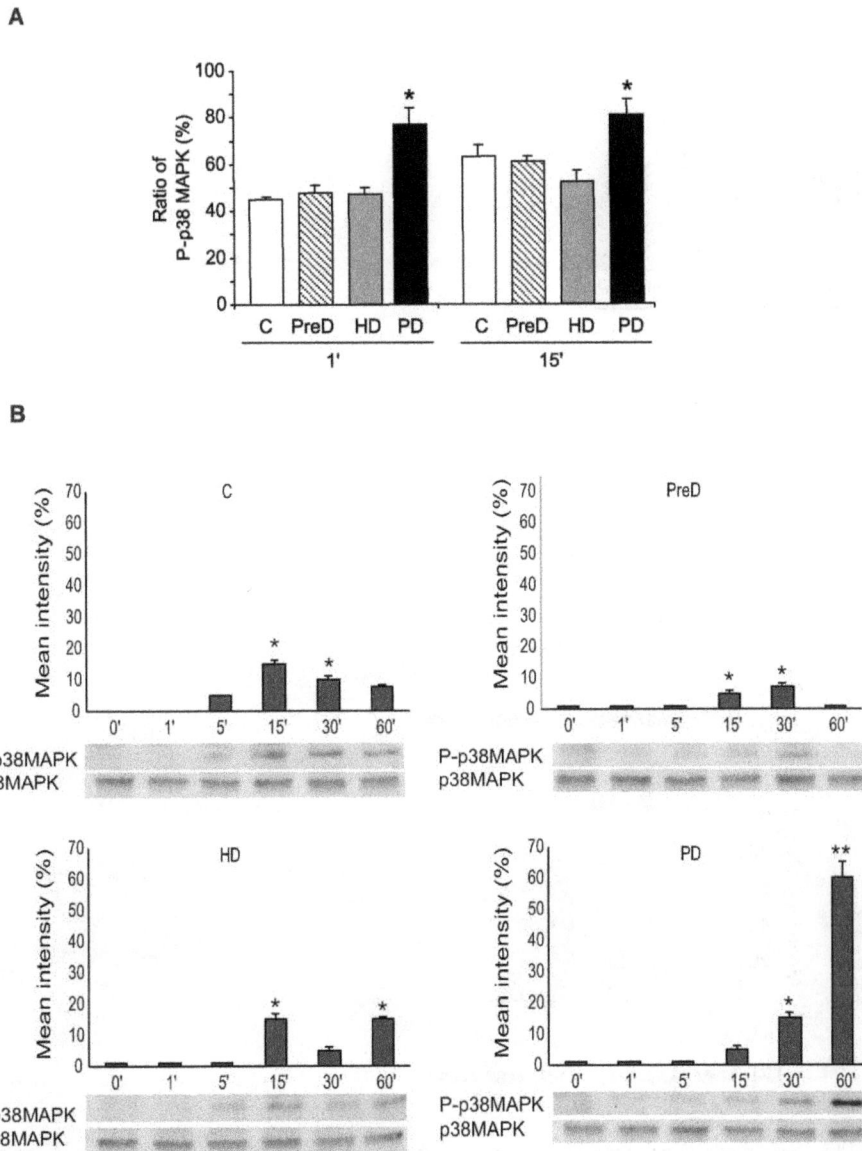

Figure 1. Effect of uremic media on the activation of p38MAPK signaling pathway. A. Ratios of phosphorylated p38 MAPK relative to the total protein, obtained in EC after 1 and 15 min of incubation with pooled sera from control donors (C), and predialysis (PreD), hemodialysis (HD), and peritoneal dialysis (PD) groups of patients. Data are corrected for cell number and are represented as mean±SEM (n = 6); *p<0.05 when compared with the other groups. **B.** EC were incubated at different time points with pooled sera from the same groups (C, PreD, HD, and PD, as indicated), and then assayed for phospho-p38 MAPK in cytosolic fractions by Western blot analysis. Images are representative of 6 different experiments and bar diagrams represent the mean intensity of phosphorylation (*p<0.05, **p<0.001).

could be attributed, at least in part, to the glucose and its degradation products present in the PD dialysis fluids.

Endothelial activation and damage could be the earliest indicator of subclinical cardiovascular disease. In the laboratory, measurement of plasma levels of different molecules and/or other elements, either discharged or up-regulated in an activated endothelium, could be useful to assess endothelial damage and activation [20,21]. Considering that to date there is no universal marker of endothelial damage, we have evaluated different indicators. Soluble adhesion receptors were evaluated by a multiplex system and showed significant activation of the endothelium in all uremic patients, being more notable in the PreD and PD groups. In relation to VWF plasma levels, our present data is consistent with previous observations in hemodia-

lyzed patients [7] being significantly higher in all the uremic patients than in controls. However, the short range in which values are included might explain the lack of differences found between the studied groups. Levels of circulating endothelial cells (CEC) have been described to correlate well with VWF plasma levels [22]. There is previous evidence generated in HD patients of increased CEC and their association with future cardiovascular events [10,23]. In our present study, blood CEC counts were higher in all the uremic patients when compared to the control group, especially in the group of peritoneal dialysis.

The analysis of plasma markers of endothelial damage indicates that the toxic environment of uremia causes inflammation on the endothelium, as observed in the non dialyzed CKD patients. This inflammatory effect is also seen in patients under both types of

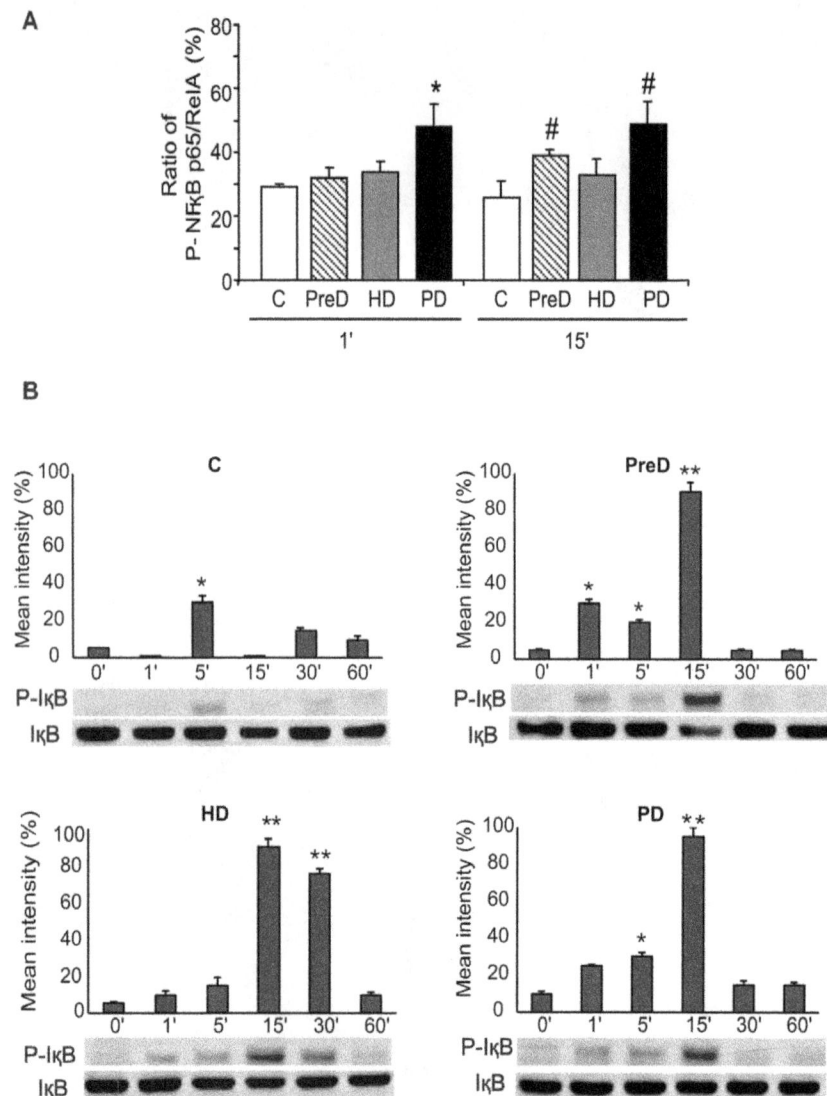

Figure 2. Effect of uremic media on the activation of NFκB p65/RelA signaling pathway. A. Ratios of phosphorylated NFκB p65/RelA relative to the total protein, obtained in EC after 1 and 15 min of incubation with pooled sera from control donors (C), and predialysis (PreD), hemodialysis (HD), and peritoneal dialysis (PD) groups of patients. Data are corrected for cell number and are represented as mean±SEM (n=6); *p<0.05 when compared with the other groups; #p<0.05 when compared with the control group. **B.** EC pretreated (for 30 min at 37°C) with N-acetyl-leucyl-leucyl-norleucinal (ALLN, 50 µg/ml) were incubated at different time points with pooled sera from the same groups (C, PreD, HD, and PD, as indicated), and then assayed for phospho-IκBα in cytosolic fractions by Western blot analysis. Images are representative of 6 different experiments and bar diagrams represent the mean intensity of phosphorylation (*p<0.05, **p<0.001).

RRT. From the results obtained, it can be predicted that PD exhibits the most deleterious effect on the endothelium and, interestingly, current HD techniques have diminished the harmful effect previously ascribed to this treatment.

Previous studies by our group and others were mostly performed in hemodialyzed patients. Results have demonstrated the existence of endothelial activation and damage in CKD both *in vivo* and *in vitro*. Plasma levels of endothelium-derived proteins [7], some of them vasoactive factors, are increased in these patients [24]. Endothelium-dependent vasodilation, the gold-standard method to assess endothelial function *in vivo*, is also decreased in these patients [25]. Exposure of cultured EC to sera from hemodialyzed patients accelerates cell cycle and proliferation, with a more prothrombotic extracellular matrix and a proinflammatory phenotype with a higher expression of cell adhesion

molecules [13,12], which represents one of the earliest pathological changes in immune and inflammatory diseases such as atherosclerosis [26]. Moreover, a proteomic characterization of these changes demonstrated a differential expression of proteins associated with inflammation and oxidative stress in cells exposed to the uremic condition, related to the NFκB signaling pathway [19]. In fact, exposure of endothelial cells in culture to sera from hemodialyzed patients induces activation of p38 MAPK [12] and of NFκB [19]. In hemodialyzed patients there is presence of the uremic toxics but also of those components released by blood cells that become activated by the procedure itself. However, results from the present study indicate that there is not an additional deleterious effect of hemodialysis over that observed in the predialysis condition. Probably, the generalized use of more biocompatible dialysis membranes and ultrapure water, among

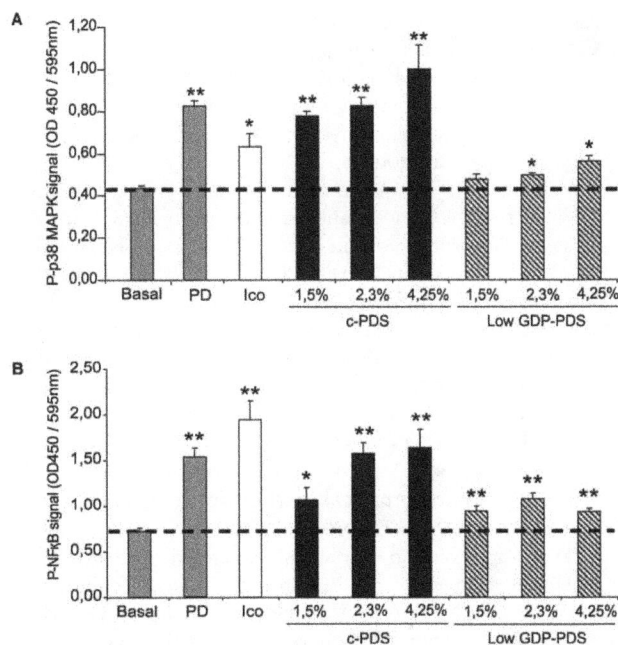

Figure 3. Effect of different peritoneal dialysis fluids on the activation of p38MAPK and NFκB p65/RelA signaling pathways. Levels of phosphorylated p38 MAPK (A) and NFκB p65/RelA (B), represented as phospho-p38 MAPK and phospho-NFκB signal at 450/595 nm, were evaluated in EC after 15 min of incubation with the pooled sera from the PD group and with the different peritoneal dialysis solutions: icodextrin (Ico) (7.5%), conventional (c-PDS) and low GDP (Low GDP-PDS) peritoneal dialysis solutions (at the concentrations of glucose of 1.5%, 2.3%, and 4.25%). Data were plotted after correction for cell number and are represented as mean±SEM (n = 6); *p<0.05 and **p<0.01 when compared with basal levels of phosphorylation.

other advances, has reduced blood cell stress with less contribution of proinflammatory cytokines. Interestingly, PreD patients showed a more significant inflammatory state than HD patients. These results are not fully in agreement with those by Merino et al. [27]. In their study, PD seems to exhibit a lower damaging condition on the endothelium than HD and predialysis. Differences between both studies may be due to the different experimental approaches applied but especially to the fact that in our study patients with CKD did not have evidence of previous cardiovascular disease and other known cardiovascular risk factors.

The present study provides the first evidence that sera from PD patients have a greater activating effect on p38 MAPK and NFκB, two intracellular key markers of inflammation and cell damage. The p38 MAPK protein kinases affect a variety of intracellular responses, with well-recognized roles in inflammation, cell-cycle regulation, cell death, development, differentiation, senescence and tumorigenesis [28]. NFκB seems to act by regulating the expression of several genes involved in tumorigenesis, including anti-apoptotic proteins, cyclooxygenase-2, matrix metalloproteinase-9, genes encoding adhesion molecules, chemokines, and inflammatory cytokines; and cell cycle regulatory genes [29]. Therefore, both p38 MAPK and NFκB participate in the proinflammatory responses and exhibit a clear role in the development of inflammatory and immunological diseases.

According to the USRDS 2011 Annual Data Report, mortality rates of dialyzed patients have declined in the last years probably reflecting changes in catheter utilization, improved cardiovascular disease care, and changes in infectious complications. However,

cardiovascular disease is still the major cause of the limited life expectancy in patients on substitutive therapies [30,31].

Patients under peritoneal dialysis are often hypertensive and sometimes volume overloaded [32], which is related to endothelial damage in PD patients [33]. Glucose is absorbed to a large extent from the dialysate, and conventional PD results in an almost unique metabolic situation involving continuous 24-hour absorption of glucose. One common and important side effect of this treatment is weight gain and accumulation of body fat stores [34,35]. These patients develop hyperlipidemia, with high levels of low-density lipoprotein and triglycerides. Advanced glycation end-products (AGEs), which are believed to promote atherosclerosis through interaction with endothelial receptors [36], are commonly accumulated in CKD patients due to decreased renal clearance, could be overproduced in PD patients due to the high exposure to glucose and glucose degradation products (GDP). Bioincompatibility of conventional glucose-based peritoneal dialysis fluids (PDF) has been partially attributed to the presence of GDP generated during heat sterilization of PDF [37,38], which are thought to contribute to cellular dysfunction and membrane damage during peritoneal dialysis [39,35,40]. In accordance with these previous results, our present study shows that the glucose load and the presence of GDP could play a role in the development of endothelial damage among these patients. Icodextrin is a colloid osmotic agent, derived from maltodextrin, used as aqueous solution for peritoneal dialysis. The osmotic activity of icodextrin keeps the solution inside the peritoneum for 10 to 16 hours without being significantly metabolized. Due to its chemical characteristics, Icodextrin reduces the burden of glucose overexposure. From this perspective, the activating effect of Icodextrin on the transcription factor (and to a lesser extent on the inflammation-dependent protein p38 MAPK) is difficult to explain. It can however not be excluded that the pH of the Icodextrin solution could exert a damaging effect on the endothelium in our in vitro studies.

From our present results it can be concluded that there is endothelial activation and damage associated with CKD, as demonstrated by the increased presence of plasma markers and by the in vitro studies in cultured endothelial cells. The uremic state seems to be a major cause of endothelial damage, probably through the activation of transcription factors, such as NFκB, which are related to inflammation. However, while improved hemodialysis procedures do not seem to have an additional deleterious effect, our different experimental approaches applied indicate that peritoneal dialysis seems to exert a more intense proinflamatory action on the endothelium that could be due, at least in part, to the increased glucose load. Studies to elucidate the potential molecular mechanisms involved should be the aim of future investigation.

Materials and Methods

Ethics statement

Written informed consent was obtained for blood utilization from every healthy donor and patient included in the study. The study was approved by the ethical committee of the Hospital Clinic (2011/6238) and was carried out according to the principles of the Declaration of Helsinki.

Experimental Design

We have applied both an *ex vivo* approach to analyze the presence of soluble plasma biomarkers of endothelial activation and damage and an *in vitro* approach to explore the activation of key signaling pathways related to inflammation in cultured endothelial cells exposed to sera from uremic patients.

In order to investigate the relative contribution of uremia and substitutive therapies, studies were carried out in four different groups: i) 15 healthy donors (control group), ii) 11 patients under conservative treatment (PreD group), iii) 15 patients undergoing hemodialysis (HD group), and iv) 9 patients under peritoneal dialysis (PD group). Patients with diabetes and/or dyslipidemia, and smokers were excluded.

In subsequent experiments, endothelial cells were exposed to conventional and low GDP peritoneal dialysis solutions with different concentrations of glucose (1.5%, 2.3%, and 4.25%), and to Icodextrin (7.5%), to explore their effect on the signaling pathways under study.

The present study has some limitations, mainly due to its nature: this is a cross-sectional observational study in which the sample population is small. However, the ex vivo measurements were performed in duplicate and confirmed by different techniques. The in vitro studies were performed in triplicate, using pooled sera from each group of patients to minimize variations, and also confirmed by two different experimental approaches.

Patients and sample collection

PreD samples were obtained from 11 (7 men and 4 women) non dialyzed patients with CKD (stage IV and V), age 62.4 ± 11.2 (mean $\pm$ SD), glomerular filtration rate 19.0 ± 7.8 ml/min/ 1.73 m^2, with glomerulonephritis (3), interstitial nephropathy (3), renal hypoplasia (1), and unknown (4). HD group consisted of 8 men and 7 women, age 55.2 ± 14.5, residual renal function 0 ml/min, and time on dialysis 55.9 ± 70.5 months. Causes of renal failure in these patients were glomerulonephritis (4), polycystic kidney disease (3), systemic lupus erythematosus (1), hemolytic uremic syndrome (1), bilateral nephrectomy (1), obstructive kidney disease (1), and unknown (4). All HD patients were dialyzed with biocompatible membranes, ultrapure water, for ≥ 4 hours, with a Kt/V ≥ 1.3. Samples were always obtained before the HD session. In the PD group, 5 men and 4 women with polycystic kidney disease (2), nephrosclerosis (2), and unknown (5) were included, age 61.4 ± 20.4, residual renal function 5.3 ± 4.8 ml/min, and time on dialysis 16.1 ± 6.2 months. PD patients only used biocompatible solutions with low levels of GDP: 5 Bicavera^{TM} (Fresenius, Spain), 2 Physioneal^{TM} (Baxter, Spain), 2 Gambrosol Trio^{TM} (Gambro, Spain) and 3 patients used Extraneal^{TM} (Baxter, Spain). The glucose concentration used or the indication for icodextrin (Extraneal^{TM}) was based on the patient's hydration status and peritoneal transport characteristics. None of the PD patients had had a peritonitis episode in the previous 2 months. See table 1 for patients data.

Diabetic patients or patients with dyslipidemia and/or previous cardiovascular disease and smokers were excluded. Most of the patients had no vascular disease as a cause of CKD. Samples from healthy donors were obtained as controls (n = 15, 7 male and 8 women, mean age 61.4 ± 20.4).

Plasma and sera samples were obtained from each patient by centrifugation of citrated blood ($800 \times g$, 15 min) and non anticoagulated blood ($3000 \times g$, 15 min), respectively, and stored at $-20°C$ until use.

Analysis of soluble markers of endothelial activation and damage

Plasma levels of VCAM-1, ICAM-1, PECAM-1, E-SELECTIN and P-SELECTIN were quantified by flow cytometry (Flowcytomix, Bender MedSystems; LabClinics S.A, Barcelona, Spain). This system employs capture antibodies coupled to fluorescent poly-

styrol beads of different sizes. A dual-laser flow cytometer (FACScan, Becton-Dickinson, Mountain View, Ca, USA) identifies the beads based upon their size and fluorescence intensity, and then quantifies the amount of antigen by measuring fluorescence emitted from Streptavidin-Phycoerythrin (PE) associated with a biotinylated detector antibody.

Circulating EC were measured by the flow cytometry method, in which whole blood was labelled with monoclonal antibodies tagged with fluorochromes (anti-CD45-PerCP, anti-CD146-FITC, anti-CD31-PE, anti-CD133-APC) (Chemicon Int, BD Pharmingen, Miltenyi Biotech, Becton & Dickinson).

VWF was evaluated by ELISA (American Diagnostica, Grifols SA, Barcelona, Spain). ADAMTS-13 activity was analyzed in citrated plasma by a fluorescence resonance energy transfer assay using a truncated synthetic 73-amino-acid VWF peptide as a substrate (FRETS-VWF73 assay) [41].

Culture of human umbilical vein endothelial cells

Primary cultures of EC were isolated from human umbilical cords veins, according to a previously described method [42], by collagenase treatment (0.2% in phosphate buffered saline, PBS, 15 min, 37°C) (Boehringer Mannheim, Mannheim, Germany). Cells were grown with culture medium (Mem 199; Gibco BRL, Life Technologies, Scotland, UK) supplemented with 100 U/ml penicillin, 50 mg/ml streptomycin and 20% pooled human serum. EC were grown at 37°C in a 5% CO_2 humidified incubator. The culture medium was changed every 48 h. After the second passage, EC were subcultured for 24 h on 0.1% gelatin-coated 96-well plates or on 0.1% gelatin-coated 6-well plates. Cells were used before reaching confluency.

Activation of the p38 MAPK and NFκB signaling pathways in endothelial cells

The activation of the p38 MAPK and NFκB p65/ReIA signaling pathways was assessed in cultured EC by two methods: a phosphospecific antibody cell-based ELISA, and immunoblotting.

To assess activation of p38 MAPK and NFκB by the phosphospecific antibody cell-based ELISA, endothelial cells were seeded in 96-well plates. After 24 h, confluent cells were serum starved during 4 h before experiments were performed by replacing their growth media with media containing 2% pooled human serum. This experimental procedure ensures basal levels of protein activity. Cells were then incubated for 1, 5, and 15 min with the 4 different pooled sera. The activation (phosphorylation) was evaluated by the cellular activation of signaling ELISA (CASE) kit superArray (SABiosciences, Tebu-bio Lab, Spain). The kit includes a complete antibody-based detection system for colorimetric quantification of the relative amount of phosphorylated protein and total target protein [43]. Detection of total and phosphorylated protein expression was determined according to the manufacturer's protocol and the levels obtained were corrected for cell number.

The activation of each of these signaling pathways was confirmed by immunoblotting as a reference method. EC were lysed with Laemmli buffer (125 mmol/l of Tris-HCl, 2% SDS, 5% glycerol, and 0.003% bromophenol blue), sonicated for 15 seconds to shear DNA and reduce viscosity, and heated to 90°C for 5 min. Protein concentrations of the supernatants were determined using Coomassie Plus (Pierce) as recommended by the manufacturer [44]. Samples were resolved by using 8% SDS-PAGE and proteins were transferred to nitrocellulose membranes, which were probed with specific antibodies to p38 MAPK phosphorylated at Thr180 and Tyr182, and to phosphorylated IκB (Cell Signaling Technology Inc, Frankfurt, Germany). Considering that translocation of NFκB to the nucleus is preceded by the phosphorylation and degradation of IκB, we analyzed the phosphorylation of the IκB protein in the presence of N-acetyl-leucyl-leucyl-norleucinal (ALLN) which prevents its degradation by the 26S proteasome [45]. Then, membranes were incubated with a peroxidase-conjugated anti-rabbit immunoglobulin G and developed using the chemiluminiscence technique. The presence of proteins was confirmed using specific antibodies. Densitometric analysis was performed to quantify the intensity of phosphorylation (ImageJ, National Institutes of Health, Bethesda, Maryland, USA).

Effect of the peritoneal dialysis fluids on p38 MAPK and NFκB signaling pathways

The effect of Icodextrin (Extraneal, Baxter, Spain), conventional peritoneal dialysis solutions (Stay-Safe 1.5%, Stay-Safe 2.3%, Stay-Safe 4.25% from Fresenius Medical Care, Spain), and low GDP peritoneal dialysis solutions (BicaVera 1.5%, BicaVera 2.3%, BicaVera 4.25% from Fresenius Medical Care, Spain) on the activation of p38 MAPK and NFκB in cultured endothelial cells was also assessed.

The amount of activated (phosphorylated) p38 MAPK and NFκB p65/ReIA was quantified in cultured endothelial cells after 15 min of incubation by using the Cellular Activation of Signaling ELISA (CASE^{TM}) kit superarray (SABiosciences, Tebu-bio Lab, Spain).

Cell viability was assessed in cultures exposed to the solution under study by the uptake of the vital dye Trypan blue (0.4% in PBS), according to standardized protocols for cell culturing and maintenance, and also by the MTT method. Cell viability was never lower than 90%.

Statistics

Results are expressed as mean ± standard error of the mean (SEM) and as ratios of phosphorylated protein with respect to the total protein values. Statistical analysis was performed with raw data using the Student's t-test for unpaired samples and ANOVA. Results were considered statistically significant when $p < 0.05$. The SPSS statistical package 17.0.0 (SPSS Inc, Chicago, IL) was used for all analyses.

Acknowledgments

We wish to thank the staff of the Hospital of Sant Joan de Déu and Hospital de la Maternitat, Barcelona for providing the umbilical cords, and Marc Pino, Fulgencio Navalón, and Mercè Pérez Gumbau for their technical assistance in this study.

Author Contributions

Conceived and designed the experiments: CC MP GE MDR. Performed the experiments: CC MP PM. Analyzed the data: CC MP PM GE MDR. Contributed reagents/materials/analysis tools: GE MDR. Wrote the paper: CC MDR. Conducted patient recruitment: AC MV. Provided intellectual content to the work and revised the article: AC MV XB GE AMG.

References

1. Gordge MP, Neild GH (1991) Platelet function in uraemia. Platelets 2: 115–123.
2. Herbelin A, Urena P, Nguyen AT, Zingraff J, Descamps-Latscha B (1991) Elevated circulating levels of interleukin-6 in patients with chronic renal failure. Kidney Int 39: 954–960.
3. Pertosa G, Gesualdo L, Tarantino EA, Ranieri E, Bottalico D et al. (1993) Influence of hemodialysis on interleukin-6 production and gene expression by peripheral blood mononuclear cells. Kidney Int Suppl 39: S149–S153.
4. Ringoir S (1997) An update on uremic toxins. Kidney Int Suppl 62: S2–S4.
5. Zemel D, Krediet RT (1996) Cytokine patterns in the effluent of continuous ambulatory peritoneal dialysis: relationship to peritoneal permeability. Blood Purif 14: 198–216.
6. Cines DB, Pollak ES, Buck CA, Loscalzo J, Zimmerman GA et al. (1998) Endothelial cells in physiology and in the pathophysiology of vascular disorders. Blood 91: 3527–3561.
7. Gris JC, Branger B, Vecina F, al Sabadani B, Fourcade J et al. (1994) Increased cardiovascular risk factors and features of endothelial activation and dysfunction in dialyzed uremic patients. Kidney Int 46: 807–813.
8. van Guldener C, Lambert J, Janssen MJ, Donker AJ, Stehouwer CD (1997) Endothelium-dependent vasodilatation and distensibility of large arteries in chronic haemodialysis patients. Nephrol Dial Transplant 12 Suppl 2: 14–18.
9. Zimmermann J, Herrlinger S, Pruy A, Metzger T, Wanner C (1999) Inflammation enhances cardiovascular risk and mortality in hemodialysis patients. Kidney Int 55: 648–658.
10. Koc M, Bihorac A, Segal MS (2003) Circulating endothelial cells as potential markers of the state of the endothelium in hemodialysis patients. Am J Kidney Dis 42: 704–712.
11. Serradell M, Diaz-Ricart M, Cases A, Zurbano MJ, Aznar-Salatti J et al. (2001) Uremic medium disturbs the hemostatic balance of cultured human endothelial cells. Thromb Haemost 86: 1099–1105.
12. Serradell M, Diaz-Ricart M, Cases A, Zurbano MJ, Lopez-Pedret J et al. (2002) Uremic medium causes expression, redistribution and shedding of adhesion molecules in cultured endothelial cells. Haematologica 87: 1053–1061.
13. Serradell M, Diaz-Ricart M, Cases A, Petriz J, Ordinas A et al. (2003) Uraemic medium accelerates proliferation but does not induce apoptosis of endothelial cells in culture. Nephrol Dial Transplant 18: 1079–1085.
14. Lindner A, Charra B, Sherrard DJ, Scribner BH (1974) Accelerated atherosclerosis in prolonged maintenance hemodialysis. N Engl J Med 290: 697–701.
15. Levey AS, Eknoyan G (1999) Cardiovascular disease in chronic renal disease. Nephrol Dial Transplant 14: 828–833.
16. Eberst ME, Berkowitz LR (1994) Hemostasis in renal disease: pathophysiology and management. Am J Med 96: 168–179.
17. Di Angelantonio E, Chowdhury R, Sarwar N, Aspelund T, Danesh J et al. (2010) Chronic kidney disease and risk of major cardiovascular disease and non-vascular mortality: prospective population based cohort study. BMJ 341: c4986.
18. Aznar-Salatti J, Escolar G, Cases A, Gomez-Ortiz G, Anton P et al. (1995) Uraemic medium causes endothelial cell dysfunction characterized by an alteration of the properties of its subendothelial matrix. Nephrol Dial Transplant 10: 2199–2204.
19. Carbo C, Arderiu G, Escolar G, Fuste B, Cases A et al. (2008) Differential expression of proteins from cultured endothelial cells exposed to uremic versus normal serum. Am J Kidney Dis 51: 603–612.
20. Blann A, Apostolakis S, Shantsila E, Lip GYH (2009) The evaluation of the endothelium: recent concepts. Haematologica 94 (extra 1): 149–155.
21. Constans J, Conri C (2006) Circulating markers of endothelial function in cardiovascular disease. Clin Chim Acta 368: 33–47.
22. Blann AD, Woywodt A, Bertolini F, Bull TM, Buyon JP et al. (2005) Circulating endothelial cells. Biomarker of vascular disease. Thromb Haemost 93: 228–235.
23. Koc M, Richards HB, Bihorac A, Ross EA, Schold JD et al. (2005) Circulating endothelial cells are associated with future vascular events in hemodialysis patients. Kidney Int 67: 1078–1083.
24. Koyama H, Tabata T, Nishzawa Y, Inoue T, Morii H et al. (1989) Plasma endothelin levels in patients with uraemia. Lancet 1: 991–992.
25. Passauer J, Bussemaker E, Range U, Plug M, Gross P (2000) Evidence in vivo showing increase of baseline nitric oxide generation and impairment of endothelium-dependent vasodilation in normotensive patients on chronic hemodialysis. J Am Soc Nephrol 11: 1726–1734.
26. Price DT, Loscalzo J (1999) Cellular adhesion molecules and atherogenesis. Am J Med 107: 85–97.
27. Merino A, Portoles J, Selgas R, Ojeda R, Buendia P et al. (2010) Effect of different dialysis modalities on microinflammatory status and endothelial damage. Clin J Am Soc Nephrol 5: 227–234.
28. Coulthard LR, White DE, Jones DL, McDermott MF, Burchill SA (2009) p38(MAPK): stress responses from molecular mechanisms to therapeutics. Trends Mol Med 15: 369–379.
29. Kumar A, Takada Y, Boriek AM, Aggarwal BB (2004) Nuclear factor-kappaB: its role in health and disease. J Mol Med 82: 434–448.
30. USRDS 2011 Annual Data Report (2011) Atlas of Chronic Kidney Disease and End-Stage Renal Disease in the United States: Morbidity & mortality.
31. Johnson DW, Dent H, Hawley CM, McDonald SP, Rosman JB et al. (2009) Association of dialysis modality and cardiovascular mortality in incident dialysis patients. Clin J Am Soc Nephrol 4: 1620–1628.
32. Konings CJ, Kooman JP, Schonck M, Dammers R, Cheriex E et al. (2002) Fluid status, blood pressure, and cardiovascular abnormalities in patients on peritoneal dialysis. Perit Dial Int 22: 477–487.

33. Cheng LT, Gao YL, Qin C, Tian JP, Gu Y et al. (2008) Volume overhydration is related to endothelial dysfunction in continuous ambulatory peritoneal dialysis patients. Perit Dial Int 28: 397–402.

34. Nordfors L, Heimburger O, Lonnqvist F, Lindholm B, Helmrich J et al. (2000) Fat tissue accumulation during peritoneal dialysis is associated with a polymorphism in uncoupling protein 2. Kidney Int 57: 1713–1719.

35. Pecoits-Filho R, Stenvinkel P, Wang AY, Heimburger O, Lindholm B (2004) Chronic inflammation in peritoneal dialysis: the search for the holy grail? Perit Dial Int 24: 327–339.

36. Himmelfarb J, Stenvinkel P, Ikizler TA, Hakim RM (2002) The elephant in uremia: oxidant stress as a unifying concept of cardiovascular disease in uremia. Kidney Int 62: 1524–1538.

37. Muller-Krebs S, Kihm LP, Zeier B, Gross ML, Deppisch R et al. (2008) Renal toxicity mediated by glucose degradation products in a rat model of advanced renal failure. Eur J Clin Invest 38: 296–305.

38. Passlick-Deetjen J, Lage C, Jorres A (2001) Continuous flow peritoneal dialysis: solution formulation and biocompatibility. Semin Dial 14: 384–387.

39. Morgan LW, Wieslander A, Davies M, Horiuchi T, Ohta Y et al. (2003) Glucose degradation products (GDP) retard remesothelialization independently of D-glucose concentration. Kidney Int 64: 1854–1866.

40. Witowski J, Korybalska K, Wisniewska J, Breborowicz A, Gahl GM et al. (2000) Effect of glucose degradation products on human peritoneal mesothelial cell function. J Am Soc Nephrol 11: 729–739.

41. Kokame K, Nobe Y, Kokubo Y, Okayama A, Miyata T (2005) FRETS-VWF73, a first fluorogenic substrate for ADAMTS13 assay. Br J Haematol 129: 93–100.

42. Jaffe EA, Nachman RL, Becker CG, Minick CR (1973) Culture of human endothelial cells derived from umbilical veins. Identification by morphologic and immunologic criteria. J Clin Invest 52: 2745–2756.

43. Versteeg HH, Nijhuis E, van den Brink GR, Evertzen M, Pynaert GN et al. (2000) A new phosphospecific cell-based ELISA for p42/p44 mitogen-activated protein kinase (MAPK), p38 MAPK, protein kinase B and cAMP-response-element-binding protein. Biochem J 350 Pt 3: 717–722.

44. Bradford MM (1976) A rapid and sensitive method for the quantitation of microgram quantities of protein utilizing the principle of protein-dye binding. Anal Biochem 72: 248–254.

45. Sung B, Ahn KS, Aggarwal BB (2010) Noscapine, a benzylisoquinoline alkaloid, sensitizes leukemic cells to chemotherapeutic agents and cytokines by modulating the NF-kappaB signaling pathway. Cancer Res 70: 3259–3268.

Prevalence and Risk Factors of Fluid Overload in Southern Chinese Continuous Ambulatory Peritoneal Dialysis Patients

Qunying Guo[9], **Chunyan Yi**[9], **Jianying Li, Xiaofeng Wu, Xiao Yang, Xueqing Yu***

Department of Nephrology, The First Affiliated Hospital, Sun Yat-sen University, Guangzhou, Guangdong, China

Abstract

Background: Fluid overload is frequently present in CAPD patients and one of important predictors of mortality. The aim of this study is to investigate the prevalence and associated risk factors in a cohort study of Southern Chinese CAPD patients.

Methods: The patients (receiving CAPD 3 months and more) in our center were investigated from January 1, 2008 to December 31, 2009. Multi-frequency bioelectrical impedance analysis was used to assess the patient's body composition and fluid status.

Results: A total of 307 CAPD patients (43% male, mean age 47.8 ± 15.3 years) were enrolled, with a median duration of PD 14.6 (5.9–30.9) months. Fluid overload (defined by Extracellular water/Total body water (ECW/TBW)≥0.40) was present in 205 (66.8%) patients. Univariate analysis indicated that ECW/TBW were inversely associated with body mass index ($r = -0.11$, $P = 0.047$), subjective global assessment score ($r = -0.11$, $P = 0.004$), body fat mass ($r = -0.15$, $P = 0.05$), serum albumin ($r = -0.32$, $P<0.001$), creatinine ($r = -0.14$, $P = 0.02$), potassium ($r = -0.15$, $P = 0.02$), and residual urine output ($r = -0.14$, $P = 0.01$), positively associated with age ($r = 0.27$, $P<0.001$), Chalrlson Comorbidity Index score ($r = 0.29$, $P<0.001$), and systolic blood pressure ($r = 0.22$, $P<0.001$). Multivariate linear regression showed that lower serum albumin ($\beta = -0.223$, $P<0.001$), lower body fat mass ($\beta = -0.166$, $P = 0.033$), old age ($\beta = 0.268$, $P<0.001$), higher systolic blood pressure ($\beta = 0.16$, $P = 0.006$), less residual urine output ($\beta = -0.116$, $P = 0.042$), and lower serum potassium ($\beta = -0.126$, $P = 0.03$) were independently associated with higher ECW/TBW. After 1 year of follow-up, the cardiac event rate was significantly higher in the patients with fluid overload (17.1% vs 6.9%, $P = 0.023$) than that of the normal hydrated patients.

Conclusions: The prevalence of fluid overload was high in CAPD patients. Fluid overload in CAPD patients were independently associated with protein-energy wasting, old age, and decreased residual urine output. Furthermore, CAPD patients with fluid overload had higher cardiac event rate than that of normal hydrated patents.

Editor: Utpal Sen, University of Louisville, United States of America

Funding: This work was supported by a grant from Key Project of Chinese Ministry of Health Clinical Disciplines ([2010]493). The funders had no role in study design, data collection and analysis, decision to publish, or preparation of the manuscript.

Competing Interests: The authors have declared that no competing interests exist.

* E-mail: yuxq@mail.sysu.edu.cn

[9] These authors contributed equally to this work.

Introduction

Fluid overload is a common complication of peritoneal dialysis [1], which is closely related to hypertension [2,3], cardiac dysfunction [4,5], inflammation [6], and mortality in dialysis patients [7,8]. In PD patients, measures of improving fluid status include attempt by dialysis prescription to optimize sodium and water removal, emphasis limits on sodium and water intake, and administration diuretics to enhance residual urine output. However, the crucial barrier to improve fluid management is the limitation of indentifying early or occult overhydration, but not the lack of strategies to enhance fluid removal [9].

Usually physicians estimate hydration status by clinical parameters, such as extremities edema, weight gain or increased blood pressure [10], which provide a useful, but imprecise picture of fluid status. Multi-frequency bioelectrical impedance analysis (BIA) is the most extensively studied technique to assess hydration in patients. It involves measurements at a large number of frequencies, with mathematical modeling of the data to estimate ECW (theoretic resistance at a frequency of zero) and TBW (theoretic resistance at infinite frequency), and ECW being the marker of hydration [11]. Recent studies demonstrate it is of potential value to provide precise and sensitive method for detecting longitudinal changes in hydration [9,12,13].

Protein-energy wasting is a major negative prognostic factor in dialysis patients, which may worsen patient outcome by aggravating existing inflammation, accelerating atherosclerosis and increasing susceptibility to infection [14]. Although it was reported that serum albumin, as a nutritional marker, correlated well with multi frequency BIA parameters [15], whether protein-energy wasting is the main contributor to fluid overload in PD patients

Table 1. Clinical, demographic and laboratory characteristics in CAPD patients with fluid overload and normal status.

	All patients 3	ECW/TBW ≥0.4	ECW/TBW<0.4	*P* value
	N = 307	N = 205	N = 102	
Baseline demographics				
Male (%)	132/307 (43%)3	82/205 (40%)	50/102 (49%)	P = 0.133
Age (years)	47.8±15.3	50.4±15.7	42.7±13.2	P<0.001**
Duration of CAPD (months)	14.6 (5.9 -30.9)	14.0 (5.9-30.4)	15.1 (5.4-32.6)	P = 0.538
BMI (kg/m²)	22.7±3.9	22.9±3.8	22.6±3.9	P = 0.497
Diabetes (%)	49/307 (16%)	39/205 (19%)	10/102 (9.8%)	P = 0.039*
Systolic blood pressure (mmHg)	137±22	140±22	132±22	P = 0.007**
Residual urine volume (ml/24 hours)	522±459	500±450	565±477	P = 0.254
D/Pcr	0.68±0.11	0.69±0.11	0.67±0.11	P = 0.96
RRF (ml/min·1.73 m²)	1.66 (0.31-3.28)	1.57 (0.42-3.25)	1.77 (0.23-3.54)	P = 0.977
SGA score≤5 percentage (%)	120/307 (39%)	90/205 (44%)	30/102 (29%)	P = 0.018*
CVD (%)	232/307 (76%)	166/205 (81%)	66/102 (65%)	P = 0.003**
CCI score	4 (3 - 6)	4 (3 - 6)	3 (3 - 5)	P = 0.02*
ECW (L)	13.9±3.1	14.1±3.2	13.4±2.7	P = 0.09
ICW (L)	20.8±4.5	20.5±4.6	21.3±4.3	P = 0.932
ECW/Height	0.085±0.17	0.087±0.018	0.082±0.014	P = 0.032*
ECW/TBW	0.40±0.13	0.41±0.01	0.39±0.01	P<0.0001**
PD prescription				
Solution glucose concentration (%)	1.5 (1.5-1.8)	1.5 (1.5-1.83)	1.5 (1.5-1.75)	P = 0.05*
KT/V	2.1 (1.8-2.6)	2.2 (1.8-2.6)	2.1 (1.7-2.5)	P = 0.567
Ultrafiltration (ml/24 hours)	496.1±475.58	483±468	520±493	P = 0.531
Salt restriction (yes/no)	177/130	116/89	61/41	P = 0.945
Biochemical markers				
HsCRP (mg/L)	2.0 (0.8-8.3)	2.23 (0.97-9.36)	1.71 (0.64-5.07)	P = 0.08
Creatinine (umol/L)	923±353	868±336	1032±362	P = 0.001**
Albumin (g/L)	39 (36-42)	38 (35-41)	41 (38-43)	P<0.001**
Transferrin (g/L)	2.3 (1.9-2.6)	2.2 (1.9-2.6)	2.4 (2.1-2.6)	P = 0.016*
Phosphate (mmol/L)	1.67±0.58	1.61±0.54	1.77±0.63	P = 0.03*
Potassium (mmol/L)	3.8 (3.3-4.2)	3.7 (3.3-4.1)	4.0 (3.4-4.4)	P = 0.02*
Carbon dioxide (mmol/L)	25±4	26±4	25±3	P = 0.01**
Glucose (mmol/L)	4.5 (3.9-5.3)	4.6 (4.1-5.7)	4.3 (3.8-4.8)	P = 0.006**
Medications				
Number of anti-hypertension drugs	2 (1-3)	2 (1-3)	2 (1-3)	P = 0.517
calcium channel blockers	199/307 (65%)	144/205 (70%)	55/102 (54%)	P = 0.26
Diuresis (%)	19/307 (6%)	12/205 (6%)	7/102 (7%)	P = 0.591
Dose of diuretics (mg/day)	80 (40, 100)	80 (40, 120)	40 (20, 80)	P=0.062

Notes: *P<0.05, **P<0.01. SGA = subjective global assessment; CVD = cardiovascular disease; CCI = Charlson Comorbidity Index; ECW = extracellular water; ICW = intracellular water; TBW = total body water; hsCRP = high-sensitivity C-reactive protein; BMI = body mass index; RRF = Residual renal function.

remains unclear. The present study attempted to assess the prevalence and correlation factors of fluid overload in the southern Chinese CAPD patients and investigate the relationship between fluid overload and malnutrition.

Methods

Objectives

This was a cross-sectional, observational, single center study. We hypothesized that protein-energy wasting was a main contributor to fluid overload in PD patients. Thus the primary aim of this study was to measure the hydration status in prevalent CAPD patients and investigate the association of fluid status with protein-energy wasting, also patient demographics, biochemical markers, PD prescription, and medications.

Participants

The patients inclusion criteria were as follows: (1) undergoing CAPD ≥3 month; (2) age >18 years; (3) signed informed consent form. The exclusion criteria were as follows: (1) patients with pacemakers; (2) patients with amputation; (3) patients who were not able to accomplish the analysis of body composition in

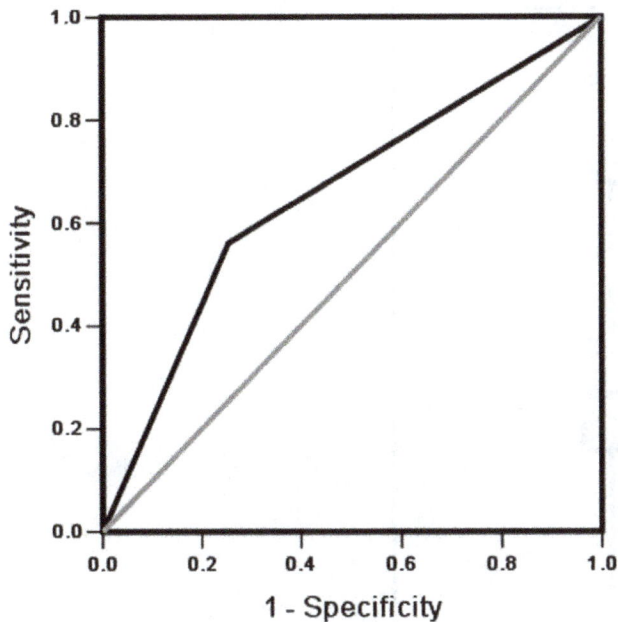

Figure 1. ROC analysis of edema for fluid overload (AUC = 0.653, sensitivity 0.562, specificity 0.745, P<0.001).

standing position for 3 minutes. Totally 585 patients were followed up regularly at the clinic from Jan 1 2008 to Dec 31, 2009. 160 patients refused to participate in this study. 118 patients were excluded from this study according to the exclusion criteria. Finally 307 PD patients were recruited.

Ethics

The study protocols were approved by the Ethics Committee of The First Affiliated Hospital of Sun Yat-sen University. Informed consent was obtained from each patient.

Investigations Undertaken

Patients were evaluated during a routine clinical visit, from January 1, 2008 to December 31, 2009.

Patients provided a 24-hour collection of urine and effluent, completed on the morning of the study visit. Then the fluid was analyzed for volume, urea, and creatinine content; Kt/V and residual renal function (RRF) were calculated using PD Adequest software (Baxter Healthcare, USA). D/Pcr was determined based on results of the last available PET test preceding the BIA measurement. Ultrafiltration and residual urine output were calculated from the patient's charts as a daily mean of ultrafiltration and urine obtained during the last week preceding the measurement. Solution glucose concentration (%) was calculated by dividing the daily total amount of glucose in dialysis solution by solution volume. At the same time, the data of patient demographic information, PD prescription, medications were collected.

Sitting blood pressure was measured using equipment that meets certification criteria, and recorded as the mean of two consecutive measurements with at least 2 minutes interval.

Blood was taken from patients to measure the following biochemical markers: hsCRP, hemoglobin, creatinine, albumin, transferrin, total cholesterol, triglyceride, serum phosphate, serum calcium, intact-PTH, serum sodium, serum chloride, serum potassium, carbon dioxide, serum glucose.

All the patients were regularly followed up and educated to restrict salt intake of approximate 5 to 6 gram per day. Patient-

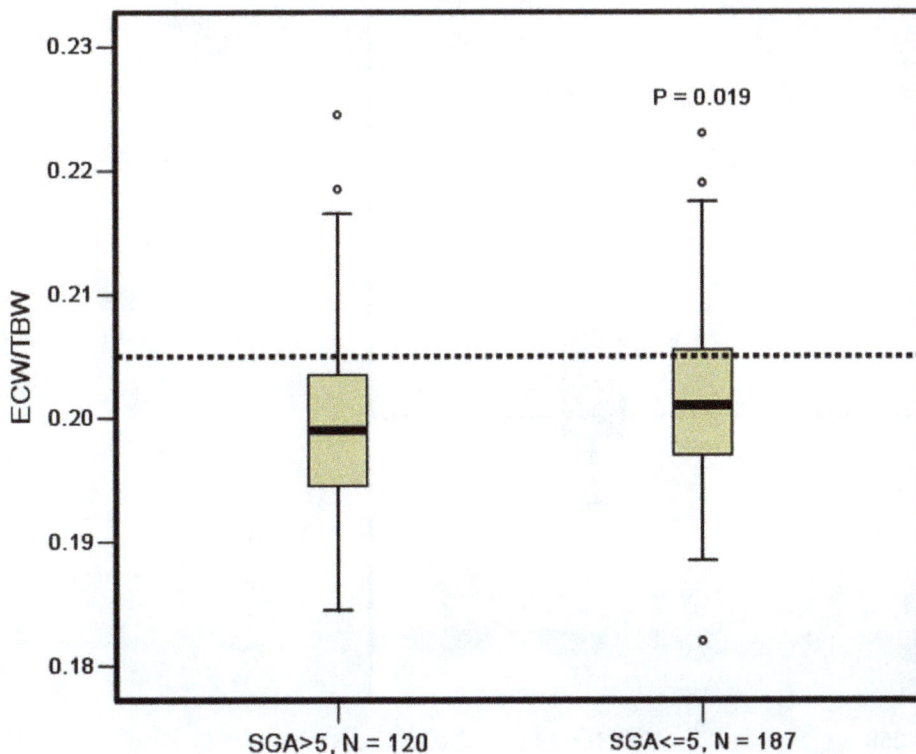

Figure 2. ECW/TBW in the CAPD patients with and without malnutrition. *, P<0.05; SGA, subjective global assessment.

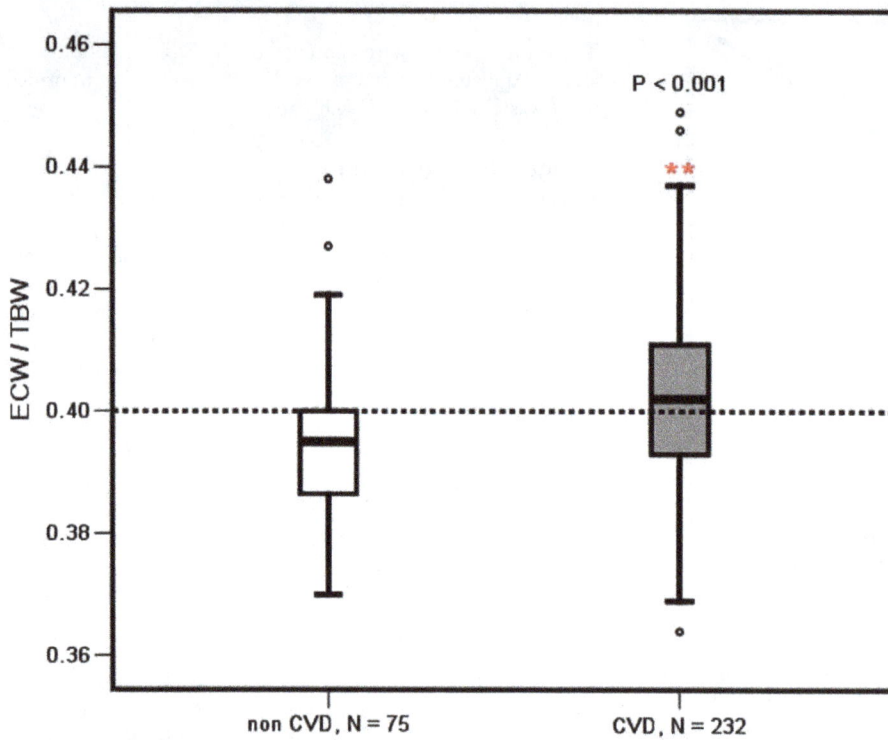

Figure 3. ECW/TBW in the CAPD patients with and without CVD. **, P<0.01; CVD, cardiovascular disease.

outcome, cardiac event rate, and residual renal function change after 1 year of follow-up were also recorded. Cardiac event was defined as myocardial infarction, angina, and congestive heart failure.

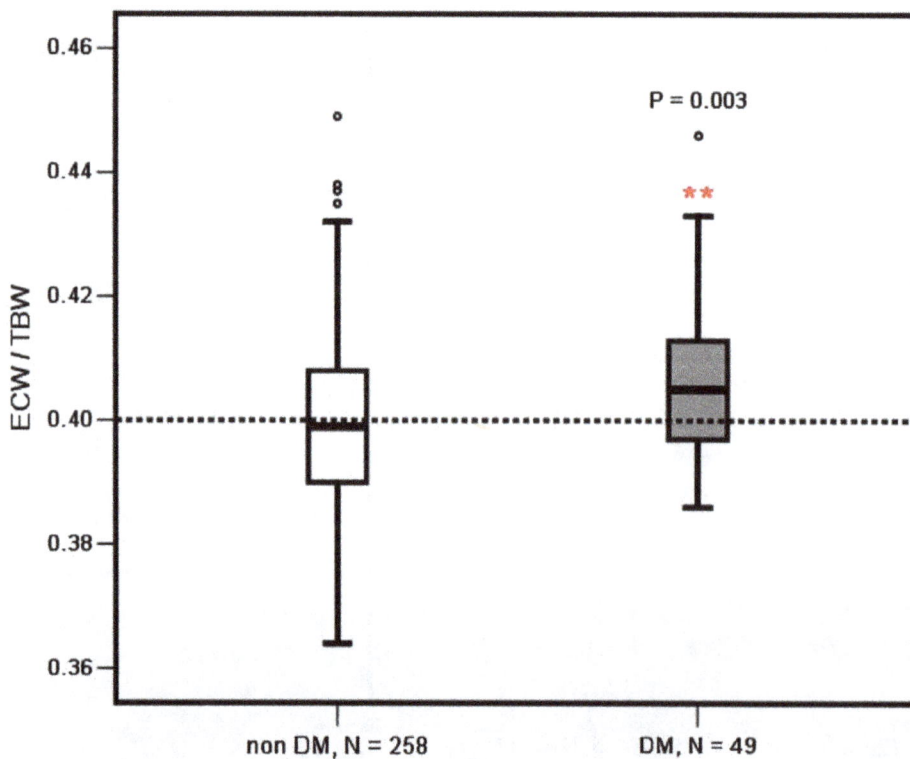

Figure 4. ECW/TBW in the diabetic and non-diabetic CAPD patients. **, P<0.01; DM: diabetes mellitus.

Table 2. Variables correlation with ECW, ECW/height, ECW/TBW.

	ECW	ECW/height	ECW/TBW
Age (years)	−0.03	0.02	0.27**
BMI (kg/m²)	0.52**	0.69**	−0.11*
Duration of CAPD (months)	0.22**	0.21**	0.03
Systolic blood pressure (mmHg)	0.21**	0.21**	0.22**
Ultrafiltration (ml/24 hours)	0.13*	0.12	0.04
Residual urine volume (ml/24 hours)	−0.11	−0.11	−0.14*
D/Pcr	0.10	0.10	0.13
RRF (ml/min·1.73 m2)	−0.17**	−0.15*	−0.11
KT/V	−0.30**	−0.24**	−0.06
SGA score	0.08	0.07	−0.17**
CCI score	0.03	0.08	0.29**
Edema[a]	0.15*	0.17**	0.39**
Body fat mass (kg)	−0.11	−0.07	−0.15*
Solution glucose concentration (%)	0.16**	0.13*	0.20**
hsCRP (mg/L)	0.06	0.06	0.13
Albumin (g/L)	−0.09	−0.12*	−0.32**
Creatinine (µmol/L)	0.31**	0.25**	−0.14*
Potassium (mmol/L)	0.16**	0.14*	−0.15*
Carbon dioxide (mmol/L)	−0.00	0.01	0.15*
Glucose (mmol/L)	0.01	0.02	0.25**

Notes: *P<0.05, **P<0.01. SGA = subjective global assessment; CVD = cardiovascular disease; CCI = Charlson Comorbidity Index; ECW = extracellular water; TBW = total body water; hsCRP = high-sensitivity C-reactive protein; BMI = body mass index; RRF = Residual renal function; a, Edema was assessed by physical examination.

Bioimpedance Analysis

TBW, ECW, intracellular water (ICW), and body composition was measured by multi-frequency bioelectrical impedance model InBody 720 (Biospace, Seoul, Korea). InBody 720 uses state –of – the-art technology, and 8-point tactile electrode system that measures the total and segmental impedance and phase angle of alternating electric current at six different frequencies (1 kHz, 5 kHz, 50 kHz, 250 kHz, 500 kHz, and 1000 kHz). Peritoneal dialysis fluid was not drained from the abdomen as it has been previously shown no significant effect on BIA measures [2,16,17]. Impedance measurements were made with the subject standing in an upright position, on foot electrodes in the platform of the instrument. The subject stood on the four foot electrodes: two oval shape electrodes and two heel shape electrodes, and gripped the two Palm-and Thumb electrodes in order to yield two thumb electrodes and two palm electrodes, without shoes or excess clothing. The skin and the electrodes were pre-cleaned using the specific electrolyte tissue according to the manufacturer's instructions. Prior to this, height was recorded to the nearest 0.1 cm. All the subjects were instructed to fast and to avoid exercise 8 h before measurement and had been resting for at least 30 min before measurement. All the body composition data were performed in the instrument by inner software and typed in the result sheet immediately after measuring. The software provides a plot of reactive and resistive components of the measured impedance at each frequency, as well as body weight, fat-free mass (FFM), TBW, ICW, ECW, segmental fluid distribution, fat mass (FM), body cell mass (BCM) and body mass index (BMI). This tool has been assessed in normal populations, renal transplant patients, hemodialysis patients, and PD patients, and closely correlates with the gold standard measurement by isotope dilution [18,19,20,21,22].

In this study, the ratio of ECW/TBW ≥0.4 was used to define overhydration, which was based on a fluid status measurement in 6520 normal healthy Koreans. The threshold of 0.4 represented mean +2SD, i.e. >95th percentile for Asian normal people.

Measurement of Nutrition Status

Subjective Global Assessment (SGA) was performed by one experienced dialysis nurse blinded to all clinical and biochemical variables of the patients. The method is based on patient's history and physical examination as described by Detsky [23]. The history focuses on gastrointestinal symptoms (anorexia, nausea, vomiting, and diarrhea) and weight loss in the preceding 6 months. The physical examination is graded by muscle wasting, loss of subcutaneous fat and the presence of ankle edema. The nutritional status was scored on the 7-point scale of the SGA. SGA scores of 5 or lower were defined as malnutrition.

Measurement of Comorbidity

The comorbidity score of each patient was determined according to the Chalrlson Comorbidity Index (CCI). The CCI is one of the most commonly used comorbidity models which based on comorbid conditions with varying assigned weights, resulting in a composite score. The CCI was calculated by assigning a weight of 2 to diabetes, stroke, renal insufficiency, and malignancy, and a weight of 1 to the other comorbidities [24,25]. Cardiovascular disease (CVD) was defined as myocardial infarction, angina, or history of congestive heart failure, cerebrovascular event, and peripheral vascular disease. Of all the patients, 10 patients had myocardial infarctions, 71 patients suffered from congestive heart-failure, 56 patients had clinical signs of peripheral atherothrombotic vascular disease and 23 patients suffered from cerebrovascular disease. Seven patients had been diagnosed with chronic lung disease, 3 had moderate or severe liver illness, 1 had gastrointestinal ulcer, and 4 patients suffered from malignant tumor.

Statistical Analyses

The patient's characteristics were presented as mean ± SD for continuous variables, and percentages and frequencies for categorical variables. The independent sample t-test was used for normally distributed continuous variables between overhydrated (ECW/TBW≥0.4) and normal hydrated (ECW/TBW<0.4) patients. A comparison of non-normally distributed continuous variables was performed using Mann-Whitney U-test. For categorical variables, the Chi-square test was used. The bivariate correlation test was performed to examine the associations of demographic and biochemical data with ECW, ECW/height, and ECW/TBW. Spearman's correlation coefficients were used for non-normally distributed variables and Pearson's correlation coefficients were used for normally distributed variables. Factors that reached statistical significance were selected for further multivariable analyses. As the ECW/TBW data was normally distributed in this study, multiple linear regressions were performed for multivariate analysis to explore the significant risk

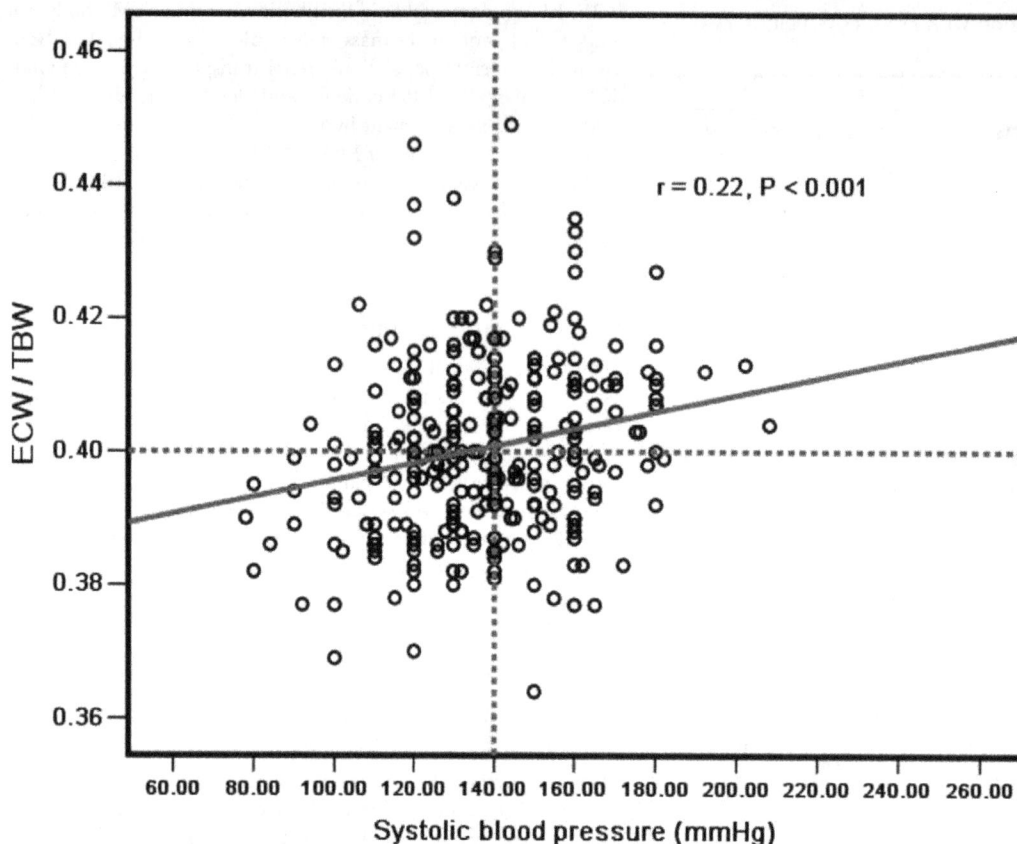

Figure 5. ECW/TBW was positively correlated with systolic blood pressure (mmHg).

factors of ECW/TBW. All calculation was performed with SPSS 13.0. *P* value of less than 0.05 was considered to be significant.

Results

Prevalence of Fluid Overload (Defined by ECW/TBW≥0.40) and Edema (by Physical Examination)

A total of 307 CAPD patients (43% male) were enrolled, their mean age was 47.8±15.3 years old, with a median PD duration of 14.6 (5.9-30.9) months. Clinical, demographic and laboratory characteristics of the 307 CAPD patients were shown in Table 1. Fluid overload was present in 205 (66.8%) CAPD patients, while edema (which was assessed by physical examination) was present in 138 (138/307, 45%) CAPD patients (*P*<0.001). Of note, 88 (88/169, 52%) patients without edema was diagnosed as fluid overload by BIA. While in the 138 CAPD patients who was clinically diagnosed as edema, 26 (26/138, 19%) patients were not fluid overload according to the BIA measurement (data not shown).

Of the 278 non-studied patients, 66% were male, 18% diabetic patients. Their mean age was 53. 2±16.0 years old, with a median PD duration of 1.73 (1.37-7.20) months. Compared with the non-studied patients, the studied patients were younger, had obvious lower male patients proportion, longer PD duration, and lower residual urine volume (data not shown). While the proportion of diabetic patients, and the proportion of patients with edema (46% vs 44%) by physical examination was comparable in the studied and non-studied patients.

Receiver – Operating Characteristic Curve (ROC) Analysis of Edema

As shown in Figure 1, we used ROC analysis to calculate the sensitivity and specificity of edema (by physical examination) as a diagnostic tool to diagnose fluid overload (defined by ECW/TBW ≥0.40) in 307 CAPD patients (area under the concentration curve, AUC = 0.653, sensitivity 0.562, specificity 0.745, P<0.001).

Characteristics of CAPD Patients with Fluid Overload

The clinical, demographic and laboratory characteristics were compared between the CAPD patients with fluid overload and patients without overhydration as shown in Table 1. Compared with normal hydrated patients, patients with fluid overload were older (50.4±15.7 vs 42.7±13.2 years, *P*<0.001), had higher diabetic percentage (19% vs 9.8%, *P = 0.039*), higher malnourished percentage (SGA score ≤5) (44% vs 29%, *P = 0.018*), higher CVD percentage (81% vs 65%, *P = 0.003*), higher CCI score (4 vs 3, *P = 0.02*), and higher systolic blood pressure (140±22 vs 132±22 mmHg, *P = 0.007*), but had lower serum albumin level (38 (35–41) vs 41 (38–43) g/L, *P*<0.001), lower serum potassium (3.7 (3.3–4.1) vs 4.0 (3.4–4.4) mmol/L, *P = 0.018*), lower serum creatinine (868±336 vs 1032±362 μmol/L, *P = 0.001*). There was no significant difference in the proportion of calcium channel blockers using (70% vs 54%, P = 0.26) and diuretics using (6% vs 7%, P = 0.59) in both two groups of patients. All the patients in this study used only one kind of loop diuretics (furosemide), and the dosage of furosemide was not significantly different between the two groups (80 (40, 120) vs 40 (20, 80), P = 0.062) (as shown in Table 1).

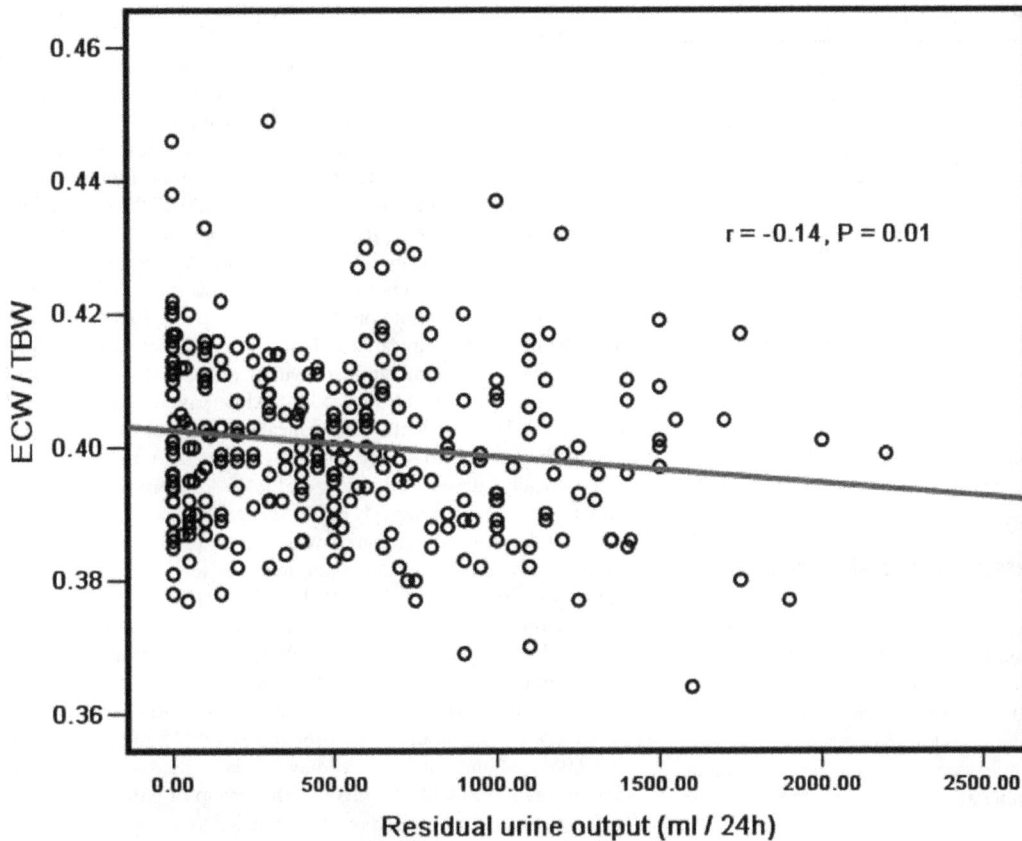

r = -0.14, P = 0.01

Figure 6. ECW/TBW was negatively correlated with residual urine output (ml/24 h).

Fluid Status in Different Subgroups of Patients

The ECW/TBW ratio of malnourished patients, CVD patients, and diabetic patients was significantly higher than that of the patients without malnutrition (0.403 ± 0.013 vs 0.399 ± 0.013, $P = 0.019$), non CVD patients (0.402 ± 0.013 vs 0.396 ± 0.011, $P < 0.001$), and non diabetic patients (0.406 ± 0.012 vs 0.399 ± 0.013, $P = 0.003$), respectively, as shown in Figures 2, 3, and 4.

Univariate Correlations for ECW/TBW in CAPD Patients

Univariate correlation analysis indicated that ECW/TBW were inversely associated with BMI ($r = -0.11$, $P = 0.047$), SGA score ($r = -0.17$, $P = 0.004$), body fat mass ($r = -0.15$, $P = 0.05$), serum albumin ($r = -0.32$, $P < 0.001$), serum creatinine ($r = -0.14$, $P = 0.02$), serum potassium ($r = -0.15$, $P = 0.02$), and residual urine output ($r = -0.14$, $P = 0.01$), but positively associated with age ($r = 0.27$, $P < 0.001$), CCI score ($r = 0.29$, $P < 0.001$), solution glucose concentration ($r = 0.20$, $P < 0.001$), and systolic blood

Table 3. Predictors of ECW/TBW in CAPD patients by multivariate linear regression analysis.

	Unstandardized Coefficients (B)	Standardized Coefficients (Beta)	P value	95% Confidence Interval for B
Age (years)	0.000	0.268	<0.001**	0.000–0.000
Sex	0.002	0.058	0.309	−0.001–0.005
BMI	0.000	−0.085	0.253	−0.001–0.000
Diabetes	0.003	0.073	0.254	−0.002–0.007
CCI	0.000	0.066	0.363	−0.001–0.001
Systolic blood pressure (mmHg)	9.80E-005	0.160	0.006**	0.000–0.000
Residual urine volume (mL)	−3.4E-006	−0.116	0.042*	0.000–0.000
Albumin (g/L)	−0.001	−0.223	<0.001**	−0.001–0.000
Body fat mass (kg)	0.000	−0.166	0.033*	−0.001–0.000
Potassium (mmol/L)	−0.002	−0.126	0.03*	−0.001–0.000

Notes: *P<0.05, **P<0.01. CCI = Charlson Comorbidity Index; ECW = extracellular water; TBW = total body water; BMI = body mass index.

Table 4. Clinical outcome at 1 year follow-up.

	ECW/TBW ≥0.4	ECW/TBW <0.4	P value
	N = 205	N = 102	
1- year patient survival (%)	93.2%	98.0%	0.086
1- year technique survival (%)	90.2%	95.1%	0.179
CVD mortality	4.4%	2.0%	0.302
Cardiac event rate (%)	17.1%	6.9%	0.023*

Notes: *P<0.05; CVD = cardiovascular disease.

pressure (r = 0.22, P<0.001), but not hs-CRP, ultrafiltration, KT/V, D/Pcr, diuretic or anti-hypertension drugs using, as shown in Table 2, Figures 5 and 6.

Multivariate Linear Regression Analysis for Predictors of ECW/TBW in CAPD Patients

In multivariate linear regression, only old age (β = 0.268, P<0.001), lower serum albumin (β = −0.223, P<0.001), lower body fat mass (β = −0.166, P=0.033), higher systolic blood pressure (β = 0.16, P=0.006), less residual urine output (β = −0.116, P=0.042), and lower serum potassium (β = −0.126, P=0.03) were independently associated with higher ECW/TBW (as shown in Table 3).

Clinical Outcome after One Year of Follow-up

After one year of follow-up, 16 (5.2%) patients died, 8 (2.6%) patients transferred to hemodialysis, 22 (7.2%) patients received kidney transplantation, 1 (0.3%) patient lost of follow-up. As shown in the Table 4, the 1- year patient survival rate in the normal hydrated patients is higher than that of the overhydrated patients (98.0% vs 93.2%, Log Rank = 0.086), but not significantly. Also, there was no significant difference of 1- year technique survival rate between the two groups of patients (90.2% and 95.1%, Log Rank = 0.179). Nevertheless the cardiac event rate was significantly higher (17.1% vs 6.9%, P=0.023) in the patients with fluid overload than that of the patients with normal hydration. While no significant difference in the CVD mortality was found between the two groups of patients (2.0% vs 4.4%, Log Rank = 0.302). In addition, no difference was found in the decrease of residual renal function in 1 year in the patients with overhydration and that of the patients without overhydration (0.45 vs 0.26 ml/min·1.73 m^2, P=0.603).

Seventy-nine patients had persistent overhydration, 187 patients had intermittent overhydration, while 41 patients were maintained euvolaemic over the 1 year follow-up period. There was no significant difference in the decrease of residual renal function in the patients who were persistently overhydrated and those that were maintained euvolaemic over the follow-up period (0.75 vs 0.26 ml/min·1.73 m^2, P=0.089).

Discussion

In the present study, the prevalence and risk factors of fluid status were investigated in a cohort study of CAPD patients. We found that the prevalence of fluid overload by bioimpedance analysis in CAPD patients was 66.8%. Fluid overload in CAPD patients were independently associated with protein-energy wasting, old age, higher systolic blood pressure, hypokalemia,

and decreased residual urine volume, but not peritoneal transport characteristics and inflammation.

In PD patients, practitioners rely most on routine physical examination, observation of body weight, blood pressure, and fluid output to diagnose fluid overload [10], which provide a useful, but imprecise picture of fluid status. BIA is the most extensively studied and most promising technique for routine monitoring of fluid status and nutrition in dialysis patients [26,27,28,29,30]. The present study showed the prevalence of fluid overload by bioimpedance analysis in CAPD patients was 66.8% in this study, which was notably higher than the diagnosis rate of 45% by the routine physical examination. Our results support BIA can be use to indentify some clinical occult fluid overload patients before notable clinical edema appear, which enables the appropriate therapeutic changes. Of the 138 CAPD patients with clinical edema, 26 (19%) patients were clinically diagnosed as edema, but not in fluid overload status according to the BIA measurement. Theoretically, under-evaluation of ECW/TBW may happen to athletes, who have relatively more skeletal muscle cells, and less extracellular water. Compared with the other 112 patients who were diagnosed as both edema and fluid overload by BIA, these 26 patients were younger (44.7±12.1 vs 51.7±15.5, P=0.033), had lower proportion of DM (7.7% vs 25%, P=0.054) and less CVD history (58.3% vs 85.8%, P=0.002). More importantly, they also had significantly higher skeletal muscle mass (27.2±5.1 vs 24.7±5.8, P=0.043), thus more intracellular water (22.4±3.9 vs 20.6±4.4, P=0.06) and body protein mass (9.7±1.7 vs 8.9±1.9, P=0.056). Thus these data may explain the reason of the underestimation of ECW/TBW in this group of patients.

We clearly demonstrated our hypothesis that a close relationship existed between protein-energy wasting and overhydration in a cohort of CAPD patients. As showed in the study, the overhydrated patients had significantly higher malnourished percentage, lower serum albumin and creatinine level than that of the normal hydrated patients. Univariate analysis showed the ECW/TBW ratio was inversely associated with BMI, SGA score, body fat mass, serum albumin, and creatinine. Further multivariate analysis confirmed that lower serum albumin and body fat mass were independently associated with overhydration. As it is well known that serum albumin, serum creatinine, BMI, body fat mass, and SGA are good surrogate markers of protein-energy wasting [31], a PD patient developing protein-energy malnutrition may gradually acquire ECW accumulation to balance loss of body cell mass or fat mass. Lower serum albumin level of malnourished patients not only caused a reduced colloid osmotic pressure and certainly aggravated the fluid retention in the tissue space, but also was a consequence of hemodilution due to fluid overload. Although worsening nutrition status may contribute to deteriorating fluid retention, whether improving nutritional status could help to improve fluid overload in dialysis patients needs further research.

Another interesting finding from this study was that decreased residual urine volume, but not ultrafiltration, RRF, or overall solute clearance (KT/V), play a possible pathogenic role in volume overload independent of diuretic usage and other confounders. Indeed, a close look at the reanalysis of the CANUSA data reveals that it was not the additional solute clearance obtained by renal function, but the urinary volume excreted that was the driving force for the relative risk of death, pointing to the fact that "volume status" is more important than small solute clearance [32,33]. The similar finding was reported by Ates et al [34], their finding suggests that removal of sodium and fluid is a predictor of mortality in PD patients, whereas Kt/V and total creatinine clearance are not risk factors. Our finding is contradictory with the report from the European Body Composition Monitoring Study Cohort [2], which showed that neither urinary output nor ultrafiltration contributed to the fluid balance. The reason of this discrepancy is not clear. We speculate that these different findings may relate to the high percentage of polyglucose usage (63.7%) and automated PD (APD) modality (53.1%) in these European group of patients, while only CAPD modality with glucose solution was performed in our patients. Indeed, APD is associated with lower sodium removal and may cause a more rapid loss of residual renal function [35,36,37], both of which may lead to an increase in extracellular fluid in these patients. However, Davison SN et al. recently compared extracellular fluid volume (ECFV) in patients who received CAPD and cycler-assisted peritoneal dialysis (CCPD) with fewer night cycles and icodextrin using for long daytime, no difference in the ratio of ECFV/TBW was found in these two groups of patients [38].

Fluid overload contributes to the development of hypertension in PD patients [2,3,39]. We also demonstrated a direct correlation between systolic blood pressure and tissue hydration as other authors reported [2]. It is well known that systolic blood pressure is a high risk factor for CVD and CVD caused death. Our findings also showed that the CAPD patients with overhydration had higher CVD percentage than that in patients without over-hydration, while the CAPD patients with CVD were more fluid overloaded than the non CVD patients. Moreover, the over-hydrated CAPD patients had a higher cardiac event rate and tended to have a poor patient survival than that of the normal hydrated CAPD patents in this study. The relationship among overhydration, systolic blood pressure, and CVD as well as the role of all these three factors in the pathogenesis of mortality need further investigation in PD patients. On the other hand, a sub-stantial proportion of patients did not follow this paradigm. Some PD patients had a normal blood pressure despite being fluid overloaded. These patients either suffer from congestive heart failure, or had a lower total peripheral resistance [2,3,40]. Some PD patients had uncontrolled hypertension despite normal tissue hydration. It is postulated that they are probably patients suffered from vascular stiffness or having a higher total peripheral resistance [2,3]. Of note, thirty-two (10.4%) patients in our study were over hydrated and normotensive but taking more than 2 anti-hypertensive drugs. Compared with the other normotensive patients, these 32 patients had a lower residual urine output (data no shown, $P = 0.044$), and used higher glucose concentration solution ($P = 0.011$), which suggested us to strengthen fluid removal in these patients to achieve the aim of maintaining normal blood pressure without useage of antihypertensive agents [41].

Although Konings CJ et al demonstrated that fluid status was related to peritoneal transport characteristics [42], we failed to demonstrate this relationship in our study. This result is consistent with Van Biese et al [2], who found a weak link between them, and disappearing in the multivariate analysis. Nevertheless, peritoneal transport status can help us understanding the mechanism of ultrafiltration failure and choosing appropriated management. After recognizing the high prevalence of fluid overload and related factors in the CAPD patients, we suggest that improving patient's malnutrition, protecting residual renal function and increasing residual urine output may improve patient's fluid status. Actually, all the associations between fluid overload and modifiable risk factors shown in our study may enhance clinical opportunities to improve morbidity and mortality in CAPD patients by identifying early overhydration and adopting measures to improve fluid status. Moreover, our survey supported that the BIA measurement could be used as a simple bedside screening tool in clinical evaluation of fluid overload in CAPD patients.

Limitation

The limitations of this report should also be noted. This is a single center cross-sectional study, and the definition of fluid overload comes from the BIA device manufacturer but lack of Chinese healthy control data. Also, patients' sodium intake restriction was only educated by the staff but not calculated accurately in this study. Further studies are needed to confirm the causal factors of fluid overload and impact of fluid control guided by BIA on residual renal function, nutrition, and cardiovascular function in CAPD patients.

Conclusion

In conclusion, fluid overload is common in CAPD patients. Bioimpedance analysis monitoring can help to identify early and occult fluid overload in CAPD patients. Fluid overload is independently associated with the protein-energy wasting, old age, higher systolic blood pressure, reduced residual urine volume, and hypokalemia in CAPD patients. CAPD patients with fluid overload have a higher cardiac event rate after 1 year and tend to have poor 1- patient survival than that of the normal hydrated CAPD patents. Further study is needed to evaluate whether monitoring fluid balance can improve residual renal function, nutrition and patient outcome.

Acknowledgments

We would like to thank the patients and personnel involved in the creation of this cohort. Also, we are indebted to our research staff at Peritoneal Dialysis Unit, The First Affiliated Hospital of Sun Yat-sen University (Dr. Haiping Mao, Jianxiong Lin, Liqiong Hu, Xiaoli Yu, Lina Zhu, Xiaodan Zhang, Peiyi Cao, Xiaoyan Lin, and Shaobin Zhang).

Author Contributions

Conceived and designed the experiments: XQY QYG. Performed the experiments: QYG CYY JYL XFW. Analyzed the data: QYG CYY XQY. Contributed reagents/materials/analysis tools: XQY QYG JYL XY. Wrote the paper: QYG CYY XQY.

References

1. Lo WK, Bargman JM, Burkart J, Krediet RT, Pollock C, et al. (2006) Guideline on targets for solute and fluid removal in adult patients on chronic peritoneal dialysis. Perit Dial Int 26: 520–522.

2. Van Biesen W, Williams JD, Covic AC, Fan S, Claes K, et al. (2011) Fluid status in peritoneal dialysis patients: the European Body Composition Monitoring (EuroBCM) study cohort. PLoS One 6: e17148.

3. Cheng LT, Tian JP, Tang LJ, Chen HM, Gu Y, et al. (2008) Why is there significant overlap in volume status between hypertensive and normotensive patients on dialysis? Am J Nephrol 28: 508–516.

4. Konings CJ, Kooman JP, Schonck M, Dammers R, Cheriex E, et al. (2002) Fluid status, blood pressure, and cardiovascular abnormalities in patients on peritoneal dialysis. Perit Dial Int 22: 477–487.

5. Enia G, Mallamaci F, Benedetto FA, Panuccio V, Parlongo S, et al. (2001) Long-term CAPD patients are volume expanded and display more severe left ventricular hypertrophy than haemodialysis patients. Nephrol Dial Transplant 16: 1459–1464.

6. Demirci MS, Demirci C, Ozdogan O, Kircelli F, Akcicek F, et al. (2011) Relations between malnutrition-inflammation-atherosclerosis and volume status. The usefulness of bioimpedance analysis in peritoneal dialysis patients. Nephrol Dial Transplant 26: 1708–1716.

7. Paniagua R, Ventura MD, Avila-Diaz M, Hinojosa-Heredia H, Mendez-Duran A, et al. (2010) NT-proBNP, fluid volume overload and dialysis modality are independent predictors of mortality in ESRD patients. Nephrol Dial Transplant 25: 551–557.

8. Chen W, Gu Y, Han QF, Wang T (2008) Contrasting clinical outcomes between different modes of peritoneal dialysis regimens: two center experiences in China. Kidney Int Suppl: S56–62.

9. Woodrow G (2007) Methodology of assessment of fluid status and ultrafiltration problems. Perit Dial Int 27 Suppl 2: S143–147.

10. Cocchi R, Degli Esposti E, Fabbri A, Lucatello A, Sturani A, et al. (1999) Prevalence of hypertension in patients on peritoneal dialysis: results of an Italian multicentre study. Nephrol Dial Transplant 14: 1536–1540.

11. Matthie J, Zarowitz B, De Lorenzo A, Andreoli A, Katzarski K, et al. (1998) Analytic assessment of the various bioimpedance methods used to estimate body water. J Appl Physiol 84: 1801–1816.

12. Moissl UM, Wabel P, Chamney PW, Bosaeus I, Levin NW, et al. (2006) Body fluid volume determination via body composition spectroscopy in health and disease. Physiol Meas 27: 921–933.

13. Wabel P, Chamney P, Moissl U, Jirka T (2009) Importance of whole-body bioimpedance spectroscopy for the management of fluid balance. Blood Purif 27: 75–80.

14. Pecoits-Filho R, Lindholm B, Stenvinkel P (2002) The malnutrition, inflammation, and atherosclerosis (MIA) syndrome – the heart of the matter. Nephrol Dial Transplant 17 Suppl 11: 28–31.

15. John B, Tan BK, Dainty S, Spanel P, Smith D, et al. (2010) Plasma volume, albumin, and fluid status in peritoneal dialysis patients. Clin J Am Soc Nephrol 5: 1463–1470.

16. Boudville NC, Cordy P, Millman K, Fairbairn L, Sharma A, et al. (2007) Blood pressure, volume, and sodium control in an automated peritoneal dialysis population. Perit Dial Int 27: 537–543.

17. Rallison LR, Kushner RF, Penn D, Schoeller DA (1993) Errors in estimating peritoneal fluid by bioelectrical impedance analysis and total body electrical conductivity. J Am Coll Nutr 12: 66–72.

18. National Institutes of Health Technology Assessment Conference and Workshops (1996) Bioelectrical impedance analysis in body composition measurement: National Institutes of Health Technology Assessment Conference Statement. Am J Clin Nutr 64: 524S–532S.

19. van den Ham EC, Kooman JP, Christiaans MH, Nieman FH, Van Kreel BK, et al. (1999) Body composition in renal transplant patients: bioimpedance analysis compared to isotope dilution, dual energy X-ray absorptiometry, and anthropometry. J Am Soc Nephrol 10: 1067–1079.

20. Chertow GM, Lowrie EG, Wilmore DW, Gonzalez J, Lew NL, et al. (1995) Nutritional assessment with bioelectrical impedance analysis in maintenance hemodialysis patients. J Am Soc Nephrol 6: 75–81.

21. Jones CH, Smye SW, Newstead CG, Will EJ, Davison AM (1998) Extracellular fluid volume determined by bioelectric impedance and serum albumin in CAPD patients. Nephrol Dial Transplant 13: 393–397.

22. Cooper BA, Aslani A, Ryan M, Zhu FY, Ibels LS, et al. (2000) Comparing different methods of assessing body composition in end-stage renal failure. Kidney Int 58: 408–416.

23. Detsky AS, McLaughlin JR, Baker JP, Johnston N, Whittaker S, et al. (2008) What is subjective global assessment of nutritional status? 1987. Classical article. Nutr Hosp 23: 400–407.

24. Volk ML, Hernandez JC, Lok AS, Marrero JA (2007) Modified Charlson comorbidity index for predicting survival after liver transplantation. Liver Transpl 13: 1515–1520.

25. Yong DS, Kwok AO, Wong DM, Suen MH, Chen WT, et al. (2009) Symptom burden and quality of life in end-stage renal disease: a study of 179 patients on dialysis and palliative care. Palliat Med 23: 111–119.

26. Wizemann V, Wabel P, Chamney P, Zaluska W, Moissl U, et al. (2009) The mortality risk of overhydration in haemodialysis patients. Nephrol Dial Transplant 24: 1574–1579.

27. Wizemann V, Rode C, Wabel P (2008) Whole-body spectroscopy (BCM) in the assessment of normovolemia in hemodialysis patients. Contrib Nephrol 161: 115–118.

28. Passauer J, Petrov H, Schleser A, Leicht J, Pucalka K (2010) Evaluation of clinical dry weight assessment in haemodialysis patients using bioimpedance spectroscopy: a cross-sectional study. Nephrol Dial Transplant 25: 545–551.

29. Machek P, Jirka T, Moissl U, Chamney P, Wabel P (2010) Guided optimization of fluid status in haemodialysis patients. Nephrol Dial Transplant 25: 538–544.

30. Devolder I, Verleysen A, Vijt D, Vanholder R, Van Biesen W (2010) Body composition, hydration, and related parameters in hemodialysis versus peritoneal dialysis patients. Perit Dial Int 30: 208–214.

31. Fouque D, Kalantar-Zadeh K, Kopple J, Cano N, Chauveau P, et al. (2008) A proposed nomenclature and diagnostic criteria for protein-energy wasting in acute and chronic kidney disease. Kidney Int 73: 391–398.

32. Van Biesen W, Lameire N, Verbeke F, Vanholder R (2008) Residual renal function and volume status in peritoneal dialysis patients: a conflict of interest? J Nephrol 21: 299–304.

33. Bargman JM, Thorpe KE, Churchill DN (2001) Relative contribution of residual renal function and peritoneal clearance to adequacy of dialysis: a reanalysis of the CANUSA study. J Am Soc Nephrol 12: 2158–2162.

34. Ates K, Nergizoglu G, Keven K, Sen A, Kutlay S, et al. (2001) Effect of fluid and sodium removal on mortality in peritoneal dialysis patients. Kidney Int 60: 767–776.

35. Rodriguez-Carmona A, Fontan MP (2002) Sodium removal in patients undergoing CAPD and automated peritoneal dialysis. Perit Dial Int 22: 705–713.

36. Rodriguez-Carmona A, Perez-Fontan M, Garca-Naveiro R, Villaverde P, Peteiro J (2004) Compared time profiles of ultrafiltration, sodium removal, and renal function in incident CAPD and automated peritoneal dialysis patients. Am J Kidney Dis 44: 132–145.

37. Ortega O, Gallar P, Carreno A, Gutierrez M, Rodriguez I, et al. (2001) Peritoneal sodium mass removal in continuous ambulatory peritoneal dialysis and automated peritoneal dialysis: influence on blood pressure control. Am J Nephrol 21: 189–193.

38. Davison SN, Jhangri GS, Jindal K, Pannu N (2009) Comparison of volume overload with cycler-assisted versus continuous ambulatory peritoneal dialysis. Clin J Am Soc Nephrol 4: 1044–1050.

39. Chen W, Cheng LT, Wang T (2007) Salt and fluid intake in the development of hypertension in peritoneal dialysis patients. Ren Fail 29: 427–432.

40. Covic A, Haydar AA, Bhamra-Ariza P, Gusbeth-Tatomir P, Goldsmith DJ (2005) Aortic pulse wave velocity and arterial wave reflections predict the extent and severity of coronary artery disease in chronic kidney disease patients. J Nephrol 18: 388–396.

41. Lameire N, Van Biesen W (2001) Importance of blood pressure and volume control in peritoneal dialysis patients. Perit Dial Int 21: 206–211.

42. Konings CJ, Kooman JP, Schonck M, Struijk DG, Gladziwa U, et al. (2003) Fluid status in CAPD patients is related to peritoneal transport and residual renal function: evidence from a longitudinal study. Nephrol Dial Transplant 18: 797–803.

Good Glycemic Control is Associated with Better Survival in Diabetic Patients on Peritoneal Dialysis

Dong Eun Yoo, Jung Tak Park, Hyung Jung Oh, Seung Jun Kim, Mi Jung Lee, Dong Ho Shin, Seung Hyeok Han, Tae-Hyun Yoo, Kyu Hun Choi, Shin-Wook Kang*

Department of Internal Medicine, College of Medicine, Brain Korea 21 for Medical Science, Severance Biomedical Science Institute, Yonsei University, Seoul, Korea

Abstract

Background: The effect of glycemic control after starting peritoneal dialysis (PD) on the survival of diabetic PD patients has largely been unexplored, especially in Asian population.

Methods: We conducted a prospective observational study, in which 140 incident PD patients with diabetes were recruited. Patients were divided into tertiles according to the means of quarterly HbA1C levels measured during the first year after starting PD. We examined the association between HbA1C and all-cause mortality using Cox proportional hazards models.

Results: The mean age was 58.7 years, 59.3% were male, and the mean follow-up duration was 3.5 years (range 0.4–9.5 years). The mean HbA1C levels were 6.3%, 7.1%, and 8.5% in the 1st, 2nd, and 3rd tertiles, respectively. Compared to the 1st tertile, the all-cause mortality rates were higher in the 2nd [hazard ratio (HR), 4.16; 95% confidence interval (CI), 0.91–18.94; p = 0.065] and significantly higher in the 3rd (HR, 13.16; 95% CI, 2.67–64.92; p = 0.002) tertiles (p for trend = 0.005), after adjusting for confounding factors. Cardiovascular mortality, however, did not differ significantly among the tertiles (p for trend = 0.682). In contrast, non-cardiovascular deaths, most of which were caused by infection, were more frequent in the 2nd (HR, 7.67; 95% CI, 0.68–86.37; p = 0.099) and the 3rd (HR, 51.24; 95% CI, 3.85–681.35; p = 0.003) tertiles than the 1st tertile (p for trend = 0.007).

Conclusions: Poor glycemic control is associated with high mortality rates in diabetic PD patients, suggesting that better glycemic control may improve the outcomes of these patients.

Editor: Shree Ram Singh, National Cancer Institute, United States of America

Funding: This work was supported by the Brain Korea 21 Project for Medical Science, Yonsei University, by the National Research Foundation of Korea grant funded by the Korea government (MEST) (No. 2011-0030711), and by a grant of the Korea Healthcare Technology Research & Development Project, Ministry of Health and Welfare, Republic of Korea (A102065). The funders had no role in study design, data collection and analysis, decision to publish, or preparation of the manuscript.

Competing Interests: The authors have declared that no competing interests exist.

* E-mail: kswkidney@yuhs.ac

Introduction

Diabetes mellitus (DM) is the leading cause of end-stage renal disease (ESRD) worldwide, accounting for more than 40% of incident dialysis patients in the United States [1]. To delay diabetic nephropathy from progressing and to improve outcomes for DM patients, a multidisciplinary approach is currently recommended, including glycemic control [2].

Accumulating evidences have shown that tight glycemic control prevents the development and progression of diabetic complications in both type 1 and type 2 DM patients [3–5]. In addition, high blood glucose concentrations were found to be associated with increased incidence of cardiovascular disease in diabetic patients [6]. Moreover, HbA1C levels were revealed as an independent risk factor for coronary heart disease in diabetic patients [7]. Since cardiovascular diseases are the most common cause of death in DM patients, it has been surmised that strict glucose control may be favorable to the outcome in these patients.

However, recent several randomized controlled trials have failed to demonstrate any beneficial effects of strict glycemic control on the cardiovascular morbidity and mortality in type 2 DM patients without advanced renal failure [8–10].

While many previous studies have excluded diabetic patients with advanced renal failure, only a few investigations have explored the impact of glycemic control on the prognosis of DM patients on dialysis, with inconsistent results [11–14]. An American report using a database from a large dialysis organization showed a significant correlation between the levels of HbA1C and prognosis in diabetic patients on hemodialysis (HD) [13], while another recent Canadian study found that higher blood glucose and HbA1C levels were not associated with mortality in maintenance HD patients with DM [14]. Different from HD, peritoneal dialysis (PD) results in a large amount of glucose load that is continuously absorbed from the dialysate. Therefore, glycemic control may be more difficult, and the impact of strict glycemic control on the clinical outcomes may be more obvious in diabetic PD patients, but definite evidence is furthermore lacking in these patients. To date, only one study has investigated the relationship between glycemic control after starting PD and the clinical outcomes in type 2 diabetic PD patients, in which only a few Asians were included [15]. Although there has been a study conducted in Asian population to show the association between glycemic control and patient outcomes, glycemic control before starting dialysis was used as an indicator of glycemic control [16]. In this study, we tried to determine whether glycemic control after starting PD was associated with all-cause and cardiovascular mortality in Asian diabetic PD patients.

Methods

Ethics statement

This study was approved by the Institutional Review Board for human research at Yonsei University College of Medicine, and all participants provided their written informed consent prior to study entry.

Study setting and participants

For this prospective observational study, we recruited 145 incident continuous ambulatory PD patients with DM from a single Korean dialysis center, and followed them at Yonsei University Health System in Seoul, Korea. Enrollment of patients was conducted from Jan 2001 until December 2008. The diagnosis of DM at the initiation of PD was based on the diagnostic criteria of the American Diabetes Association [17]. We excluded patients who were younger than 20 years old (n = 1), had a history of malignancy (n = 1), a history of receiving a kidney transplant (n = 1), or a history of HD for more than three months (n = 1). Patients who failed to maintain PD for more than three months were also excluded (n = 1).

Data Collection

To assess glycemic control, monthly preprandial blood glucose and quarterly HbA1C levels were collected during the first year after starting PD. However, to exclude the possibility of undue hyperglycemia, the HbA1C levels were omitted from mean HbA1C levels when measured during acute illness or when taking medications such as glucocorticoid that can affect blood glucose concentrations. Blood glucose concentrations were determined by the hexokinase-UV method and HbA1C levels were measured by high-performance liquid chromatography. The mean preprandial blood glucose and HbA1C values were used for this analysis.

The following demographic and clinical data were collected for each patient at the beginning of PD: age, gender, height, weight, body mass index (BMI), primary renal disease, duration of DM, smoking status, and comorbid conditions including hypertension, chronic lung disease, chronic liver disease, cardiovascular disease (CVD), and other serious medical illnesses. CVD included coronary artery disease, peripheral vascular disease, and cerebrovascular disease. The Charlson comorbidity index (CCI) score was used to quantify comorbid conditions [18]. Information on blood pressure and antihypertensive medications was collected at 3 months after beginning PD, when the patients' volume status had stabilized. The management of hyperglycemia was categorized into 4 groups; no medication, oral hypoglycemic agents alone, insulin alone, and combined treatment (oral hypoglycemic agents and insulin). The following laboratory data were also measured from blood samples taken 3 months after beginning PD: hemoglobin, white blood cell count, blood urea nitrogen, creatinine, albumin, calcium, phosphorus, intact parathyroid hormone (iPTH), total cholesterol, uric acid, bicarbonate, and high sensitivity c-reactive protein (hsCRP). Residual GFR was calculated as the average of urea and creatinine clearance from a 24-hour urine collection. Kt/V_{urea} was determined from the total urea nitrogen loss in the spent dialysate using the Watson equation [19], and normalized protein catabolic rate (nPCR) [20] was assessed for nutritional status.

Outcomes

Patients were classified into tertile groups, based on their average HbA1Cs during the first year after beginning PD, and prospectively followed from enrollment until death, transfer to an alternative dialysis method, or Dec 2010. Patients who transferred to HD or transplantation were censored for the patient survival analysis. The primary and secondary outcomes for all analyses were all-cause and cardiovascular mortality, respectively.

Statistical analysis

Statistical analysis was performed using SPSS version 13.0 (SPSS, Inc., Chicago, Illinois, USA). Data were basically expressed as mean ± standard deviation (SD) or percentages. Due to the log-normal distributions of hsCRP and iPTH, natural log values were used for analyses. Geometric means for all log-normally distributed continuous variables were calculated and reported with geometric SD. Results were analyzed using ANOVA or chi-square tests for comparisons. Significant differences detected by ANOVA were further confirmed by the Student's t-tests with the Bonferroni corrections. The relationships between HbA1C and preprandial blood glucose or log-transformed hsCRP (log hsCRP) levels were determined by Pearson's correlation analysis. Cox proportional hazards analysis was performed on variables revealed to be significant by univariate analysis to define the effect of HbA1C levels on mortality. A case-mix model was performed after adjusting for age, gender, year of PD start, CCI score. In the fully-adjusted model, mean arterial pressure (MAP), serum creatinine, albumin, and log hsCRP levels were further adjusted in addition to all variables used in the case-mix model. P-values less than 0.05 were considered statistically significant.

Results

Baseline characteristics and laboratory findings of patients

Of the 810 patients who began PD between January 2001 and December 2008, 145 patients had DM. After excluding 5 patients, a total of 140 patients were finally recruited in this study. The baseline characteristics of the study patients are shown in Table 1. The mean age was 58.7 years, 59.3% were male, and the mean follow-up duration was 3.5 years (range 0.4–9.5 years). The primary renal diseases were diabetic nephropathy (85.0%), chronic glomerulonephritis (7.1%), and hypertensive nephrosclerosis (4.3%) in order. Hypertension and CVD were accompanied in 139 (99.3%) and 44 (31.4%) patients, respectively. The mean systolic and diastolic blood pressures were 133.9±19.4 and 77.5±11.5 mmHg, respectively, and 75.7% of patients were taking RAS blockades. The frequency distribution of HbA1C values for all study patients is shown in Figure 1, and 47.1% of patients were within the recommended target HbA1C (less than 7%). Hypoglycemia occurred at the frequency of 1.1 events per 100 patient-year.

During the follow-up, 23 (16.4%) patients died, 28 (20.0%) were transferred to HD, and 7 (5.0%) received a kidney transplant. Cardiovascular disease (39.1%) and infection (39.1%) were the most common causes of death. Among death due to infection, PD-related infection such as PD peritonitis accounted for only 22.2% of all infection-related death, while non-PD-related causes, including pneumonia, wound infection, and necrotizing colitis, contributed to the majority of infection-related death (77.8%).

Table 1. Comparision of demographic, clinical, and laboratory characteristics in each tertile.

		I (5.15–6.7)	II (6.8–7.5)	III (7.6–13.25)	P
	n=140	n=46	n=47	n=47	
Age, years (SD)	58.7±10.6	57.2±11.5	59.2±9.2	59.6±11.0	0.493
Male gender	83 (59.3%)	33 (71.7%)	30 (63.8%)	20 (42.6%)	0.012
Follow-up duration, years	3.5±2.0	3.6±1.9	3.9±2.0	3.0±1.9	0.095
Diabetes as the cause of ESRD	119 (85.0%)	37 (80.4%)	40 (85.1%)	42 (89.4%)	0.105
CVD	44 (31.4%)	18 (39.1%)	10 (21.3%)	16 (34.0%)	0.160
CCI score	5.8±1.4	5.6±1.4	5.8±1.2	6.0±1.7	0.352
Year of starting PD					0.306
2001~2004	45 (32.1%)	12 (26.1%)	14 (29.8%)	19 (40.4%)	
2005~2008	95 (67.9%)	34 (73.9%)	33 (70.2%)	28 (59.6%)	
BMI (kg/m^2)	23.2±2.7	23.4±3.0	23.4±2.4	22.8±2.8	0.489
Systolic BP (mmHg)	133.9±19.4	134.1±19.2	135.2±21.2	132.4±17.9	0.796
Diastolic BP (mmHg)	77.5±11.5	77.8±11.0	78.2±11.0	76.6±12.6	0.778
Methods of glycemic control					0.135
Insulin	55 (39.3%)	17 (37.0%)	18 (38.3%)	20 (42.6%)	
Oral hypoglycemic agent	59 (42.1%)	24 (52.2%)	20 (42.6%)	15 (31.9%)	
Combined	19 (13.6%)	3 (6.5%)	5 (10.6%)	11 (23.4%)	
No control	7 (5.0%)	2 (4.3%)	4 (8.5%)	1 (2.1%)	
Hypoglycemic event*	1.1	0.9	1.1	1.2	0.250
Hemoglobin (g/dL)	11.0±1.7	11.0±1.8	11.1±1.8	10.9±1.5	0.842
HbA1C (%)	7.3±1.1	6.3±0.3	7.1±0.3	8.5±1.1	<0.001
Preprandial glucose (mg/dL)	145.3±50.3	104.9±22.6	136.2±16.6	194.0±52.2	<0.001
Creatinine (mg/dL)	6.6±2.4	6.9±2.6	6.9±2.7	6.0±1.9	0.100
Albumin (g/dL)	3.3±0.5	3.4±0.4	3.4±0.4	3.1±0.5$^{(I,II)}$	0.003
Total cholesterol (mg/dL)	184.1±44.6	178.7±45.6	180.2±38.1	193.3±49.0	0.220
Bicarbonate (mmol/L)	27.7±3.1	27.7±3.0	27.6±3.2	28.0±3.3	0.821
Calcium (mg/dL)	8.9±0.9	8.9±1.0	9.1±0.8	8.9±0.9	0.411
Phosphorus (mg/dL)	4.2±1.0	4.4±1.0	4.2±0.9	4.0±0.9	0.125
iPTH (pg/mL)#	74.9±3.5	98.2±4.1	70.0±3.5	59.3±2.9	0.245
hsCRP (mg/L)#	1.57±5.38	1.60±5.37	1.31±5.02	1.83±5.85	0.654
Total Kt/V$_{urea}$	2.48±0.62	2.37±0.61	2.54±0.68	2.55±0.58	0.450
RRF (ml/min/1.73 m^2)	4.62±3.20	4.59±2.49	4.50±3.88	4.76±3.38	0.953
nPCR (g/kg/day)	0.97±0.21	0.95±0.21	1.04±0.21	0.94±0.20	0.120

Data are presented as mean ± SD or n (%).
#expressed as geometric mean ± geometric SD. ESRD, end-stage renal disease; CVD, cardiovascular disease; CCI, Charlson comorbidity index; PD, peritoneal dialysis; BMI, body mass index; BP, blood pressure; iPTH, intact parathyroid hormone; hsCRP, high-sensitivity C-reacitve protein; RRF, residual renal function; nPCR, normalized protein catabolic rate.
*per 100-patient year.

Correlation between preprandial blood glucose and HbA1C

Pearson's correlation analysis revealed a significant correlation between preprandial blood glucose and HbA1C concentrations, as shown in Figure 2 (r = 0.622, p<0.001). Using a linear regression model, the following formula was extracted:

$$HbA1C(\%) = preprandial\ serum\ glucose(mg/dL) \times 0.016 + 5.377$$

On the other hand, there was no significant association between HbA1C and log hsCRP levels (r = 0.029, p = 0.744).

Comparisons of clinical and biochemical parameters among patients according to HbA1C levels

To explore whether patients with good and poor glycemic control had different clinical and biochemical parameters, the study subjects were divided into tertile groups according to their mean of HbA1C levels. The mean HbA1C levels in the 1st, 2nd, and 3rd tertiles were 6.3% (range, 5.2–6.7), 7.1% (6.8–7.5), and 8.5% (7.6–13.3), respectively. The percentage of patients in each tertile with HbA1C levels within the levels recommended by the American Diabetes Association [2] were 100%, 42.6%, and 0% in the 1st, 2nd, and 3rd tertiles, respectively. The proportion of male patients was significantly higher in the 1st and 2nd tertiles than in the 3rd tertile (p<0.05). Serum albumin was significantly lower in

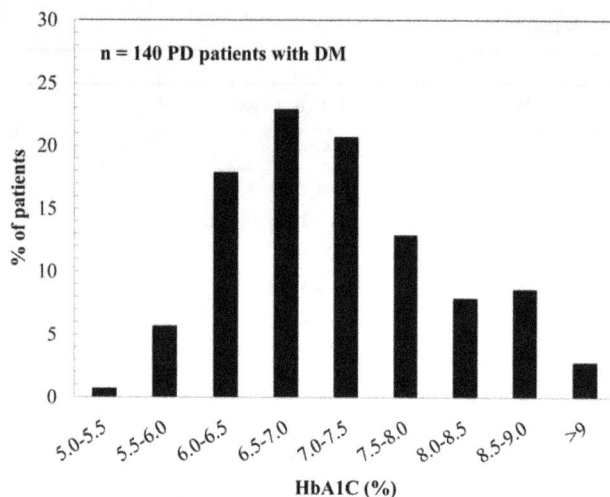

Figure 1. The frequency distribution of HbA1C values for all study patients.

the 3rd tertile than the 1st tertile (p<0.05). In contrast, there were no significant differences among the three tertiles in age, proportion of diabetes as the cause of ESRD, CCI score, BMI, systolic and diastolic blood pressure, hemoglobin, creatinine, calcium, phosphorus, total cholesterol, log-transformed iPTH, and log hsCRP levels. Residual renal function, Kt/V_{urea}, and nPCR were also comparable among the three groups. In addition, there was no difference in the frequencies of hypoglycemic events among tertiles (Table 1).

Causes of death among patients according to HbA1C levels

The causes of death for each tertile are shown in Table 2. Overall, cardiovascular disease and infection were the most common causes of death (18.5 per 1000-patient-year for each). However, while deaths from cardiovascular diseases occurred at similar frequencies across tertiles, deaths from infection increased according to increasing HbA1C tertiles. Therefore, compare to the 1st tertile, all-cause mortality increased in the 2nd tertile and even

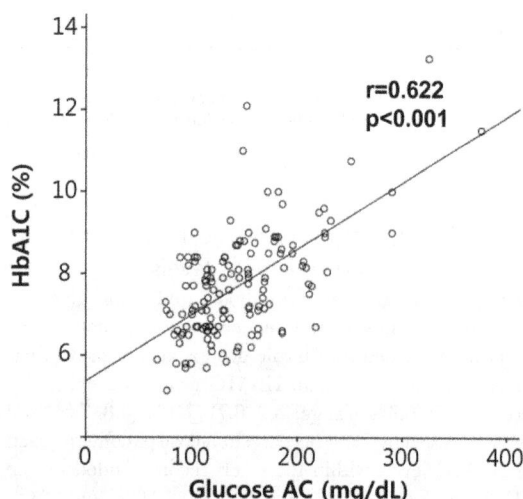

Figure 2. Bivariate correlation analysis between HbA1C and preprandial glucose (Glucose AC).

Table 2. Differences in the cause of death among tertiles.

Cause of death	I	II	III	Total
Cardiovascular disease	12.2	22.0	21.3	18.5
Infection	0	16.5	42.6	18.5
Other (Malignancy, Bleeding)	6.1	11.0	7.1	8.2
All-cause	18.3	49.5	71.0	45.2

per 1000-patient-year.

more increased in the 3rd tertile. While cardiovascular disease was the most common cause of death in the 1st (12.2 per 1000-patient year) and 2nd (22.0 per 1000-patient-year) tertiles, infection was the leading cause of death in the 3rd tertile (42.6 per 1000-patient-year).

Factors influencing all-cause mortality

In univariate Cox proportional hazards analysis, age [hazard ratio (HR), 1.07 per 1 year; 95% confidence interval (CI), 1.02–1.13; p = 0.01], CCI score (HR, 1.82 per 1 point; 95% CI, 1.24–2.67; p<0.01), and log hsCRP (HR, 1.43 per 1 unit; 95% CI, 1.10–1.87; p<0.01) were significantly associated with all-cause mortality in diabetic PD patients, whereas there were significant inverse correlations between all-cause mortality and variables such as MAP (HR, 0.95 per 1 mmHg; 95% CI, 0.92–0.99; p = 0.013) and serum creatinine [HR, 0.83 per 1 mg/dL; 95% CI, 0.68–0.99; p = 0.045].

Impact of HbA1C levels on all-cause mortality

Although all-cause mortality in the 3rd tertile group was significantly higher than in the 1st tertile (HR, 4.18; 95% CI, 1.15–15.21; p = 0.030), higher HbA1C levels were not associated with all-cause mortality in the unadjusted Cox proportional hazards analysis (p for trend = 0.089) (Table 3 and Figure 3). Using case-mix and fully-adjusted models, however, there was a significant association between the mean HbA1C levels and all-cause mortality (p for trend, 0.020 and 0.005, respectively). In the case-mix model, there were 2.22- and 6.08-fold increases in the risk of all-cause mortality in the 2nd (95% CI, 0.58–8.41; p = 0.243) and the 3rd tertiles (95% CI, 1.58–23.49; p = 0.009), respectively, compared to the 1st tertile. The risk of all-cause mortality increased further in the 2nd (HR, 4.16; 95% CI, 0.91–18.94; p = 0.065) and 3rd tertiles (HR, 13.16; 95% CI, 2.67–64.92; p = 0.002) using the fully-adjusted model.

Impact of HbA1C levels on cardiovascular mortality

The risk of cardiovascular mortality was comparable among the three tertiles in the unadjusted, case-mix, and fully-adjusted models (p for trend, 0.731, 0.532, and 0.682, respectively) (Table 3 and Figure 3).

Impact of HbA1C on non-cardiovascular mortality

The risk of non-cardiovascular mortality increased in the 2nd (HR, 4.16; 95% CI, 0.49–35.65; p = 0.194) and 3rd tertiles (HR, 8.31; 95% CI, 1.02–51.57; p = 0.048) compared to the 1st tertile, but this trend failed to reach statistical significance (p for trend, 0.107). In the case-mix model, there were 3.01- and 13.03-fold increases in the risk of non-cardiovascular mortality in the 2nd (95% CI, 0.34–26.78; p = 0.323) and the 3rd tertiles (95% CI, 1.47–85.34; p = 0.021), respectively, compared to the 1st tertile (p for trend = 0.029). The risk of non-cardiovascular mortality

Table 3. Risk of all-cause, cardiovascular, and non-cardiovascular mortality among tertiles (n = 140).

Model	All-cause HR (95% CI)	Cardiovascular HR (95% CI)	Non-cardiovascular HR (95% CI)
Unadjusted	P for trends 0.089	P for trends 0.731	P for trends 0.107
Tertile I	1.00	1.00	1.00
Tertile II	2.55 (0.69–9.41)	1.74 (0.32–9.54)	4.16 (0.49–35.65)
Tertile III	4.18 (1.15–15.21)	2.02 (0.33–12.17)	8.31 (1.02–51.57)
Case-mix	P for trends 0.020	P for trends 0.532	P for trends 0.029
Tertile I	1.00	1.00	1.00
Tertile II	2.22 (0.58–8.41)	1.76 (0.30–10.21)	3.01 (0.34–26.78)
Tertile III	6.08 (1.58–23.49)	3.09 (0.43–22.28)	13.03 (1.47–85.34)
Fully-adjusted	P for trends 0.005	P for trends 0.682	P for trends 0.007
Tertile I	1.00	1.00	1.00
Tertile II	4.16 (0.91–18.94)	2.80 (0.28–28.40)	7.67 (0.68–86.37)
Tertile III	13.16 (2.67–64.92)	2.46 (0.15–39.67)	51.24 (3.85–340.35)

Case-mix model is adjusted for age, gender, year of PD start, Charlson comorbidity index score. Fully-adjusted model is adjusted for mean arterial pressure, albumin, serum creatinine, and log-transformed hsCRP, in addition to all variables which were used in case-mix model.

significantly increased further in the 2nd (HR, 7.67; 95% CI, 0.68–86.37; p = 0.099) and 3rd tertiles (HR, 51.24; 95% CI, 3.85–340.35; p = 0.003) using the fully-adjusted model (p for trend = 0.007), as shown in Table 3 and Figure 3.

Impact of HbA1C on clinical outcomes in diabetic PD patients, whose etiology of ESRD was diabetic nephropathy

To elucidate whether the impact of glycemic control on clinical outcomes was comparable in diabetic PD patients whose etiology of ESRD was diabetic nephropathy, we performed additional analysis with the data of these patients (n = 119). The risk of all-cause mortality was not significantly increased in the 2nd (HR, 1.40; 95% CI, 0.35–5.60; p = 0.638) and 3rd tertiles (HR, 3.69; 95% CI, 0.99–13.70; p = 0.051) compared to the 1st tertile in the unadjusted model (p for trend = 0.065). In the case-mix model, however, there were 1.2- and 4.68-fold increases in the risk of all-cause mortality in the 2nd (95% CI, 0.29–5.05; p = 0.328) and 3rd tertiles (95% CI, 1.19–18.44; p = 0.028), respectively, compared to the 1st tertile (p for trend = 0.023). The risk of all-cause mortality increased further in the 2nd (HR, 3.30; 95% CI, 0.57–19.28; p = 0.185) and 3rd tertiles (HR, 12.71; 95% CI, 2.23–42.39; p = 0.004) using the fully-adjusted model (p for trend = 0.010). Meanwhile, there was a significant increase in the risk of non-cardiovascular mortality in the 2nd (HR, 4.62; 95% CI, 0.33–44.42; p = 0.255) and 3rd tertiles (HR, 33.92; 95% CI, 2.80–120.22; p = 0.003) relative to the 1st tertile using the fully-adjusted model (p for trend = 0.006), while the risk of cardiovascular mortality was comparable among the three tertiles in the unadjusted, case-mix, and fully-adjusted models (p for trend, 0.898, 0.920, and 0.498, respectively) (Table 4).

Discussion

In this prospective observational study on 140 incident diabetic PD patients from a single center, we found that poor glycemic control was associated with increased risk of mortality in diabetic PD patients, after adjusting for confounding factors. However, there were no differences in cardiovascular mortality rates among patients with different levels of glycemic control. These findings suggest that diabetic patients on PD could benefit from strict glycemic control, even if such control may not decrease cardiovascular mortality.

Tight glycemic control has been demonstrated to prevent the development and progression of microvascular complications and to be associated with reduced risk of coronary heart disease in diabetic patients [3–5]. In addition, previous studies have shown that high blood glucose concentrations are associated with increased incidence of cardiovascular diseases in patients with DM [6,7]. Based on these findings, it has been supposed that strict glucose control could exert a beneficial impact on the survival and cardiovascular outcome in diabetic patients, drawing up current guidelines of a target HbA1C level of 7.0% or less for most DM patients. Against these expectations, however, several recent studies showed that there was no beneficial effect of tight glycemic control on the cardiovascular morbidity and mortality in type 2 DM patients without advanced renal failure [8–10].

Findings regarding the impact of glycemic control on the outcomes of DM patients on dialysis have also been inconsistent. An analysis of 23,618 American diabetic HD patients showed that the adjusted risk for all-cause mortality in patients with HbA1C ≥10.0% was 1.41-higher than patients with HbA1C in the 5–6% range [13]. Most previous studies including East Asian diabetic patients on HD also found that poor glycemic control was associated with reduced surivival, which agrees with the results of our study [11,21]. In contrast, a recent study by Shurraw et al [14] showed that higher blood glucose and HbA1C levels were not associated with mortality in 1,484 incident HD patients in Canada. These conflicitng results may be attributed to the differences in ethnicity, body size, the duration of dialysis, and the definition of good glycemic control.

Meanwhile, there has been only one study conducted among PD patients, and it has revealed that poor glycemic control was associated with poor survival in diabetic PD patients [15]. However, few Asian patients were included in that study, and the impact of glycemic control on patient outcomes among Asian diabetic PD patients is still unclear. Although another report by Wu et al [16], which was conducted among Asian PD patients, revealed that glycemic control before starting dialysis was a predictor of survival for type 2 diabetic patients on PD, the importance of glycemic control after starting dialysis was not evaluated. Since PD fluid contains extremely high concentrations of glucose, we hypothesized that the glycemic control in PD patients would be different from the predialysis state. Therefore, we determined glycemic control by using average HbA1C levels during the 1st year after beginning PD, which were supposed to better reflect overall serum glucose concentrations. To exclude the possibility of improper hyperglycemia, moreover, the HbA1C levels around the time of acute illness or when taking medications that could affect serum glucose concentrations were omitted from the mean HbA1C levels.

In this study, poor glycemic control was associated with deleterious outcomes but not cardiovascular mortality which is the most common cause of death in ESRD patients undergoing dialysis. Consistent with these results, most previous studies have failed to demonstrate that good glycemic control improves cardiovascular survival in patients with long duration of DM [8–10]. Since most diabetic ESRD patients already have advanced microvascular and macrovascular complications, there might be a "point of no return", after which patient outcomes are not affected

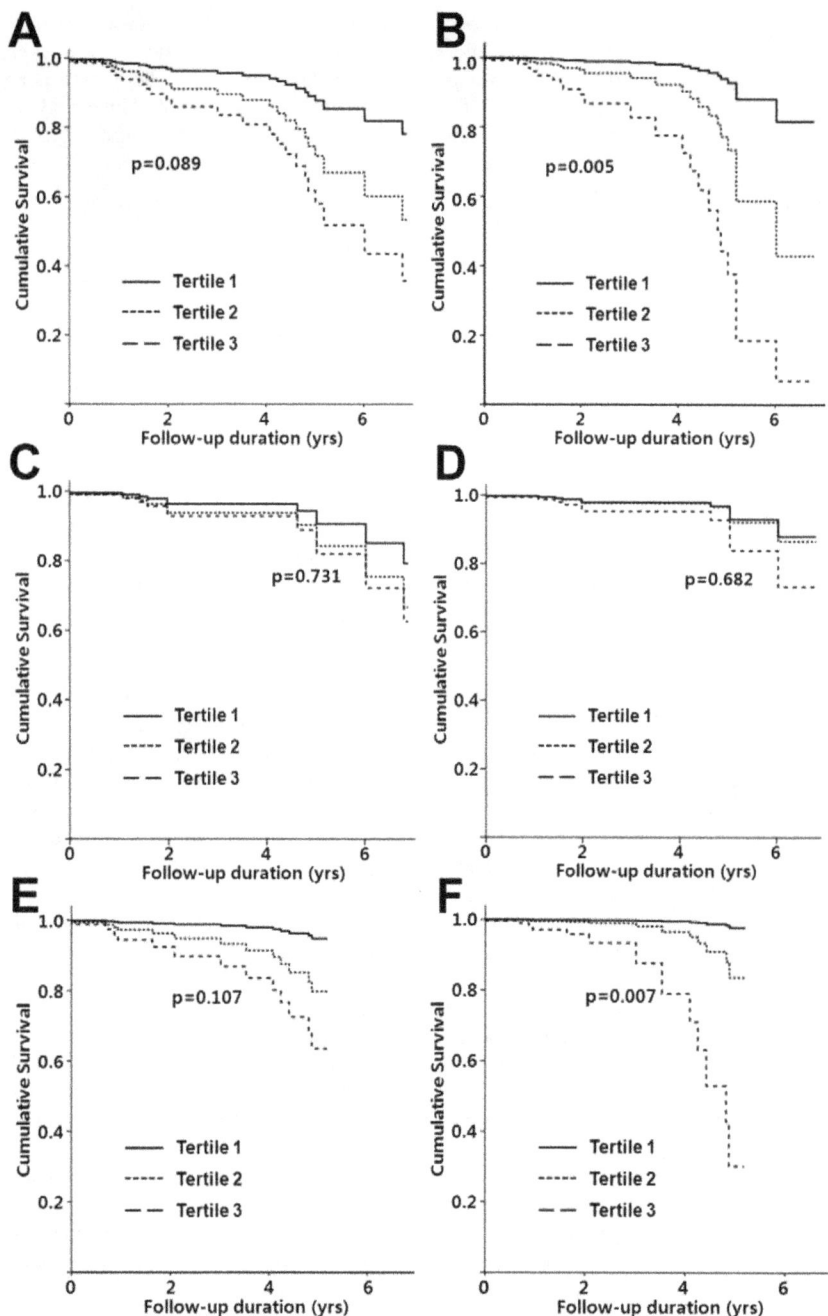

Figure 3. Comparison of cumulative survival among tertiles, plotted by Cox proportional hazards analysis. (A–B) Comparison of all-cause mortality among tertiles in unadjusted (A) and fully-adjusted model (B). (C–D) Comparison of cardiovascular mortality among tertiles in unadjusted (C) and fully-adjusted model (D). (E–F) Comparison of non-cardiovascular mortality among tertiles in unadjusted (E) and fully-adjusted model (F).

by strict glycemic control. Is it also relevant for diabetic ESRD patients whose primary renal diagnosis is not diabetic nephropathy? To answer this issue, we performed an additional subgroup analysis in patients whose primary renal disease was diabetic nephropathy. In result, the all-cause and non-cardiovascular mortality was also significantly higher in the 3rd tertile group compared to the 1st tertile group, whereas the risk of cardiovascular mortality was not different among groups, which were similar to the results with all diabetic PD patients. Therefore, it is surmised that "point of no return" theory can be applied at least to

PD patients in whom the etiology of ESRD was diabetic nephropathy. Meanwhile, a previous American report [13] observed a significantly higher cardiovascular mortality in patients with HbA1C ≥10.0%, while the rates were comparable among patients with HbA1C levels between 5.0% and 10.0%, suggesting that only extremely uncontrolled hyperglycemia may affect cardiovascular outcomes. Only 4 patients (2.8%) in our study sample had mean HbA1C levels greater than 10.0%, and therefore this effect might not be reflected in our study. There is also another possibility that "survival bias" could be involved in

Table 4. Risk of all-cause, cardiovascular, and non-cardiovascular mortality among tertiles in patients whose etiology of ESRD was diabetic nephropathy (n = 119).

Model	All-cause HR (95% CI)	Cardiovascular HR (95% CI)	Non-cardiovascular HR (95% CI)
Unadjusted	P for trends 0.065	P for trends 0.898	P for trends 0.107
Tertile I	1.00	1.00	1.00
Tertile II	1.40 (0.35–5.60)	1.13 (0.19–6.80)	4.16 (0.49–35.65)
Tertile III	3.69 (0.99–13.70)	0.65 (0.06–7.57)	8.31 (1.02–67.57)
Case-mix	P for trends 0.023	P for trends 0.920	P for trends 0.013
Tertile I	1.00	1.00	1.00
Tertile II	1.21 (0.29–5.05)	1.47 (0.23–9.56)	1.43 (0.14–14.47)
Tertile III	4.68 (1.19–18.44)	1.40 (0.10–19.97)	9.22 (1.10–77.37)
Fully-adjusted	P for trends 0.010	P for trends 0.498	P for trends 0.005
Tertile I	1.00	1.00	1.00
Tertile II	3.30 (0.57–19.28)	1.29 (0.28–14.54)	4.62 (0.33–44.42)
Tertile III	12.71 (2.23–42.39)	0.60 (0.10–28.57)	33.92 (2.80–120.22)

Case-mix model is adjusted for age, gender, year of PD start, Charlson comorbidity index score. Fully-adjusted model is adjusted for mean arterial pressure, albumin, serum creatinine, and log-transformed hsCRP, in addition to all variables which were used in case-mix model.

strict glycemic control more difficult in PD patients. These local and systemic hyperglycemic conditions have been suggested to be able to modify cytokine production and phagocytotic activity of immune cells by several mechansims, including hyperosmotic stress [24]. Furthermore, the production of advanced glycation endproducts can increase under hyperglycemic conditions, resulting in increased interaction between advanced glycation endproducts and their receptors, which can in turn increase inflammatory response [25].

Several shortcomings of this study should be discussed. First, as a single center study, it is subject to the biases inherent to this study design. In addition, 145 patients out of the total incident PD patients (n = 810) had diabetes, which corresponds to only 18% of incident PD patients. Considering the fact that 35 to 40% of incident ESRD patients in Korea from 2001 to 2009 had diabetes [26], we could not completely affirm that there was no selection bias even though it was not intentional. We surmise that the discrepancy in the proportion of DM patients between incident HD and PD patients in our institute may be partially attributed to our physician's tendency to hesitate to perform PD in DM patients, especially in whom predialysis blood glucose control was not appropriate. In fact, only 2.8% of this study subjects had mean HbA1C greater than 10.0%, which was much lower than 6.6% of enrolled patients in an American report [15]. Second, besides serum glucose and HbA1C levels, laboratory values at 3 months after starting PD were used for analyses in most cases. Therefore, the changes of confounding factors during the follow-up were not reflected. Third, diabetic ESRD patients, whose cause of ESRD was not diabetic nephropathy, could have different response to poor glycemic control. However, due to a small number of these patients (n = 21), subgroup analysis was not able to be performed for this issue. Lastly, there are some limitations for using HbA1C levels as a surrogate marker of glycemic control in dialysis patients. However, tests for better surrogate markers such as glycoalbumin are not widely performed and have been available in our institute only after 2009.

In conclusion, this study demonstrated that poor glycemic control was associated with higher all-cause mortality, mainly non-cardiovascular mortality represented by infection-related deaths, in diabetic PD patients. These findings suggest that better glycemic control may improve the outcome of these patients. Clinical trials are needed to better examine the impact of strict glycemic control on survival in diabetic PD patients.

the results of cardiovascular mortality. In our study subjects, CVD was less in tertile II (21.3%), as compared with tertile I (39.1%) and tertile III (34.0%). One explanation to this observation is that patients with moderate glycemic control died of cardiovascular events even before starting PD and reaching at poorer glycemic states, and those who have reached to the 3rd tertile survived from any cardiovascular events.

This study revealed that patients with poor glycemic control had significantly higher non-cardiovascular mortality, mainly due to infection. Similarly, a Taiwanese study [16] and another Korean study on diabetic PD patients [22] also found that the proportion of mortality from infection was high and comparable to that from cardiovascular diseases in their subjects, which raises several questions. Why is there a difference in the proportion of mortality from infection between diabetic HD and PD patients? Why infection-related mortality is influenced by the degree of glycemic control? While the answers are not clear, mounting evidence has shown that diabetic PD patients may be more vulnerable to infections. Frequently exchanging PD fluid could eliminate or dilute phagocytes and immunoglobulins normally present in the peritoneal cavity. In fact, the amount of removed immunoglobulin G and C3 through PD is reported to be significantly greater in DM than non-diabetic patients [23]. Moreover, hypertonic glucose solution used for PD could make patients susceptible to infection, especially in diabetic patients. It is well known that 60 to 80% of glucose in dialysate is systemically absorbed by diffusion and lymphatic absorption during a 6-hour dwell, which makes

Acknowledgments

The authors acknowledge our gratitude to the patients who participated in this study. The abstract of this study was presented as a poster at the American Society of Nephrology Annual Meeting 2011, Philadelphia, PA, U.S.A.

Author Contributions

Conceived and designed the experiments: DEY JTP. Analyzed the data: SHH T-HY KHC. Contributed reagents/materials/analysis tools: HJO SJK MJL DHS. Wrote the paper: DEY S-WK.

References

1. United States Renal Data System (2010) Atlas of End-Stage Renal Disease in the United States - Introduction. Am J Kidney Dis 52: S212.
2. American Diabetes Association (2011) Standards of medical care in diabetes–2011. Diabetes Care 34 Suppl 1: S11–61.
3. The Diabetes Control and Complications Trial Research Group (1993) The effect of intensive treatment of diabetes on the development and progression of

long-term complications in insulin-dependent diabetes mellitus. N Engl J Med 329: 977–986.
4. UK Prospective Diabetes Study Group (1998) Intensive blood-glucose control with sulphonylureas or insulin compared with conventional treatment and risk of complications in patients with type 2 diabetes (UKPDS 33). UK Prospective Diabetes Study (UKPDS) Group. Lancet 352: 837–853.

5. Ohkubo Y, Kishikawa H, Araki E, Miyata T, Isami S, et al. (1995) Intensive insulin therapy prevents the progression of diabetic microvascular complications in Japanese patients with non-insulin-dependent diabetes mellitus: a randomized prospective 6-year study. Diabetes Res Clin Pract 28: 103–117.

6. Wei M, Gaskill SP, Haffner SM, Stern MP (1998) Effects of diabetes and level of glycemia on all-cause and cardiovascular mortality. The San Antonio Heart Study. Diabetes Care 21: 1167–1172.

7. Selvin E, Marinopoulos S, Berkenblit G, Rami T, Brancati FL, et al. (2004) Meta-analysis: glycosylated hemoglobin and cardiovascular disease in diabetes mellitus. Ann Intern Med 141: 421–431.

8. Gerstein HC, Miller ME, Byington RP, Goff DC, Jr., Bigger JT, et al. (2008) Effects of intensive glucose lowering in type 2 diabetes. N Engl J Med 358: 2545–2559.

9. Duckworth W, Abraira C, Moritz T, Reda D, Emanuele N, et al. (2009) Glucose control and vascular complications in veterans with type 2 diabetes. N Engl J Med 360: 129–139.

10. Patel A, MacMahon S, Chalmers J, Neal B, Billot L, et al. (2008) Intensive blood glucose control and vascular outcomes in patients with type 2 diabetes. N Engl J Med 358: 2560–2572.

11. Oomichi T, Emoto M, Tabata T, Morioka T, Tsujimoto Y, et al. (2006) Impact of glycemic control on survival of diabetic patients on chronic regular hemodialysis: a 7-year observational study. Diabetes Care 29: 1496–1500.

12. Williams ME, Lacson E, Jr., Teng M, Ofsthun N, Lazarus JM (2006) Hemodialyzed type I and type II diabetic patients in the US: Characteristics, glycemic control, and survival. Kidney Int 70: 1503–1509.

13. Kalantar-Zadeh K, Kopple JD, Regidor DL, Jing J, Shinaberger CS, et al. (2007) A1C and survival in maintenance hemodialysis patients. Diabetes Care 30: 1049–1055.

14. Shurraw S, Majumdar SR, Thadhani R, Wiebe N, Tonelli M (2010) Glycemic control and the risk of death in 1,484 patients receiving maintenance hemodialysis. Am J Kidney Dis 55: 875–884.

15. Duong U, Mehrotra R, Molnar MZ, Noori N, Kovesdy CP, et al. (2011) Glycemic control and survival in peritoneal dialysis patients with diabetes mellitus. Clin J Am Soc Nephrol 6: 1041–1048.

16. Wu MS, Yu CC, Wu CH, Haung JY, Leu ML, et al. (1999) Pre-dialysis glycemic control is an independent predictor of mortality in type II diabetic patients on continuous ambulatory peritoneal dialysis. Perit Dial Int 19 Suppl 2: S179–183.

17. Genuth S, Alberti KG, Bennett P, Buse J, Defronzo R, et al. (2003) Follow-up report on the diagnosis of diabetes mellitus. Diabetes Care 26: 3160–3167.

18. Charlson ME, Pompei P, Ales KL, MacKenzie CR (1987) A new method of classifying prognostic comorbidity in longitudinal studies: development and validation. J Chronic Dis 40: 373–383.

19. Watson PE, Watson ID, Batt RD (1980) Total body water volumes for adult males and females estimated from simple anthropometric measurements. Am J Clin Nutr 33: 27–39.

20. Blagg CR (1991) Importance of nutrition in dialysis patients. Am J Kidney Dis 17: 458–461.

21. Morioka T, Emoto M, Tabata T, Shoji T, Tahara H, et al. (2001) Glycemic control is a predictor of survival for diabetic patients on hemodialysis. Diabetes Care 24: 909–913.

22. Chung SH, Han DC, Noh H, Jeon JS, Kwon SH, et al. (2010) Risk factors for mortality in diabetic peritoneal dialysis patients. Nephrol Dial Transplant 25: 3742–3748.

23. Krediet RT, Zuyderhoudt FM, Boeschoten EW, Arisz L (1986) Peritoneal permeability to proteins in diabetic and non-diabetic continuous ambulatory peritoneal dialysis patients. Nephron 42: 133–140.

24. Wade CE (2008) Hyperglycemia may alter cytokine production and phagocytosis by means other than hyperosmotic stress. Crit Care 12: 182.

25. Bopp C, Bierhaus A, Hofer S, Bouchon A, Nawroth PP, et al. (2008) Bench-to-bedside review: The inflammation-perpetuating pattern-recognition receptor RAGE as a therapeutic target in sepsis. Crit Care 12: 201.

26. Jin DC (2011) Current status of dialysis therapy in Korea. Korean J Intern Med 26: 123–131.

Lean Body Mass Predicts Long-Term Survival in Chinese Patients on Peritoneal Dialysis

Jenq-Wen Huang[1], Yu-Chung Lien[4], Hon-Yen Wu[1,5], Chung-Jen Yen[1], Chun-Chun Pan[3], Tsai-Wei Hung[3], Chi-Ting Su[6], Chih-Kang Chiang[1,2], Hui-Teng Cheng[7]*, Kuan-Yu Hung[1]*

1 Department of Internal Medicine, National Taiwan University College of Medicine and Hospital, Taipei, Taiwan, 2 Department of Integrated Diagnostics and Therapeutics, National Taiwan University College of Medicine and Hospital, Taipei, Taiwan, 3 Department of Nursing, National Taiwan University College of Medicine and Hospital, Taipei, Taiwan, 4 Department of Internal Medicine, Buddhist Tzu Chi General Hospital, Taipei Branch, New Taipei City, Taiwan, 5 Department of Internal Medicine, Far Eastern Memorial Hospital, New Taipei City, Taiwan, 6 Department of Internal Medicine, National Taiwan University College of Medicine and Hospital, Yun-Lin Branch, Yun-Lin County, Taiwan, 7 Department of Internal Medicine, National Taiwan University College of Medicine and Hospital, Hsin-Chu Branch, Hsin Chu City, Taiwan

Abstract

Background: Reduced lean body mass (LBM) is one of the main indicators in malnutrition inflammation syndrome among patients on dialysis. However, the influence of LBM on peritoneal dialysis (PD) patients' outcomes and the factors related to increasing LBM are seldom reported.

Methods: We enrolled 103 incident PD patients between 2002 and 2003, and followed them until December 2011. Clinical characteristics, PD-associated parameters, residual renal function, and serum chemistry profiles of each patient were collected at 1 month and 1 year after initiating PD. LBM was estimated using creatinine index corrected with body weight. Multiple linear regression analysis, Kaplan–Meier survival analysis, and Cox regression proportional hazard analysis were used to define independent variables and compare survival between groups.

Results: Using the median LBM value (70% for men and 64% for women), patients were divided into group 1 (n = 52; low LBM) and group 2 (n = 51; high LBM). Group 1 patients had higher rates of peritonitis (1.6 vs. 1.1/100 patient months; $p < 0.05$) and hospitalization (14.6 vs. 9.7/100 patient months; $p < 0.05$). Group 1 patients also had shorter overall survival and technique survival ($p < 0.01$). Each percentage point increase in LBM reduced the hazard ratio for mortality by 8% after adjustment for diabetes, age, sex, and body mass index (BMI). Changes in residual renal function and protein catabolic rate were independently associated with changes in LBM in the first year of PD.

Conclusions: LBM serves as a good parameter in addition to BMI to predict the survival of patients on PD. Preserving residual renal function and increasing protein intake can increase LBM.

Editor: Emmanuel A. Burdmann, University of Sao Paulo Medical School, Brazil

Funding: The authors have no support or funding to report.

Competing Interests: The authors have declared that no competing interests exist.

* E-mail: kyhung@ntu.edu.tw (KYH); cheng78@hotmail.com (HTC)

Introduction

Protein–energy wasting (PEW) presents as low serum albumin and serum cholesterol levels, low body mass index (BMI), and reduced dietary protein intake [1]. In the general population, this condition is often associated with metabolic stresses and an inadequate diet. However, in patients with chronic kidney disease (CKD), loss of lean body mass (LBM) relates to reduced nutrient intake [1] and consistently high mortality [2,3]. In patients on hemodialysis (HD), lower LBM negatively influences survival, as does age [4]. Other studies that followed patients up to 20 more months also showed that LBM predicted survival among PD patients [5–7], indicating the importance of LBM in this population. However, the factors affecting LBM changes remain unclear.

LBM can be measured using the creatinine index derived from creatinine kinetics. Creatinine clearance from dialysate and urine,

in addition to creatinine degradation, represent patient dietary skeletal muscle protein intake and muscle mass [8]. The creatinine index can be used to accurately estimate fat-free body mass in dialysis patients [6,9,10,11].

The current study enrolled incident PD patients and measured their LBM at 1 month and 1 year after initiating PD, then followed their clinical outcomes for >8 years. The aims of this study were to investigate the impact of LBM on patient outcomes and the factors that are associated with LBM changes. This study demonstrates that LBM significantly affects PD patient survival and establishes the factors that may increase LBM.

Methods

Patients

Patients who started PD as a chronic renal replacement therapy between January 2002 and December 2003 were enrolled in this study. PD clearance and residual renal function were measured 1 month and 1 year after PD initiation. Follow-up continued until December 2011.

Clinical Characteristics and Follow-up

Clinical characteristics and dialysis parameters were reviewed from the medical records and included body mass index (BMI), peritoneal equilibration test (PET) results, adequacy Kt/V, residual renal function (renal KT/V), and normalized protein catabolic rate (nPCR). The results of regular serum chemistry studies including blood urea nitrogen (BUN), creatinine, albumin, total cholesterol (CHO), and triglycerides (TG), and total iron binding capacity (TIBC) were also reviewed. These data were collected at the initial evaluation 1 month and 1 year after PD initiation. LBM was evaluated using the creatinine index at these 2 time points. The change between the data at 1 month and at 1 year was calculated using the following formula:

change in LBM = $100 \times (LBM_{1y} - LBM_{1m})/LBM_{1m}$.

After initiation of PD, patients were followed prospectively for the occurrence of hospitalization, peritonitis, technique failure, and mortality. Patients who received transplants were censored in assessments of technique failure and mortality rates.

Ethical Considerations

All medical records and individual laboratory data were reviewed in this study. The study was also approved by the ethics committee of National Taiwan University Hospital under NTUH-REC No. 201205010RIC.

Calculation of Creatinine Index and Lean Body Mass

The creatinine index is measured as the sum of creatinine removed from the body (measured as the creatinine removed in dialysate, ultrafiltrate, and urine), any increase in the body creatinine pool, and the creatinine degradation rate [11]. This study assumed that the creatinine levels in patients on PD were stable, so no change in the body creatinine pool was included in the creatinine index calculation. Thus, the creatinine index was simplified to the formula [12]:

Creatinine index (mg/24 h) = Effluent creatinine+urine creatinine) (mg/24 h)+creatinine degradation (mg/24 h).

Creatinine degradation was further estimated using the following equation:

Creatinine degradation (mg/24 h) = 0.38 dL/kg/24 h × serum creatinine (mg/dL) × body weight (kg).

The creatinine index can be used to estimate edema-free LBM using the equation [13]:

Edema-free lean body mass (kg) = (0.029 kg/mg/24 h) × creatinine index (mg/24 h) +7.38 kg.

The calculated LBM corrected with individual body weight (BW) as the percentage of BW.

Statistical Analysis

All variables are reported as mean ± SD (or with 95% confidence intervals where appropriate) for continuous variables and as frequencies or percentages for categorical variables. Student's *t* test was used for analysis between groups where appropriate. Differences in frequency were tested using Chi square analysis. Relationships between variables were tested using Pearson correlation. The independent determinants of any variable were analyzed using multiple linear regression analysis. The adjusted variables were stated in each analysis. Change-score analysis was used to examine how the change in LBM was affected by the changes in other covariates after 1 year of PD. The baseline

LBM measurement was added into the multiple linear regression model of change-score analysis as a control covariate. The incidence of peritonitis was compared using Poisson analysis. Kaplan–Meier survival analysis and Cox regression proportional hazard analysis were used to analyze survival rates between groups and predictors for survival, respectively. p Values <0.05 were considered significant. The statistical analyses were performed using SPSS 13.0 for Windows (SPSS Inc., IL, USA).

Results

LBM in Patients on PD

A total of 115 incident PD patients were enrolled in the current study between January 2002 and December 2003 entered the current study. During the first year on PD, 12 patients dropped out (3 died, 3 underwent transplants, and 6 were transferred to HD). The remaining 103 patients were categorized into 2 groups according to median LBM values of 70% in men and 64% women evaluated at 1 month after PD initiation. Group 1 included 52 patients with low LBM, and group 2 included 51 patients with high LBM. Clinical characteristics were compared between the 2 groups. Compared with group 2 patients, group 1 patients were older, had a higher incidence of diabetes mellitus (DM), and had lower serum albumin levels and nPCR (Table 1). The use of PD modality did not differ between these 2 groups.

Predictors of LBM

The relationship between LBM and other nutritional and clinical parameters was further analyzed using Pearson correlation. LBM was negatively correlated with age, BMI, and fasting blood glucose levels and was positively correlated with BUN, creatinine, and albumin levels as well as TIBC and nPCR (Table 2). Peritoneal clearance and residual renal function were irrelevant to LBM.

From the above results, we concluded that nutrition was clearly associated with LBM. We further analyzed the independent determinants for LBM using multiple linear regression analysis. Age, DM, and BUN levels were negatively associated with LBM (Table 3). On the other hand, male gender, serum creatinine level, renal KT/V, and nPCR were positively associated with LBM. These independent determinants contributed to high predictability ($R^2 = 0.828$; Table 3).

LBM and Patient Outcomes

To clarify the impact of LBM on patient survival, the differences in outcomes between the 2 groups, including technique failure, mortality, and morbidity, were further analyzed. Both mean patient follow-up duration and time on PD were longer in group 2 patients (Table 4). The incidences of peritonitis and hospitalization and the duration of hospital stay were higher in group 1 patients. In addition, group 2 patients had a lower mortality rate, higher transplant rate, and higher PD duration. Kaplan–Meier survival analysis revealed that group 2 patients had longer patient (p<0.001, Figure 1) and technique survival (p<0.01, Figure 1).

Cox regression proportional hazard analysis was applied to determine the hazard ratio of LBM for mortality and technique failure. In univariate analysis, each percentage point increase in LBM reduced the hazard ratio for technique failure and mortality by 8% and 10%, respectively (Model 1; Tables 5 and 6). In multivariate analysis, LBM remained an independent factor for reducing the hazard ratio for technique failure, as did age and sex (Model 2, Table 5), even after controlling for DM and residual renal function (Model 3, Table 5). LBM also consistently reduced the hazard ratio for mortality after controlling for age and DM

Table 1. Comparison of clinical, nutritional, and clearance parameters between patients on peritoneal dialysis with low LBM (group 1) and high LBM (group 2).

	Group 1 (n = 52)	Group 2 (n = 51)
Age*	65±12	52±14
Men	24	25
DM*	14	1
APD	24	22
BMI (kg/m²)*	22.2±3.3	21.0±2.6
1Y BMI (kg/m²)*	23.8±3.6	22.0±2.6
nPCR (g/kg BW/day)*	1.06±0.24	1.16±0.20
1Y nPCR (g/kg BW/day)*	1.00±0.24	1.15±0.22
BUN (mg/dL)*	59±17	60±17
1Y BUN (mg/dL)	59±16	64±15
Creatinine (mg/dL)*	7.8±2.8	9.6±2.5
1Y Cre (mg/dL)	10.1±3.3	11.4±3.3
Albumin (g/dL)*	3.7±0.4	4.0±0.4
1Y albumin (g/dL)*	3.9±0.5	4.1±0.4
Cholesterol (mg/dL)*	191±53	216±48
1Y cholesterol (mg/dL)	213±51	222±44
Triglyceride (mg/dL)	154±116	132±59
1Y triglyceride (mg/dL)	229±147	191±163
TIBC*	221±56	245±43
1Y TIBC	240±57	251±31
Peritoneal Kt/V	1.74±0.37	1.76±0.36
1Y Peritoneal Kt/V	1.89±0.30	1.83±0.35
Renal Kt/V	0.56±0.43	0.68±0.40
1Y Renal Kt/V*	0.29±0.38	0.47±0.41
Total Kt/V	2.30±0.48	2.44±0.46
1Y Total Kt/V	2.18±0.37	2.30±0.36
Peritoneal WCCR (L/week)	38.4±8.5	40.0±7.4
1Y Peritoneal WCCR (L/week)	41.3±8.8	41.0±8.3
Renal WCCR (L/week)	31.9±23.8	32.5±20.7
1Y Renal WCCR (L/week)	15.2±17.5	21.7±20.3
Standard WCCR (L/week)	75.4±24.6	80.1±21.1
1Y standard WCCR (L/week)*	59.2±18.6	68.2±19.9
LBM (%)*	58±8	76±8
1Y LBM (%)*	59±11	74±12

*p<0.05 using Student's *t* test for continuous variables or the Chi-square test for categorical variables.
1Y: the value evaluated 1 year after initiating peritoneal dialysis, APD: automated peritoneal dialysis with a cycler, BMI: body mass index, BUN: blood urea nitrogen, LBM: % of lean body mass corrected with body weight, nPCR: normalized protein catabolic rate, TIBC: total iron binding capacity, WCCR: weekly creatinine clearance.

Table 2. Correlation between LBM and other clinical characteristics in all patients on peritoneal dialysis.

	LBM	p
Age	−0.59	<0.001
BMI	−0.20	0.04
Renal KT/V	0.09	0.39
Peritoneal KT/V	−0.07	0.49
Total KT/V	0.02	0.81
Renal WCCR	0.02	0.80
Peritoneal WCCR	0.10	0.29
Standardized WCCR	0.08	0.40
4 Hr D/P Cre	0.09	0.36
BUN	0.33	<0.001
Creatinine	0.57	<0.001
Glucose	−0.47	<0.001
Albumin	0.37	<0.001
Cholesterol	0.13	0.20
Triglyceride	−0.11	0.26
TIBC	0.31	<0.01
nPCR	0.47	<0.001

BMI: body mass index, BUN: blood urea nitrogen, LBM: % of lean body mass corrected with body weight, nPCR: normalized protein catabolic rate, TIBC: total iron binding capacity, WCCR: weekly creatinine clearance.

first month of PD treatment and 1 year later were further analyzed. Changes in LBM were inversely correlated with changes in BMI and directly correlated with changes in nPCR, creatinine levels, renal KT/V, and total KT/V at 1 year (Table 7). In change-score analysis with multiple linear regression analysis, nPCR, renal KT/V, creatinine levels, BUN, age, and baseline LBM changes were associated with changes in LBM with a high predictability of 0.712 (Table 8).

Discussion

In this study, we followed a PD population for 8 years and showed that higher LBM predicts longer technique survival and

Table 3. Independent predictors for LBM with multiple linear regression analysis among patients on peritoneal dialysis.

	B±SE	p
Constant	23±6	<0.001
DM	−3.7±1.6	<0.05
Age	−0.2±0.1	<0.001
Men	6.4±1.2	<0.001
Creatinine	3.3±0.3	<0.001
Renal Kt/V	7.5±1.5	<0.001
nPCR (per 0.1 g/kg/day)	3.9±0.4	<0.001
BUN	−0.4±0.1	<0.001
R²	0.828	

BUN: blood urea nitrogen, LBM: % of lean body mass corrected with body weight, nPCR: normalized protein catabolic rate.

status (Model 2, Table 6), even after the addition of sex and residual renal function as variables (Model 3, Table 6). In Model 3, with control of several other variables, each percent increase in LBM was shown to reduce risk of mortality by 8%.

Factors Associated with Changes in LBM

Because LBM was shown to be important to the outcomes of patients on PD, the factors influencing LBM changes between the

A

Accumulating rate

B.

Accumulating rate

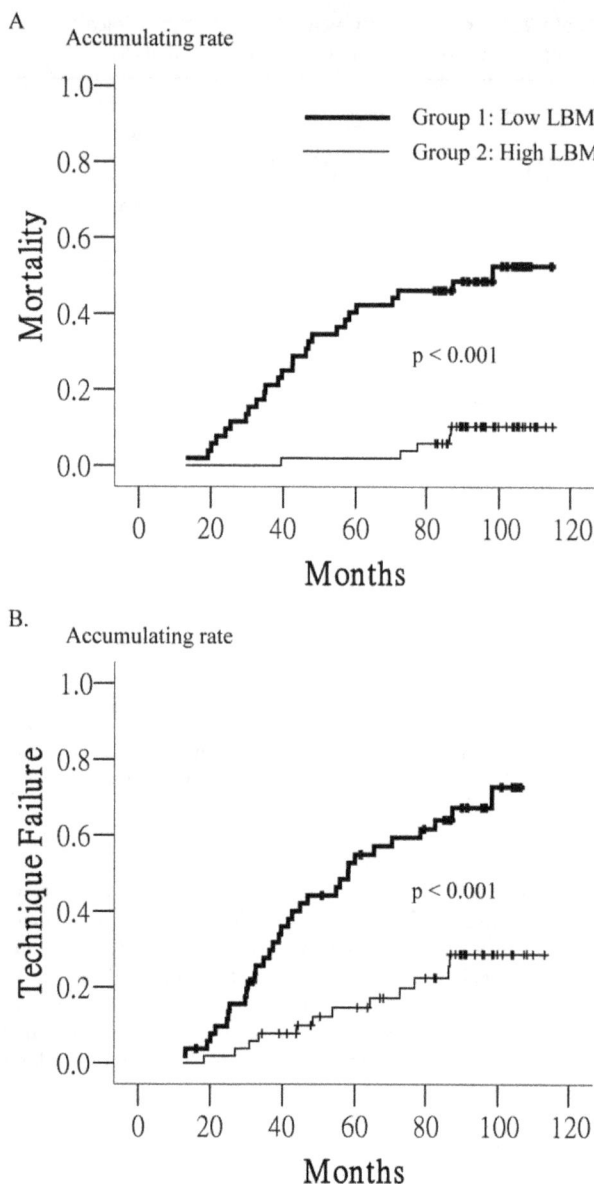

Figure 1. Lean Body Mass and Survival. Patients with low LBM (group 1) had shorter patient survival (A) and technique survival (B) than patients with high LBM (group 2) according to Kaplan–Meier survival analysis.

Table 4. Comparison of variable target outcomes between patients on peritoneal dialysis with low LBM (group 1) and high LBM (group 2).

	Group 1 (n = 52)	Group 2 (n = 51)
Mean time on PD (M)*	57±30	75±26
Mean patient follow-up (M)*	71±31	95±12
Peritonitis/100 M*	1.6	1.1
Hospitalization days/100 M*	71	25
Hospitalization/100 M*	14.6	9.7
Outcome*		
Death	19	4
Transfer to HD	15	9
Transplant	4	15
PD	14	23

*p<0.05 using Student's *t* test for continuous variables and Poisson analysis for incidence or Chi-square test for categorical variables.

mortality, but LBM reduced mortality risk in women only and not in men [16]. Several studies showed that high LBM predicts a better outcome among patients on PD in short-term follow-up [5–7,17]. In our study, which followed patients for up to 8 years, patients with low LBM had poorer survival and higher morbidity rates (Figure 1, Table 4). Incremental changes in both LBM and BMI reduced the hazard ratio for mortality, an effect that persisted after controlling for age, DM, and sex in Cox regression analysis (Table 6). Our findings further support that both LBM and BMI independently predict survival in patients on dialysis as demonstrated previously [15].

Serum albumin level is a well-known predictor for survival of patients on dialysis, although the relationships between LBM and albumin levels remain unclear. LBM represents somatic protein storage, while serum albumin level represents visceral protein. There was previously only a weak and even negative association

Table 5. Hazard ratio for dialysis technique failure according to Cox regression proportional hazard analysis using data at peritoneal dialysis initiation.

Technique failure			
Model 1	**HR**	**95% CI for HR**	**p**
LBM	0.92	0.89~0.94	<0.001
Model 2			
LBM	0.93	0.91~0.97	<0.001
Age	1.04	1.01~1.07	0.01
Men	2.22	1.21~4.08	0.01
Model 3			
LBM	0.94	0.91~0.98	<0.01
Age	1.04	1.01~1.07	0.02
Men	1.90	1.00~3.62	0.05
DM	1.81	0.75~4.35	0.19
Renal KtV	1.14	0.53~2.47	0.74

CI: confidence interval, DM: diabetes mellitus, HR: hazard ratio, LBM: % of lean body mass corrected with body weight.

overall patient survival. Changes in LBM were directly correlated with changes in nPCR, residual renal function, and serum creatinine and BUN levels. These results support that increasing protein intake and preserving residual renal function increase LBM, which would prolong patient survival.

High BMI is associated with increased survival in most patients on dialysis. However, this association cannot be applied to Asian patients on dialysis [14]. Different body components may have variable effects on the outcomes of patients on dialysis. LBM represents a non-fat component, but the role of LBM in this "reverse epidemiology" has remained unclear. Some authors have reported that LBM is not associated with this reverse outcome [14], but others have reported that LBM should be added to BMI to improve its predictive power [15]. Another study in patients on HD showed that increased fat mass reduced the hazard ratio for

Table 6. Hazard ratio for mortality according to Cox regression proportional hazard analysis in all peritoneal dialysis patients.

Mortality			
Model 1	**HR**	**95% CI for HR**	**p**
LBM	0.90	0.87~0.93	<0.001
Model 2			
LBM	0.93	0.89~0.98	<0.01
DM	3.44	1.30~9.10	0.01
Age	1.05	1.02~1.09	<0.01
BMI	0.83	0.70~1.00	0.05
BUN	1.05	1.00~1.09	0.03
nPCR (per 0.1 g/kg/day)	0.68	0.48~0.97	0.03
Model 3			
LBM	0.92	0.88~0.97	<0.01
DM	3.02	1.07~8.48	0.04
Age	1.05	1.00~1.09	0.03
BMI	0.82	0.68~0.99	0.04
BUN	1.04	0.99~1.09	0.11
nPCR (per 0.1 g/Kg/day)	0.73	0.50~1.1	0.11
Men	1.74	0.66~4.55	0.26
Renal KtV	1.06	0.40~2.87	0.90

BMI: body mass index, BUN: blood urea nitrogen, DM: diabetes mellitus, LBM: % of lean body mass corrected with body weight, nPCR: normalized protein catabolic rate.

Table 7. Correlation between changes in LBM and changes in other parameters at 1 year.

	Changes in LBM	**p**
Age	−0.14	0.15
BMI	−0.25	0.01
nPCR	0.46	<0.001
Albumin	−0.04	0.69
TIBC	−0.07	0.49
Creatinine	0.44	<0.001
Glucose	−0.07	0.49
BUN	0.22	0.02
KtV	0.27	<0.01
Peritoneal KtV	0.17	0.08
Renal KtV	0.20	0.04

Change in each parameter is the change at 1 year divided by the initial value. BMI: body mass index, BUN: blood urea nitrogen, LBM: % of lean body mass corrected with body weight, nPCR: normalized protein catabolic rate, TIBC: total iron binding capacity.

LBM can be conveniently estimated using the equation for creatinine index in patients on PD because all variables represented in that equation are measured regularly in dialysis adequacy evaluation. The influence of overhydration and obesity are reduced in this method, which can provide a more reliable estimate of LBM than can other formulae [20]. Although the creatinine kinetics and PD dose shared similar variables, our results did not show any correlation between PD dose and LBM (Table 2). The association between change in residual renal function and in LBM might link to some pathogenesis caused by loss of renal function in the follow-up period.

An important strength of our study was its long follow-up period of 8–9 years. Its potential limitations include: First, the restricted case number and the lack of physical activity evaluation, which would be another factor for increasing LBM. Second, as seen in other observational studies, we cannot account for unmeasured or residual confounding variables. Finally, because our patients' BMI values were 21–22 kg/m^2, the confounding factor of obesity could not be adequately assessed.

In conclusion, low LBM is associated with higher mortality in

Table 8. Independent predictors for changes in LBM at 1 year of PD according to change-score analysis.

	B±SE	**p**
Constant	26.78±9.25	0.005
Change in nPCR	0.51±0.05	<0.001
Change in renal KtV	0.06±0.01	<0.001
Change in creatinine	0.33±0.03	<0.001
Change in BUN	−0.24±0.03	<0.001
Age	−0.23±0.07	0.002
LBM baseline	−0.24±0.08	0.006
R^2	0.712	

Change in each parameter was the change at 1 year divided by the initial value. BUN: blood urea nitrogen, LBM: % of lean body mass corrected with body weight, nPCR: normalized protein catabolic rate.

between serum albumin and LBM in patients on HD [18]. In our study, LBM was positively correlated with serum creatinine and serum albumin levels in the PD population as shown previously [9]. In addition, LBM was also positively correlated with BUN and nPCR in the present study (Table 2). However, in multiple linear regression analysis, albumin lost its significance to predict LBM (Table 3). As a protein storage marker, LBM was not a substitute for albumin; rather, it provided a different representation of protein mass.

Because low LBM is a strong predictor of mortality in patients on PD, efforts to increase LBM should be valuable. Therefore, factors associated with LBM changes should be monitored to guide further management of patients on PD. Increased levels of physical activity and total daily protein intake are associated with higher LBM in patients on HD [18]. A study of patients on PD also showed that daily protein intake is positively correlated with LBM and associated with survival [17]. In our study, changes in LBM were positively correlated with changes in nPCR, creatinine, and renal KT/V and were negatively correlated with changes in BMI (Table 7). In other words, LBM increased as BMI decreased. Reducing body fat might reduce inflammation and increase LBM [18]. However, in patients on HD, higher fat mass is also associated with better survival [16,19] as in the present study of patients with PD (Table 6; Models 2 and 3). This obesity paradox creates a dilemma for advising obese patients on dialysis to reduce body weight. Increased protein intake and preservation of renal function were both modifiable independent factors associated with increasing LBM and served as 2 main targets in caring for patients on PD.

patients on PD. Increasing protein intake and preserving residual renal function can increase LBM. Although these findings need to be confirmed by further studies, they may have important clinical implications regarding protein energy intake and weight reduction policy in patients on PD.

Author Contributions

Conceived and designed the experiments: JWH KYH. Performed the experiments: JWH YCL HYW CJY CCP TWH CTS CKC HTC. Analyzed the data: JWH YCL HYW CJY CCP TWH. Contributed reagents/materials/analysis tools: JWH YCL HYW CJY CCP TWH. Wrote the paper: JWH.

References

1. Fouque D, Kalantar-Zadeh K, Kopple J, Cano N, Chauveau P, et al. (2008) A proposed nomenclature and diagnostic criteria for protein-energy wasting in acute and chronic kidney disease. Kidney Int 73: 391–398.
2. Kovesdy CP, Kalantar-Zadeh K. (2009) Why is protein-energy wasting associated with mortality in chronic kidney disease? Semin Nephrol 29: 3–14.
3. Rambod M, Bross R, Zitterkoph J, Benner D, Pithia J, et al.(2009) Association of malnutrition-inflammation score with quality of life and mortality in hemodialysis patients: A 5-year prospective cohort study. Am J Kidney Dis 53: 298–309.
4. De Lima JJ, Sesso R, Abensur H, Lopes HF, Giorgi MC, et al(1995) Predictors of mortality in long-term haemodialysis patients with a low prevalence of comorbid conditions. Nephrol Dial Transplant 10: 1708–1713.
5. Trivedi H, Tan SH, Prowant B, Sherman A, Voinescu CG, et al. (2005) Predictors of death in patients on peritoneal dialysis: The missouri peritoneal dialysis study. Am J Nephrol 25: 466–473.
6. Dong J, Li YJ, Lu XH, Gan HP, Zuo L, et al. (2008) Correlations of lean body mass with nutritional indicators and mortality in patients on peritoneal dialysis. Kidney Int 73: 334–340.
7. Szeto CC, Wong TY, Leung CB, Wang AY, Law MC, et al. (2000) Importance of dialysis adequacy in mortality and morbidity of chinese capd patients. Kidney Int 58: 400–407.
8. (2000) Clinical practice guidelines for nutrition in chronic renal failure. K/doqi, national kidney foundation. Am J Kidney Dis 35: S1–140.
9. Keshaviah PR, Nolph KD, Moore HL, Prowant B, Emerson PF, et al. (1994) Lean body mass estimation by creatinine kinetics. J Am Soc Nephrol 4: 1475–1485.
10. Borovnicar DJ, Wong KC, Kerr PG, Stroud DB, Xiong DW, et al. (1996) Total body protein status assessed by different estimates of fat-free mass in adult peritoneal dialysis patients. Eur J Clin Nutr 50: 607–616.
11. Bhatla B, Moore H, Emerson P, Keshaviah P, Prowant B, et al. (1995) Lean body mass estimation by creatinine kinetics, bioimpedance, and dual energy x-ray absorptiometry in patients on continuous ambulatory peritoneal dialysis. ASAIO J 41: M442–446.
12. Mitch WE, Collier VU, Walser M. (1980) Creatinine metabolism in chronic renal failure. Clin Sci (Lond) 58: 327–335.
13. Forbes GB, Bruining GJ. (1976) Urinary creatinine excretion and lean body mass. Am J Clin Nutr 29: 1359–1366.
14. Johansen KL, Young B, Kaysen GA, Chertow GM, (2004) Association of body size with outcomes among patients beginning dialysis. Am J Clin Nutr 80: 324–332.
15. Moreau-Gaudry X, Guebre-Egziabher F, Jean G, Genet L, Lataillade D, et al. (2011) Serum creatinine improves body mass index survival prediction in hemodialysis patients: A 1-year prospective cohort analysis from the arnos study. J Ren Nutr 21: 369–375.
16. Noori N, Kovesdy CP, Dukkipati R, Kim Y, Duong U, et al. (2010) Survival predictability of lean and fat mass in men and women undergoing maintenance hemodialysis. Am J Clin Nutr 92: 1060–1070.
17. Dong J, Li Y, Xu Y, Xu R. (2011) Daily protein intake and survival in patients on peritoneal dialysis. Nephrol Dial Transplant 26: 3715–3721.
18. Majchrzak KM, Pupim LB, Sundell M, Ikizler TA.(2007) Body composition and physical activity in end-stage renal disease. J Ren Nutr 17: 196–204.
19. Huang CX, Tighiouart H, Beddhu S, Cheung AK, Dwyer JT, et al. (2010) Both low muscle mass and low fat are associated with higher all-cause mortality in hemodialysis patients. Kidney Int 77: 624–629.
20. Tzamaloukas AH, Murata GH, Piraino B, Raj DS, VanderJagt DJ, et al. (2010) Sources of variation in estimates of lean body mass by creatinine kinetics and by methods based on body water or body mass index in patients on continuous peritoneal dialysis. J Ren Nutr 20: 91–100.

Impact of Individual and Environmental Socioeconomic Status on Peritoneal Dialysis Outcomes

Rong Xu[1], Qing-Feng Han[2], Tong-Ying Zhu[3], Ye-Ping Ren[4], Jiang-Hua Chen[5], Hui-Ping Zhao[6], Meng-Hua Chen[7], Jie Dong[1]*, Yue Wang[2], Chuan-Ming Hao[3], Rui Zhang[4], Xiao-Hui Zhang[5], Mei Wang[6], Na Tian[7], Hai-Yan Wang[1]

1 Renal Division, Department of Medicine, Peking University First Hospital, Institute of Nephrology, Peking University, Key Laboratory of Renal Disease, Ministry of Health, Key Laboratory of Renal Disease, Ministry of Education, Beijing, China, 2 Department of Nephrology, Peking University Third Hospital, Beijing, China, 3 Department of Nephrology, Huashan Hospital of Fudan University, Shanghai, China, 4 Department of Nephrology, Second Affiliated Hospital of Harbin Medical University, Heilongjiang, China, 5 Kidney Disease Center, The First Affiliated Hospital, College of Medicine, Zhejiang University, Hangzhou, China, 6 Department of Nephrology, Peking University People's Hospital, Beijing, China, 7 Department of Nephrology, General Hospital of Ningxia Medical University, Ningxia, China

Abstract

Objectives: We aimed to explore the impacts of individual and environmental socioeconomic status (SES) on the outcome of peritoneal dialysis (PD) in regions with significant SES disparity, through a retrospective multicenter cohort in China.

Methods: Overall, 2,171 incident patients from seven PD centers were included. Individual SES was evaluated from yearly household income per person and education level. Environmental SES was represented by regional gross domestic product (GDP) per capita and medical resources. Undeveloped regions were defined as those with regional GDP lower than the median. All-cause and cardiovascular death and initial peritonitis were recorded as outcome events.

Results: Poorer PD patients or those who lived in undeveloped areas were younger and less-educated and bore a heavier burden of medical expenses. They had lower hemoglobin and serum albumin at baseline. Low income independently predicted the highest risks for all-cause or cardiovascular death and initial peritonitis compared with medium and high income. The interaction effect between individual education and regional GDP was determined. In undeveloped regions, patients with an elementary school education or lower were at significantly higher risk for all-cause death but not cardiovascular death or initial peritonitis compared with those who attended high school or had a higher diploma. Regional GDP was not associated with any outcome events.

Conclusion: Low personal income independently influenced all-cause and cardiovascular death, and initial peritonitis in PD patients. Education level predicted all-cause death only for patients in undeveloped regions. For PD patients in these high risk situations, integrated care before dialysis and well-constructed PD training programs might be helpful.

Editor: Matthias Eberl, Cardiff University School of Medicine, United Kingdom

Funding: This study is supported by Baxer Clinical Research Award from Baxter Corp, China and ISN Research Award from ISN GO R&P Committee. The funders had no role in study design, data collection and analysis, decision to publish, or preparation of the manuscript.

Competing Interests: The authors have the following interests. This work was supported in part by the Baxer Clinical Research Award of Baxter Corp. There are no patents, products in development or marketed products to declare. This does not alter authors' adherence to all the PLOS ONE policies on sharing data and materials, as detailed online in the guide for authors.

* E-mail: dongjie@medmail.com.cn

Introduction

Recently, the China National Survey of Chronic Kidney Disease Working Group reported that the prevalence of chronic kidney disease was 10.8%, close to that in Western countries [1]. It is predicted that end stage renal disease (ESRD) will increase rapidly and become highly prevalent [2]. In China, medical insurance will be extended to cover all ESRD patients as proposed in a government working report in 2012 (http://english.gov.cn/official/2012-03/15/content_2092737.htm). Because peritoneal dialysis (PD) is less expensive [3], has a comparable survival rate [4,5] and can confer a better quality of life than hemodialysis (HD)

[6,7], a series of healthcare policies have been considered to increase the penetration of PD (http://www.moh.gov.cn/publicfiles/business/htmlfiles/chenz/pldjh/201107/52373.htm). At present, the possibility of popularizing PD treatment for ESRD patients urgently needs to be explored.

As a home-care therapy, PD requires patients to self-monitor and self-manage their treatment [8,9,10], abilities that are closely associated with socioeconomic status (SES) [11,12]. SES has been investigated for its association with the outcomes of treatment in the general population and in patients with chronic kidney disease at the individual [13,14,15,16,17] and environmental

[13,15,16,17,18] level. A few large-scale multi-center cohort studies have also explored this issue in PD patients and shown inconsistencies in the impact of individual [19,20,21,22,23] and environmental [21,22,24,25,26,27] SES on PD outcome. In China, we have experienced great economic development in the last 20 years, with an increase in gross domestic product (GDP) of around 10% per year, but there are imbalances between regions. Individual income and education levels also vary markedly within regions and probably lead to diverse availability of medical facilities and health-care services. Given this situation, a specific model is needed to determine whether variations in individual or environmental SES influence PD outcome. Moreover, the interaction between individual and environmental SES on PD outcome, which has never been studied in a dialysis population, should be explored.

This multicenter large-scale retrospective cohort study will be helpful in providing evidence for clinicians deciding whether PD is suitable for individuals with differing SES, and for health policymakers exploring potential strategies for establishing PD programs in regions with varying SES in China and other developing countries.

Methods

Center Enrollment

Centers with professional PD doctors and nurses and well-developed databases maintained for least 3 years, recording baseline characteristics and follow-up data for Chinese patient every 1~3 months, participated in this study voluntarily. Nine centers were qualified, and seven of these, accouting for about 70% of all incident patients attending the nine centers, agreed to participate. The included PD centers were located in five different provinces and four geographical regions (north, northeast, northwest, and east) of China. Data from each center were collected within a strict quality control framework and further inspected and optimized to ensure the integrity and accuracy of the database. All study investigators and staff members completed a training program that taught them the methods and processes of the study. A manual of detailed instructions for data collection was distributed. The ethics committee of Peking University First Hospital approved the study.

Subject Selection

All incident patients receiving chronic PD between the date of intact database creation and August 2011 were enrolled into this study. After starting PD, each patient signed informed consent agreeing to the use of their demographic and laboratory data in future studies. All subjects began the PD program within 1 month after catheter implantation and were given lactate-buffered glucose dialysate with a twin-bag connection system (Baxter Healthcare, Guangzhou, China). Patients who had been on PD for less than 3 months were excluded, as in previous studies [20,21].

Table 1. Baseline characteristics according to individual income.

		Individual income			P
	Total	Low (<¥20,000, i.e., <$3160)	Medium (¥20,000-¥40,000, i.e., $3160~$6320)	High (>¥40,000, i.e., >$6320)	
Proportion (%)	100	36.5	39.8	23.7	----
Age>65yrs (%)	41.5	33.0	39.8	46.0	<0.001
Male (%)	49.5	46.8	51.6	51.1	0.10
Body mass index (kg/m²)	22.9±3.6	22.8±3.7	23.1±3.6	23.0±3.5	0.27
DM (%)	37.6	34.7	39.7	39.9	0.13
CGN (%)	34.9	37.6	34.4	30.7	0.18
CVD (%)	40.9%	37.5	44.9	40.9	0.01
High school or above (%)	44.3	33.9	45.0	67.7	<0.001
Proportion of individual income used for medical expenses *>50% (%)	48.4	76.6	33.5	17.2	<0.001
Rural residence (%)	19.5	27.3	17.2	6.1	<0.001
Live alone (%)	3.1	3.0	3.3	2.6	0.17
Distance from hospital (KM)	20(8~80)	32(10~150)	20(7~79)	12(6~32)	<0.001
Frequent visitors ** (%)	85.4	82.4	88.8	88.3	<0.001
Live in undeveloped region (%)	55.9	64.7	55.2	38.6	<0.001
Hemoglobin (g/L)	103.9±19.2	100.8±19.0	106.8±18.9	106.5±18.9	<0.001
Serum albumin (g/L)	35.5±5.3	34.9±5.5	36.0±5.2	36.3±4.7	<0.001
RRF (ml/min)	4.67(3.52–6.09)	4.67(3.41–6.15)	4.70(3.57–6.06)	4.58(3.70–6.10)	0.74
Baseline dialysis dosage (ml)	5874±2009	5809±1987	5947±2001	5868±2095	0.49
Total kt/v	1.96(1.65–2.37)	1.95(1.61–2.38)	1.95(1.65–2.38)	1.97(1.70–2.33)	0.90

DM: diabetes mellitus; CGN: chronic glomerulonephritis; CVD: cardiovascular disease; RRF: residual renal function. *Proportion of individual income used for medical expenses was calculated as the percentage of yearly household income per person used each year for yearly self-paid medical expenses. **Frequent visitors were those who visited a doctor at least once every 3 months.

Table 2. Baseline characteristics according to regional GDP.

	Regional GDP		P
	undeveloped (GDP per capital <¥95000 i.e $15009)	Developed (GDP per capital ≥¥95000 i.e $15009)	
Age>65yrs (%)	30.6	53.2	<0.001
Male %	50.1%	47.3%	0.21
Body mass index (kg/m²)	22.9±3.6	23.2±3.6	0.08
DM (%)	34.1	45.6	<0.001
CGN (%)	37.7	26.8	<0.001
CVD (%)	40.2	43.2	0.19
Low individual income (%)	48.3%	33.7%	<0.001
High school or above (%)	38.7	52.9	<0.001
Proportion of individual income used for medical expenses*>50% (%)	57.6	30.5	<0.001
Rural residence (%)	28.9	2.0	<0.001
Live alone (%)	2.9	3.4	0.76
Distance to hospital (KM)	40(20~130)	6.8(3.7~11.6)	<0.001
Frequent visitors ** (%)	85.0	92.2	<0.001
Hemoglobin (g/L)	103.2±19.1	106.3±18.4	<0.001
Serum albumin (g/L)	35.8±5.5	35.2±4.9	0.02
RRF (ml/min)	4.70(3.52–6.05)	4.61(3.52–6.05)	0.91
Baseline dialysis dosage (ml)	5900±1939	5909±2104	0.94
Total kt/v	1.94(1.63–2.37)	1.98(1.67–2.37)	0.54
Registered doctors per thousand inhabitants	4.5±2.3	6.2±1.7	<0.001
Available hospital beds per thousand inhabitants	7.7±5.1	7.8±3.0	0.49

DM: diabetes mellitus; CGN: chronic glomerulonephritis; CVD: cardiovascular disease; RRF: residual renal function.
*Proportion of individual income used for medical expenses was calculated as the percentage of yearly household income per person used each year for yearly self-paid medical expenses.
**Frequent visitors were those who visited a doctor at least once every 3 months.

Data Collection

Demographic and clinical data including age, gender, body mass index (BMI), primary renal disease, history of cardiovascular disease (CVD), and presence of diabetes mellitus (DM) were collected at baseline. CVD was recorded if one of the following conditions was present: angina, class III/IV congestive heart failure (New York Heart Association), transient ischemic attack, history of myocardial infarction or cerebrovascular accident, or peripheral arterial disease [28]. Baseline biochemistry data including hemoglobin and serum albumin were calculated as the mean of measurements made during the first 3 months. Dialysis adequacy and residual renal function (RRF) were measured during the first 6 months. RRF was defined as the mean of residual creatinine clearance and residual urea clearance. Dialysis adequacy was determined from the total Kt/V and total creatinine clearance. Center size was also recorded according to the number of enrolled patients from each center.

SES data were collected for each patient. Individual income level was defined as the yearly household income per person and was divided into low (<¥20,000, <$3160,), medium (¥20,000–40,000, $3160–6320) and high (>¥40,000, >$6320); because most of the subjects were from urban areas, these groups were defined according to the average income for the urban population in 2011, obtained from the Bureau of Statistics (http://www.bjstats.gov.cn/nj/main/2011-tjnj/index.htm). The exchange rate of the US dollar ($) to the Chinese Yuan (¥) was set at 6.3293 on November

1, 2011. Education levels were recorded according to diplomas obtained based on school level, that is, elementary school or lower, middle school, high school, or above high school. Other individual SES data included the proportion of individual income used for medical expenses (the percentage of yearly household income per person spent each year on self-paid medical expenses), occupation, rural or urban residence, living alone or not, travel distance from the PD center, and frequency of visits to the PD center. A frequent visitor was defined as someone who saw a doctor at least once every 3 months. Regional SES included regional GDP per capita and regional medical resources such as number of registered doctors and available hospital beds per inhabitant. Data were obtained from the Bureau of Statistics in each province; Beijing data were downloaded from http://www.bjstats.gov.cn/nj/main/2011-tjnj/index.htm. Regions were divided into undeveloped regions and developed according to the median of regional GDP per capita (¥95000, $15009).

Definition of Outcome Events

The Primary outcome was all-cause death or cardiovascular death. Cardiovascular death was defined as death due to myocardial infarction, congestive heart failure, cerebral bleeding, cerebral infarction, arrhythmia, or peripheral arterial disease, or sudden death. The secondary outcome was initial peritonitis, which was diagnosed according to International Society for Peritoneal Dialysis 2010 guidelines [29]. In all analyses, we

Table 3. Detailed clinical outcome of the study population.

Peritoneal dialysis outcome	n(%)
Death	553
cardiovascular disease	210(38.0%)
myocardial infarction	*46*
congestive heart failure	*41*
cerebral bleeding	*30*
cerebral infarction	*29*
arrhythmia	*10*
peripheral arterial disease	*3*
Sudden death	*20*
undefined causes	*31*
infection	140(25.3%)
malignancy	66(11.9%)
gastrointestinal bleeding	23(4.2%)
malnutrition	27(4.9%)
miscellaneous	25(4.5%)
undefined	62(2.9%)
Transfer to hemodialysis	168
peritoneal dialysis related infection	77(45.8%)
leakage	13(7.7%)
hernia	5(3.0%)
catheter disposition	4(2.4%)
ultrafiltration failure	9(5.4%)
severe congestive heart failure	3(1.8%)
dialysis inadequacy	15(8.9%)
miscellaneous	30(17.9%)
undefined	12(7.1%)

censored follow-up at transferring to HD, loss to follow-up, renal transplantation, or the end of the study (November 1, 2011).

Statistical Analysis

Continuous data were presented as means with standard deviation except for distance to PD center, RRF, and total Kt/V, which were presented as the median (interquartile range) because of high skew. Categorical variables were presented as proportions. Relevant characteristics were compared between different individual income groups and between different education groups, respectively. Patient data were compared using the t-test or the analysis of variance F-test for normally distributed continuous variables, the chi-square test for categorical variables, or the Mann–Whitney U test for skewed continuous variables.

To determine predictors of outcome events, univariable Cox regression models were first constructed to explore individually the potential risk factors for all-cause death including demographic and bioclinical data, individual income, education level, and regional GDP per capita. Risk factors identified from univariable Cox regression models were included in multivariable analyses with all-cause death, CVD death and initial peritonitis as events. In multivariable analysis, stratified Cox regression models with center size as the stratified factor were employed to adjust for center effects. The center effect was reflected not only in disparity of center size (ranging from 78 patients to 815 patients), which has been demonstrated to be an independent predictor of PD outcome [30,31,32], but also in differences in practice patterns and biochemical assays between centers, which differed from the regional effect. The regional effect was defined by regional GDP per capita and reflected differences in SES between regions. To determine whether individual income or education level interacted with regional GDP per capita, we explored their two-way interaction effects on the likelihood of patient survival and peritonitis-free survival. When an interactive effect was observed, subgroup analysis was performed.

We reported the multivariable adjusted hazard ratios (HRs) with 95% confidence interval (CI). All probabilities were two-

Table 4. Predicting the roles of individual income and education level in all-cause death, cardiovascular death, and initial peritonitis.

	All cause death		Cardiovascular death		Initial peritonitis	
	adjusted HR* (95% CI)	P	adjusted HR* (95% CI)	P	adjusted HR* (95% CI)	P
Individual income group						
Low (<¥20,000, i.e., <$3160)	Ref		Ref		Ref	
Medium (¥20,000–¥40,000, i.e., $3160~$6320)	0.62(0.48–0.79)	<0.001	0.60(0.41–0.90)	0.012	0.91(0.71–1.16)	0.44
High (>¥40,000, i.e., >$6320)	0.44(0.33–0.61)	<0.001	0.47(0.29–0.76)	0.002	0.69(0.50–0.94)	0.02
Education level						
Elementary or lower	Ref		Ref		Ref	
Middle school	0.76(0.58–1.01)	0.06	0.81(0.53–1.26)	0.36	0.97(0.72–1.30)	0.84
High school	0.78(0.57–1.06)	0.12	0.79(0.49–1.28)	0.34	0.95(0.69–1.32)	0.77
Higher than high school	0.68(0.50–0.93)	0.02	0.54(0.32–0.91)	0.02	0.84(0.60–1.18)	0.31
Regional socioeconomic status						
Undeveloped region (GDP per capita <¥95,000 i.e $15,009)	Ref		Ref		Ref	
Developed region (GDP per capita ≥¥95,000 i.e $15,009)	0.88(0.70–1.12)	0.30	0.73(0.51–1.04)	0.09	1.11(0.88–1.42)	0.38

*Adjusted for confounders such as age, gender, body mass index, diabetes, cardiovascular disease, hemoglobin, serum albumin, and residual renal function, and stratified by center size.

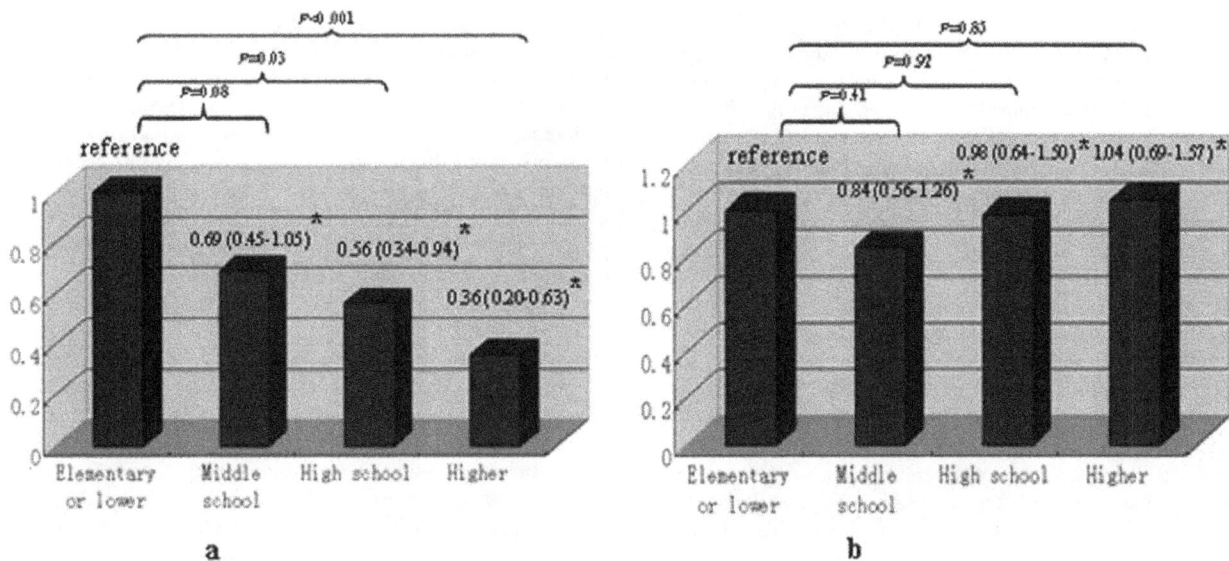

Figure 1. Subgroup analysis of predicted role of education level in all-cause death according to regional economic status. *Adjusted hazard ratio with 95% confidence interval (adjusted for confounders such as age, gender, body mass index, diabetes, cardiovascular disease, hemoglobin, serum albumin, and residual renal function, and stratified by center size) **Undeveloped region: gross domestic product (GDP) per capita <¥95,000 ($15,009); developed region: GDP per capita≥¥95,000 ($15,009).

tailed, and the level of significance was set at 0.05. Statistical analyses were performed using SPSS for Windows software version 13.0 (SPSS Inc., Chicago, IL).

Results

Baseline Characteristics

Data from 2409 patients were collected. One hundred and forty-five patients were excluded because they began the PD program before the date of intact database creation or more than 1 month after catheter implantation. Another 93 patients who had been receiving PD for less than 3 months were also excluded. The included 2171 patients had a mean age of 58.0±15.5 years and BMI 22.9±3.6 kg/m^2; 37.6% were diabetic and CVD was present in 40.9% of the subjects at baseline. Chronic glomerulonephritis (CGN) was the most common cause of ESRD (34.9%), followed by diabetic nephropathy and hypertensive nephropathy. The proportions of patients with low, median and high income were 36.5%, 39.8% and 23.7% respectively; 44.3% had a diploma from high school or above. There was significant regional economic disparity across the whole cohort, with GDP per capita ranging from the 10th percentile at ¥24,768 ($3913) to the 90th percentile at ¥175,495 ($27,722). Undeveloped regions were areas with GDP per capita lower than the median (¥95,000, $15,009) and had fewer registered doctors than developed regions but comparable numbers of available hospital beds per thousand inhabitants (4.5±2.3 vs 6.2±1.7, P<0.001 for doctors; 7.7±5.1 vs 7.8±3.0, P = 0.49 for beds).

Socioeconomic and Clinic Characteristics

Patients with low individual income were less likely to be elderly (33.0%) and have a history of CVD (37.5%). The lowest individual incomes were associated with the lowest education level and highest proportion of individual income used for medical expenses. The poorest patients were also more likely to live in rural areas and undeveloped regions at the greatest distances from hospital. Accordingly, the percentage of frequent visitors was lowest in the

low individual income group. At baseline, hemoglobin and serum albumin were lowest in the low individual income group. However, gender, BMI, prevalence of DM and CGN, living alone, RRF, baseline dialysis dose, and total Kt/V did not differ significantly between income groups (**Table 1**).

Patients who lived in undeveloped regions were significantly younger, poorer, and less educated and lived further from hospital. There were more cases of diabetes and fewer cases of CGN in this group. Hemoglobin and serum albumin were lower, but RRF and dialysis dose were comparable to those in developed regions. Undeveloped regions had fewer registered doctors per thousand inhabitants than developed regions. These data are shown in **Table 2**.

Follow-up and Outcome

The median follow-up time was 27.7(15.5–45) months. As shown in Table 3, among 553 patients who died, 210 deaths (38%) were due to CVD and 140 (25.3%) to infection; other causes were malignancy, gastrointestinal bleeding, malnutrition, miscellaneous, and undefined. Of the 210 patients who died from CVD, the leading cause was myocardial infarction (46 cases, 21.9%); other causes were congestive heart failure, cerebral bleeding, cerebral infarction, arrhythmia, peripheral arterial disease, sudden death, and undefined. One hundred and sixty-eight patients were transferred to HD, most due to PD-associated infection (77 cases, 45.8%); other reasons were leakage, hernia, catheter disposition, ultrafiltration failure, severe congestive heart failure, inadequacy of dialysis, miscellaneous, and undefined.

The time to first-episode peritonitis was 23.7 (11.9–40.4) months. Four hundred and fifty-five episodes of initial peritonitis occurred during the study period; 160 episodes (35.2%) were due to Gram-positive organisms, 94 (20.7%) to Gram-negative organisms, and six (1.3%) to fungi; 12 (2.6%) were polymicrobial, 130 (28.6%) were culture negative and 53 had no culture result (11.6%).

Association between SES and Outcome

On univariable Cox regression analysis, individual income and education level but not regional GDP per capita were significantly associated with all-cause death. The predicted role of these factors were further explored by multivariable Cox regression analysis. Age, BMI, DM, CVD, hemoglobin, serum albumin, RRF, and center size were also found to be significantly associated with all-cause death on univariable Cox regression analysis. After stratification by center and controlling for all of these confounders and gender, compared with the low income group, the adjusted HRs for all-cause death in the medium and high income group were 0.62 (95%CI 0.48–0.79, P<0.001) and 0.44 (95%CI 0.33–0.61, P<0.001) respectively. Medium income and high income were also associated with significantly lower risks for cardiovascular death, with adjusted HRs of 0.60 (95%CI 0.41–0.90 P=0.012) and 0.47 (95%CI 0.29–0.76, P=0.002) respectively. The high income group, but not the medium income group had a significantly lower risk for initial peritonitis, with an adjusted HR of 0.69 (95%CI 0.50–0.94, P=0.02) compared with the low income group (**Table 4**).

Compared with patients with an elementary school education or lower, patients with higher education levels did not show a constant trend toward lower risk for all-cause death. Only a diploma above the high school level predicted significantly lower risk for all-cause death, with an adjusted HR of 0.68 (95%CI 0.50–0.93, P=0.02), and for cardiovascular death, with an adjusted HR of 0.54 (95%CI 0.32–0.91, P=0.02). Otherwise, education level had no effect on cardiovascular death or initial peritonitis (**Table 4**).

Compared with patients living in undeveloped regions, patients in developed regions had similar risk of cardiovascular or all-cause death and initial peritonitis, even after controlling for all of above mentioned confounders such as age, proportion of patients with diabetes, serum albumin, and so on (**Table 4**).

In addition, we explored the interactive effect between individual income, education level and regional GDP per capita. We found that individual education but not income level had a significant interactive effect with regional GDP per capita on all-cause death (adjusted HR 0.79, 95% CI 0.65–0.97, P=0.024), and this influence was further explored after stratifying the patients according to regional development. In undeveloped regions, an education level of high school or above predicted a significantly lower risk for all-cause death compared with elementary school or lower, with adjusted HRs of 0.56 (95% CI 0.34–0.94, P=0.03) and 0.36 (95% CI 0.20–0.63, P<0.001), respectively. In developed regions, education level did not predict all-cause death (**Fig. 1**). No interaction effects were observed between individual income or education and regional GDP in terms of cardiovascular death and initial peritonitis.

Discussion

From this first large-scale multi-center cohort of incident Chinese PD patients, we found that individual rather than regional income independently predicted all-cause death, cardiovascular death, and initial peritonitis. Education level was only significantly associated with all-cause death in undeveloped regions but not in developed regions. An interaction effect of individual education level and environmental SES is reported for the first time.

Consistent with former studies [19,33,34,35], lower individual income emerged as an independently significant risk indicator for death and initial peritonitis. Although poorer patients were younger and had less comorbidity, they bore a heavier burden of medical expenses and had access to fewer medical resources,

which strongly supports increasing the personal medical coverage rate for PD patients in China. Of note, poorer patients were prone to be anemic and malnourished at baseline, probably due to inadequate health care and late referral to nephrologists before the development of ESRD. Given that the standard chronic kidney disease program is helpful in retarding progression to ESRD and improving complications such as anemia, malnutrition and bone mineral disease [36,37], the timing of and strategies used for medical support before dialysis in China need to be urgently investigated. We note that effective medical support aids the establishment of successful PD programs for disadvantaged minorities [38,39].

By contrast, no impact of regional GDP per capita on PD outcome was observed, the opposite of previous findings showing an independently negative effect of regional SES on outcome in chronic disease [15,16,17]. One potential reason for our finding is that, in the undeveloped regions in our study, the patients were younger, there were fewer cases of diabetes, and baseline serum albumin levels were higher than in the developed regions. Given that age, diabetes and serum albumin have been recognized as the strongest predictors by most studies [40,41,42], these favorable individual factors in our study possibly offset the disadvantages of regional SES. A similar finding was obtained in a study from the USA [24], in which the risk of technique failure was significantly lower in remote-dwelling patients than in those living closer to the hospital, because the former were younger and had fewer complications from diabetes. However, no association between regional SES and cardiovascular or all-cause death or initial peritonitis was observed, even after adjustment for age, proportion of patients with diabetes, serum albumin, and so on. We hypothesize that unknown confounding factors related to regional SES are also associated with PD outcome. In addition, only baseline characteristics, and not the change trend in clinical variables, were analyzed for the prediction of outcome during follow-up. This choice may have influenced the reliability of our results.

Our analysis indicates that education level had no effect on risk of initial peritonitis. This result is consistent with the analysis of a US regional ESRD registry in which 1595 new PD patients were observed over 2 years [23], but is contrary to recently published data from Brazil and Canada [21,22]. One possible explanation is that our selected centers had professional PD doctors/nurses and well-constructed training programs. Patients and their home-care helpers were often trained simultaneously, which probably led to stronger family support [43]. Whether better compliance in Asian people [44,45] plays a role in this phenomemon is unclear. However, lower education level still significantly predicted death in undeveloped regions. The causes for this finding are unknown, but it has been shown that PD networks linking developed and developing units might be a means of improving the quality of therapy [46]. Whether the establishment of a standardized PD program in undeveloped regions will benefit less-educated patients needs to be investigated. More trials are also needed to explore new strategies for improving the efficacy of training for less-educated patients.

Our large-scale multicenter PD cohort gave us a valuable opportunity to explore the association of SES and outcome at both the individual and the environmental level. Our results will be helpful for PD clinicians and health policy-makers in generating appropriate strategies to improve the use of PD in developing countries such as China. Compared with former studies, this study has the advantage of more detailed information on individual SES. The enrollment of representative centers in a rapidly developing country with huge diversity in regional economic development is also a merit. The interactive effect between individual and regional SES has never been investigated in a dialysis population.

This study has some limitations. First, based on estimates of the size of the dialysis population (no registry data available as yet), only about 10% of PD patients in China were enrolled in the study and thus we cannot confirm the generalizability of our results. However, all incident patients were enrolled from 'core' PD centers of medical school-affiliated hospitals and came from provinces and counties with varied level of SES and penetration rate of PD therapy. Therefore, it is reasonable to conclude that the range of SES of our study population reflects the overall situation to a certain degree. A national dialysis registry has been initiated recently, so more representative data will be obtained in future years. We Hope our study will provide useful cues for the analysis of national data in the future. Second, individual SES is a general index and many SES-related physiological and non-physiological factors were not measured. We cannot verify whether worse nutritional status, deficient pre-dialysis care, less access to standardized training courses, or poor compliance contributed to the worse outcome observed in poorer patients. Regional SES-related information such as local hygiene status, availability of medical services and social support systems was not assessed in detail. Third, we should be aware of the possibility of ascertainment bias (4.1% of eligible patients were not included), vintage bias (different centers created their databases at different times), and residual confounding and recall bias because of the retrospective nature of this study. Furthermore, an observational study cannot demonstrate cause–effect relationships.

In conclusion, our findings strongly support the present health-care strategies implemented by the Chinese government to improve the medical coverage rate for ESRD patients. Our data also suggest that, under the present training program, the risk for peritonitis in less-educated patients is comparable with that in patients with higher diplomas. A series of strategies should be applied to improve the quality of treatment for poorer patients and less-educated patients in undeveloped region. Constructing an integrated care system for chronic kidney disease patients to prevent various complications and developing PD networks to standardize training programs may be potential approaches to improving the quality of therapy.

Acknowledgments

The authors express their appreciation to the patients, doctors, and nursing staff of the peritoneal dialysis center of Peking University First Hospital, Division of Nephrology of Peking University Third Hospital, Division of Nephrology of Huashan Hospital, Fudan University, Division of Nephrology of the second affiliated hospital of Harbin Medical University, Division of Nephrology of Peking University People's Hospital, Division of Nephrology of the first affiliated hospital of Zhejiang University School of Medicine, Division of Nephrology of General Hospital of NingXia Medical University, for their participation in this study. The authors also thank ELIXIGEN (Shanghai) Corp. for native English speaking proofreading of the manuscript.

Author Contributions

Conceived and designed the experiments: HYW JD. Performed the experiments: RX QFH YPR TYZ JHC HPZ MHC YW CMH RZ XHZ MW NT. Analyzed the data: RX. Wrote the paper: RX JD.

References

1. Zhang L, Wang F, Wang L, Wang W, Liu B, et al. (2012) Prevalence of chronic kidney disease in China: a cross-sectional survey. Lancet 379: 815–822.
2. Zuo L, Wang M (2006) Current status of hemodialysis treatment in Beijing, China. Ethn Dis 16: S2–31–34.
3. Klarenbach S, Manns B (2009) Economic evaluation of dialysis therapies. Semin Nephrol 29: 524–532.
4. Weinhandl ED, Foley RN, Gilbertson DT, Arneson TJ, Snyder JJ, et al. (2010) Propensity-matched mortality comparison of incident hemodialysis and peritoneal dialysis patients. J Am Soc Nephrol 21: 499–506.
5. ANZDATA website. The 30th Annual Report (2007). available: http://www.anzdata.org.au/anzdata/AnzdataReport/30thReport/Ch03Deaths.pdf.Accessed 2012 Oct 30.
6. Juergensen E, Wuerth D, Finkelstein SH, Juergensen PH, Bekui A, et al. (2006) Hemodialysis and peritoneal dialysis: patients' assessment of their satisfaction with therapy and the impact of the therapy on their lives. Clin J Am Soc Nephrol 1: 1191–1196.
7. Brown EA, Johansson L, Farrington K, Gallagher H, Sensky T, et al. (2010) Broadening Options for Long-term Dialysis in the Elderly (BOLDE): differences in quality of life on peritoneal dialysis compared to haemodialysis for older patients. Nephrol Dial Transplant 25: 3755–3763.
8. Oliver MJ, Garg AX, Blake PG, Johnson JF, Verrelli M, et al. (2010) Impact of contraindications, barriers to self-care and support on incident peritoneal dialysis utilization. Nephrol Dial Transplant 25: 2737–2744.
9. Jager KJ, Korevaar JC, Dekker FW, Krediet RT, Boeschoten EW (2004) The effect of contraindications and patient preference on dialysis modality selection in ESRD patients in The Netherlands. Am J Kidney Dis 43: 891–899.
10. Oliver MJ, Quinn RR, Richardson EP, Kiss AJ, Lamping DL, et al. (2007) Home care assistance and the utilization of peritoneal dialysis. Kidney Int 71: 673–678.
11. Adams AS, Mah C, Soumerai SB, Zhang F, Barton MB, et al. (2003) Barriers to self-monitoring of blood glucose among adults with diabetes in an HMO: a cross sectional study. BMC Health Serv Res 3: 6.
12. Goldman DP, Smith JP (2002) Can patient self-management help explain the SES health gradient? Proc Natl Acad Sci U S A 99: 10929–10934.
13. Kennedy BP, Kawachi I, Glass R, Prothrow-Stith D (1998) Income distribution, socioeconomic status, and self rated health in the United States: multilevel analysis. BMJ 317: 917–921.
14. Goldfarb-Rumyantzev AS, Rout P, Sandhu GS, Khattak M, Tang H, et al. (2010) Association between social adaptability index and survival of patients with chronic kidney disease. Nephrol Dial Transplant 25: 3672–3681.

15. Merkin SS, Roux AV, Coresh J, Fried LF, Jackson SA, et al. (2007) Individual and neighborhood socioeconomic status and progressive chronic kidney disease in an elderly population: The Cardiovascular Health Study. Soc Sci Med 65: 809–821.
16. Wee LE, Koh GC (2012) Individual and neighborhood social factors of hypertension management in a low-socioeconomic status population: a community-based case-control study in Singapore. Hypertens Res 35: 295–303.
17. Chichlowska KL, Rose KM, Diez-Roux AV, Golden SH, McNeill AM, et al. (2008) Individual and neighborhood socioeconomic status characteristics and prevalence of metabolic syndrome: the Atherosclerosis Risk in Communities (ARIC) Study. Psychosom Med 70: 986–992.
18. Volkova N, McClellan W, Klein M, Flanders D, Kleinbaum D, et al. (2008) Neighborhood poverty and racial differences in ESRD incidence. J Am Soc Nephrol 19: 356–364.
19. Sanabria M, Munoz J, Trillos C, Hernandez G, Latorre C, et al. (2008) Dialysis outcomes in Colombia (DOC) study: a comparison of patient survival on peritoneal dialysis vs hemodialysis in Colombia. Kidney Int Suppl: S165–172.
20. de Andrade Bastos K, Qureshi AR, Lopes AA, Fernandes N, Barbosa LM, et al. (2011) Family income and survival in Brazilian Peritoneal Dialysis Multicenter Study Patients (BRAZPD): time to revisit a myth? Clin J Am Soc Nephrol 6: 1676–1683.
21. Martin LC, Caramori JC, Fernandes N, Divino-Filho JC, Pecoits-Filho R, et al. (2011) Geographic and educational factors and risk of the first peritonitis episode in Brazilian Peritoneal Dialysis study (BRAZPD) patients. Clin J Am Soc Nephrol 6: 1944–1951.
22. Chidambaram M, Bargman JM, Quinn RR, Austin PC, Hux JE, et al. (2011) Patient and physician predictors of peritoneal dialysis technique failure: a population based, retrospective cohort study. Perit Dial Int 31: 565–573.
23. Farias MG, Soucie JM, McClellan W, Mitch WE (1994) Race and the risk of peritonitis: an analysis of factors associated with the initial episode. Kidney Int 46: 1392–1396.
24. Tonelli M, Hemmelgarn B, Culleton B, Klarenbach S, Gill JS, et al. (2007) Mortality of Canadians treated by peritoneal dialysis in remote locations. Kidney Int 72: 1023–1028.
25. Caskey FJ, Roderick P, Steenkamp R, Nitsch D, Thomas K, et al. (2006) Social deprivation and survival on renal replacement therapy in England and Wales. Kidney Int 70: 2134–2140.
26. Lim WH, Boudville N, McDonald SP, Gorham G, Johnson DW, et al. (2011) Remote indigenous peritoneal dialysis patients have higher risk of peritonitis, technique failure, all-cause and peritonitis-related mortality. Nephrol Dial Transplant 26: 3366–3372.

27. Mehrotra R, Story K, Guest S, Fedunyszyn M (2011) Neighborhood Location, Rurality, Geography, and Outcomes of Peritoneal Dialysis Patients in the United States. Perit Dial Int.

28. Smith SC, Jr., Jackson R, Pearson TA, Fuster V, Yusuf S, et al. (2004) Principles for national and regional guidelines on cardiovascular disease prevention: a scientific statement from the World Heart and Stroke Forum. Circulation 109: 3112–3121.

29. Li PK, Szeto CC, Piraino B, Bernardini J, Figueiredo AE, et al. (2010) Peritoneal dialysis-related infections recommendations: 2010 update. Perit Dial Int 30: 393–423.

30. Afolalu B, Troidle L, Osayimwen O, Bhargava J, Kitsen J, et al. (2009) Technique failure and center size in a large cohort of peritoneal dialysis patients in a defined geographic area. Perit Dial Int 29: 292–296.

31. Mujais S, Story K (2006) Peritoneal dialysis in the US: evaluation of outcomes in contemporary cohorts. Kidney Int Suppl: S21–26.

32. Schaubel DE, Blake PG, Fenton SS (2001) Effect of renal center characteristics on mortality and technique failure on peritoneal dialysis. Kidney Int 60: 1517–1524.

33. Rubin J, Kirchner K, Ray R, Bower JD (1985) Demographic factors associated with dialysis technique failures among patients undergoing continuous ambulatory peritoneal dialysis. Arch Intern Med 145: 1041–1044.

34. Rubin J, Ray R, Barnes T, Teal N, Hellems E, et al. (1983) Peritonitis in continuous ambulatory peritoneal dialysis patients. Am J Kidney Dis 2: 602–609.

35. Raaijmakers R, Gajjar P, Schroder C, Nourse P (2010) Peritonitis in children on peritoneal dialysis in Cape Town, South Africa: epidemiology and risks. Pediatr Nephrol 25: 2149–2157.

36. D Batlle PR, M J Soler (2006) Progress in retarding the progression of advanced chronic kidney disease: Grounds for optimism. Kidney International: S40–S44.

37. Pereira BJ (2000) Optimization of pre-ESRD care: the key to improved dialysis outcomes. Kidney Int 57: 351–365.

38. Carruthers DM, Whishaw JM, Thomas M, Thatcher G (1996) Planes, kangaroos, and the CAPD manual. Perit Dial Int 16 Suppl 1: S452–454.

39. Carruthers D, Warr K (2004) Supporting peritoneal dialysis in remote Australia. Nephrology (Carlton) 9 Suppl 4: S129–133.

40. Avram MM, Goldwasser P, Erroa M, Fein PA (1994) Predictors of survival in continuous ambulatory peritoneal dialysis patients: the importance of pre-albumin and other nutritional and metabolic markers. Am J Kidney Dis 23: 91–98.

41. Blake PG, Flowerdew G, Blake RM, Oreopoulos DG (1993) Serum albumin in patients on continuous ambulatory peritoneal dialysis–predictors and correlations with outcomes. J Am Soc Nephrol 3: 1501–1507.

42. Leinig CE, Moraes T, Ribeiro S, Riella MC, Olandoski M, et al. (2011) Predictive value of malnutrition markers for mortality in peritoneal dialysis patients. J Ren Nutr 21: 176–183.

43. Xu R, Zhuo M, Yang Z, Dong J (2012) Experiences with assisted peritoneal dialysis in China. Perit Dial Int 32: 94–101.

44. Blake PG, Korbet SM, Blake R, Bargman JM, Burkart JM, et al. (2000) A multicenter study of noncompliance with continuous ambulatory peritoneal dialysis exchanges in US and Canadian patients. Am J Kidney Dis 35: 506–514.

45. Taira DA, Gelber RP, Davis J, Gronley K, Chung RS, et al. (2007) Antihypertensive adherence and drug class among Asian Pacific Americans. Ethn Health 12: 265–281.

46. Yang X, Mao HP, Guo QY, Yu XQ (2011) Successfully managing a rapidly growing peritoneal dialysis program in Southern China. Chin Med J (Engl) 124: 2696–2700.

9

Higher Peritoneal Protein Clearance as a Risk Factor for Cardiovascular Disease in Peritoneal Dialysis Patient

Tae Ik Chang, Ea Wha Kang, Yong Kyu Lee, Sug Kyun Shin*

Department of Internal Medicine, NHIC Medical Center, Ilsan Hospital, Goyangshi, Gyeonggi–do, Republic of Korea

Abstract

Background and Aims: Although a number of studies have been published on peritoneal protein clearance (PrCl) and its association with patient outcomes, the results have been inconsistent. Therefore, the intent of this study was to evaluate the impact of PrCl on cardiovascular disease (CVD) and mortality in peritoneal dialysis (PD) patients.

Methods: This prospective observational study included a total of 540 incident patients who started PD at NHIC Ilsan Hospital, Korea from January 2000 to December 2009. Two different types of analyses such as intention-to-treat and as-treated were used.

Results: Correlation analyses revealed that PrCl was positively correlated with diabetes, pulse pressure, C–reactive protein (CRP) level, dialysate/plasma creatinine ratio (D/P cr) at 4 h, and peritoneal Kt/V urea. PrCl was inversely correlated with serum albumin and triglyceride levels. On multivariate analysis, serum albumin, pulse pressure, D/P cr at 4 h, and peritoneal Kt/V urea were found to be independent determinants of PrCl. A total of 129 (23.9%) patients in intention-to-treat analysis and 117 (21.7%) patients in as-treated analysis developed new cardiovascular events. Time to occurrence of cardiovascular event was significantly longer in patients with a value of PrCl below the median (89.4 ml/day). In multivariate analysis, older age, presence of diabetes or previous CVD, and higher PrCl were independent predictors of cardiovascular events. Patients above the median value of PrCl had a significantly lower rate of survival than those below the median. However, a higher PrCl was not associated with increased mortality in multivariate Cox analysis.

Conclusions: A higher PrCl is a risk for occurrence of cardiovascular event, but not mortality in PD patients. Large randomized clinical trials are warranted to confirm this finding.

Editor: Utpal Sen, University of Louisville, United States of America

Funding: The authors have no support or funding to report.

Competing Interests: The authors have declared that no competing interests exist.

* E-mail: sskyun@hotmail.com

Introduction

Peritoneal dialysis (PD) is an established treatment modality in end-stage renal disease (ESRD) patients and approximately 150000 patients are being maintained on PD worldwide [1]. In Korea, PD was introduced in the early 1980s and has been performed in many centers so far. Currently, more than 7500 Korean patients are maintained on PD. Recently, there have been significant improvements in patient outcomes due to advances such as the optimization of the adequacy of dialysis, management of blood pressure and anemia, and the maintenance of biochemical parameters within the target range. However, their morbidities and mortality have been much higher than those of the general population. Specifically, cardiovascular disease (CVD) is the most important cause of hospitalization and death in this population. Therefore, the management of CVD is one of the primary goals in treating patients with ESRD on PD [2]. Although the pathogenesis of CVD in PD patients is complicated and not completely understood, non-traditional as well as traditional risk factors such as diabetes, hypertension, smoking, and dyslipidemia are all associated with the high prevalence of CVD in PD patients [3]. Chronic inflammation and malnutrition are risk factors

specifically related to ESRD patients on chronic PD which play a pivotal role in the development of CVD in these patients [4].

Although waste products are cleared during dialysis treatment, nutrients are also lost into the dialysate. Patients on PD may lose approximately 9–12 g of total protein and 6–8 g of albumin daily through the peritoneal membrane [5,6]. Variability in peritoneal protein loss both within and between patients is high, which can be explained by the dependency of protein transport on both the effective peritoneal surface area (the number of mainly small pores) and the intrinsic size-selective permeability (the diameter of the large pores) [7]. Protein loss during dialysis is usually compensated for by an increase in albumin synthesis in PD patients [8]. However, this process can be suppressed in cases of coexisting inflammation and malnutrition. In addition, the type of peritoneal membrane transport might influence the amount of protein loss. Protein loss is much greater in patients with a fast peritoneal solute transport rate than in those with a low solute transport rate [9]. Fast peritoneal solute transport rates have also been associated with hypoalbuminemia [10], inflammation [11], mortality, and technique failure [12–14] in some studies, but this is not always the case [15–17].

During the last decade, a number of studies have been published on peritoneal protein clearance (PrCl) and its association with outcomes in PD patients [18–25]. In some studies, PrCl has been shown to be associated with a higher prevalence of CVD and increased mortality in PD patients [18–22]. However, other studies have found no association between PrCl and an increased in cardiovascular events or mortality [23–25]. Therefore, the intent of this study was to investigate the impact of PrCl on mortality and the occurrence of cardiovascular events and to identify the determinants of PrCl in a large prospective cohort of incident patients who were on PD for at least six months.

Methods

Ethics statement

The study was carried out in accordance with the Declaration of Helsinki and approved by the Institutional Review Board of Ilsan Hospital Clinical Trial Center. We obtained informed written consent from all participants involved in our study.

Patients and data collection

We considered all of 620 patients who started PD at NHIC Ilsan hospital, one of the largest PD centers in Korea, from January 2000 to December 2009. We then excluded patients that were younger than 18 years of age at initiation of PD, patients that had less than 6 months of follow-up, and patients that had been on hemodialysis or received a kidney transplant before PD. Patients that recovered kidney function or started PD for other reasons, such as acute renal failure or congestive heart failure, were also excluded from the analysis. Therefore, this prospective observational study included a total of 540 incident patients finally. All of the patients underwent a peritoneal equilibration test, measurement of dialysis adequacy, and a 24-h dialysate PrCl analysis within three months of PD initiation. Demographic and clinical data were collected at the beginning of PD. The data recorded included age, gender, body mass index (BMI) calculated as weight/(height)^2, duration of PD, cause of ESRD, prevalence of diabetes and CVD, blood pressure, and patient outcomes. Laboratory data obtained at the time of dialysis adequacy measurement were considered baseline values and included blood urea nitrogen, serum creatinine, total cholesterol, serum triglyceride, serum albumin concentrations, serum C-reactive protein (CRP) levels, Kt/V urea, percentage of lean body mass (%LBM), normalized protein catabolic rate (nPCR), residual glomerular filtration rate (GFR), and 24-h residual urine volume. Residual GFR was calculated as the average urea and creatinine clearance from a 24-h urine collection [26].

Peritoneal dialysate protein losses were measured from the collection of 24-h peritoneal dialysate effluent by the pyrogallol red method. Serum and dialysate concentrations of urea, creatinine, glucose, and albumin were all measured by a colorimetric method (UniCel DXC 800; Beckman Coulter, Inc., California, USA). To calculate PrCl, the total 24-h dialysate protein loss was divided by a validated correction factor (serum albumin/0.4783) which has been used in other previous studies [22,23]. PrCl was expressed as ml of plasma cleared per day.

Statistical analysis

All values are expressed as mean ± standard deviation or percentages. Statistical analyses were performed using SPSS for Windows version 13.0 (SPSS, Inc., Chicago, IL, USA). Data were analyzed using Student's t-test and the chi-square test. The relationship between PrCl and continuous variables was examined by Pearson's correlation coefficient, and categorical variables were examined using Spearman's R test. Multiple linear regression analysis was performed to identify the determinants of PrCl using two different models with or without serum albumin because of the fact that serum albumin levels inevitably interfered in the estimation of PrCl. Primary outcomes were death and newly developed cardiovascular events, which were defined as coronary artery disease (angioplasty, coronary artery bypass graft, myocardial infarction, or angina), cerebrovascular disease (transient ischemic attack, stroke, or carotid endarterectomy), and peripheral artery disease (revascularization or amputation). We used both intention-to-treat and as-treated analyses. In the former, we followed patients from the date of dialysis initiation to the earlier of death or December 31, 2011. In the latter, we followed patients from the date of dialysis initiation to the earlier of death, change to hemodialysis (88 patients), renal transplantation (36 patients), loss to follow-up (29 patients), or December 31, 2011. To determine risk factors for cardiovascular events and mortality, multivariate Cox regression was performed, and all significant covariates from the univariate analysis were included. Survival was also examined by comparing patients above and below the median value of PrCl using the Kaplan-Meier method and the log-rank test. A p-value of less than 0.05 was considered statistically significant.

Results

Demographic and clinical data

Table 1 details baseline characteristics of the 540 incident PD patients. The mean age of the patients was 59 years (range 20 to 88 years), 53.7.1% were males, and patients were on PD for a mean of 50 months (range 6 to 142 months). The prevalence of diabetes and CVD was 53.3% and 28%, respectively. Total 24-h peritoneal protein loss was 6.7±4.4 g/day and the mean PrCl was 107.3±82.8 ml/day (median 89.4 ml/day, range 22.7 to 617.7 ml/day).

Gender, prevalence of CVD, and residual renal function (RRF) were not different between the groups when patients were divided into two groups (low and high) based on the median levels of baseline PrCl. Age (60.4±13.5 versus 57.8±14.4 years, P=0.026), prevalence of diabetes (58.8 versus 47.8%, P=0.01), serum log$_{10}$CRP level (−0.79±0.79 versus −0.95±0.71 mg/dL, P=0.022), D/P cr at 4 h (0.72±0.18 versus 0.64±0.16, P<0.001), and peritoneal Kt/V (1.5±0.6 versus 1.4±0.5, P=0.044) were significantly higher, while serum triglyceride (137.3±85.5 versus 163.9±95.2 mg/dL, P=0.001) and albumin levels (2.9±0.5 versus 3.4±0.5 g/dL, P<0.001), and nPCR (0.95±0.24 versus 1.01±0.27 g/Kg/day, P=0.004) were significantly lower in the high PrCl group compared to the low PrCl group.

Factors associated with peritoneal protein clearance

Correlation analyses were performed to identify factors associated with PrCl. PrCl was positively correlated with the presence of diabetes ($\gamma = 0.1$, $P=0.005$), pulse pressure ($\gamma = 0.11$, $P=0.016$), log$_{10}$CRP level ($\gamma = 0.096$, $P=0.033$), D/Pcr at 4 h ($\gamma = 0.13$, $P=0.004$), and peritoneal Kt/V urea ($\gamma = 0.22$, $P<0.001$), whereas it was inversely correlated with serum albumin concentration ($\gamma = -0.37$, $P<0.001$), and triglyceride level ($\gamma = -0.09$, $P=0.038$). In contrast, there was no correlation between age, gender, BMI, presence of preexisting CVD, RRF, nPCR or %LBM and PrCl. On multivariate linear regression analysis, serum albumin, D/Pcr, peritoneal Kt/V urea, and pulse pressure were independently associated with PrCl (Table 2; Model 1). In model 2, in which albumin was excluded, D/Pcr, peritoneal Kt/V urea, and pulse pressure remained in the model with the additional

Table 1. Baseline characteristics of the study subjects (n = 540).

Age (years)	59.1	±	14.0
Gender (Male)	290		(53.7)
Body mass index (kg/m^2)	22.8	±	6.2
Pulse pressure (mmHg)	56.6	±	17.5
Follow-up duration (months)	50.2	±	33.9
Underlying renal disease			
Diabetes mellitus	258		(47.8)
Hypertension	155		(28.7)
Chronic glomerulonephritis	76		(14.1)
Polycystic kidney disease	9		(1.7)
Others	15		(2.8)
Unknown	27		(5.0)
Presence of diabetes mellitus	288		(53.3)
Presence of prior cardiovascular disease	151		(28.0)
Laboratory findings			
Serum albumin (g/dL)	3.2	±	1.6
Total cholesterol (mg/dL)	183.6	±	48.6
Triglyceride (mg/dL)	150.6	±	91.4
CRP (mg/dL)	0.7	±	2.6
Peritoneal transport (D/P cr at 4 h)	0.68		0.18
Dialysis adequacy			
Peritoneal Kt/V urea	1.5	±	0.6
24-h dialysate protein loss (g)	6.7	±	4.4
24-h PrCl (mL)	107.3	±	82.8
24-h residual urine volume (mL)	1083.9	±	719.1
Residual GFR (mL/min/1.73 m^2)	6.1	±	5.2
nPCR (g/Kg/day)	1.0	±	0.3
Lean body mass (% body weight)	66.0	±	28.5

Data are expressed as mean ± standard deviation or number of patients (percent).
CRP, C-reactive protein; D/P cr, dialysate/plasma creatinine ratio; PrCl, peritoneal protein clearance; GFR, residual glomerular filtration rate; nPCR, normalized protein catabolic rate.

Table 2. Multivariate associations between peritoneal protein clearance and patient characteristics[a].

	Model 1		Model 2	
	β	P-value	β	P-value
Serum albumin (g/dL)	−0.310	<0.001	-	-
D/P cr at 4 h	0.134	0.002	0.194	<0.001
Peritoneal Kt/V urea	0.311	<0.001	0.314	<0.001
Pulse pressure (mmHg)	0.085	0.046	0.094	0.037
Presence of diabetes	0.084	0.062	0.169	<0.001
Log$_{10}$CRP (mg/dL)	0.070	0.106	0.111	0.014
Triglyceride (mg/dL)	0.001	0.998	−0.048	0.278

[a]Model 1 includes albumin; model 2 excludes serum albumin.
CRP, C-reactive protein; D/P cr, dialysate/plasma creatinine ratio.

measured total peritoneal protein loss, not only the calculated clearance. Even when we considered absolute peritoneal protein amount with or without correction to body surface area, an association with increased cardiovascular events persisted (details not shown).

Predictors of mortality

In intention-to-treat analysis, 203 (37.6%) deaths were recorded, and the median survival period was 42 months (range 6 to 142.2 months). CVD (37.9%) was the most common cause of death in this study, followed by infection (32.0%), unknown cause (22.7%), and others (7.4%). Additionally, in as-treated analysis, 187 (21.7%) deaths were recorded. In both intension-to-treat and as-treated analyses, patients above the median value of PrCl had a significantly lower rate of survival than those below the median (Figure 2). In the univariate Cox proportional hazards model, age, presence of diabetes or CVD, serum albumin concentration, Log$_{10}$CRP level, peritoneal Kt/V urea, nPCR, %LBM, RRF, and PrCl were significantly associated with mortality. However, gender, BMI, pulse pressure, serum triglyceride level, and small solute transport status (D/Pcr at 4 h) were not associated with mortality. In multivariate analysis, older age, presence of diabetes or prior CVD, and hypoalbuminemia were independent predictors of mortality, whereas RRF was also identified as a significant risk factor for mortality in as-treated analysis (Table 4).

Discussion

This study, which included a total of 540 incident PD patients, is the largest one published to date on peritoneal transport of total protein and its association with patient outcomes in terms of cardiovascular events and mortality. The results demonstrated that a higher PrCl is a risk factor for occurrence of cardiovascular event, but not mortality in patients treated with PD.

Peritoneal protein clearance in PD patients reflects protein leakage across the large pores, which is equivalent to large-pore flow (JvL). Although a number of studies have been published on PrCl and its association with patient outcomes, the results have been inconsistent, and no consensus has been reached on the relationship and significance of PrCl in the development of

inclusion of diabetes and increased serum CRP levels (Table 2; Model 2).

Predictors of cardiovascular events

In intention-to-treat analysis, 129 (23.9%) patients developed new cardiovascular events, which included coronary artery disease (73 patients, 56.6%), cerebrovascular disease (44 patients, 34.1%), and peripheral artery disease (12 patients, 9.3%). Additionally, in as-treated analysis, 117 (21.7%) patients developed new cardiovascular events. In both intention-to-treat and as-treated analyses, time to occurrence of cardiovascular event was significantly longer in patients with a value of PrCl below the median (Figure 1). In the univariate Cox proportional hazards model, age, presence of diabetes or preexisting CVD, serum albumin concentration, %LBM, and PrCl were significantly associated with cardiovascular events, whereas CRP level, peritoneal Kt/V urea, nPCR, and RRF were not associated with cardiovascular events. In multivariate analysis, older age, presence of diabetes or previous CVD, and higher PrCl were independent predictors of cardiovascular events (Table 3). Furthermore, we performed additional analysis using

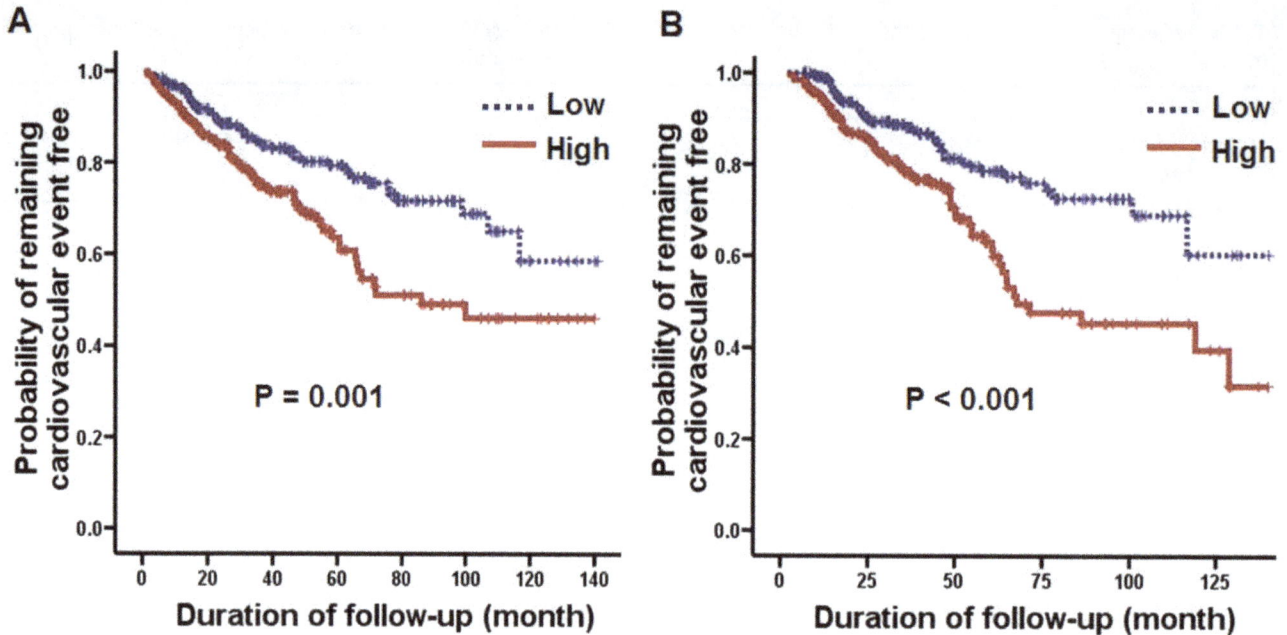

Figure 1. Kaplan-Meier plots of the probability of remaining cardiovascular event-free based on the median level (89.4 ml/day) of baseline peritoneal protein. (A) Intention-to-treat analysis. (B) As-treated analysis.

subsequent cardiovascular events and death in PD patients [18–25]. Szeto *et al.* [18] showed that patients starting PD with active CVD had higher protein and albumin levels in the peritoneal effluent, and cardiovascular events were more frequent in patients with greater peritoneal albumin losses. The authors postulated that peritoneal protein losses or PrCl could be an independent cardiovascular risk factor, and is likely associated with high mortality in PD patients. In addition, Heaf *et al.* [20] found that JvL is related to hypoalbuminemia and mortality after PD initiation, and Van Biesen *et al.* [21] found that a higher JvL, when corrected for membrane area parameter (A0/Δx), is a marker of inflammation and is related to decreased patient survival. Another recent study by Peal *et al.* [22] revealed that increased PrCl at the start of PD is a predictor of death independent of baseline small solute transport status, serum albumin, age, and comorbidity. All of the above studies support the hypothesis that protein leakage across the membrane may be a manifestation of local or systemic inflammation as likely as

microalbuminuria, which is another manifestation of capillary protein leakage, and is recognized as an endothelial dysfunction marker [27]. In contrast to the aforementioned studies, no association between PrCl and an increase in cardiovascular events or mortality was found in other studies [23–25]. Sanchez-Villanueva *et al.* [23] showed that PrCl is significantly and independently related to the presence of peripheral artery disease, but failed to demonstrate the association of PrCl with mortality or subsequent cardiovascular events. In addition, a recent study by Balafa *et al.* [25], which was the largest published to date, reported that PrCl was not an independent predictor of mortality. The authors postulated that the association of increased albumin leakage with inflammation is only consequence of the availability of an increased number of large pores and is not related to endothelial dysfunction or CVD. This discrepancy between findings is likely due to differences in study design, the number of enrolled patients, patient characteristics, timing and methods of

Table 3. Multivariate Cox regression analysis for cardiovascular events.

	Intention to Treat			As Treated		
	HR	(95% CI)	*P*-value	HR	(95% CI)	*P*-value
Age (years)	1.02	(1.00–1.03)	0.022	1.02	(1.01–1.04)	0.012
Presence of diabetes	1.96	(1.33–2.86)	0.001	1.95	(1.29–2.94)	0.002
Presence of prior CVD	1.67	(1.14–2.44)	0.008	1.72	(1.15–2.57)	0.009
Serum albumin (g/dL)	0.85	(0.59–1.22)	0.374	0.74	(0.51–1.08)	0.743
Lean body mass (% body weight)	0.99	(0.98–1.01)	0.388	0.99	(0.98–1.01)	0.367
PrCl (per 10 ml/day increase)	1.02	(1.00–1.03)	0.041	1.02	(1.00–1.04)	0.025

HR, hazard ratio; CI, confidence interval; CVD, cardiovascular disease; nPCR, normalized protein catabolic rate; PrCl, peritoneal protein clearance.

A

B

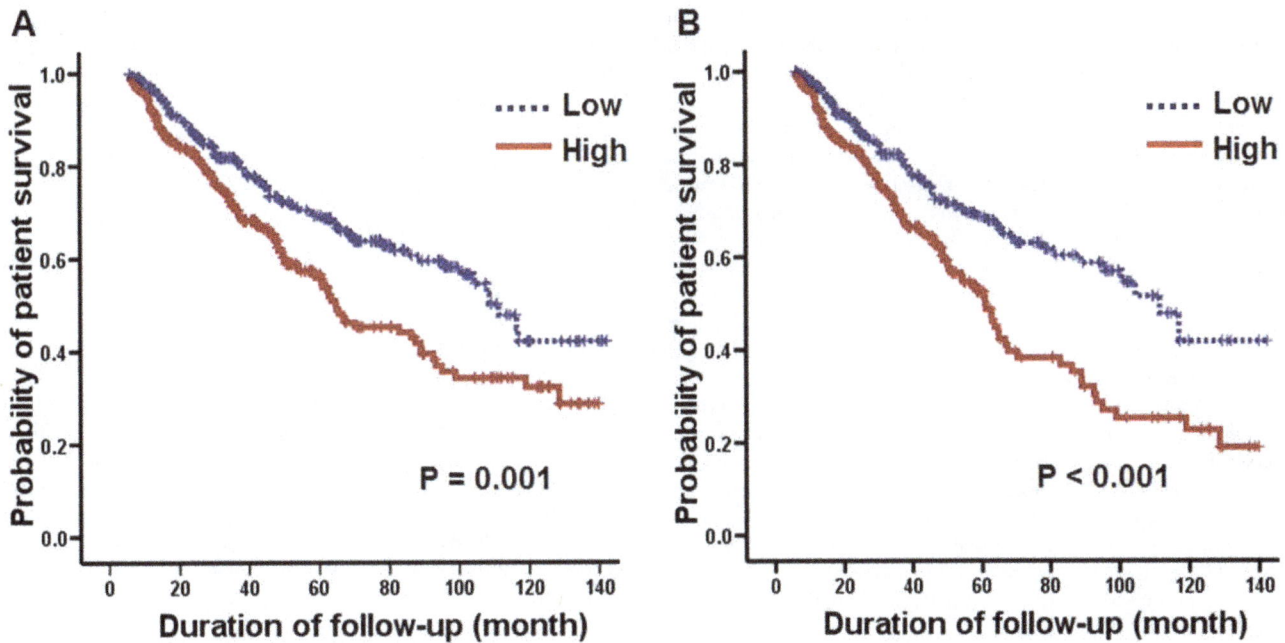

Figure 2. Kaplan-Meier plots for patient survival based on the median level (89.4 ml/day) of baseline peritoneal protein clearance. (A) Intention-to-treat analysis. (B) As-treated analysis.

measuring PrCl, and variables included in the multivariate analysis.

This study of long term (up to 142 month) clinical outcomes of a large cohort of patients treated with PD provides strong evidence of that a higher PrCl is a risk factor for occurrence of cardiovascular event in these patients. These findings were observed consistently in both intention-to-treat and as-treated analyses. Even when we considered absolute protein losses corrected to body surface area, an association with reduced survival of remaining cardiovascular event-free persisted. On the other hand, our study on mortality does not significantly demonstrate differences according to initial PrCl. We, however, reconfirmed that older age, presence of diabetes or previous CVD, hypoalbuminemia, and lower RRF, all of which are well-known risk factors, are independent predictors of mortality in PD patients. The underlying mechanisms for these poor outcomes in patients with higher PrCl are unclear. One possible explanation could be the link between CVD and endothelial dysfunction as evidenced by microalbuminuria [27]. Here, we found that higher peritoneal protein losses or PrCl were significantly associated with lower serum albumin concentrations, which might reflect a high inflammatory and poor nutritional status [28,29] and a higher pulse pressure, which might reflect arterial stiffness and systemic vascular damage [30]. In addition, higher serum CRP values, which were available in 494 patients in this study, was also associated with higher PrCl, which although did not reach statistical significance on multivariate analysis. In line with our results, a recent cross-sectional study of prevalent PD patients from

Table 4. Multivariate Cox regression analysis for mortality.

	Intention to Treat			As Treated		
	HR	(95% CI)	P-value	HR	(95% CI)	P-value
Age (years)	1.06	(1.04–1.08)	<0.001	1.07	(1.05–1.08)	<0.001
Presence of diabetes	1.56	(1.11–2.19)	0.010	1.58	(1.10–2.25)	0.012
Presence of prior CVD	1.61	(1.17–2.22)	0.004	1.70	(1.21–2.37)	0.002
Serum albumin (g/dL)	0.50	(0.37–0.68)	<0.001	0.48	(0.35–0.66)	<0.001
$Log_{10}CRP$ (mg/dL)	1.20	(0.97–1.48)	0.102	1.19	(0.96–1.47)	0.112
Peritoneal Kt/V urea	1.29	(0.95–1.77)	0.108	1.12	(0.81–1.57)	0.491
nPCR (g/Kg/day)	0.80	(0.38–1.67)	0.550	0.91	(0.43–1.95)	0.813
Lean body mass (% body weight)	0.99	(0.98–1.01)	0.317	1.00	(0.98–1.01)	0.632
Residual GFR (mL/min/1.73 m^2)	0.96	(0.92–1.01)	0.106	0.93	(0.88–0.98)	0.005
PrCl (per 10 ml/day increase)	1.00	(1.00–1.00)	0.425	1.01	(0.99–1.03)	0.260

HR, hazard ratio; CI, confidence interval; CVD, cardiovascular disease; CRP, C-reactive protein; nPCR, normalized protein catabolic rate; GFR, residual glomerular filtration rate; PrCl, peritoneal protein clearance.

Korea [31] showed that PrCl exhibited a positive correlation with both heart-to-femoral pulse wave velocity implicating arterial stiffness and peripheral vascular calcium scores, which is representative of vascular calcification. Along with systemic inflammation, local inflammation may also contribute to CVD for those on PD. With high dialysate leukocyte count and IL-6 concentration, the peritoneal protein or albumin leakage has been considered to be one of these intra-peritoneal inflammation-related factors in PD patients [18,32]. Taken together, we surmised that PrCl could represent systemic or local vascular damage and endothelial dysfunction in PD patients. Another possible factor to note is that patients with a higher PrCl might have poor nutritional status. In our results, BMI, nPCR, and serum triglyceride concentration were significantly lower in patients above the median PrCl value irrespective of the presence of hypoalbuminemia. Other nutritional markers such as total cholesterol and %LBM were also lower in patients with a higher PrCl, although the differences were not statistically significant. Based on these findings, it might be possible to postulate that these poor outcomes of patients with higher PrCl are mediated, at least partially, by the poor preserved nutritional status seen with protein–energy wasting, which has been shown to be an important predictor of morbidity and mortality in PD patients [33–35]. However, other mechanisms that remain to be explored may also play a role.

The strengths of this study are the large number of patients, the long duration of follow-up, and the adjustment for multiple potentially confounding covariates such as serum CRP. Potential limitations are the single-center design of the study and the fact that data from a full panel of peritoneal inflammation markers were not available. The lack of urinary protein excretion measurements limited the testing of possible relationships between urinary and peritoneal protein losses as a result of the common pathway of endothelial dysfunction.

Conclusions

This study showed that baseline PrCl is a risk factor for occurrence of cardiovascular event, but not mortality in patients on PD. These results suggest that protein leakage across the membrane may be a manifestation of a systemic or local inflammation and poor nutritional status, serving as a surrogate marker for the increased morbidity seen with malnutrition, inflammation, and atherosclerosis syndrome. A large, prospective study is required to further elucidate the association between PrCl and inflammatory or nutritional status in PD patients. Further investigations focusing on the description of changes in PrCl with time on treatment and the associated prognostic significance are also warranted.

Author Contributions

Conceived and designed the experiments: TIC SKS. Performed the experiments: TIC EWK. Analyzed the data: TIC YKL. Contributed reagents/materials/analysis tools: TIC SKS. Wrote the paper: TIC.

References

1. Grassmann A, Gioberge S, Moeller S, Brown G (2005) ESRD patients in 2004: global overview of patient numbers, treatment modalities and associated trends Nephrol Dial Transplant 20: 2587–2593.
2. Krediet RT, Balafa O (2010) Cardiovascular risk in the peritoneal dialysis patient. Nat Rev Nephrol.6:451–460.
3. Zoccali C (2006) Traditional and emerging cardiovascular and renal risk factors: an epidemiologic perspective. Kidney Int 70:26–33.
4. Pecoits-Filho R, Lindholm B, Stenvinkel P (2002) The malnutrition, inflammation, and atherosclerosis (MIA) syndrome – the heart of the matter. Nephrol Dial Transplant 17[Suppl 11]: S28–S31.
5. Dukkipati R, Kopple JD (2009) Causes and prevention of protein-energy wasting in chronic kidney failure. Semin Nephrol 29: 39–49.
6. Blumenkrantz MJ, Gahl GM, Kopple JD, Kamdar AV, Jones MR, et al. (1981) Protein losses during peritoneal dialysis. Kidney Int 19:593–602.
7. Rippe B (1993) A three-pore model of peritoneal transport. Perit Dial Int 13[Suppl 2]: S35–S38.
8. Kaysen GA (1998) Meta-analysis: Biological basis of hypoalbuminaemia in ESRD. J Am Soc Nephrol 9: 2368–2376.
9. Kathuria P, Moore HL, Khanna R, Twardowski ZJ, Goel S, et al. (1997) Effect of dialysis modality and membrane transport characteristics on dialysate protein losses of patients on peritoneal dialysis. Perit Dial Int 17: 449–454.
10. Margetts PJ, McMullin J, Rabbat CG, Churchill DN (2000) Peritoneal membrane transport and hypoalbuminemia: Cause or effect? Perit Dial Int 20: 14–18.
11. Wang T, Heimburger O, Cheng HH, Bergstrom J, Lindholm B (1999) Does a high peritoneal transport rate reflect a state of chronic inflammation? Perit Dial Int 19: 17–22.
12. Churchill DN, Thorpe KE, Nolph KD, Keshaviah PR, Oreopoulos DG, et al. (1998) Increased peritoneal membrane transport is associated with decreased patient and technique survival for continuous peritoneal dialysis patients. The Canada-USA (CANUSA) Peritoneal Dialysis Study Group. J Am Soc Nephrol 9: 1285–1292.
13. Rumpsfeld M, McDonald SP, Johnson DW (2006) Higher peritoneal transport status is associated with higher mortality and technique failure in the Australian and New Zealand peritoneal dialysis patient populations. J Am Soc Nephrol 17: 271–278.
14. Brimble KS, Walker M, Margetts PJ, Kundhal KK, Rabbat CG (2006) Meta-analysis: Peritoneal membrane transport, mortality, and technique failure in peritoneal dialysis. J Am Soc Nephrol 17: 2591–2598.
15. Wiggins KJ, McDonald SP, Brown FG, Rosman JB, Johnson DW (2007) High membrane transport status on peritoneal dialysis is not associated with reduced survival following transfer to haemodialysis. Nephrol Dial Transplant 22: 3005–3012.
16. Johnson DW, Hawley CM, McDonald SP, Brown FG, Rosman JB, et al. (2010) Superior survival of high transporters treated with automated versus continuous ambulatory peritoneal dialysis. Nephrol Dial Transplant 25: 1973–1979.
17. Rodrigues AS, Almeida M, Fonseca I, Martins M, Carvalho MJ, et al. (2006) Peritoneal fast transport in incident peritoneal dialysis patients is not consistently associated with systemic inflammation. Nephrol Dial Transplant 21: 763–769.
18. Szeto CC, Chow KM, Lam CW, Cheung R, Kwan BC, et al. (2005) Peritoneal albumin excretion is a strong predictor of cardiovascular events in peritoneal dialysis patients: A prospective cohort study. Perit Dial Int 25: 445–452.
19. Nakamoto H, Imai H, Kawanishi H, Nakamoto M, Minakuchi J, et al. (2002) Effect of diabetes on peritoneal function assessed by personal dialysis capacity test in patients undergoing CAPD. Am J Kidney Dis 40: 1045–1054.
20. Heaf JG, Sarac S, Afzal S (2005) A high peritoneal large pore fluid flux causes hypoalbuminaemia and is a risk factor for death in peritoneal dialysis patients. Nephrol Dial Transplant 20: 2194–2201.
21. Van Biesen W, Van der Tol A, Veys N, Dequidt C, Vijt D, et al. (2006) The personal dialysis capacity test is superior to the peritoneal equilibration test to discriminate inflammation as the cause of fast transport status in peritoneal dialysis patients. Clin J Am Soc Nephrol 1:269–274.
22. Perl J, Huckvale K, Chellar M, John B, Davies SJ (2009) Peritoneal protein clearance and not peritoneal membrane transport status predicts survival in a contemporary cohort of peritoneal dialysis patients. Clin J Am Soc Nephrol 4: 1201–1206.
23. Elsurer R, Afsar B, Sezer S, Ozdemir FN, Haberal M (2009) Peritoneal albumin leakage: 2 year prospective cardiovascular event occurrence and patient survival analysis. Nephrology (Carlton) 14: 712–715.
24. Sanchez-Villanueva R, Bajo A, Del Peso G, Fernandez-Reyes MJ, Gonzalez E, et al. (2009) Higher daily peritoneal protein clearance when initiating peritoneal dialysis is independently associated with peripheral arterial disease (PAD): A possible new marker of systemic endothelial dysfunction? Nephrol Dial Transplant 24: 1009–1014.
25. Balafa O, Halbesma N, Struijk DG, Dekker FW, Krediet RT (2011) Peritoneal albumin and protein losses do not predict outcome in peritoneal dialysis patients. Clin J Am Soc Nephrol 6: 561–566.
26. Nolph KD, Moore HL, Prowant B, Meyer M, Twardowski ZJ, et al. (1993) Cross sectional assessment of weekly urea and creatinine clearances and indices of nutrition in continuous ambulatory peritoneal dialysis patients. Perit Dial Int 13: 178–183.
27. Weir MR (2007) Microalbuminuria and cardiovascular disease. Clin J Am Soc Nephrol 2: 581–590.
28. De Mutsert R, Grootendorst DC, Indemans F, Boeschoten EW, Krediet R, et al. (2009) Association between serum albumin and mortality in dialysis patients is partly explained by inflammation, and not by malnutrition. J Ren Nutr 19: 127–135.

29. Friedman AN, Fadem SZ (2010) Reassessment of albumin as a nutritional marker in kidney disease. J Am Soc Nephrol 21: 223–230.
30. Malone AF, Reddan DN (2010) Pulse pressure. Why is it important? Perit Dial Int 30: 265–268.
31. Lee H, Hwang YH, Jung JY, Na KY, Kim HS, et al. (2009) Comparison of vascular calcification scoring systems using plain radiographs to predict vascular stiffness in peritoneal dialysis patients. Nephrology (Carlton) 16: 656–662.
32. Oh KH, Jung JY, Yoon MO, Song A, Lee H, et al. (2010) Intra-peritoneal interleukin-6 system is a potent determinant of the baseline peritoneal solute transport in incident peritoneal dialysis patients. Nephrol Dial Transplant 25:1639–1646.
33. Kopple JD (1994) Effect of nutrition on morbidity and mortality in maintenance dialysis patients. Am J Kidney Dis 24: 1002–1009.
34. Canada-USA (CANUSA) Peritoneal Dialysis Study Group (1996) Adequacy of dialysis and nutrition in continuous peritoneal dialysis: association with clinical outcomes. J Am Soc Nephrol 7: 198–207.
35. Han SH, Han DS (2012) Nutrition in patients on peritoneal dialysis. Nat Rev Nephrol 8: 163–175.

10

Back to Basics: Pitting Edema and the Optimization of Hypertension Treatment in Incident Peritoneal Dialysis Patients (BRAZPD)

Sebastião R. Ferreira-Filho[1,2]*, Gilberto R. Machado[1,2], Valéria C. Ferreira[1], Carlos F. M. A. Rodrigues[1], Thyago Proença de Moraes[3], José C. Divino-Filho[4], Marcia Olandoski[3], Christopher McIntyre[5], Roberto Pecoits-Filho[3], on behalf of the BRAZPD study investigators

1 Nefroclínica de Uberlândia, Minas Gerais, Brazil, **2** Federal University of Uberlândia, Minas Gerais, Brazil, **3** Center for Health and Biological Sciences, Pontifícia Universidade Católica do Paraná, Curitiba, Brazil, **4** Baxter Healthcare, Division of Baxter Novum and Renal Medicine, CLINTEC, Karolinska Institute, Stockholm, Sweden, **5** Faculty of Medicine & Health Sciences, University of Nottingham, Nottingham, United Kingdom,

Abstract

Systemic arterial hypertension is an important risk factor for cardiovascular disease that is frequently observed in populations with declining renal function. Initiation of renal replacement therapy at least partially decreases signs of fluid overload; however, high blood pressure levels persist in the majority of patients after dialysis initiation. Hypervolemia due to water retention predisposes peritoneal dialysis (PD) patients to hypertension and can clinically manifest in several forms, including peripheral edema. The approaches to detect edema, which include methods such as bioimpedance, inferior vena cava diameter and biomarkers, are not always available to physicians worldwide. For clinical examinations, the presence of pitting located in the lower extremities and/or over the sacrum to diagnose the presence of peripheral edema in their patients are frequently utulized. We evaluated the impact of edema on the control of blood pressure of incident PD patients during the first year of dialysis treatment. Patients were recruited from 114 Brazilian dialysis centers that were participating in the BRAZPD study for a total of 1089 incident patients. Peripheral edema was diagnosed by the presence of pitting after finger pressure was applied to the edematous area. Patients were divided into 2 groups: those with and without edema according to the monthly medical evaluation. Blood arterial pressure, body mass index, the number of antihypertensive drugs and comorbidities were analyzed. We observed an initial BP reduction in the first five months and a stabilization of blood pressure levels from five to twelve months. The edematous group exhibited higher blood pressure levels than the group without edema during the follow-up. The results strongly indicate that the presence of a simple and easily detectable clinical sign of peripheral edema is a very relevant tool that could be used to re-evaluate not only the patient's clinical hypertensive status but also the PD prescription and patient compliance.

Editor: Emmanuel A. Burdmann, University of Sao Paulo Medical School, Brazil

Funding: The authors have no funding or support to report.

Competing Interests: Baxter Healthcare sponsored this study. During the data collection and analysis, JCDF was employed by Baxter. RPF received a consulting fee and speaker honorarium from Baxter Healthcare. There are no patents, products in development or marketed products to declare. This does not alter the authors' adherence to all the PLoS ONE policies on sharing data and materials, as detailed online in the guide for authors.

* E-mail: sebahferreira@gmail.com

Introduction

Cardiovascular disease is the most common cause of morbidity and mortality in patients with chronic kidney disease (CKD) [1–3]. Systemic arterial hypertension (SAH) is an important risk factor for cardiovascular disease and is frequently observed in this population along with a decline of renal function [4]. Although overload and renal replacement therapy (RRT) with dialysis usually improve fluid balance and partially remove uremic toxins, high blood pressure levels may persist after the initiation of dialysis, and hypertension is present in the majority of both peritoneal and hemodialysis patients [5,6].

The reduction in blood pressure levels observed in peritoneal dialysis (PD) patients can be attributed to the continuous effective control of fluid balance and, consequently, extracellular volume [7]; however, this reduction is not always sustained. In fact, higher than normal blood pressure levels are observed in many patients during dialysis therapy, mainly due to the limitations in achieving normal fluid status [8–10]. Hypervolemia due to water retention predisposes PD patients to hypertension [11,12] and can manifest clinically in several forms, including peripheral edema [9]. Detecting occult edema often involves the measurement of metrics such as bioimpedance, inferior vena cava diameter and biomarkers, but these methods are not available to all physicians. To detect edema in their patients, many doctors have at their disposal only the presence of pitting located in the lower extremities and/or over the sacrum.

Despite the fact that some patients present SAH independently of volemic status, it is recognized that hypervolemia, with or without the presence of edema, is one of the principal factors responsible for the resistance of PD patients to SAH treatment [13,14]. Blood pressure normalization often requires modifications to the ultrafiltration target, an increase in sodium removal, a decrease in fluid and sodium intake, blood sugar control and/or an increase in the number of prescribed hypertension drugs [6,7,15,21]. Considering that the expansion of extracellular volume can occur during dialysis and that peripheral edema detectable on a physical exam can be the result of a hypervolemic state [13], little is known about the correlations between pitting edema and blood pressure control in hypertensive patients receiving PD treatment.

We hypothesized that the presence of pitting edema is associated with the worsening of SAH, which leads to the cardiovascular impact observed in fluid-overloaded patients. Thus, in the present study, we evaluated the impact of peripheral edema on hypertensive control in incident PD patients with SAH during the first year of dialysis treatment.

Methods

Each consecutive incident patient recruited from 114 Brazilian dialysis centers participating in the BRAZPD study from December 2004 through October 2007 was included, totaling 3439 patients. Incident patients were defined as patients who originated from pre-dialysis conservative treatment or HD, who started treatment with PD during the study period and who remained on the therapy for at least 90 days. In Brazil, 60% of the patients start treatment in APD and 40% in CAPD. Details of the BRAZPD study design and characteristics of the cohort are described elsewhere [16]. Briefly, after being selected to participate in the study, each clinic submitted the project to its local ethics committee (the protocol was approved by the ethics committees of Federal University of Uberlandia), and all patients signed an informed consent. Physician and nurses at each dialysis center were trained by the study monitors to use the clinical research software *PDnet*, which was designed specifically to collect data for this study. From a total of 3439 incident patients, 239 were excluded because they were less than 18 years old, 1650 were excluded for not completing 12 full months of follow up (i.e., patients who missed at least one medical evaluation monthly for 12 consecutive months, or who dropped out due to hemodialysis, transplant or death), 430 were excluded because they were normotensive with or without previously using any antihypertensive drugs and because they did not have peripheral edema at the beginning of the PD treatment, and 31 were excluded due to missing data. After exclusion criteria were applied, 1089 hypertensive patients were included in the analysis.

The variables analyzed included anthropomorphic data, comorbidities, systolic arterial pressure (SAP), diastolic arterial pressure (DAP), mean arterial pressure (MAP), erythropoietin use, PD modality (CAPD or APD), and physical examination. During the physical examination, peripheral edema was characterized by the presence of pitting after finger pressure was applied to the edematous area for at least five seconds. The nephrologists graded pitting edema on a scale from 1+ to 4+. The urea and plasma creatinine, serum potassium, and hemoglobin values of the patients were measured to be used as annual means.

For all patients, the dialysis nurse or the nephrologist measured blood pressure during their monthly visits to the dialysis clinic. For the diagnosis of systemic hypertension, the following WHO/ISH criteria were applied: SAP≥140 mmHg and/or DAP≥90 mmHg, with or without the use of hypertensive medication. SAP levels were verified using an oscillating method. Mean arterial pressure was calculated using the formula MAP=(2DAP+SAP)/3. The number of anti-hypertensive drug classes used monthly by the patients (NAC) was also reported. The classes considered were

diuretics, beta-blockers, ACE inhibitors, angiotensin II receptor blockers, centrally and peripherally acting alpha-blockers, and calcium channel blockers. Each class listed was counted as one unit, and the NAC represented the mathematical mean of the number of anti-hypertensive drug classes used per patient for each subgroup.

After the exclusion criteria were applied, the final sample consisted of 1089 hypertensive patients. These patients were subdivided into those with (E+) and without (E−) clinically detectable pitting edema, according to the monthly medical evaluation at both the beginning of the observation period and during the twelve months of follow up. The number of patients in each subgroup varied monthly depending on the presentation of edema at that particular evaluation (Figure 1). In order to analyze the trend for edema and high blood pressure levels, we also monitored for 12 months the patients classified E+ and E− based on the first month classification.

Statistical Analysis

Categorical variables are presented as frequencies and percentages. Continuous variables are presented as the mean ± standard deviation (mean ± SD). In the figures, continuous variables are presented as the mean ± standard error. The chi-squared test and analysis of variance (ANOVA), with repeat measures and measures of position and distribution, were utilized for the comparison between the E+ and E− subgroups. The parallelism analysis of both groups was performed to verify the trends and similarities between the groups, for the initial defined groups at month 1. For all analyses, a p-value of <0.05 was considered statistically significant. All statistical analyses were performed using SPSS version 8.0 (Chicago, IL, USA).

Results

Descriptive data at baseline PD treatment level (after the first month on PD) for all patients included in this study are shown in Table 1. The mean patient age was 58.2±15.3 years, and more than half (56.9%) of the patients were female. The mean SBP was 156.7±18.7 mmHg, the mean DBP was 90.0±12.7 mmHg, and the mean MAP was 112.2±12.8 mmHg. The mean body mass index (BMI) was 25.4±5.0 kg/m². The correlation between BMI and the number of patients with edema was negative and significant (r = −0.83). The increase of blood pressure (SBP, DBP and MAP) correlated with the number of patients with

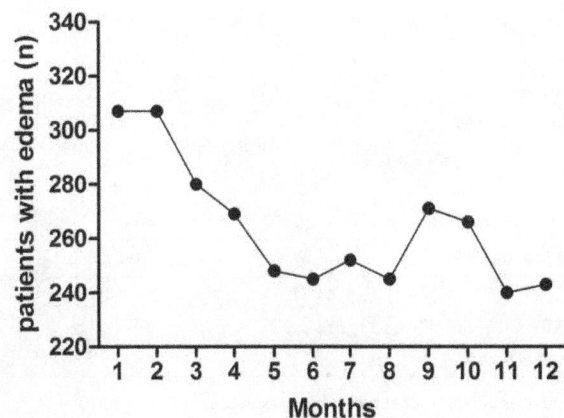

Figure 1. Number of patients/month with clinically detectible edema.

edema: 0.76; 0.69 and 0.52 respectively (p<0.001).Overall, 42.6% of study participants were diabetic, and the mean number of anti-hypertensive class drugs (NAC) used was 2.1 ± 1.0 drugs/patient. Forty-three percent of patients were on APD using Home-choice[TM] (Baxter Healthcare) as the cycler, and all patients were prescribed only glucose-based PD solutions (Dianeal, Baxter Healthcare).

Analysis of groups divided by the presence of clinically detectible edema

Subgroup analysis of patients with clinically detectible edema (E+)

During the study, subgroup E+ (n = 307) presented a decrease in SAP between the 1st and 5th month (from 159.5 ± 19.6 to 150.0 ± 25.3 mmHg, $p<0.05$), and SAP remained constant from the 5th month until the end of the study (151.2 ± 30.3 mmHg, $p>0.05$). DAP did not change significantly between the 1st and 12th month (from 90.7 ± 13.3 to 89.0 ± 17.7 mmHg, $p>0.05$). SAP decreased significantly between the 1st and 5th month (from 113.7 ± 13.4 to 108.0 ± 17.2 mmHg, $p<0.05$), and MAP remained constant from the 5th month through the 12th month (109.7 ± 19.8 mmHg, $p>0.05$). NAC did not change between the 1st and 12th months (from 2.3 ± 1.0 to 2.2 ± 1.0 drugs/patient,

$p>0.05$). The number of patients with edema decreased between the 2nd and 6th months from 307 to 245 individuals; this number varied through the end of the evaluation period, at which point 243 patients were clinically diagnosed with edema (Figure 1). BMI

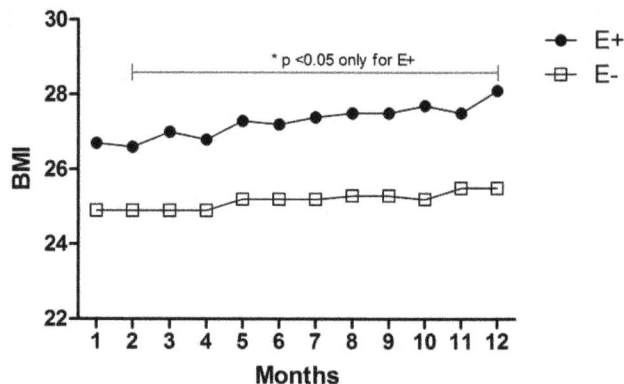

Figure 2. Twelve-month evolution of the body mass index (BMI) in the patient cohort.

Table 1. Demographic, clinical and laboratory characteristics of patients at the baseline evaluation.

Variable	Total population	Patients with edema (E+)	without edema (E−)	P value
Number of patients (n)	1089	307	782	<0.001
Age (year)	58.2±15.3	59. 6±14.3	57.7±15.6*	0.03
Female (%)	56.9	55.7	57.4	0.61
Diabetes (%)	42.6	56.0	37.3*	<0.0001
Race (%)				
Asian	2.7	3.2	2.8	0.92
White	61.7	61.6	61.1	0.96
Black	35.6	35.2	36.1	0.93
Height (cm)	161.6±10.0	161.6±10.5	161.7±9.8	0.44
Weight (Kg)	66.7±15.0	69.8±14.5	65.5±15.1*	<0.0001
Body mass index (Kg/m2)	25.4±5.0	26.7±5.1	24.9±4.9*	<0.0001
SAP (mmHg)	156.7±18.7	159.5±19.6	155.6±18.2*	0.001
DAP (mmHg)	90.0±12.7	90.7±13.3	89.7±12.5	0.11
MAP (mmHg)	112.2±12.8	113.7±13.4	111.7±12.6*	0.01
NCA	2.1±1.0	2.3±1.0	2.0±0.7*	<0.0001
Erythropoietin (%)	44.0	51.0	41.2*	0.003
CAPD/APD (%)	57.0/43.0	63.5/36.5	55.5*/44.5*	0.01/0.02
Conservative treatment (%)	56.2	60.4	54.7	0.093
Serum Albumin (g/dL)(n)	3.6±0.69	3.54±0.78	3.64±0.64	0.295
Hemodialysis previously (%)	44.5	44.4	44.6	0.933
Serum urea (mg/dl)	101.2±24.8	124.5±26.2	101.8±24.9	0.34
Serum creatinine (mg/dl)	8.0±3.1	7.8±3.1	8.1±3.1	0.12
Serum potassium (mEq/L)	4.3±0.6	4.3±0.6	4.4±0.6	0.08
Haemoglobin (g/dl)	11.5±4.0	11.4±3.7	11.5±4.1	0.44

NCA, number of classes of anti-hypertensives in use;
*(E−) vs (E+);
SAP: systolic arterial pressure; DAP: diastolic arterial pressure;
MAP: mean arterial pressure.

increased from the 2nd to the 12th month of evaluation (from 26.7±5.1 to 28.1±5.6 kg/m2, $p<0.05$) (Figure 2).

Subgroup analysis of patients without clinically detectible edema (E−)

Subgroup E− (n = 782) presented a significant decrease in SAP between the 1st and 5th month (from 155.6±18.2 to 142.7±24.2 mmHg, $p<0.05$). After this initial period, SAP remained constant until the end of the study period (141.2±26.6 mmHg, $p>0.05$). DAP did not change between the 1st and 12th months (89.7±12.5 to 84.7±15.8 mmHg, $p>0.05$). MAP decreased significantly between the 1st and 5th months (from 111.7±12.6 to 104.1±15.8 mmHg, $p<0.05$) and then remained constant from the 5th month through the 12th month (103.6±17.9 mmHg, $P>0.05$). NAC did not vary throughout the study period; the mean at the 1st month was 2.0±0.7, and the mean at the 12th month was 2.1±1.1 ($p>0.05$). For subgroup E−, there was no difference in BMI during the 12 months of follow-up (Figures 3 and 4)).

Comparison between the two subgroups of patients

The descriptive characteristics of the two subgroups defined by the presence of edema at the start of dialysis are shown in Table 1. At baseline, subgroup E+ consisted of 307 patients and E− consisted of 782 patients; however, these numbers varied according to monthly clinical evaluations (Figure 1). When only the patients classified E+ and E− in the first month were monitored, the results confirmed the monthly patient classification. E+ and E− move in the same way for the SBP (p = 0.654) although with different mean profiles (p = 0.001). In other words, E+ group showed higher SAP values than E-group during the 12 months period. For the DAP and MAP the trend and mean profile did not show statistical diferences (Figure 4). A comparison of subgroups E+ and E− at the start of treatment (Table 1) revealed significant differences with respect to age (59.6±14.3 vs. 57.7±15.6 years, respectively; p<0.03), BMI (26.7±5.1 vs. 24.9±4.9 kg/m2, respectively; p<0.0001), SAP (159.5±19.6 vs. 155.6±18.2 mmHg, respectively; P<0.001), MAP (113.7±13.4 vs. 111.7±12.6 mmHg, respectively; P<0.01), NAC (2.3±1.0 vs. 2.0±0.7 drugs/patient, respectively; P<0.05) and erythropoietin use (51.0 vs. 41.2%, respectively; P = 0.003). In both subgroups, there were a greater percentage of patients on APD than on CAPD (63.5/36.5 vs. 55.5/44.5%, respectively; p<0.01/0.02). The percentage of patients with diabetes mellitus was greater in subgroup E+ than in subgroup E− (56.0 vs. 37.3%, respectively;

P<0.0001), and the number of patients with a history of cardiovascular disease at the start of PD was not significantly different between the two groups (Table 1). SAP, MAP, NAC, and BMI were significantly different between the two subgroups (E+ and E−) in the analysis of the entire follow up period (p<0.05).

Discussion

It is well known that the expansion of extracellular volume with or without detectible edema is one of the principal factors responsible for the increase in SAP in patients with CKD [3,9]. In the present study, we observed that SAP and MAP of both subgroups presented a significant decrease in values in the first five months after starting PD therapy and stabilization of these values through the end of the observation period. This behavior was also conferred by Menon et al. [17], who reported a reduction in systemic pressures at the start of PD and, contrary to our data, detected an increase in blood pressure levels after 6–12 months on PD. On the other hand, Saldanha et al. [7] reported a decrease in blood pressure levels during PD treatment over 5 years, which was associated with the concomitant increase in the number of anti-hypertensive drugs used. In the present study, the initial decline observed in the E+ and E− groups could be attributed to a reduction in extracellular volume as a result of PD [8,18] because NAC did not change during this period. However, it should be noted that NAC represents a number of anti-hypertensive classes of drugs, which allows for the possibility of variations in the measurement of anti-hypertensive drugs within the same class. On the other hand, NAC maintenance can reflect a non-worsening of SAH in these patients and/or the medical preference to use these drugs for other therapeutic goals such as cardio-protection and/or preservation of residual renal function. Despite the initial decline in arterial blood pressure levels observed in our study, they did not decrease to values within the normal limits; SAP levels were above 140 mmHg during the entire study period. There are other reasons that could explain in the relative control of blood pressure levels in both groups, which are increase activity of the sympathetic nervous system, increase endothelium-derived vaso-constrictors, vascular calcification and activation of the renin-angiotensin system.

Upon separate analysis of the E+ and E− groups, we observed a monthly variation throughout the study period in the number of patients. This variation was a consequence of bi-directional flow between these groups. Despite this, the number of patients in the E+ subgroup decreased significantly after 12 months, from 307 to 243 patients (Figure 1). Among the E+ subgroup, SAP and MAP levels decreased from baseline until the 5th month, at which time they stabilized until the 12th month (Figure 3 and 4), while DAP did not change significantly during the entire period. In our study, patients with edema exhibited greater blood pressure levels (SAP and MAP) than those observed in the E− subgroup (Figure 3 and 4). Gunal et al. [12] and Katzarski et al. [19] demonstrated that volume overload is an important factor in resistance to SAH treatment for dialysis patients, while Ates et al. [20] showed that SBP and DBP were negatively correlated with total fluid and sodium removal, as well as with sodium restriction. The increase of blood pressure values was correlated with the number of patients with edema. This association shows that the patients who belonged to the E+ had higher blood pressure levels than those of group E− (Figure 5).

Our data demonstrated that the NAC in the E+ subgroup, despite not varying throughout the study, was significantly greater than in the E− subgroup during the months evaluated. This observation may suggest a greater difficulty in SAH control in the

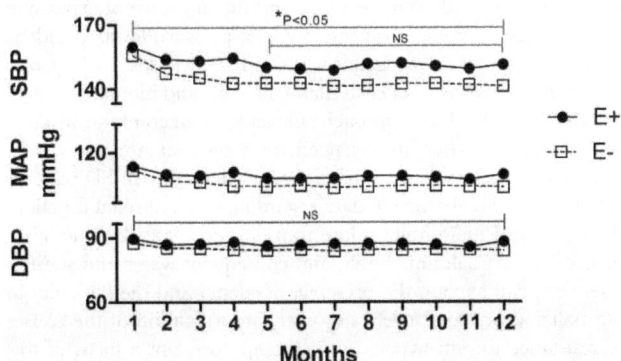

Figure 3. Systolic (SBP), Diastolic (DBP) and Mean Arterial Pressures (MAP) in incident PD patients during 12 months of follow up.

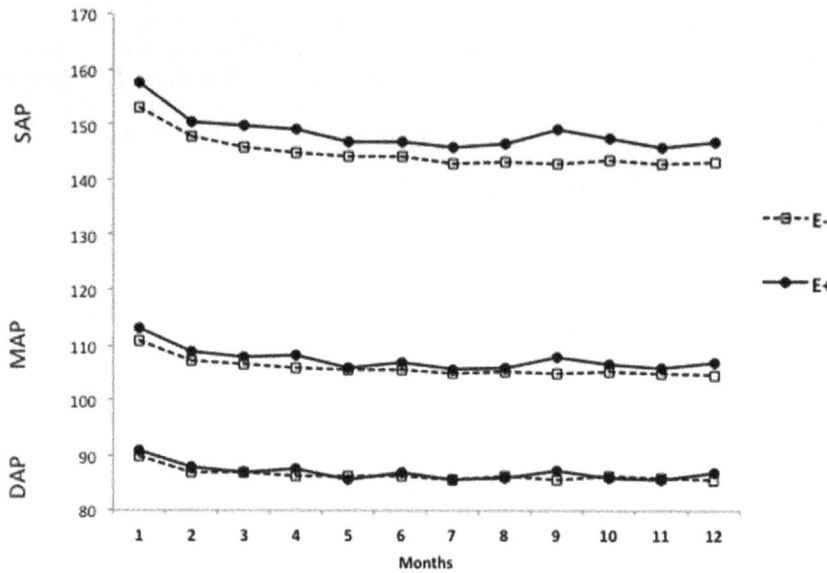

Figure 4. The initial groups (first month) were followed for 12 months.

E+ group. Furthermore, BMI in the E+ group increased progressively over the 12 month period. A strong and negative correlation between BMI and the number of patients with edema was observed. This association could be explained in two ways: a worsening of the edema status during PD therapy or a real gain of body mass. We believe that future studies with adequate designs will help to answer this question.

The progressive increase in body weight, likely caused to a large extent by the presence of edema, can be attributed to a water and salt imbalance, the patient's failure to follow medical recommendations, and/or an inadequate PD prescription. The progressive increase in body weight among PD patients might also be attributed to a gain of fat mass due to glucose absorption from the peritoneal cavity, as the patients may have been prescribed more hypertonic PD solutions to improve UF.

In the E− subgroup, blood pressure patterns followed the trend observed in the E+ group and decreased in the first months of PD before subsequently stabilizing (Figure 3). In the E− group, blood pressure levels were lower than those observed in the E+ group during the entire observation period, whereas the NAC in the E− group did not vary significantly during the study period. However, blood pressure values did not reach the normal recommended levels. In general, there are several associated factors that make normalization of blood pressure levels difficult to attain in PD patients, including the presence of diabetes mellitus, aging, and the use of erythropoietin [11,14,18]. This was observed in the present study in the E+ group, in which the patients were significantly older and the percentage of patients with diabetes mellitus was significantly greater than in the E− group (Table 1). The significantly larger number of E+ patients who were treated with CAPD as opposed to APD may reflect an inadequate PD prescription, as many of these CAPD patients may be high transporters and/or have UF problems in the long run. Therefore, these patients should have been switched to APD. However, during the observation period, Extraneal was not available in Brazil. Moreover, blood pressures above the normal values could be caused by therapeutic inertia, where soft reasoning often leads to avoidance of intensified therapy by the medical staff [21].

The present study presents several limitations. Edema evaluation cannot be easily standardized, and the influence of expansion or retraction of volume on the systemic pressure levels could be better analyzed if it was evaluated by other methods, such as bioimpedance, inferior vena cava diameter [22], and biomarkers such as ANP [22,23]. This approach, however, is uncommon in daily medical practice due to the need for tools that are not always available. In addition, the analysis of fluid retention in PD patients is limited by the absence of data regarding residual renal function, the peritoneal membrane solute transport type and UF measurements [9]. Hypoalbuminemia, and consequent water and sodium retention, can explain the presence of edema and the difficulty in normalizing pressure levels; however, an evaluation of the causes of resistance to anti-hypertension therapy was not a focus of this study. It is important to note that the results of this observational study reflect PD practices in Brazil, which may be similar to treatment practices in a large number of countries around the world.

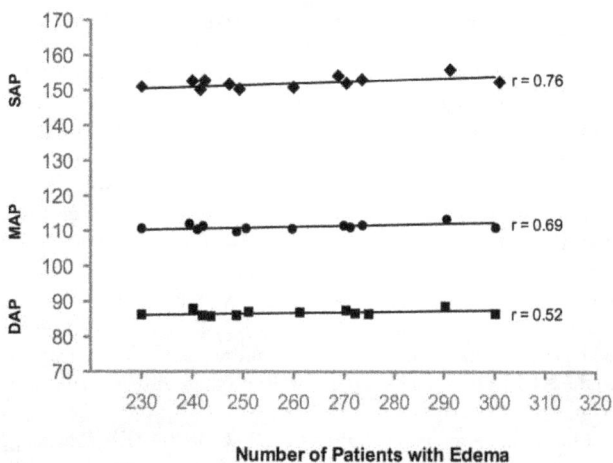

Figure 5. The increase in blood pressure levels correlates positively to the number of patients with edema.

Hypertensive CKD patients experienced a significant reduction in blood pressure levels after the initiation of PD, which was more pronounced in the first few months of therapy. However, most patients do not achieve normalization during the first year of treatment. This difficulty in reducing arterial blood pressure to normal levels is aggravated by the presence of edema, which points to a pivotal role of fluid overload in the hypertension of CKD patients on dialysis. The presence of clinically detectible pitting edema can be a useful clinical sign that could be used to guide the optimization of SAH treatment in patients undergoing continuous peritoneal dialysis.

In summary, volume status is of major importance to outcomes in patients undergoing PD. The lack of a robust edema evaluation and the limited availability of BIA and other objective measures of quantifying volume status make clinicians highly dependent on clinical evaluation. Clinically detectable pitting edema remains the most readily used clinical assessment tool. This study is the first to give a large-scale systematic description of pitting edema in the context of arterial hypertension in PD patients and to assess the effects of edema resolution in blood pressure values with PD initiation.

The results presented here strongly indicate that the presence of such a simple and easily detected clinical sign as pitting edema should be considered to be a relevant observational tool to assess a patient's clinical status, PD prescription and compliance with treatment. The term "back to basics" could mean, "examine your patients, look for edema and observe the blood pressure" and to do this sophisticated technologies are not needed.

Author Contributions

Conceived and designed the experiments: SRFF GRM RPF. Performed the experiments: GRM SRFF. Analyzed the data: SRFF GRM VCF CFMAR CM TPM MO JCDF. Wrote the paper: SRFF GRM. These authors contributed with important points in the discussion: JCDF.

References

1. Lynn KL, McGregor DO, Moesbergen T, Buttimore AL, Inkster JA, et al. (2002) Hypertension as a determinant of survival for patients treated with home dialysis. Kidney Int 62: 2281–2287.
2. Levey AS, Beto JA, Coronado BE, Eknoyan G, Foley RN, et al. (1998) Controlling the epidemic of cardiovascular disease in chronic renal disease: what do we know? What do we need to learn? Where do we go from here? National Kidney Foundation Task Force on Cardiovascular Disease. Am J Kidney Dis 32: 853–906.
3. van Dijk PC, Jager KJ, de Charro F, Collart F, Cornet R, et al. (2001) Renal replacement therapy in Europe: the results of a collaborative effort by the ERA-EDTA registry and six national or regional registries. Nephrol Dial Transplant 16: 1120–1129.
4. Barri YM (2008) Hypertension and kidney disease: a deadly connection. Current hypertension reports 10: 39–45.
5. Foley RN, Parfrey PS, Sarnak MJ (1998) Clinical epidemiology of cardiovascular disease in chronic renal disease. Am J Kidney Dis 32: S112–119.
6. Cocchi R, Degli Esposti E, Fabbri A, Lucatello A, Sturani A, et al. (1999) Prevalence of hypertension in patients on peritoneal dialysis: results of an Italian multicentre study. Nephrol Dial Transplant 14: 1536–1540.
7. Saldanha LF, Weiler EW, Gonick HC (1993) Effect of continuous ambulatory peritoneal dialysis on blood pressure control. Am J Kidney Dis 21: 184–188.
8. Lameire N (1993) Cardiovascular risk factors and blood pressure control in continuous ambulatory peritoneal dialysis. Perit Dial Int 13 Suppl 2: S394–395.
9. Tzamaloukas AH, Saddler MC, Murata GH, Malhotra D, Sena P, et al. (1995) Symptomatic fluid retention in patients on continuous peritoneal dialysis. J Am Soc Nephrol 6: 198–206.
10. Tang W, Cheng LT, Lu XH, Wang T (2009) Effect of nutrition on arterial stiffness in peritoneal dialysis patients. American journal of nephrology 30: 120–125.
11. Rahman M, Dixit A, Donley V, Gupta S, Hanslik T, et al. (1999) Factors associated with inadequate blood pressure control in hypertensive hemodialysis patients. American journal of kidney diseases : the official journal of the National Kidney Foundation 33: 498–506.
12. Gunal AI, Duman S, Ozkahya M, Toz H, Asci G, et al. (2001) Strict volume control normalizes hypertension in peritoneal dialysis patients. American journal

of kidney diseases : the official journal of the National Kidney Foundation 37: 588–593.
13. Van Biesen W, Verbeke F, Devolder I, Vanholder R (2008) The relation between salt, volume, and hypertension: clinical evidence for forgotten but still valid basic physiology. Perit Dial Int 28: 596–600.
14. Fishbane S, Natke E, Maesaka JK (1996) Role of volume overload in dialysis-refractory hypertension. Am J Kidney Dis 28: 257–261.
15. Slingeneyer A, Canaud B, Mion C (1983) Permanent loss of ultrafiltration capacity of the peritoneum in long-term peritoneal dialysis: an epidemiological study. Nephron 33: 133–138.
16. Fernandes N, Bastos MG, Cassi HV, Machado NL, Ribeiro JA, et al. (2008) The Brazilian Peritoneal Dialysis Multicenter Study (BRAZPD) : characterization of the cohort. Kidney Int Suppl: S145–151.
17. Menon MK, Naimark DM, Bargman JM, Vas SI, Oreopoulos DG (2001) Long-term blood pressure control in a cohort of peritoneal dialysis patients and its association with residual renal function. Nephrol Dial Transplant 16: 2207–2213.
18. Mailloux LU, Haley WE (1998) Hypertension in the ESRD patient: pathophysiology, therapy, outcomes, and future directions. Am J Kidney Dis 32: 705–719.
19. Katzarski KS, Charra B, Luik AJ, Nisell J, Divino Filho JC, et al. (1999) Fluid state and blood pressure control in patients treated with long and short haemodialysis. Nephrology, dialysis, transplantation : official publication of the European Dialysis and Transplant Association - European Renal Association 14: 369–375.
20. Ates K, Nergizoglu G, Keven K, Sen A, Kutlay S, et al. (2001) Effect of fluid and sodium removal on mortality in peritoneal dialysis patients. Kidney international 60: 767–776.
21. Basile J (2009) Clinical Inertia and Blood Pressure Goal Attainment. The Journal of Clinical Hypertension 11.
22. Leunissen KM, Kouw P, Kooman JP, Cheriex EC, deVries PM, et al. (1993) New techniques to determine fluid status in hemodialyzed patients. Kidney Int Suppl 41: S50–56.
23. Lang SM, Wolfram G, Gerzer R, Schiffl H (1999) Characterization of subtypes of hypertension in CAPD patients by cyclic guanosine monophosphate. Perit Dial Int 19: 143–147.

Seeking Clarity within Cloudy Effluents: Differentiating Fungal from Bacterial Peritonitis in Peritoneal Dialysis Patients

Ruchir Chavada[1], Jen Kok[2], Sebastiaan van Hal[1], Sharon C-A. Chen[2]*

1 Department of Microbiology and Infectious Diseases, Sydney South West Pathology Service, Liverpool Hospital, Liverpool, Australia, **2** Centre for Infectious Diseases and Microbiology Laboratory Services, Institute of Clinical Pathology and Medical Research, Westmead Hospital, Westmead, Australia

Abstract

Background: Fungal peritonitis is a serious complication of peritoneal dialysis (PD) therapy with the majority of patients ceasing PD permanently. The aims of this study were to identify risk factors and clinical associations that may discriminate between fungal from bacterial peritonitis.

Methods: We retrospectively identified episodes of fungal peritonitis from 2001–2010 in PD patients at Liverpool and Westmead Hospitals (Australia). Fungal peritonitis cases were matched in a 1:2 ratio with patients with bacterial peritonitis from each institution's dialysis registry, occurring closest in time to the fungal episode. Patient demographic, clinical and outcome data were obtained from the medical records.

Results: Thirty-nine episodes of fungal peritonitis (rate of 0.02 episodes per patient-year of dialysis) were matched with 78 episodes of bacterial peritonitis. *Candida* species were the commonest pathogens (35/39; 90% episodes) with *Candida albicans* (37%), *Candida parapsilosis* (32%) and *Candida glabrata* (13%) the most frequently isolated species. Compared to bacterial peritonitis, fungal peritonitis patients had received PD for significantly longer (1133 vs. 775 catheter-days; $p = 0.016$), were more likely to have had previous episodes of bacterial peritonitis (51% vs. 10%; $p = 0.01$), and to have received prior antibacterial therapy (51% vs. 10%; $p = 0.01$). Patients with fungal peritonitis were less likely to have fever and abdominal pain on presentation, but had higher rates of PD catheter removal (79% vs. 22%; $p < 0.005$), and permanent transfer to haemodialysis (87% vs. 24%; $p < 0.005$). Hospital length of stay was significantly longer in patients with fungal peritonitis (26.1 days vs. 12.6 days; $p = 0.017$), but the all-cause 30-day mortality rate was similar in both groups. Fluconazole was a suitable empiric antifungal agent; with no *Candida* resistance detected.

Conclusion: Prompt recognition of clinical risk factors, initiation of antifungal therapy and removal of PD catheters are key considerations in optimising outcomes.

Editor: Brad Spellberg, Los Angeles Biomedical Research Institute, United States of America

Funding: The authors have no funding or support to declare.

Competing Interests: The authors have declared that no competing interests exist.

* E-mail: sharon.chen@swahs.health.nsw.gov.au

Introduction

Patients with end stage kidney disease (ESKD) undergoing dialysis are at increased risk of infections, with infection-related hospitalisation rates 31–68% higher than patients without kidney disease [1]. The route of dialysis determines the principal dialysis-associated infection type; peritonitis occurs almost exclusively in peritoneal dialysis (PD) patients. PD peritonitis is common (annual rates of ~0.6 episodes per patient-year in the United States and Australia) [1,2] and accounts for up to 16% of all deaths in PD patients [3]. Most peritonitis episodes are due to bacteria, with fungi causing only 2–10% of cases [4–6]. Although uncommon compared with bacterial peritonitis, fungal peritonitis is associated with higher mortality rates (5%–53% vs. 0.7%–15%) [4,7] and often results in permanent discontinuation of PD with high morbidity [4,8].

Management of PD peritonitis requires initiation of empiric antimicrobial therapy directed against Gram-positive and Gram-negative, organisms [3], whilst awaiting definitive identification and susceptibility data of the aetiologic pathogen. For fungal peritonitis, the guidelines also emphasise the importance of prompt catheter removal to reduce the high attendant morbidity and mortality [3]. Since laboratory results are often non-specific and mycological information may be delayed, it is important to recognise risk factors, clinical features and laboratory variables that discriminate fungal, from bacterial, peritonitis to guide early initiation of targeted antifungal therapy.

Herein, we examine clinical and epidemiological data from a multicentre case control study of PD patients to identify unique risk factors and clinical associations of fungal, compared to bacterial, peritonitis episodes.

Results

A total of 1568 PD peritonitis episodes occurred in 2075 patients over the 9-year study period (rate of 1 episode every 15 patient-month or ~0.8 episodes every patient-year). Thirty-nine (2.5%) episodes (in 39 patients) were due to fungi (rate of 0.02 episodes every patient-year). The median age of patients with fungal peritonitis was 64 years (range 51–77); 51% were female. Most episodes occurred in patients with their first PD catheter following mean PD duration of 1133 catheter-days (interquartile range 466–1710). All patients were receiving CAPD.

Causative fungal pathogen

Candida species accounted for 35 of 39 (90%) fungal peritonitis episodes (Table 1). The remaining four episodes were caused by *Trichosporon beigelii*, *Rhodotorula mucilaginosa*, *Curvularia lunata* and *Prototheca wickerhamii* (one episode each). Thirty-three of fungal peritonitis episodes were monomicrobial, and six, polymicrobial (three episodes were caused by two different *Candida* species and in three other episodes, infection was caused by both a *Candida* and bacterium).

Thirty-eight *Candida* isolates were recovered. Fourteen of 38 (37%) of *Candida* isolates were *Candida albicans*; 12 (32%) were *Candida parapsilosis*; five (13%), *Candida glabrata*; and three (8%), *Candida tropicalis*. There was a single episode each due to *Candida famata* and *Candida guilliermondii*. Two *Candida* isolates were not speciated (Table 1). Blood cultures performed in 27 fungal episodes isolated *C. glabrata* once in a patient with *C. glabrata* peritonitis. Two patients had concurrent/prior exit site infections with the same fungus recovered in the preceding five and 12 days, respectively, of their peritonitis episodes.

In vitro antifungal susceptibility testing performed on 36 speciated *Candida* isolates using Sensititre YeastOne (TREK Diagnostic Systems, Inc., Cleveland, OH) and/or Etest (AB BIODISK, Solna, Sweeden), demonstrated fluconazole MICs of ≤4 µg/ml (n = 32), 8 µg/ml (n = 2) and 16 µg/ml (n = 2) [9].

Table 1. Fungal isolates in thirty nine episodes of fungal peritonitis.

Fungal species	[a]No. of isolates (%)
[b]*Candida* species (n = 38)	
Candida albicans	14 (37%)
Candida parapsilosis	12 (32%)
Candida glabrata	5 (13%)
Candida tropicalis	3 (8%)
Candida famata	1 (2.5%)
Candida guilliermondii	1 (2.5%)
Non-speciated Candida	2 (5%)
Non-*Candida* species (n = 4)	
Trichosporon beigelii	1
Rhodotorula mucilaginosa	1
Curvularia lunata	1
Prototheca wickerhamii	1

[a]Forty-two isolates were responsible for 39 episodes of fungal peritonitis; percentages are relative to total *Candida* isolates (n = 38).
[b]Thirty-eight *Candida* isolates (29 monomicrobial episodes with 29 *Candida* isolates and 6 polymicrobial episodes with 9 *Candida* isolates [3 dual *Candida* infections and 3 mixed *Candida*/bacterial infections]).

Amphotericin MICs available for 36 isolates were 0.032 µg/ml (n = 1); 0.12 µg/ml (n = 4); 0.125 µg/ml (n = 3); 0.25 µg/ml (n = 8); 0.38 µg/ml (n = 1); 0.5 µg/ml (n = 13); and 1 µg/ml (n = 6). Caspofungin MICs available for 24 isolates were 0.03 µg/ml (n = 3); 0.06 µg/ml (n = 8); 0.12 µg/ml (n = 3); 0.25 µg/ml (n = 4); and 0.5 µg/ml (n = 6).

Comparison of fungal and bacterial peritonitis

Patient demographics, major co-morbidities, risk factors, clinical features and laboratory parameters associated with fungal, and bacterial, peritonitis episodes are summarised in Table 2. Underlying co-morbidities and causes of ESKD were similar in both patient groups; the single patient with ESKD due to systemic lupus erythematosus had fungal peritonitis (Table 2). Episodes of fungal peritonitis were associated with significantly longer duration of PD (1133 vs. 775 catheter-days, p = 0.016), greater likelihood of previous bacterial peritonitis (51% vs. 10%, p = 0.01) and receipt of prior antibacterial agents (51% vs. 10%, p = 0.01). Conversely, patients with bacterial peritonitis were more likely to have been anaemic and suffer hyperparathyroidism, as reflected by more frequent use of erythropoiesis-stimulating (p < 0.005), and calcimimetic agents (p = 0.02) respectively (Table 2).

Fever and abdominal pain were more common in bacterial compared to fungal peritonitis (54% vs. 26%, p < 0.05 and 99% vs. 85%, p < 0.05 respectively), while there was a trend towards fungal peritonitis if hypotension was present. Gram stain of peritoneal fluid showed the presence of yeast in 8/25 (32%) episodes; in 15 cases, no organisms were seen and in two, only bacteria were visualised although cultures subsequently yielded both *Candida* and bacterial infection. Other laboratory parameters in fungal and bacterial peritonitis were in general, similar although the median peripheral blood white cell count was higher in fungal peritonitis (p = 0.05) (Table 2).

Treatment and outcomes

Fluconazole was the main antifungal agent prescribed in fungal peritonitis (33 or 82% of cases); six patients received intravenous fluconazole monotherapy for the duration of the treatment course whilst 27 received intravenous, followed by oral therapy. Liposomal amphotericin B monotherapy was given in 11% of episodes (one each of *R. mucilaginosa*, *P. wickerhamii*, *C. glabrata* and *C. parapsilosa* peritonitis). Voriconazole (oral) and caspofungin (intravenous) at recommended doses were given in one instance each of *C. lunata* and *C. tropicalis*/*C. glabrata* infection, respectively. Flucytosine was not prescribed. Patients with fungal peritonitis received antifungal therapy for a mean duration of 24 days (vs. 11 days of antibacterial therapy in bacterial peritonitis episodes; p = 0.017). The majority of fungal peritonitis patients were treated in hospital and had a mean length of stay of 26.1 days compared with 12.6 days for bacterial infections (p = 0.017). Fungal episodes were also associated with higher rates of PD catheter removal (79% vs. 22%, p < 0.005) and permanent cessation of PD (87% vs. 24%, p < 0.005); reasons for catheter retainment were death (n = 3 patients), refusal of removal (n = 2) and decision for palliative treatment (n = 3).

The all-cause 30-day mortality was similar in both peritonitis groups (15% vs. 14%, p = 0.853), as was the need for infection-related surgery (these included adhesiolysis, colectomy post perforation and resection with primary anastomosis) during catheter removal (18% vs. 15%, p = 0.79; Table 2). By univariate analysis, factors associated with increased mortality in patients with fungal peritonitis were age >65 years (p = 0.009), previous bacterial peritonitis (p = 0.02) and polymicrobial infection (p = 0.011) (Table 3). Conversely, PD catheter removal was

Table 2. Comparison of patients with fungal versus bacterial peritonitis.

Characteristics	Fungal Peritonitis n = 39 (%)	Bacterial Peritonitis (n = 78 (%)	P value
Median age (years ± SD)	64±13	61±13	0.20
Female	20 (51)	36 (46)	0.74
Diabetes mellitus	18 (46)	41 (53)	0.64
Ischaemic heart disease	16 (38)	35 (46)	0.84
Solid organ tumour	5 (8)	4 (4)	0.76
Aetiology ESKD			
Diabetes mellitus	18(46)	41(53)	0.64
Chronic Glomerulonephritis	7(18)	14(18)	0.79
Hypertension	5(13)	12(15)	0.80
Polycystic kidney disease	3 (8)	2(3)	0.33
Systemic lupus erythematosus	1	0	-
Other[a]	6(15)	9(12)	0.77
Markers of ESKD severity			
Anaemia	16 (41)	64 (82)	<0.005
Hyperparathyroidism	6 (15)	29 (37)	0.02
Duration of dialysis (catheter days)	1133	775	0.016
Prior bacterial peritonitis episodes	20 (51)	8 (10)	0.01
Receipt of antibacterial therapy within the preceding 30 days	20 (51)	8 (10)	0.01
Clinical/Laboratory findings			
Abdominal pain	33 (85)	77 (99)	0.04
Fever	10 (26)	42 (54)	<0.01
Hypotension	12 (31)	11 (14)	0.06
Median blood WCC (cells×10^9/L)	12	10	0.05
Median effluent WCC (cells×10^6/L)	2094	7973	0.16
Median CRP (mg/L)	190	179	0.73
Outcomes at 30 days			
Technique failure	34 (87)	19 (24)	<0.005
Infection related surgery	7 (18)	12 (15)	0.79
All-cause mortality	6 (15)	11 (14)	0.85

[a]Includes cancer chemotherapy-induced, analgesic nephropathy, chronic pyelonephritis, renal calculi disease. ESKD = end stage kidney disease.

Table 3. Variables associated with mortality in patients with fungal peritonitis.

Variables	Died n = 6 (%)	Survived n = 33 (%)	P value
Univariate analysis			
Sex (Female)	3 (50)	17 (52)	0.09
Mean age (years ± SD)	77±5	62±13	0.01
Diabetes mellitus	3 (50)	15 (45)	0.83
Anaemia	4 (67)	22 (67)	0.34
Hyperparathyroidism	1 (17)	5 (15)	0.92
Previous peritonitis	6 (100)	14 (42)	0.02
Peritoneal dialysis catheter removed	2 (33)	29 (88)	0.01
Polymicrobial infection	3 (50)	3 (9)	0.01

associated with increased survival (p = 0.013); 67% (4/6) of deaths occurred in patients with persistent sepsis from retained catheters.

Discussion

Fungal peritonitis in PD patients remains an important clinical entity with significant morbidity and implications for the continuation of PD. In contrast to bacterial peritonitis, the majority of patients with fungal peritonitis cease PD permanently and commence haemodialysis. Heightened awareness and early recognition of fungal peritonitis is central to optimise patient care as well as preserving the existing renal replacement therapy option. In the present study, we have identified (relative to bacterial infection) a number of clinical variables that may assist clinicians in differentiating fungal from bacterial infection.

The proportion of peritonitis episodes caused by fungi in our study (2.5%) is lower than that reported in a previous Australian study (4.5%) [4]; however, this proportion may vary across different regions in Australia (0–15%), with the highest rates reported in indigenous populations in Western Australia (WA) and the Northern Territory (NT) [4]. The proportion of fungal peritonitis that was observed in our largely non-indigenous population of metropolitan New South Wales was similar to the rate reported in Australian states other than WA and NT (0–3.5%) [4]. Overall, the rate of fungal peritonitis (0.02 episodes per patient-year) was also lower than that previously observed (0.03 episodes per patient-year) [4].

A key finding of the present study was that a relatively prolonged duration of PD was significantly associated with increased risk for developing fungal peritonitis, an observation not previously reported. Fungal contamination of peritoneal fluid may result from inadequate sterile technique when connecting PD catheters to dialysate bags, exit site and catheter tunnel infections, intestinal perforation or fistulae track formation [10]. However, the relative protracted timeframe in which fungal peritonitis occurred in our study argues against inadequate sterile technique, particularly in the immediate period following commencement of PD. We postulate that this association may be in fact due to the late recognition of fungal peritonitis or because of the high rates of PD catheter retention following previous bacterial peritonitis episodes.

Diabetes mellitus was not a risk factor for fungal peritonitis in the present study, as have been previously noted [11,12]. Consistent with the findings of others, prior bacterial peritonitis and receipt of antibacterial therapy in the preceding 30 days were associated with the development of fungal peritonitis [8,13]. Fungal peritonitis may have been initially misdiagnosed as bacterial peritonitis prior to laboratory confirmation of the former, prompting the prescription of empirical antibacterial therapy. On the other hand, the change in intestinal flora as a result of antibacterial therapy promotes the proliferation and transmural migration of fungi across the intestinal mucosa, increasing the risk of fungal peritonitis in the peritoneal cavity [6,8,14]. Previous reports have noted that secondary fungal peritonitis can be prevented by prophylactic antifungal use (fluconazole or nystatin) in patients receiving antibacterial therapy [15,16], but this is not a strategy that is widely adopted in PD centres within Australia [4], including ours. The benefits of antifungal prophylaxis have not been clearly defined [3] and could lead to emergence of more antifungal-resistant species as previously noted in other populations [3,17]. In contrast to bacterial peritonitis, anaemia and hyperparathyroidism were not significantly associated with fungal peritonitis (Table 1) consistent with previous studies [18,19]. However, we were unable to examine the potential effects of varying dosing regimens of erythropoeitin-stimulating agents with either bacterial or fungal peritonitis; this remains to be studied in future surveys.

Although observational studies have suggested that the clinical signs in fungal peritonitis are similar to those of bacterial infection [8], few studies have systematically compared the clinical presentation in these two entities. We observed that whilst abdominal pain is almost universal in bacterial peritonitis, the relative absence of abdominal pain and fever despite a cloudy effluent raises the greater likelihood of fungal peritonitis. Previous reports have documented fever and abdominal pain in 36% and 68% of patients with fungal peritonitis respectively [6] (cf. with 26% and 85% in the present study, Table 2). Sensitivity of gram stain is low in fungal peritonitis [3] due to the relatively large volume of fluid examined and presumably low fungal load; we visualised yeasts in only a third of instances in our study. Yet Gram stain of peritoneal fluid is recommended by the International Society for Peritoneal Dialysis in the management of PD peritonitis since the visualisation of yeasts allows prompt initiation of antifungal therapy [3].

In the present study, Candida species were the commonest cause of fungal peritonitis, with C. albicans, C. parapsilosis and C. glabrata

the most often isolated (37%, 32% and 13% of Candida isolates respectively). Our data is similar to that of other studies where non-albicans Candida species were more common than C. albicans [4,6,8]. Guidelines recommend systemic amphotericin and flucytosine as empiric antifungal therapy whilst awaiting identification and susceptibility of the aetiologic fungus [3]. Given that no Candida isolates were resistant to fluconazole in our study, this azole agent is an appropriate alternate empiric antifungal agent, pending species identification and susceptibility. In one large series, fluconazole monotherapy was used in 90% of fungal peritonitis cases; however, the impact of this strategy is uncertain as microbiological data on causative species and susceptibility were not presented [4]. An echinocandin (e.g. caspofungin) may be required to treat azole-resistant yeasts such as C. krusei or C. glabrata peritonitis [9]. Hence, where possible, all Candida isolates should be identified to species level, and antifungal susceptibility testing done to guide therapy. Although non-yeast fungi are occasionally reported to cause fungal peritonitis, Candida species still account for the majority of cases [4,6,8]. The newer azoles, voriconazole and posaconazole may be alternatives to amphotericin B when filamentous fungi are cultured [3]. Systematic study of larger numbers of patients are required to determine their position in the treatment of fungal peritonitis.

The overall mortality rate of fungal peritonitis has been reported to be 9–60%; with increased age, abdominal pain (with or without fever) and retained PD catheters the most frequently identified factors predicting mortality [4,5,8,20]. In the present study, increased mortality was noted in those with retained catheters, emphasising the importance of prompt catheter removal when managing fungal peritonitis [3]. Although late (especially after 5 days following diagnosis) catheter removal has been associated with poorer survival [6,21], this was not found in this and several other studies, perhaps due to the high rates of catheter removal at the outset and prompt initiation of antifungal therapy [4,22]. This may have also accounted for the equivalent mortality rates between fungal and bacterial peritonitis that was observed, in contrast to previous reports of higher mortality rates for fungal peritonitis [3,6]. Notably, fungal peritonitis patients with polymicrobial infection were more likely to die (Table 3). Fungal peritonitis was significantly associated with longer hospital stay, removal of the PD catheter, commencement of haemodialysis and receipt of systemic antifungal therapy.

The limitations of our study include the retrospective nature of the study, the lack of PD submodality analysis (continuous ambulatory vs. automated) as other potential risk factors for fungal peritonitis, and the potential biases that may have been introduced when matching fungal to bacterial peritonitis using PD registries, and by survivor bias. Our small sample size, although not enabling multivariate analysis for risk of death and involving only two large referral institutions, is nevertheless representative of the population of patients that suffer PD-related infectious complications.

In conclusion, fungal peritonitis is a serious PD-related complication. Morbidity is high and permanent cessation of peritoneal dialysis common despite adherence to management guidelines. Prompt recognition, especially in patients who have had their catheter in situ for a prolonged period, and removal of the catheter are key considerations in optimising outcomes.

Methods

Ethics Statement

Approval was obtained from the respective Human Research Ethics Committees of the Sydney West (SCA2008/8/5.3 [2846]) and Sydney South West (QA2009/071) Area Health Services. As the study was performed retrospectively with no intervention arm, the need for patient consent was waived by the Ethics Committees.

Episodes of fungal peritonitis occurring between January 2001 to March 2010 in PD patients at Liverpool and Westmead Hospitals (Sydney, New South Wales, Australia) were retrospectively identified from both institution's microbiology laboratory information systems and medical records. An episode of peritonitis was defined as the presence of any clinical sign of peritonism (including fever, abdominal tenderness and rebound tenderness) or peritoneal fluid (effluent) leucocyte count of $>100 \times 10^6$/L with a positive microbiological culture [4].

Fungal peritonitis cases were matched in a 1:2 ratio with patients diagnosed with bacterial peritonitis from each institution's dialysis registry, occurring closest in time to the fungal episode. Denominator data obtained included the total patient-years of dialysis for the entire period.

Each patient's medical record was examined for demographic data and relevant history pertaining to ESKD (including aetiology, severity [as determined by erythropoietin-stimulating agent and phosphate binder/calcimimetic use], the date of PD commencement and duration of PD with the current catheter [inferred from the date of catheter insertion]). Data on previous peritonitis episodes, antibiotic use within the preceding 30 days, clinical symptoms and signs (e.g. fever, abdominal pain, hypotension) on presentation were also extracted, as was the presence of PD catheter exit site infection, antimicrobial therapy given, surgical procedures and hospital length of stay (if hospitalised). Laboratory

data obtained include the cellular (white cells) profile results, identification and antimicrobial susceptibility profile of all positive peritoneal fluid and blood culture isolates, haematological and biochemical parameters, and C-reactive protein. Clinical outcomes including overall (all cause) 30-day mortality and technique failure (defined as permanent cessation of PD) were recorded.

Data were analysed using SSPS statistical software (version 18.0, IBM, Chicago, IL). For univariate analyses, categorical variables were analysed using Fisher's exact test or χ^2 test and for continuous variables, the student's t-test; p values<0.05 were considered statistically significant. Multivariate analysis was not performed due to the small sample size of fungal peritonitis cases (n = 39).

Acknowledgments

The authors wish to thank the Departments of Renal Medicine at Liverpool and Westmead Hospitals, Ms. Kathy Kable for providing the numbers of patients receiving peritoneal dialysis during the study period, and Mr Brain O'Toole for assisting with statistical analysis. This work was presented in part at the 50th Interscience Conference on Antimicrobial Agents and Chemotherapy (ICAAC) meeting, Boston, September 2010.

Author Contributions

Conceived and designed the experiments: SvH SC. Performed the experiments: RC JK SvH SC. Analyzed the data: RC JK SvH SC. Contributed reagents/materials/analysis tools: RC JK SvH SC. Wrote the paper: RC JK SvH SC.

References

1. U.S. Renal Data System (2010) USRDS 2010 Annual data report: Atlas of chronic kidney disease and end-stage renal disease in the Unites States, National Institutes of Health, National Institute of Diabetes and Digestive and Kidney Diseases, Bethesda, MD. Available: http://www.usrds.org/default.asp. Accessed 2011 May 21.
2. Australia and New Zealand Dialysis and Transplant Registry 33rd Annual Report 2010 (Data to 2009) (2010) Available: http://www.anzdata.org.au/v1/report_2010.html. Accessed 2011 January 21.
3. Li PK, Szeto CC, Piraino B, Bernardini J, Figueiredo AE, et al. (2010) Peritoneal dialysis-related infections recommendations: 2010 update. Perit Dial Int 30: 393–423.
4. Miles R, Hawley CM, McDonald SP, Brown FG, Rosman JB, et al. (2009) Predictors and outcomes of fungal peritonitis in peritoneal dialysis patients. Kidney Int 76: 622–628.
5. Troidle L, Gorban-Brennan N, Kliger A, Finkelstein FO (2003) Continuous peritoneal dialysis-associated peritonitis: A review and current concepts. Semin Dial 16: 428–437.
6. Wang AY, Yu AW, Li PK, Lam PK, Leung CB, et al. (2000) Factors predicting outcome of fungal peritonitis in peritoneal dialysis: Analysis of a 9-year experience of fungal peritonitis in a single center. Am J Kidney Dis 36: 1183–1192.
7. Mujais S (2006) Microbiology and outcomes of peritonitis in North America. Kidney Int 103: S55–S62.
8. Prasad N, Gupta A (2005) Fungal peritonitis in peritoneal dialysis patients. Perit Dial Int 25: 207–222.
9. Clinical Laboratory Standards Institute (CLSI) (2010) Performance standards for antifungal susceptibility testing; sixteenth informational supplement. CLSI document M27-A3 & M27-S3. Wayne, PA.
10. Gandhi BV, Bahadur MM, Dodeja H, Aggrwal V, Thamba A, et al. (2005) Systemic fungal infections in renal diseases. J Postgrad Med 51: 30–36.
11. Matsuzkiewicz-Rowinska J (2009) Update on fungal peritonitis and its treatment. Perit Dial Int 29(suppl): S161–S165.

12. Ram R, Swarnalatha G, Neela P, Murty KV (2008) Fungal peritonitis in patients on continuous ambulatory peritoneal dialysis: a single-centre experience in India. Nephron Clin Pract 110: c207–c212.
13. Bren A (1998) Fungal peritonitis in patients on continuous ambulatory peritoneal dialysis: a report of 17 cases. Eur J Clin Microbiol Infect Dis 17: 839–843.
14. Chen C, Ho M, Yu W, Wang J (2004) Fungal peritonitis in perioneal dialysis patients: effect of fluconazole treatment and use of the twin-bag disconnect system. J Microb Immunol Infect 37: 115–120.
15. Restrepo C, Chacon J, Manjarres G (2010) Fungal peritonitis in peritoneal dialysis patients: Successful prophylaxis with fluconazole, as demonstrated by prospective randomized control trial. Perit Dial Int 30: 619–625.
16. Wong P, Lo K, Tong GM, Chan SF, Lo MW, et al. (2007) Prevention of fungal peritonitis with nystatin prophylaxis in patients receiving CAPD. Perit Dial Int 27: 531–536.
17. Pfaller MA, Diekema DJ (2010) Epidemiology of invasive candidiasis: a persistent public health problem. Clin Microbiol Rev 20: 133–163.
18. Kestenbaum B, Sampson JN, Rudser KD, Patterson DJ, Seliger SL, et al. (2005) Serum phosphate levels and mortality risk among people with chronic kidney disease. J Am Soc Nephrol 16: 520–528.
19. Mohanram A, Zhang Z, Shahinfar S, Keane WF, Brenner BM, et al. (2004) Anemia and end-stage renal disease in patients with type 2 diabetes and nephropahty. Kidney Int 66: 1131–1138.
20. Oygar DD, Altiparmak MR, Murtezaoglu A, Yalin AS, Ataman R, et al. (2009) Fungal peritonitis in peritoneal dialysis: Risk factors and prognosis. Renal Failure 31: 25–28.
21. Chang TI, Kim HW, Park JT, Lee DH, Lee JH, et al. (2011) Early catheter removal improves patient survival in peritoneal dialysis patients with fungal peritonitis: Results of ninety-four episodes of fungal peritonitis at a single centre. Perit Dial Int 31: 60–66.
22. Wong P, Lo K, Tong GM, Chan SF, Lo MW, et al. (2008) Treatment of fungal peritonitis with a combination of intravenous amphotericin B and oral flucytosine, and delayed catheter replacement in continuous ambulatory peritoneal dialysis. Perit Dial Int 28: 155–162.

12

Laparoscopic versus Open Peritoneal Dialysis Catheter Insertion

Sander M. Hagen[1], Jeffrey A. Lafranca[1], Ewout W. Steyerberg[2], Jan N. M. IJzermans[1], Frank J. M. F. Dor[1]*

1 Department of Surgery, Erasmus MC, University Medical Center, Rotterdam, The Netherlands, **2** Department of Public Health, Erasmus MC, University Medical Center, Rotterdam, The Netherlands

Abstract

Background: Peritoneal dialysis is an effective treatment for end-stage renal disease. Key to successful peritoneal dialysis is a well-functioning catheter. The different insertion techniques may be of great importance. Mostly, the standard operative approach is the open technique; however, laparoscopic insertion is increasingly popular. Catheter malfunction is reported up to 35% for the open technique and up to 13% for the laparoscopic technique. However, evidence is lacking to definitely conclude that the laparoscopic approach is to be preferred. This review and meta-analysis was carried out to investigate if one of the techniques is superior to the other.

Methods: Comprehensive searches were conducted in MEDLINE, Embase and CENTRAL (the Cochrane Library 2012, issue 10). Reference lists were searched manually. The methodology was in accordance with the Cochrane Handbook for interventional systematic reviews, and written based on the PRISMA-statement.

Results: Three randomized controlled trials and eight cohort studies were identified. Nine postoperative outcome measures were meta-analyzed; of these, seven were not different between operation techniques. Based on the meta-analysis, the proportion of migrating catheters was lower (odds ratio (OR) 0.21, confidence interval (CI) 0.07 to 0.63; P = 0.006), and the one-year catheter survival was higher in the laparoscopic group (OR 3.93, CI 1.80 to 8.57; P = 0.0006).

Conclusions: Based on these results there is some evidence in favour of the laparoscopic insertion technique for having a higher one-year catheter survival and less migration, which would be clinically relevant.

Editor: Mercedes Susan Mandell, University of Colorado, United States of America

Funding: The authors have no support or funding to report.

Competing Interests: The authors declare no competing interests.

* E-mail: f.dor@erasmusmc.nl

Introduction

Peritoneal dialysis (PD) is an effective treatment for end-stage renal disease (ESRD) [1–4]. The most important benefit of PD relative to haemodialysis is the preservation of residual renal function, which equates to improved survival during the first several years of therapy [5]. The key to successful PD is the presence of a well-functioning dialysis catheter, defined as one that facilitates free dialysis solution in- and outflow. However, several complications, such as in- and outflow obstruction, peritonitis, exit-site infections, leakage and migration, can lead to catheter removal and loss of peritoneal access [6]. Currently, different surgical techniques are in practice for PD catheter placement [6–10]. The insertion technique may have a great influence on the occurrence of complications. The literature describes a 10–35% catheter failure rate when using the open technique [11–14] and 2.8–13% catheter failures for the laparoscopic insertion technique [15–18].

The open technique is still the most frequently used technique. However, laparoscopic procedures have proven to be superior to a number of open surgical procedures, by reducing morbidity, length of hospital stay, postoperative pain and lead to a quicker convalescence [19–22]. In case of PD catheter insertion, the laparoscopic approach enables the surgeon to insert the PD catheter under direct vision and thus at the end of the operation the correct catheter position is assured, which may lead to a better and prolonged catheter function.

In the existing literature, there is no consensus about the preferred operative technique for PD catheter insertion. Our aim is to investigate whether there is a preferable method or not, when data from the literature are reviewed and analyzed systematically. In 2004, Strippoli et al. [23] performed a review of the literature up to April 2004, summarizing data comparing laparoscopic, peritoneoscopic and open insertion of PD catheters. This study only included randomized controlled trials and the primary outcome was the prevention of peritonitis. Furthermore, in 2012, Xie et al. [24] performed a review and meta-analysis of the literature. However, this study also included trials using other techniques and studying other populations. Our systematic review includes randomized controlled trials as well as cohort studies up to October 2012, describing multiple outcomes of studies comparing the laparoscopic and open technique in adults.

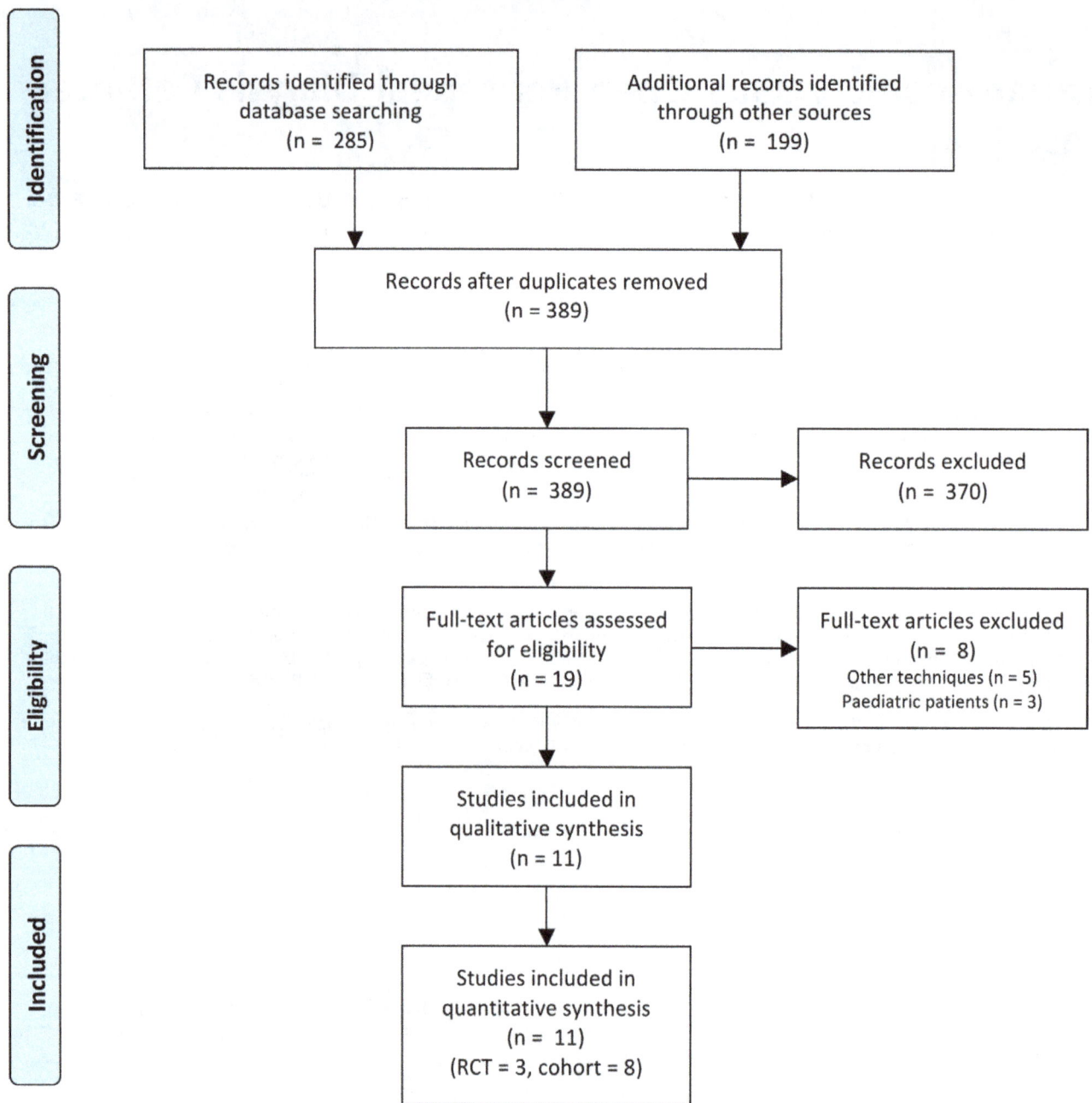

Figure 1. PRISMA flow diagram of the systematic literature search.

Methods

All aspects of the Cochrane Handbook for Interventional Systematic Reviews were followed and the study was written according to the Preferred Reporting Items for Systematic Reviews and Meta-Analyses (PRISMA) statement [25]. A review protocol was drafted before the initial search was started.

Literature Search Strategy

Comprehensive searches were carried out in MEDLINE, Embase and CENTRAL (the Cochrane Library 2012, issue 10). The search was performed for articles published up to October 2012 relevant to outcome of laparoscopic or open insertion of a PD catheter. There was no publication year or publication language restriction applied. The search-string used in PubMed was ("Peritoneal Dialysis"[Majr] AND (Laparoscopy OR laparotomy OR open)) AND ("catheters"[Majr] OR catheter). Other databases were searched with comparable terms, suitable for the specific database. Reference lists of the identified relevant studies were scrutinized for additional citations.

Literature Screening

Studies were evaluated for inclusion by two independent researchers (SMH, JAL) for relevance to the subject. A random check was performed by a supervisor (FJMFD). Study selection was accomplished through three phases of study screening. In phase 1, the following types of studies were excluded: reviews,

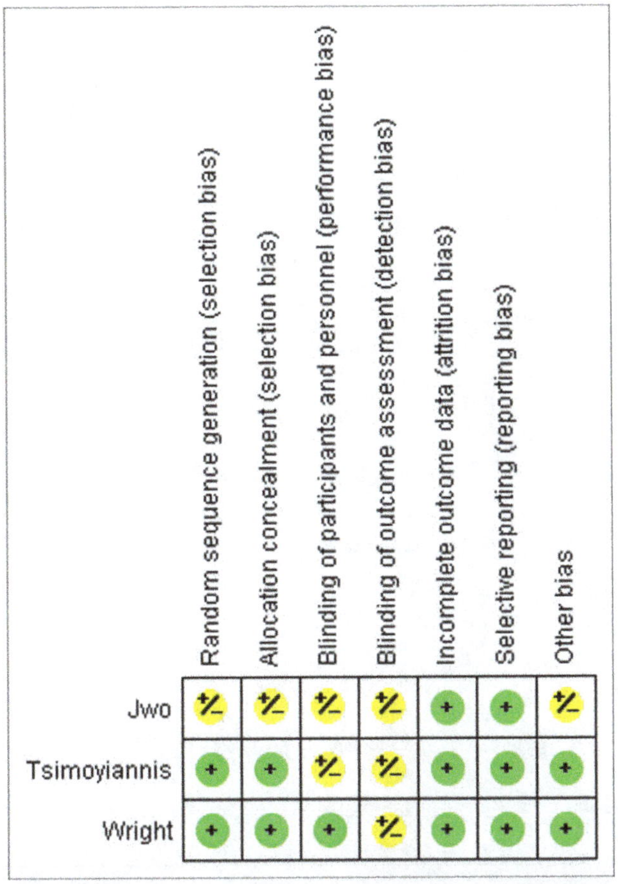

Figure 2. Risk of bias summary graph of the included studies.
The green symbol indicates that there is possibly a low level of bias, red symbolizes a possible high level of bias and a yellow symbol is presented if the risk of bias is unclear.

case-reports, letters, editorials, case-series, and papers studying non-human, infants and/or adolescents. In phase 2, abstracts were reviewed for relevance and the full-text articles were obtained. In phase 3, full-text articles were reviewed; inclusion required studies describing laparoscopic and open insertion of the PD catheter. The studies had to describe one or more of the following outcome measures to be included: incidence of peritonitis, exit-site/tunnel infection, pericanullar leakage, catheter migration, catheter removal for complications, need for revision and catheter survival. Any discrepancies in in- or exclusion were resolved by discussion between the reviewers with supervision of a third person.

Data Extraction and Critical Appraisal

The level of evidence of each paper was established following the Oxford Centre for Evidence-Based Medicine Level of Evidence scale [26,27] and by using the GRADE tool [28]. The quality and the potential of bias of the randomized controlled trials were assessed according to the Cochrane Collaboration's tool for assessing risk of bias by Higgins [29].

Statistical Analysis

Odds ratios (OR) and their 95% confidence interval (CI) were calculated from raw data using patients with an open catheter insertion as the control group. A meta-analysis was performed with complications and catheter survival as outcome measures using

Review Manager Software (RevMan, 5.1; The Nordic Cochrane Centre, Copenhagen, Denmark). Each study was weighted by sample size. Heterogeneity of treatment effects between studies was tested using the Q (heterogeneity χ^2) and the I^2 statistics. A random-effects model was used for calculating the summary estimates and 95% CI, to account for possible clinical heterogeneity. Overall effects were determined using the Z-test. In addition, the individual study effect on the results was examined by removing each study at a time to examine whether removing a particular study would significantly change the results.

Results

Of the 285 papers found after the initial search, eleven fell within the scope of the study; three randomized controlled trials [14,30,31] and eight cohort studies [32–39]. These eleven studies were represented by twelve individual references. One publication (by Crabtree et al. 2005) was excluded for describing patients that were already described in another paper in 2000 by the same group [40]. No additional studies were included after manually scrutinizing reference lists. The PRISMA [25] flow diagram for systematic reviews is presented in figure 1. The assessment of the quality of the included studies is presented in figure 2. A meta-analysis was performed using a total of eleven studies; the characteristics of these studies are presented in table 1. Definitions of the analyzed outcome measures are presented in table 2.

Infections (Peritonitis, Exit-site/Tunnel Infection)

Nine studies [14,30–32,34–36,38,39] that investigated the incidence of peritonitis after PD catheter insertion were included for meta-analysis, with a total of 541 patients. There was no statistically significant difference in the risk of developing peritonitis between treatment groups (OR 0.83, 95% CI 0.48 to 1.42; P = 0.49).

With a total of 474 patients from seven studies [14,31,32,34–36,39], the pooled incidence of exit-site/tunnel infection was calculated in the meta-analysis. There was no statistically significant difference in the risk of developing an exit-site/tunnel infection between laparoscopic or open PD catheter insertion (OR 0.80, 95% CI 0.47 to 1.37; P = 0.41). (figure 3).

Catheter-related Outcome (Migration, Leakage and Obstruction)

The incidence of PD catheter migration was described in five studies [14,30,34,38,39], with a total of 319 patients, and were used to perform a meta-analysis. Migration occurred statistically significant less frequent in the laparoscopic group (OR 0.21, 95% CI 0.07 to 0.63; P = 0.006). With nine studies [14,30–35,37–39], with a total of 826 patients, the pooled incidence of leakage was calculated. There is no statistically significant difference between the two treatment groups (OR 0.88, 95% CI 0.40 to 1.92; p = 0.74). The incidence of obstructed/dysfunctioning catheters was reported for 665 patients in six studies [31–36] and was used for meta-analysis. There was a borderline statistically significant difference in favour of the laparoscopic group in this respect between the two treatment methods (OR 0.39, 95% CI 0.14 to 1.07; P = 0.07) (figure 4).

Interventional Outcome (Surgical Intervention/Catheter Revision and Removal)

The need for a surgical intervention or catheter revision was described in four studies [32,35,37,38], with a total of 165 patients. After meta-analysis, the need for an intervention showed no difference between groups (OR 0.32, CI 0.08 to 1.26; P = 0.10)

Table 1. Characteristics of studies comparing laparoscopic and open PD catheter insertion.

Reference	Year	Country	Study type	Groups	N	Evidence
Li [39]	2011	Taiwan	Prospective cohort	Laparoscopic	50	2b
				Open	23	
Jwo [14]	2010	Taiwan	RCT	Laparoscopic	37	2b
				Open	40	
Gajjar [32]	2007	USA	Retrospective cohort	Laparoscopic	45	2b
				Open	30	
Lund [38]	2007	Denmark	Retrospective cohort	Laparoscopic	9	2b
				Open	13	
Crabtree [33]	2005	USA	Prospective cohort	Laparoscopic	278	2b
				Open	63	
Soontrapornchai [34]	2005	Thailand	Prospective cohort	Laparoscopic	50	2b
				Open	52	
Ögünç [35]	2003	Turkey	Prospective cohort	Laparoscopic	21	2b
				Open	21	
Batey [37]	2002	USA	Retrospective cohort	Laparoscopic	14	2b
				Open	12	
Tsimoyiannis [30]	2000	Greece	RCT	Laparoscopic	25	2b
				Open	25	
Wright [31]	1999	UK	RCT	Laparoscopic	24	1b
				Open	21	
Draganic [36]	1998	Australia	Retrospective cohort	Laparoscopic	30	2b
				Open	30	

RCT: Randomized controlled trial, n.a.: not applicable.

The removal of PD catheters as mentioned above was investigated in seven studies [14,30,31,35–38], including a total of 317 patients. The meta-analysis showed no statistically significant difference between the two groups. (OR 0.65, 95% CI 0.35 to 1.21; P = 0.17) (figure 5).

Overall Catheter Survival, Year 1 and 2

The probability of catheter survival at one year postoperatively was investigated in five studies [30,31,34,35,39], with a total of 307 patients. The 1-year survival of the catheters was statistically significant higher in the laparoscopic group (OR 3.93, 95% CI 1.80 to 8.57; P = 0.0006) The chance of catheter survival at two years postoperatively was described for 262 patients in four studies [31,34,35,39]. There was a borderline statistically significant difference in catheter survival at this time point (OR 2.17, CI 0.99 to 4.75; P = 0.05) (figure 6).

The quality of evidence of each study and outcome measure are presented as a summary of findings in figure 7. In this figure, the risk differences are presented, using which the numbers needed to treat (NNT) can be derived. For the statistically significant different outcome measures, the NNT are 8 (migration) and 6 (catheter survival year 1). Furthermore, as stated in the methods section, the quality of the RCTs was assessed by the Higgins-classification. No studies were excluded based on this classification. Sensitivity analysis, by removing each study separately, did not change results significantly, except for obstruction (when Ögünç [35] and/or Soontrapornchai [34] were excluded, respectively P = 0.03 and P = 0.01, cumulative P<0.0001) and catheter intervention/replacement/revision (when Batey [37] was exclud-

ed, P = 0.004). Additionally, sensitivity analysis was performed per type of study (RCT versus cohort) and no differences were found.

Discussion

This systematic review and meta-analysis reveals that the laparoscopic PD catheter insertion technique is to be preferred over the conventional open technique. Catheter survival at one year is higher in the laparoscopic group and the incidence of catheter migration is lower in this group. Furthermore, laparoscopic insertion of the PD-catheters assumingly would result in higher patient comfort, lower hospital costs and better overall PD results.

Recently, a similar meta-analysis was published by Xie et al. [24] of which the conclusion is that laparoscopic catheter placement has no superiority to open surgery. However, the authors included two studies that assessed a different technique (peritoneoscopic and percutaneous insertion) and studies including pediatric patients. In our opinion, those studies do not comply with the inclusion criteria that should be used for a meta-analysis regarding this specific topic, being aware of possible selection bias, and therefore potentially a false conclusion is drawn by the authors. In addition, the papers of Lund and Li [38,39], are not included at all.

Large case series reported no difference in the incidence of peritonitis when using the open insertion technique (2.9–31%) [41–44] or the laparoscopic technique (2.5–31%) [15,45,46]. The pooled data in this meta-analysis also shows no significant difference in the incidence of peritonitis in agreement with these studies, but there seems to be an overall trend in favour of

Table 2. List of variables/outcome measures meta-analyzed and the definitions stated by the authors.

Reference	Peritonitis	Exit-site Infection	Migration	Catheter obstruction	Leakage	Intervention/revision	Catheter removal	Catheter survival
Li [39]	Abdominal pain, cloudy effluent with white blood cell count higher than 100/mm3 and/or polymorphonuclear neutrophils larger than 50%, and identification of microorganisms	Not described	transient or prolonged, catheter malfunction during follow up and confirmed by abdominal KUB films	–	Fluid extravasation from the catheter exit-site related to dialysate infusion	–	–	'catheter dysfunction-free'
Jwo [14]	Not described	Not described	Not described	–	exit-site leak, wound leak, or extra-abdominal dialysate outflow	–	Inadequate dialysis, peritonitis, hydrocele, hydrothorax, change to HD	catheter survival excluding patients with catheter dropout due to clearly unrelated causes such as renal transplantation, renal recovery, or death from unrelated underlying diseases
Tsimoyiannis [30]	Not described	–	Not described	–	Not described	–	Peritonitis	Not described
Wright [31]	Early: <6 weeks post-op Late: >6 weeks post-op	Not described	–	Not described	Not described	–	(pseudomonas) peritonitis, ultra filtration failure, patient death	See 'removal'
Gajjar [32]	Not described	Not described	–	Not described	Early: occur within 30 days of insertion, Late: occur after 30 days of insertion	Not described	–	
Crabtree [33]	–	–	–	Not described	Not described	–	–	–
Soontrapornchai [34]	Not described	Not described	Radiological confirmation	Not described	Not described	–	–	calculated from the day of insertion to the day of revision or removal
Öğünç [35]	Early: <4 weeks post-op Late: >4 weeks post-op	Positive microbiological of an organism from peritoneal fluid on ether Gram staining or culture	–	Due to omental wrapping and/or fibrin clotting	Not described	Pericatheter leak, chronic tunnel infection, chronic exit-site infection	Relapse or resistant peritonitis, Successful transplantation, Persistent dialysate leak, exit-site infection, patient's choice, treatment failure	'Catheter failure free'
Draganic [36]	positive microbiological identification of an organism from peritoneal fluid on either Gram staining or culture	any surrounding inflammation which required additional dressings or antibiotics	–	Not described		–	Exit-site infection, peritonitis	–
Batey [37]	–	–	–	–	Not described	Migration, Occlusion	Peritonitis, infected hematoma, persistent scrotal swelling	–
Lund [38]	Not described	–	Not described	–	–	'Displacement'	'Displacement'	

KUB = kidneys, ureters and bladder.

Study or Subgroup	Laparoscopy Events	Total	Open Events	Total	Weight	Odds Ratio M-H, Random, 95% CI
1.1.1 Peritonitis						
Draganic	5	30	7	30	12.4%	0.66 [0.18, 2.36]
Gajjar	8	45	6	30	13.9%	0.86 [0.27, 2.80]
Jwo	10	37	6	40	14.7%	2.10 [0.68, 6.50]
Li	1	50	1	23	3.4%	0.45 [0.03, 7.51]
Lund	1	9	0	13	2.5%	4.76 [0.17, 130.96]
Ogünc	3	21	11	21	9.9%	0.15 [0.03, 0.67]
Soontrapornchai	16	50	13	52	20.0%	1.41 [0.59, 3.35]
Tsimoyiannis	3	25	5	20	9.2%	0.41 [0.08, 1.98]
Wright	9	21	12	24	13.9%	0.75 [0.23, 2.44]
Subtotal (95% CI)		288		253	100.0%	0.83 [0.48, 1.42]
Total events	56		61			

Heterogeneity: Tau² = 0.19; Chi² = 11.16, df = 8 (P = 0.19); I² = 28%
Test for overall effect: Z = 0.70 (P = 0.49)

Study or Subgroup	Laparoscopy Events	Total	Open Events	Total	Weight	Odds Ratio M-H, Random, 95% CI
1.1.2 Exit-site/tunnel Infection						
Draganic	5	30	5	30	15.7%	1.00 [0.26, 3.89]
Gajjar	2	45	3	30	8.4%	0.42 [0.07, 2.67]
Jwo	6	37	5	40	17.6%	1.35 [0.38, 4.88]
Li	3	50	2	23	8.3%	0.67 [0.10, 4.31]
Ogünc	6	21	10	21	17.7%	0.44 [0.12, 1.58]
Soontrapornchai	3	50	5	52	13.0%	0.60 [0.14, 2.66]
Wright	8	21	8	24	19.3%	1.23 [0.36, 4.18]
Subtotal (95% CI)		254		220	100.0%	0.80 [0.47, 1.37]
Total events	33		38			

Heterogeneity: Tau² = 0.00; Chi² = 2.72, df = 6 (P = 0.84); I² = 0%
Test for overall effect: Z = 0.82 (P = 0.41)

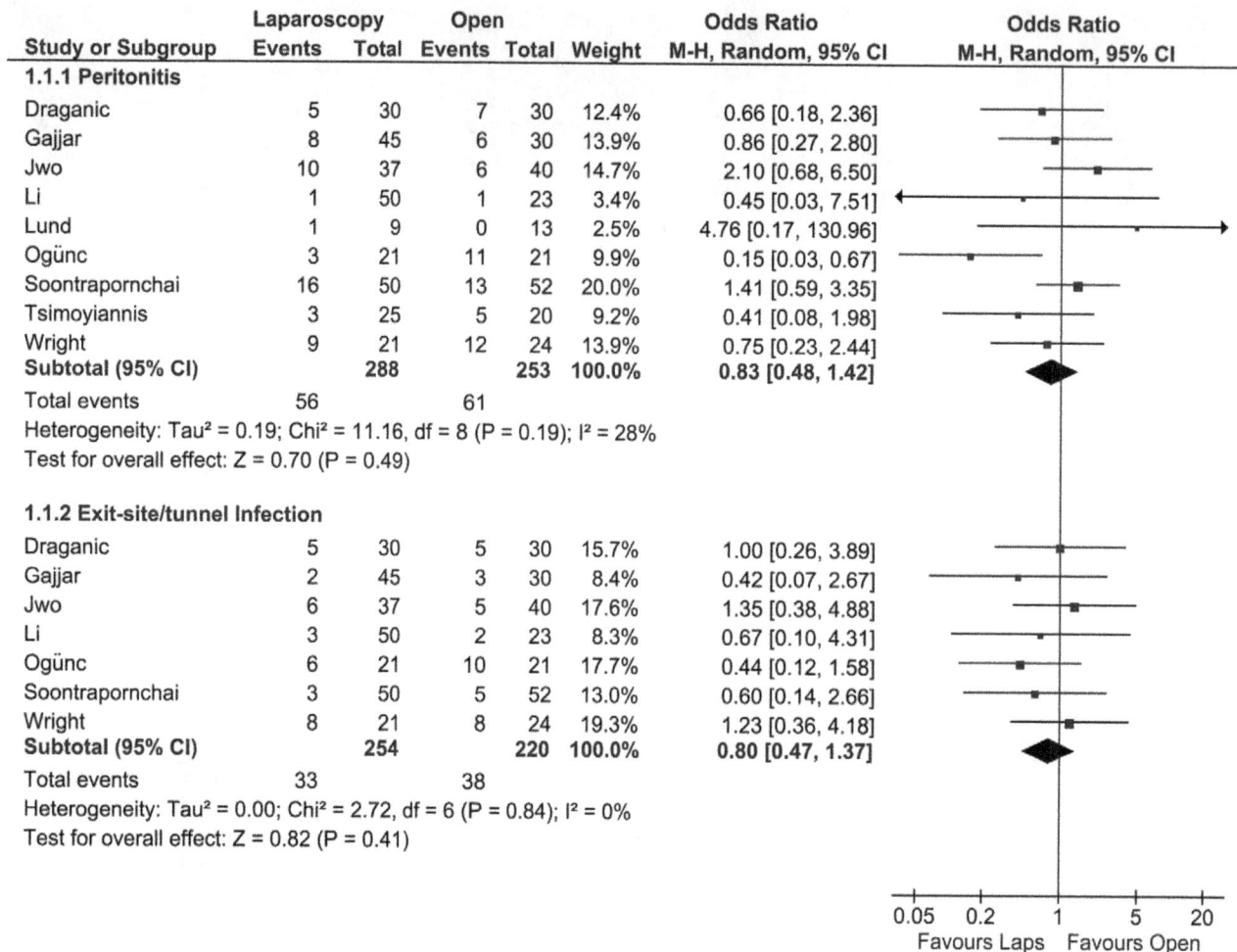

Odds Ratio M-H, Random, 95% CI
0.05 0.2 1 5 20
Favours Laps   Favours Open

Figure 3. Forest plot. Odds ratios of the incidence of peritonitis and exit-site/tunnel infection, evaluating the statistical difference between laparoscopic and open PD catheter insertion. CI: confidence interval.

laparoscopy. The variety in peritonitis incidence in different reports may partly be due to a different antibiotic (AB) prophylaxis regimen used. There is no consensus about which AB to administer and when it should be given to prevent peritonitis. The type of AB used, may influence the incidence of peritonitis [47]. Five studies [30,34,36,38,39] in our analysis made no mention of (specific) antibiotic prophylaxis, five studies [14,32,33,35,37] reported the use of cefazolin and one study [31] the use of vancomycin. However, Gadallah [48] reported in a large RCT that the use of 1 g vancomycin preoperatively significantly reduced the risk of developing peritonitis in comparison with 1 g cefazolin and no antibiotic at all. International guidelines state that the use of vancomycin is to be preferred [49].

The incidence of exit-site/tunnel infections does not differ between the laparoscopic and open insertion technique. In all cases, the PD catheter was subcutaneously tunnelled, which is thought to reduce the incidence of exit-site infections, regardless of the insertion technique [50,51]. The literature, not analyzed in this meta-analysis, suggests a higher incidence of exit-site infections in the open group (6.3–41% [41–44]) versus the laparoscopic group (2.5–18% [15,45]). The time to start the actual PD after catheter insertion may be a possible confounder regarding this issue. Authors of some of the studies included in this analysis favour immediate PD start [30,35] where others suggest a waiting period

of 3 to 5 days [36] or two weeks [31–34]. Two studies [35,36] started PD 1 week earlier in the laparoscopic group than in the open group. Therefore, a definite conclusion is not possible to be drawn. Currently, Ranganathan [52] is performing a randomized controlled trial to determine what the most appropriate time to start PD after catheter insertion might be. The correlation between exit-site infections and peritonitis remains to be elucidated.

One might reason that the influence of the surgical insertion technique on migration is different in the early phase as compared to late phase postoperatively. A subgroup analysis on this issue was desired, but there was insufficient data to perform such an analysis.

Migration is reported in case-series in 1.3–5.4% of the laparoscopically inserted PD catheters [15,27,45] and in 7.6–17.1% when using the open technique [41,44,53]. A possible advantage of the laparoscopic insertion technique might be the ability to fixate the catheter to the ventral abdominal wall. Jwo, Li, Lund, Soontrapornchai and Tsimoyiannis [14,30,34,38,39] accurately described the incidence of migration. Li, Soontrapornchai and Tsimoyiannis used a fixation technique in the laparoscopic group; they reported no migration. The overall effectiveness of laparoscopic insertion to prevent catheter migration seems clear, but the benefit of catheter fixation is still under investigation. Ashegh et al. [15] reported 1.3% migration without fixation of the

Study or Subgroup	Laparoscopy Events	Total	Open Events	Total	Weight	Odds Ratio M-H, Random, 95% CI	Odds Ratio M-H, Random, 95% CI
1.2.1 Migration							
Jwo	4	37	7	40	43.6%	0.57 [0.15, 2.14]	
Li	0	50	4	23	12.5%	0.04 [0.00, 0.83]	
Lund	1	9	4	13	18.2%	0.28 [0.03, 3.07]	
Soontrapornchai	0	50	6	52	13.0%	0.07 [0.00, 1.29]	
Tsimoyiannis	0	25	5	20	12.6%	0.06 [0.00, 1.07]	
Subtotal (95% CI)		**171**		**148**	**100.0%**	**0.21 [0.07, 0.63]**	
Total events	5		26				

Heterogeneity: Tau² = 0.29; Chi² = 4.81, df = 4 (P = 0.31); I² = 17%
Test for overall effect: Z = 2.78 (P = 0.006)

1.2.2 Leakage							
Batey	1	14	5	12	9.6%	0.11 [0.01, 1.11]	
Crabtree	5	278	1	63	11.0%	1.14 [0.13, 9.89]	
Gajjar	5	45	4	30	21.1%	0.81 [0.20, 3.31]	
Jwo	8	37	7	40	27.7%	1.30 [0.42, 4.03]	
Li	2	50	0	23	5.9%	2.42 [0.11, 52.51]	
Ogünc	1	21	0	21	5.3%	3.15 [0.12, 81.74]	
Soontrapornchai	1	50	1	52	7.0%	1.04 [0.06, 17.11]	
Tsimoyiannis	0	25	5	20	6.3%	0.06 [0.00, 1.07]	
Wright	2	21	0	24	5.9%	6.28 [0.28, 138.62]	
Subtotal (95% CI)		**541**		**285**	**100.0%**	**0.88 [0.40, 1.92]**	
Total events	25		23				

Heterogeneity: Tau² = 0.25; Chi² = 9.69, df = 8 (P = 0.29); I² = 17%
Test for overall effect: Z = 0.33 (P = 0.74)

1.2.3 Obstruction							
Crabtree	11	278	11	63	32.0%	0.19 [0.08, 0.47]	
Draganic	1	30	3	30	13.0%	0.31 [0.03, 3.17]	
Gajjar	1	45	6	30	14.3%	0.09 [0.01, 0.80]	
Ogünc	5	21	5	21	23.0%	1.00 [0.24, 4.14]	
Soontrapornchai	3	50	2	52	17.7%	1.60 [0.26, 9.98]	
Wright	0	21	0	24		Not estimable	
Subtotal (95% CI)		**445**		**220**	**100.0%**	**0.39 [0.14, 1.07]**	
Total events	21		27				

Heterogeneity: Tau² = 0.62; Chi² = 7.91, df = 4 (P = 0.10); I² = 49%
Test for overall effect: Z = 1.82 (P = 0.07)

```
   0.005   0.1    1    10   200
      Favours Laps  Favours Open
```

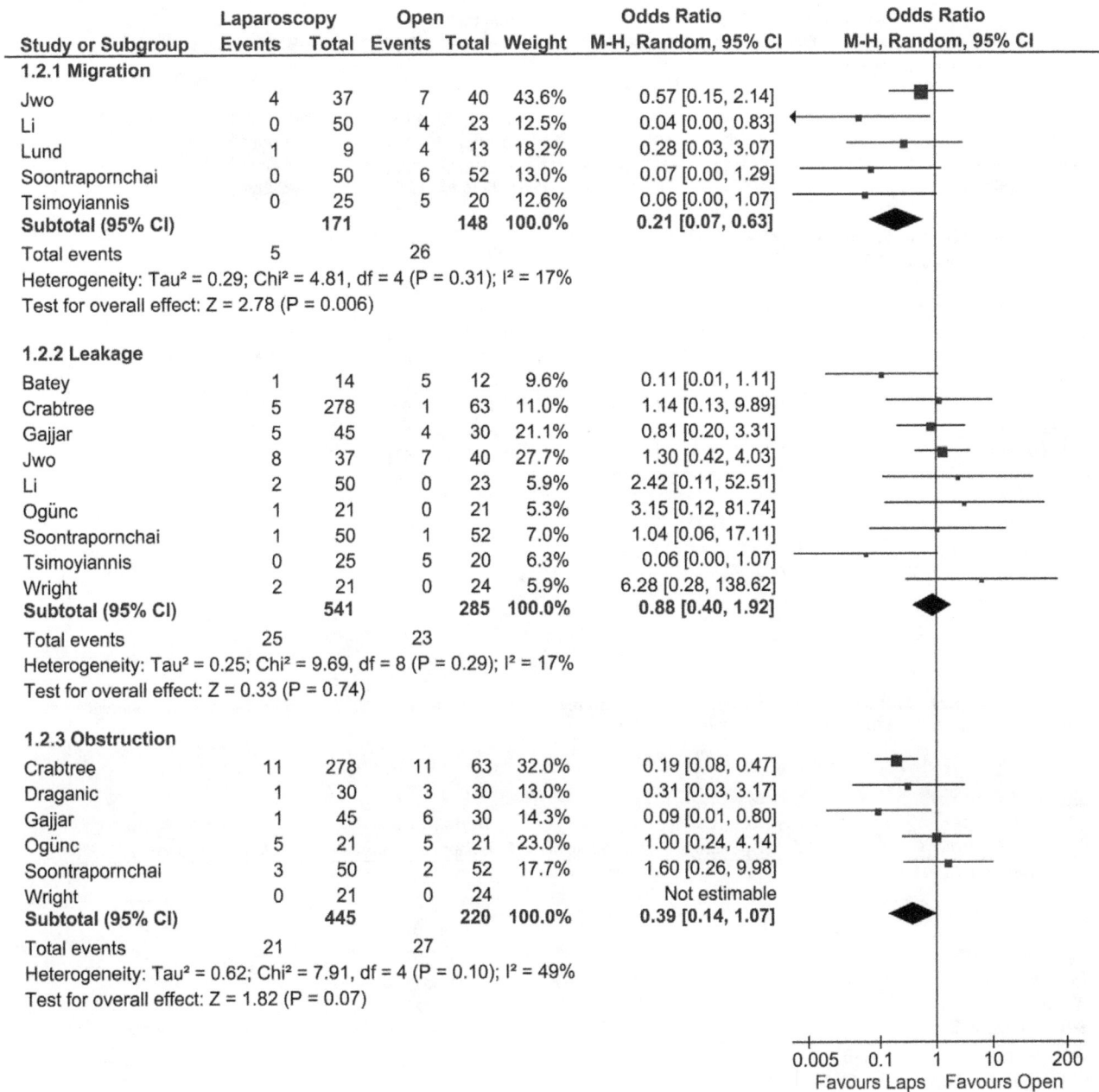

Figure 4. Forest plot. Odds ratios of the incidence of migration, leakage and obstruction, evaluating the statistical difference between laparoscopic and open PD catheter insertion. CI: confidence interval.

catheter tip and Lo et al. [27] 5.4% with fixation during laparoscopic insertion. Chen et al. [54] used a fixation technique in the open approach and reported no migration. Complication rates are reported to be comparable in case-series using fixation and no fixation [15,27,54]. Good clinical trials comparing fixation with no fixation are not available in literature. Besides the suture technique, rectus sheath tunneling might also contribute to a lower migration rate. Soontrapornchai, Ögünç and Crabtree [33–35] used this technique, but only Soontrapornchai reported the migration rate accurately and could be included for analysis.

Different types of catheters are used in the studies included in this analysis. This may bias the results of catheter obstruction/dysfunction. Also, the use of either a coiled or a straight catheter might influence the results. Swartz et al. have suggested that the use of coiled catheters reduces the incidence of catheter dysfunction [55]. The literature, not analyzed in the meta-analysis, does not show consensus at this point. Johnson et al. [41] performed a RCT to evaluate the use of a coiled and a straight catheter and reported a significantly higher one-year survival when using a straight catheter (64% vs. 75% respectively). However, Nielsen et al. [56] also performed a RCT comparing coiled and straight catheters, and reported a significantly higher one year survival of coiled catheters (77% vs. 36% respectively). Johnson inserted the catheters using the open method, where Nielsen used a percutaneous technique. The importance of the type of catheters inserted laparoscopically remains unknown at this point. The ideal type of catheter may depend on the operative insertion technique.

Study or Subgroup	Laparoscopy Events	Total	Open Events	Total	Weight	Odds Ratio M-H, Random, 95% CI	Odds Ratio M-H, Random, 95% CI
1.5.1 Intervention/replacement/revision							
Batey	3	14	1	12	21.9%	3.00 [0.27, 33.49]	
Gajjar	1	45	5	30	24.8%	0.11 [0.01, 1.03]	
Lund	0	9	4	13	15.5%	0.11 [0.01, 2.36]	
Ogünc	3	21	8	21	37.8%	0.27 [0.06, 1.22]	
Subtotal (95% CI)		**89**		**76**	**100.0%**	**0.32 [0.08, 1.26]**	
Total events	7		18				
Heterogeneity: Tau² = 0.69; Chi² = 4.66, df = 3 (P = 0.20); I² = 36%							
Test for overall effect: Z = 1.63 (P = 0.10)							
1.5.2 Catheter removal							
Batey	3	14	3	12	11.7%	0.82 [0.13, 5.08]	
Draganic	5	30	9	30	25.5%	0.47 [0.14, 1.61]	
Jwo	5	37	4	40	20.0%	1.41 [0.35, 5.69]	
Lund	1	9	0	13	3.6%	4.76 [0.17, 130.96]	
Ogünc	2	21	6	21	12.9%	0.26 [0.05, 1.50]	
Tsimoyiannis	1	25	3	20	7.1%	0.24 [0.02, 2.47]	
Wright	4	21	6	24	19.2%	0.71 [0.17, 2.94]	
Subtotal (95% CI)		**157**		**160**	**100.0%**	**0.65 [0.35, 1.21]**	
Total events	21		31				
Heterogeneity: Tau² = 0.00; Chi² = 4.66, df = 6 (P = 0.59); I² = 0%							
Test for overall effect: Z = 1.37 (P = 0.17)							

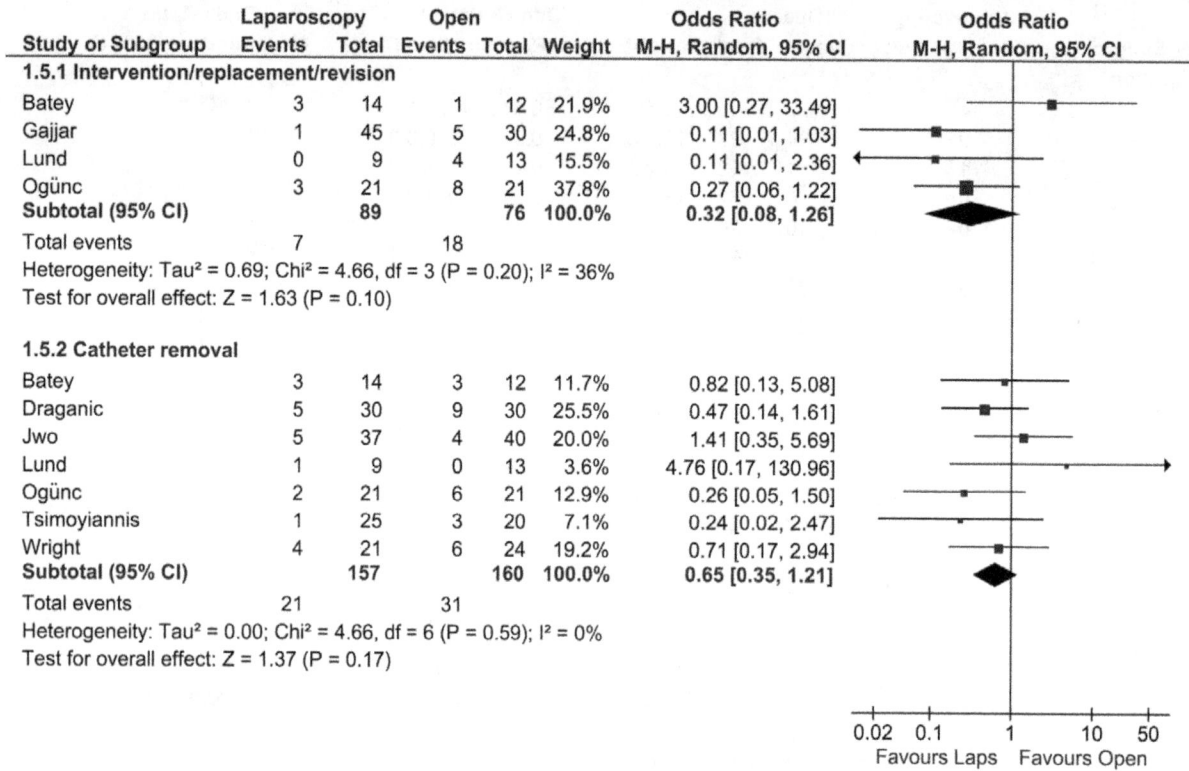

0.02   0.1   1   10   50
Favours Laps   Favours Open

Figure 5. Forest plot. Odds ratio of the incidence of intervention/revision and catheter removal, evaluating the statistical difference between laparoscopic and open PD catheter insertion. CI: confidence interval.

Study or Subgroup	Laparoscopy Events	Total	Open Events	Total	Weight	Odds Ratio M-H, Random, 95% CI	Odds Ratio M-H, Random, 95% CI
1.6.1 Catheter Survival Year 1							
Li	50	50	18	23	6.9%	30.03 [1.58, 570.06]	
Ogünc	19	21	15	21	19.2%	3.80 [0.67, 21.60]	
Soontrapornchai	45	50	34	52	45.8%	4.76 [1.61, 14.12]	
Tsimoyiannis	25	25	18	20	6.3%	6.89 [0.31, 152.19]	
Wright	18	21	20	24	21.8%	1.20 [0.24, 6.10]	
Subtotal (95% CI)		**167**		**140**	**100.0%**	**3.93 [1.80, 8.57]**	
Total events	157		105				
Heterogeneity: Tau² = 0.04; Chi² = 4.18, df = 4 (P = 0.38); I² = 4%							
Test for overall effect: Z = 3.44 (P = 0.0006)							
1.6.2 Catheter Survival Year 2							
Li	50	50	17	23	6.6%	37.51 [2.01, 700.71]	
Ogünc	8	21	5	21	24.1%	1.97 [0.52, 7.49]	
Soontrapornchai	27	50	22	52	44.4%	1.60 [0.73, 3.50]	
Wright	16	21	15	24	25.0%	1.92 [0.52, 7.05]	
Subtotal (95% CI)		**142**		**120**	**100.0%**	**2.17 [0.99, 4.75]**	
Total events	101		59				
Heterogeneity: Tau² = 0.20; Chi² = 4.36, df = 3 (P = 0.23); I² = 31%							
Test for overall effect: Z = 1.93 (P = 0.05)							

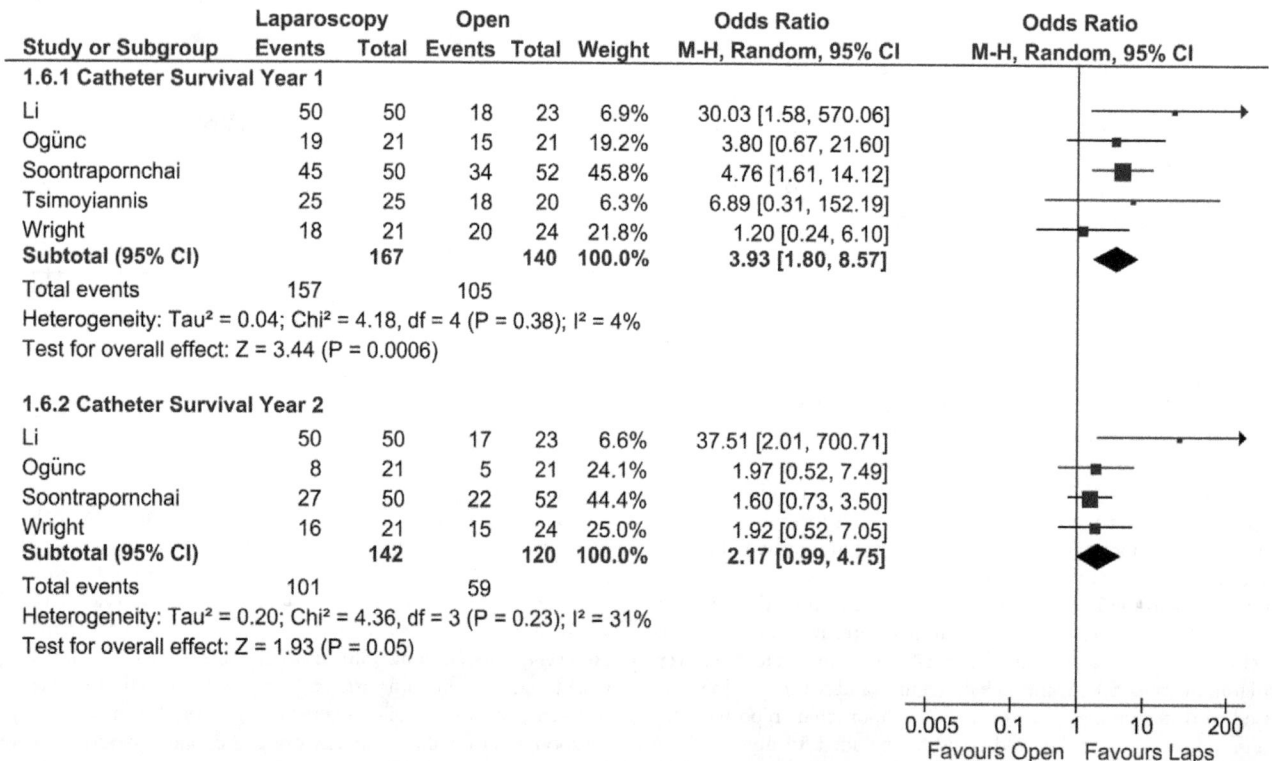

0.005   0.1   1   10   200
Favours Open   Favours Laps

Figure 6. Forest plot. Odds ratios of the catheter survival, at one year and two years after insertion, evaluating the statistical difference between laparoscopic and open PD catheter insertion. CI: confidence interval.

Laparoscopic PD catheter insertion compared to Open PD catheter insertion for End-Stage Renal Disease

Bibliography:

Outcomes	No of Participants (studies) Follow up	Quality of the evidence (GRADE)	Relative effect (95% CI)	Anticipated absolute effects — Risk with Open PD catheter insertion	Risk difference with Laparoscopic PD catheter insertion (95% CI)
Patient-related outcome - Peritonitis	541 (9 studies[1]) 1 - 55 months	⊕⊕⊕⊕ VERY LOW[2,3] due to risk of bias, imprecision	OR 0.83 (0.48 to 1.42)	Study population — 241 per 1000	32 fewer per 1000 (from 109 fewer to 70 more)
				Moderate — 233 per 1000	32 fewer per 1000 (from 106 fewer to 68 more)
Patient-related outcome - Exit-site/tunnel Infection	474 (7 studies) 1 - 55 months	⊕⊕⊕⊕ VERY LOW[2,4] due to risk of bias, imprecision	OR 0.8 (0.47 to 1.37)	Study population — 173 per 1000	30 fewer per 1000 (from 83 fewer to 50 more)
				Moderate — 125 per 1000	22 fewer per 1000 (from 62 fewer to 39 more)
Catheter-related outcome - Migration	319 (5 studies) 1 - 55 months	⊕⊕⊕⊕ HIGH[2,5] due to risk of bias, large effect	OR 0.21 (0.07 to 0.63)	Study population — 176 per 1000	133 fewer per 1000 (from 57 fewer to 161 fewer)
				Moderate — 175 per 1000	132 fewer per 1000 (from 57 fewer to 160 fewer)
Catheter-related outcome - Leakage	826 (9 studies) 1 - 55 months	⊕⊕⊕⊕ VERY LOW[2,4] due to risk of bias, imprecision	OR 0.88 (0.4 to 1.92)	Study population — 81 per 1000	9 fewer per 1000 (from 47 fewer to 64 more)
				Moderate — 19 per 1000	2 fewer per 1000 (from 11 fewer to 17 more)
Catheter-related outcome - Obstruction	665 (6 studies) 1 - 55 months	⊕⊕⊕⊕ LOW[2,5] due to risk of bias, large effect	OR 0.39 (0.14 to 1.07)	Study population — 123 per 1000	71 fewer per 1000 (from 104 fewer to 7 more)
				Moderate — 137 per 1000	79 fewer per 1000 (from 115 fewer to 8 more)
Interventional outcome - Intervention/replacement/revision	165 (4 studies) 1 - 36 months	⊕⊕⊕⊕ MODERATE[2,3,5] due to risk of bias, imprecision, large effect	OR 0.32 (0.08 to 1.26)	Study population — 237 per 1000	147 fewer per 1000 (from 213 fewer to 44 more)
				Moderate — 237 per 1000	147 fewer per 1000 (from 213 fewer to 44 more)
Interventional outcome - Catheter removal for complications	317 (7 studies) 1 - 36 months	⊕⊕⊕⊕ VERY LOW[2,4] due to risk of bias, imprecision	OR 0.65 (0.35 to 1.21)	Study population — 194 per 1000	59 fewer per 1000 (from 118 fewer to 32 more)
				Moderate — 250 per 1000	72 fewer per 1000 (from 146 fewer to 37 more)
Catheter survival - Catheter Survival Year 1	307 (5 studies) 1 - 55 months	⊕⊕⊕⊕ MODERATE[3] due to risk of bias	OR 3.93 (1.8 to 8.57)	Study population — 750 per 1000	172 more per 1000 (from 94 more to 213 more)
				Moderate — 783 per 1000	151 more per 1000 (from 84 more to 186 more)
Catheter survival - Catheter Survival Year 2	262 (4 studies) 1 - 55 months	⊕⊕⊕⊕ VERY LOW[2,3] due to risk of bias, imprecision	OR 2.17 (0.99 to 4.75)	Study population — 492 per 1000	186 more per 1000 (from 3 fewer to 330 more)
				Moderate — 524 per 1000	181 more per 1000 (from 3 fewer to 315 more)

*The basis for the assumed risk (e.g. the median control group risk across studies) is provided in footnotes. The **corresponding risk** (and its 95% confidence interval) is based on the assumed risk in the comparison group and the **relative effect** of the intervention (and its 95% CI).

CI: Confidence interval; OR: Odds ratio;
GRADE Working Group grades of evidence
High quality: Further research is very unlikely to change our confidence in the estimate of effect.
Moderate quality: Further research is likely to have an important impact on our confidence in the estimate of effect and may change the estimate.
Low quality: Further research is very likely to have an important impact on our confidence in the estimate of effect and is likely to change the estimate.
Very low quality: We are very uncertain about the estimate.

[1] 3 RCTs; Jwo, Tsimoyiannis and Wright
[2] inclusion of observational studies
[3] Event rates are lower than 300 and 95% confidence interval around the pooled estimate of effect includes both no effect and appreciable benefit
[4] 95% confidence interval around the pooled estimate of effect includes both no effect and appreciable benefit
[5] Risk ratio < 0.5

Figure 7. Summery of findings table generated by the GRADE tool.

The incidence of dialysate leakage is not significantly different between the laparoscopic and open insertion technique. As with the incidence of peritonitis, the time to start PD may also influence the occurrence of leakage. Starting PD shortly after insertion might cause an increased percentage of persistent leakage, for not allowing the peritoneum to heal properly. A possible confounder might be the number of cuffs on the catheter used. Most studies in this meta-analysis used a double-cuffed catheter, Gajjar [32] used single cuffed as well as double cuffed catheters. In the literature, comparative studies indicate no difference in outcome between double and single cuffed catheters [57,58]. However, these studies did not use the laparoscopic insertion technique. It is possible that the number of cuffs used influences the incidence of leakage when using the laparoscopic insertion technique, but not when using the open technique. However, this meta-analysis and review cannot give a solution to this problem.

In case of dysfunctioning catheters, a laparoscopic revision was successfully performed in most cases. Catheter insertion via the open technique required more interventions or revisions, although not significant (P = 0.07), which may lead to a lower patient comfort and higher costs. The results might be biased, because not all studies reported whether an intervention was performed in case of a dysfunctioning catheter. A cost-benefit analysis is recommended at this point.

Most importantly, PD catheters that were inserted using the laparoscopic technique have been demonstrated to have a significantly higher 1 year survival. Remarkably, the 2-year catheter survival is only borderline significantly different between the groups. This can be attributed to the fact that Tsimoyiannis et al. is not included in the analysis, because of a shorter follow-up than 2 years, resulting in a smaller number of analyzed patients.

Most studies analyzed in this meta-analysis, reported the survival in percentages, where a Kaplan-Meier curve is to be preferred. The reporting of proportions might have led to inaccurate survival data.

Although the incidence of most complications, except for catheter migration, individually is not significantly different between laparoscopic and open insertion, all studies combined show that laparoscopically inserted catheters tend to enable better and prolonged PD.

Limitations

In order to include sufficient patient data to draw solid conclusions, both observational and intervention studies were included. This might have lead to selection bias. In our opinion, it was more important to have a larger number of included patients than the inclusion of interventional studies only, despite the fact that cohort studies are more prone to possible bias. Furthermore, the observational studies support the findings of the RCTs, as we confirmed in our sensitivity analysis. According to the assessment using the GRADE tool, we conclude that the evidence of each individual included study varies from very low to high. However, the highest level of evidence was found for the outcome measures that showed significant differences in our analysis. One other possible limitation is that the analysis might be biased because of difference in the individual experience of the operating surgeons. Furthermore, the procedures are not always carried out by one surgeon only. Possible downside of the analyzed studies is the small number of patients in both intervention arms for some outcome measures. Small patient groups increase the chance of getting smaller or larger differences based on random chance. Despite the statistical homogeneity, some outcome measures appear to be clinically heterogeneous. This might be caused by possible center bias.

Despite these limitations, this meta-analysis is the first step in giving a definite answer as to which procedure of the two (laparoscopic or open insertion technique) might be the better procedure for reducing complications and better PD catheter survival. This systematic review and meta-analysis reveals the potential benefits of laparoscopic PD-catheter insertion. In order to be able to evaluate the true value of laparoscopy in PD-catheter insertion, a large randomized controlled trial is recommended [59].

Author Contributions

Conceived and designed the experiments: SMH JNMIJ FJMFD. Performed the experiments: SMH JAL. Analyzed the data: SMH JAL EWS FJMFD. Contributed reagents/materials/analysis tools: EWS. Wrote the paper: SMH JAL JNMIJ FJMFD.

References

1. Fenton SS, Schaubel DE, Desmeules M, Morrison HI, Mao Y, et al. (1997) Hemodialysis versus peritoneal dialysis: a comparison of adjusted mortality rates. Am J Kidney Dis. 30: 334–42.

2. Maiorca R, Vonesh EF, Cavalli P, De Vecchi A, Giangrande A, et al. (1991) A multicenter, selection-adjusted comparison of patient and technique survivals on CAPD and hemodialysis. Perit Dial Int. 11: 118–27.

3. Heaf JG, Lokkegaard H, Madsen M (2002) Initial survival advantage of peritoneal dialysis relative to haemodialysis. Nephrol Dial Transplant. 17: 112–7.

4. Termorshuizen F, Korevaar JC, Dekker FW, Van Manen JG, Boeschoten EW, et al. (2003) Hemodialysis and peritoneal dialysis: comparison of adjusted mortality rates according to the duration of dialysis: analysis of The Netherlands Cooperative Study on the Adequacy of Dialysis 2. J Am Soc Nephrol. 14: 2851–60.

5. Bargman JM, Thorpe KE, Churchill DN (2001) Relative contribution of residual renal function and peritoneal clearance to adequacy of dialysis: a reanalysis of the CANUSA study. J Am Soc Nephrol. 12: 2158–62.

6. Ash SR (2003) Chronic peritoneal dialysis catheters: overview of design, placement, and removal procedures. Semin Dial. 16: 323–34.

7. Davis AS, Reed WP (1983) A leak-free technique for open insertion of peritoneal dialysis catheters. Surg Gynecol Obstet. 157: 579–80.

8. Robison RJ, Leapman SB, Wetherington GM, Hamburger RJ, Fineberg NS, et al. (1984) Surgical considerations of continuous ambulatory peritoneal dialysis. Surgery. 96: 723–30.

9. Gadallah MF, Pervez A, el-Shahawy MA, Sorrells D, Zibari G, et al. (1999) Peritoneoscopic versus surgical placement of peritoneal dialysis catheters: a prospective randomized study on outcome. Am J Kidney Dis. 33: 118–22.

10. Poole GH, Tervit P (2000) Laparoscopic Tenckhoff catheter insertion: a prospective study of a new technique. Aust N Z J Surg. 70: 371–3.

11. Velasco Garcia MA, Garcia Urena MA, Carnero F, Fernandez Ruiz E, Remon Rodriguez C, et al. (1997) Omental entrapping of the peritoneal dialysis catheter solved by a laparoscopic approach. Perit Dial Int. 17: 194–5.

12. Crabtree JH, Fishman A (1999) Laparoscopic omentectomy for peritoneal dialysis catheter flow obstruction: a case report and review of the literature. Surg Laparosc Endosc Percutan Tech. 9: 228–33.

13. Crabtree JH, Fishman A (1999) Videolaparoscopic implantation of long-term peritoneal dialysis catheters. Surg Endosc. 13: 186–90.

14. Jwo SC, Chen KS, Lee CC, Chen HY (2010) Prospective randomized study for comparison of open surgery with laparoscopic-assisted placement of Tenckhoff peritoneal dialysis catheter—a single center experience and literature review. J Surg Res. 159: 489–96.

15. Ashegh H, Rezaii J, Esfandiari K, Tavakoli H, Abouzari M, et al. (2008) One-port laparoscopic technique for placement of Tenckhoff peritoneal dialysis catheters: report of seventy-nine procedures. Perit Dial Int. 28: 622–5.

16. Crabtree JH, Burchette RJ (2009) Effective use of laparoscopy for long-term peritoneal dialysis access. Am J Surg. 198: 135–41.

17. Ko J, Ra W, Bae T, Lee T, Kim HH, et al. (2009) Two-port laparoscopic placement of a peritoneal dialysis catheter with abdominal wall fixation. Surg Today. 39: 356–8.

18. Yan X, Zhu W, Jiang CM, Huang HF, Zhang M, et al. (2010) Clinical application of one-port laparoscopic placement of peritoneal dialysis catheters. Scand J Urol Nephrol. 44: 341–4.

19. Kok NF, Lind MY, Hansson BM, Pilzecker D, Mertens zur Borg IR, et al. (2006) Comparison of laparoscopic and mini incision open donor nephrectomy: single blind, randomised controlled clinical trial. BMJ. 333: 221.

20. Keus F, de Jong JA, Gooszen HG, van Laarhoven CJ (2006) Laparoscopic versus open cholecystectomy for patients with symptomatic cholecystolithiasis. Cochrane Database Syst Rev. CD006231.

21. Keus F, Gooszen HG, van Laarhoven CJ (2010) Open, small-incision, or laparoscopic cholecystectomy for patients with symptomatic cholecystolithiasis. An overview of Cochrane Hepato-Biliary Group reviews. Cochrane Database Syst Rev. CD008318.

22. Klarenbeek BR, Bergamaschi R, Veenhof AA, van der Peet DL, van den Broek WT, et al. (2011) Laparoscopic versus open sigmoid resection for diverticular disease: follow-up assessment of the randomized control Sigma trial. Surg Endosc. 25: 1121–6.

23. Strippoli GF, Tong A, Johnson D, Schena FP, Craig JC (2004) Catheter type, placement and insertion techniques for preventing peritonitis in peritoneal dialysis patients. Cochrane Database Syst Rev. CD004680.

24. Xie H, Zhang W, Cheng J, He Q (2012) Laparoscopic versus open catheter placement in peritoneal dialysis patients: a systematic review and meta-analysis. BMC Nephrol. 13: 69.

25. Moher D, Liberati A, Tetzlaff J, Altman DG (2009) Reprint–preferred reporting items for systematic reviews and meta-analyses: the PRISMA statement. Phys Ther. 89: 873–80.

26. OCEBM Levels of Evidence Working Group Jeremy Howick ICJLL, Paul Glasziou, Trish Greenhalgh, Carl Heneghan, Alessandro Liberati, Ivan Moschetti, Bob Phillips, Hazel Thornton, Olive Goddard and Mary Hodgkinson. OCEBM Levels of Evidence Working Group. "The Oxford 2011 Levels of Evidence". Oxford Centre for Evidence-Based Medicine.; Available: http://www.cebm.net/index.aspx?o = 5653 Accessed 2012 Oct 1.

27. Lo WK, Lui SL, Li FK, Choy BY, Lam MF, et al. (2003) A prospective randomized study on three different peritoneal dialysis catheters. Perit Dial Int. 23 Suppl 2: S127–31.

28. Brozek J, Oxman A, Schünemann H. GRADEpro. Version 3.2 for Windows ed22008.

29. Higgins JP, Altman DG, Gotzsche PC, Juni P, Moher D, et al. (2011) The Cochrane Collaboration's tool for assessing risk of bias in randomised trials. BMJ. 343: d5928.

30. Tsimoyiannis EC, Siakas P, Glantzounis G, Toli C, Sferopoulos G, et al. (2000) Laparoscopic placement of the Tenckhoff catheter for peritoneal dialysis. Surg Laparosc Endosc Percutan Tech. 10: 218–21.

31. Wright MJ, Bel'eed K, Johnson BF, Eadington DW, Sellars L, et al. (1999) Randomized prospective comparison of laparoscopic and open peritoneal dialysis catheter insertion. Perit Dial Int. 19: 372–5.

32. Gajjar AH, Rhoden DH, Kathuria P, Kaul R, Udupa AD, et al. (2007) Peritoneal dialysis catheters: laparoscopic versus traditional placement techniques and outcomes. Am J Surg. 194: 872–5; discussion 5–6.

33. Crabtree JH, Fishman A (2005) A laparoscopic method for optimal peritoneal dialysis access. Am Surg. 71: 135–43.

34. Soontrapornchai P, Simapatanapong T (2005) Comparison of open and laparoscopic secure placement of peritoneal dialysis catheters. Surg Endosc. 19: 137–9.

35. Ogunc G, Tuncer M, Ogunc D, Yardimsever M, Ersoy F (2003) Laparoscopic omental fixation technique versus open surgical placement of peritoneal dialysis catheters. Surg Endosc. 17: 1749–55.

36. Draganic B, James A, Booth M, Gani JS (1998) Comparative experience of a simple technique for laparoscopic chronic ambulatory peritoneal dialysis catheter placement. Aust N Z J Surg. 68: 735–9.

37. Batey CA, Crane JJ, Jenkins MA, Johnston TD, Munch LC (2002) Mini-laparoscopy-assisted placement of Tenckhoff catheters: an improved technique to facilitate peritoneal dialysis. J Endourol. 16: 681–4.

38. Lund L, Jonler M (2007) Peritoneal dialysis catheter placement: is laparoscopy an option? Int Urol Nephrol. 39: 625–8.

39. Li JR, Chen WM, Yang CK, Shu KH, Ou YC, et al. (2011) A novel method of laparoscopy-assisted peritoneal dialysis catheter placement. Surg Laparosc Endosc Percutan Tech. 21: 106–10.

40. Crabtree JH, Fishman A (2000) A laparoscopic approach under local anesthesia for peritoneal dialysis access. Perit Dial Int. 20: 757–65.

41. Johnson DW, Wong J, Wiggins KJ, Kirwan R, Griffin A, et al. (2006) A randomized controlled trial of coiled versus straight swan-neck Tenckhoff catheters in peritoneal dialysis patients. Am J Kidney Dis. 48: 812–21.

42. Tiong HY, Poh J, Sunderaraj K, Wu YJ, Consigliere DT (2006) Surgical complications of Tenckhoff catheters used in continuous ambulatory peritoneal dialysis. Singapore Med J. 47: 707–11.

43. Yang PJ, Lee CY, Yeh CC, Nien HC, Tsai TJ, et al. (2010) Mini-laparotomy implantation of peritoneal dialysis catheters: outcome and rescue. Perit Dial Int. 30: 513–8.

44. Liu WJ, Hooi LS (2010) Complications after tenckhoff catheter insertion: a single-centre experience using multiple operators over four years. Perit Dial Int. 30: 509–12.

45. Lu CT, Watson DI, Elias TJ, Faull RJ, Clarkson AR, et al. (2003) Laparoscopic placement of peritoneal dialysis catheters: 7 years experience. ANZ J Surg. 73: 109–11.

46. Schmidt SC, Pohle C, Langrehr JM, Schumacher G, Jacob D, et al. (2007) Laparoscopic-assisted placement of peritoneal dialysis catheters: implantation technique and results. J Laparoendosc Adv Surg Tech A. 17: 596–9.

47. Strippoli GF, Tong A, Johnson D, Schena FP, Craig JC (2004) Antimicrobial agents to prevent peritonitis in peritoneal dialysis: a systematic review of randomized controlled trials. Am J Kidney Dis. 44: 591–603.

48. Gadallah MF, Ramdeen G, Mignone J, Patel D, Mitchell L, et al. (2000) Role of preoperative antibiotic prophylaxis in preventing postoperative peritonitis in newly placed peritoneal dialysis catheters. Am J Kidney Dis. 36: 1014–9.

49. Figueiredo A, Goh BL, Jenkins S, Johnson DW, Mactier R, et al. (2010) Clinical practice guidelines for peritoneal access. Perit Dial Int. 30: 424–9.

50. Attaluri V, Lebeis C, Brethauer S, Rosenblatt S (2010) Advanced laparoscopic techniques significantly improve function of peritoneal dialysis catheters. J Am Coll Surg. 211: 699–704.

51. Prischl FC, Wallner M, Kalchmair H, Povacz F, Kramar R (1997) Initial subcutaneous embedding of the peritoneal dialysis catheter–a critical appraisal of this new implantation technique. Nephrol Dial Transplant. 12: 1661–7.

52. Ranganathan D, Baer R, Fassett RG, Williams N, Han T, et al. (2010) Randomised controlled trial to determine the appropriate time to initiate peritoneal dialysis after insertion of catheter to minimise complications (Timely PD study). BMC Nephrol. 11: 11.

53. Hwang SJ, Chang JM, Chen HC, Tsai MK, Tsai JC, et al. (1998) Smaller insertion angle of Tenckhoff catheter increases the chance of catheter migration in CAPD patients. Perit Dial Int. 18: 433–5.

54. Chen WM, Cheng CL (2007) A simple method to prevent peritoneal dialysis catheter tip migration. Perit Dial Int. 27: 554–6.

55. Swartz R, Messana J, Rocher L, Reynolds J, Starmann B, et al. (1990) The curled catheter: dependable device for percutaneous peritoneal access. Perit Dial Int. 10: 231–5.

56. Nielsen PK, Hemmingsen C, Friis SU, Ladefoged J, Olgaard K (1995) Comparison of straight and curled Tenckhoff peritoneal dialysis catheters implanted by percutaneous technique: a prospective randomized study. Perit Dial Int. 15: 18–21.

57. Eklund B, Honkanen E, Kyllonen L, Salmela K, Kala AR (1997) Peritoneal dialysis access: prospective randomized comparison of single-cuff and double-cuff straight Tenckhoff catheters. Nephrol Dial Transplant. 12: 2664–6.

58. Nessim SJ, Bargman JM, Jassal SV (2010) Relationship between double-cuff versus single-cuff peritoneal dialysis catheters and risk of peritonitis. Nephrol Dial Transplant. 25: 2310–4.

59. Hagen SM, van Alphen AM, Ijzermans JN, Dor FJ (2011) Laparoscopic versus open peritoneal dialysis catheter insertion, the LOCI-trial: a study protocol. BMC Surg. 11: 35.

13

Predictors and Prevalence of Latent Tuberculosis Infection in Patients Receiving Long-Term Hemodialysis and Peritoneal Dialysis

Chin-Chung Shu[1,2], Vin-Cent Wu[2,3], Feng-Jung Yang[4], Sung-Ching Pan[3], Tai-Shuan Lai[5], Jann-Yuan Wang[2,3]*, Jann-Tay Wang[2,3], Li-Na Lee[6]

1 Department of Traumatology, National Taiwan University Hospital, Taipei City, Taiwan, 2 College of Internal Medicine, National Taiwan University, Taipei City, Taiwan, 3 Department of Internal Medicine, National Taiwan University Hospital, Taipei City, Taiwan, 4 Department of Internal Medicine, National Taiwan University Hospital, Yun-Lin Branch, Yun-Lin County, Taiwan, 5 Department of Internal Medicine, National Taiwan University Hospital, Bei-Hu Branch, Taipei City, Taiwan, 6 Department of Laboratory Medicine, National Taiwan University Hospital, Taipei City, Taiwan

Abstract

Background: Tuberculosis is a common infectious disease in long-term dialysis patients. The prevalence of latent tuberculosis infection (LTBI) in this population is unclear, particularly in those receiving peritoneal dialysis (PD). This study investigated the prevalence of LTBI in patients receiving either hemodialysis (HD) or PD to determine predictors of LTBI and indeterminate results of interferon-gamma release assay.

Methods: Patients receiving long-term (≥3 months) HD or PD from March 2011 to February 2012 in two medical centers were prospectively enrolled. QuantiFERON-Gold in tube (QFT) test was used to determine the status of LTBI after excluding active tuberculosis. The LTBI prevalence was determined in patients receiving different dialysis modes to obtain predictors of LTBI and QFT-indeterminate results.

Results: Of 427 patients enrolled (124 PD and 303 HD), 91 (21.3%) were QFT-positive, 316 (74.0%) QFT-negative, and 20 (4.7%) QFT-indeterminate. The prevalence of LTBI was similar in the PD and HD groups. Independent predictors of LTBI were old age (OR: 1.034 [1.013–1.056] per year increment), TB history (OR: 6.467 [1.985–21.066]), and current smoker (OR: 2.675 [1.061–6.747]). Factors associated with indeterminate QFT results were HD (OR: 10.535 [1.336–83.093]), dialysis duration (OR: 1.113 [1.015–1.221] per year increment), anemia (OR: 8.760 [1.014–75.651]), and serum albumin level (OR: 0.244 [0.086–0.693] per 1 g/dL increment).

Conclusion: More than one-fifth of dialysis patients have LTBI. The LTBI prevalence is similar in PD and HD patients but is higher in the elderly, current smokers, and those with prior TB history. Such patients require closer follow-up. Repeated or alternative test may be required for malnutrition patients who received long length of HD.

Editor: Emmanuel A. Burdmann, University of Sao Paulo Medical School, Brazil

Funding: This study was funded by Institute of Biotechnology and Medicine Industry in Taiwan. The funders had no role in study design, data collection and analysis, decision to publish, or preparation of the manuscript.

Competing Interests: The authors have declared that no competing interests exist.

* E-mail: jywang@ntu.edu.tw

Introduction

Tuberculosis (TB) remains a worldwide infectious disease with high mortality. Control involves preventing further TB transmission via early diagnosis and treatment of latent TB infection (LTBI) [1]. Dialysis patients are at increased risk of tuberculosis (TB) due to attenuated cellular immunity [2]. Compared to the general population, their risk of developing active TB is 7.8–25 times higher [3–5] and their mortality rate due to TB is also higher [4–7]. Moreover, TB diagnosis in dialysis patients is usually delayed because of frequent extra-pulmonary manifestations [8,9]. Early LTBI detection and monitoring of the development of active TB in this specific group are therefore important [1]. Currently, interferon-gamma release assays (IGRAs) used to determine LTBI cases, though not 100% accurate, have been proven useful even in

immuno-compromised hosts and Bacille Calmette Guérin (BCG)-vaccinated subjects [10–12]. For patients receiving hemodialysis, the IGRA-positive rate is reportedly around 21–40% [13–15], while 6–11% of patients have indeterminate IGRA results [14–17]. However, studies focusing on patients receiving peritoneal dialysis (PD) are lacking.

Traditionally, HD patients are believed to have higher prevalence of LTBI than PD patients due to more frequent hospital visits and longer hospital stay [14]. In fact, studies supporting this argument are lacking. Understanding the predictors for LTBI and indeterminate IGRA results in the dialysis population is important in policy-making to determine the priority groups for IGRA screening [18,19]. This cross sectional study was conducted to analyze the prevalence of LTBI in patients receiving long-term HD and PD, and to examine the predictors for LTBI and indeterminate IGRA results.

Methods

This cross sectional study was conducted at National Taiwan University Hospital, a tertiary referral center in northern Taiwan, and its branch in southern Taiwan. The hospital's institutional review board approved the study. From March 2011 to February 2012, adult patients (age ≥20 years) receiving long-term (>3 months) dialysis were prospectively identified. All participants provided written informed consent. Chest radiography and clinical history were obtained to exclude active TB disease. Acid-fast smear and mycobacterial culture for three sputum samples were performed as previously described if TB was suspected [20]. Those with human immunodeficiency virus infection, liver cirrhosis of Child-Pugh class C [21], cancer or autoimmune disease receiving chemotherapy within the last three months, life expectancy of less than 6 months, and active TB within the last three years were excluded.

Peripheral blood samples were taken to detect LTBI using QuantiFERON-TB Gold In-Tube assay (QFT) (Celestis, Australia), which was performed according to the manufacturer's instructions [22]. Interferon-gamma level of the post-reaction supernatant was then measured by enzyme-linked immuno-sorbent assay (ELISA) and results were interpreted as positive, negative, or indeterminate accordingly [23,24]. In this study, LTBI was defined as a positive QFT result.

Data collection

Demographic and clinical data, including age, sex, underlying co-morbidities, prior TB history, contact history of TB, respiratory and constitutional symptoms, smoking status, and blood hemo-globin and serum albumin levels were recorded in a standardized case report form. Dialysis mode was defined as its use in the past three months prior to the QFT test. Every session of HD regularly lasted for 4 hours according to the National Kidney Foundation Kidney Disease Outcome Quality Initiative (NKF KDOQI) [25], with two-to-three sessions per week depending on the patient's residual renal function and the adequacy of dialysis. Peritoneal dialysis was recorded as continuous ambulatory peritoneal dialysis (CAPD) or automated peritoneal dialysis (APD). Hypoalbumin-emia was defined as serum albumin level <3.5 g/dL [26] and anemia as hemoglobin level <12 g/dL in males and <11 g/dL in females. Cough ≥3 weeks was defined as chronic cough. Current smoker was defined as those who had smoked >100 cigarettes, with the latest time of smoking within one month prior to the study [27].

Chest radiography findings were classified into "no lung parenchymal lesion"; "lung lesion not compatible with TB"; or "lung lesion compatible with prior TB". The lung lesion compatible with TB was defined as new patch(es) of consolidation, collapse, lymphadenopathy, mass or nodule, or cavitary lesion without other proven etiology [5]. Prior TB was defined radiographically as fibrotic infiltrates with pleural thickening or calcified nodules over the upper lung fields and other fibrotic lesions documented from previous TB disease [28].

Statistical analysis

Subjects were classified according to LTBI status for further comparison. Inter-group differences were analyzed using the student t test for numerical variables and chi-square test for categorical variables. Multivariate logistic regression analysis was used to identify factors associated with LTBI and QFT-indeter-

minate results. All potential predictors were included in the stepwise variable selection procedure. A two-sided $p<0.05$ was considered significant. All analyses were performed using the SPSS (Version 13.0, Chicago, IL).

Results

A total of 427 subjects (mean age, 61.1±13.1 years; male, 53%) with long-term dialysis (mean length of dialysis use, 4.8±4.2 years) were enrolled, including 303 HD patients and 124 PD patients (Table 1). Among HD patients, 271 (89.4%) had three sessions per week while the remaining 32 (10.6%) had two sessions per week. Among PD patients, 81 (65.3%) had CAPD and 43 (34.7%) had APD.

Compared to HD patients, PD patients were significantly younger, predominantly female, more symptomatic with chronic cough, had shorter length of dialysis duration, had lower serum albumin level, and were less likely to have pulmonary lesions on chest radiograph (18% vs. 37%; $p<0.001$). The proportion of QFT-positive patients was similar in the two groups (19% vs. 22%, $p = 0.109$).

The QFT result was positive in 91 (21.3%) patients, negative in 316 (74.0%), and indeterminate in the remaining 20 (4.7%) (Table 2). Among the 20 QFT-indeterminate results, 19 were due to weak response to mitogen and one due to strong response of negative control. The QFT tests were repeated in 14 of the 20 patients and were negative in 9, positive in 1, and indeterminate in the remaining 4.

Compared to combined group of QFT- positive and QFT-negative patients, the 20 QFT-indeterminate patients were older and less likely to be ex-smokers, received HD for a longer period, and had more dyspnea and constitutional symptoms (Table 2). They also had lower serum albumin level and a higher proportion of patients with pulmonary lesions. Multivariate logistic regression analysis revealed that dialysis duration (Odds Ratio [O.R.] 1.113, 95% C.I. 1.015–1.221 per year increment), HD (O.R. 10.535, 95% C.I. 1.336–83.093), anemia (O.R. 8.760, 95% C.I. 1.014–75.651), and serum albumin level (O.R. 0.244, 95% C.I. 0.086–0.693 per unit increment) were significant predictors of QFT-indeterminate results (Table 3). If 3.5 g/dl was used as cut-off value for serum albumin level to predict an indeterminate QFT result, sensitivity and specificity were 80% and 93%, respectively.

Patients with LTBI (QFT-positive) were older and more likely had a prior TB history compared to QFT-negative patients, by univariate analysis (Table 2). In multivariate logistic regression analysis, independent predictors of LTBI included age (O.R. 1.034, 95% C.I. 1.013–1.056, per year increment), prior TB history (O.R. 6.467, 95% C.I. 1.985–21.066), and current smoker (O.R. 6.467, 95% C.I. 1.985–21.066) (Table 4; Figure 1). The presence of underlying co-morbidity was not an independent predictor. In patients with prior TB history and those who were current smokers, the prevalence of LTBI was 57.1% and 29.6%, respectively. This prevalence increased by <15% in patients younger than 50 years old to almost 30% in those older than 80 years old.

Discussion

This is the first cross sectional study that investigated the prevalence of LTBI in a large number of patients receiving either long-term PD or HD. Using QFT as a diagnostic tool for LTBI in this immuno-compromised population, 4.7% may have an indeterminate result, especially those with anemia, hypoalbumin-emia, and who have been receiving HD for a long time. There is a high prevalence (21.3%) of LTBI in the long-term dialysis

Table 1. Clinical characteristics of patients with different modes of dialysis.

	PD group (n = 124)	HD group (n = 303)	p value
Age, year	55.4±12.3	63.5±12.7	<0.001
Male gender	54 (44%)	172 (57%)	0.013
Smoking status			
Ex-smoker	17 (14%)	65 (22%)	0.065
Current smoker	5 (4%)	22 (7%)	0.213
Dialysis duration, years	4.1±3.9	5.0±4.3	0.039
Underlying co-morbidity			
Malignancy	5 (4%)	25 (8%)	0.111
Diabetes mellitus	23 (19%)	85 (28%)	0.040
Cirrhosis of liver	3 (2%)	3 (1%)	0.255
Autoimmune disease	4 (3%)	7 (2%)	0.588
Prior TB history	1 (1%)	13 (4%)	0.066
TB exposure history	16 (13%)	23 (8%)	0.084
Symptoms at visit			
Chronic cough with sputum	36 (29%)	27 (9%)	<0.001
Dyspnea	1 (1%)	3 (1%)	0.858
Constitutional symptoms	1 (1%)	1 (1%)	0.513
Chest radiograph around visit			
Lesion, not compatible with TB	22 (18%)	110 (36%)	<0.001
Lesion, compatible with prior TB	0	3 (1%)	0.252
Anemia	99 (79%)	223 (74%)	0.174
Serum albumin, g/dL	3.9±0.4	4.1±0.4	0.002
QFT status			
Positive	24 (19%)	67 (22%)	0.528
Negative	98 (79%)	218 (72%)	0.130
Indeterminate	2 (2%)	18 (6%)	0.055

Abbreviations: PD, peritoneal dialysis; HD, hemodialysis; TB, tuberculosis; QFT, QuantiFERON-TB test.
Data are no. (%) or mean ± standard deviation.

population, especially in the elderly, current smokers, and those with prior TB history. However, the use of either PD or HD is associated with similar risks of LTBI.

Though IGRA-positive is not 100% equivalent of LTBI, it has several advantages over tuberculin skin test (TST) in terms of convenience and accuracy [10–12]. The TST has a significant limitation in Taiwan due to BCG vaccination [29] and the high prevalence of NTM disease [30]. In QFT, by incorporating positive control (mitogen) and negative control (no antigen) tubes, the true immune reaction against *Mycobacterium tuberculosis*-specific antigens can be differentiated from false-positive result due to non-specific activation and false-negative result due to immuno-suppression. Thus, IGRA is a better screening test for LTBI than TST while implementing public health policy, especially for an immune-compromised host.

Previous studies using IGRA report an LTBI prevalence of 21–40% in HD patients [13–15]. The QFT-positive rate in the present study is within this range and lower than 40%, as reported in a study conducted in south Taiwan [14]. This is probably because the incidence of TB has been decreasing in Taiwan [31]. However, the prevalence in the present study (21.3%) is similar to that reported in household contacts in large-scale studies (11~30%) [12,32] and much higher than the results of new health-care staff in the study institute at the same period (13

[5.7%] QFT-positive in 229 [unpublished data]). As such, it can be posited that dialysis patients in Taiwan have a much higher prevalence of LTBI than the general population and should be a priority group for targeted screening for active TB disease, especially IGRA-positive patients. If IGRA is unavailable, focus should be on older patients, current smokers, and those with prior TB history. Quite interestingly, the three predictors for LTBI identified in the present study are also risk factors of active TB disease [14,33,34]. Different combinations of these predictors may be useful to select the target population for preventive therapy for LTBI. However, the cost and benefit of preventive therapy in this special population should be further evaluated.

The population of chronic renal failure patients receiving long-term dialysis is increasing worldwide and TB is a commonly associated infectious disease [18,19]. It has been previously assumed that because HD patients frequently visit the HD room, they are more likely to acquire *Mycobacterium tuberculosis* infection than PD patients via airborne transmission. Only a report of PD patients in Spain has shown a comparable LTBI prevalence of 18% [35]. By simultaneously enrolling HD and PD patients, this is the first study to demonstrate similar LTBI prevalence in the two patient groups, thereby challenging the hypothesis of occult transmission in the HD room. Although the two dialysis groups are different in more ways than just dialysis place and duration, this

Table 2. Clinical characteristics of patients with different QuantiFERON-TB test (QFT) results.

	QFT-positive (n = 91)	QFT-negative (n = 316)	QFT-indeterminate (n = 20)
Age, year	64.9±11.0*	60.0±13.5	66.2±11.0#
Male gender	55 (60%)	162 (51%)	9 (45%)
Smoking status			
Ex-smoker	22 (24%)	60 (19%)	0#
Current smoker	8 (9%)	16 (5%)	3 (15%)
Dialysis duration: year	4.3±3.6	4.7±4.3	7.5±5.2#
Underlying co-morbidity			
Malignancy	10 (11%)	19 (6%)	1 (5%)
Diabetes mellitus	24 (26%)	78 (25%)	6 (30%)
Cirrhosis of liver	1 (1%)	5 (2%)	0
Autoimmune disease	2 (2%)	9 (3%)	0
Prior TB history	8 (9%)*	6 (2%)	0
TB exposure history	11 (12%)	27 (9%)	1 (5%)
Symptoms at visit			
Chronic cough with sputum	14 (15%)	47 (15%)	2 (10%)
Dyspnea	1 (1%)	1 (1%)	2 (10%)#
Constitutional symptoms	1 (1%)	0	1 (5%)#
Chest radiograph around visit			
Lesion, not compatible with TB	29 (33%)	92 (31%)	11 (55%)#
Lesion, compatible with prior TB	0	2 (1%)	1 (5%)#
Anemia	64 (70%)	240 (76%)	18 (90%)
Serum albumin, g/dL	4.1±0.3	4.0±0.4	3.7±0.4#
HD patients	67 (74%)	218 (69%)	18 (90%)

Abbreviations: HD, hemodialysis; PD, peritoneal dialysis; TB, tuberculosis.
Data are no. (%) or mean ± standard deviation.
*Significant difference ($p<0.05$) between QFT-positive and QFT-negative groups.
#Significant difference ($p<0.05$) between QFT-indeterminate and the combined QFT-negative and QFT-positive groups.

Table 3. Multivariate logistic regression for indeterminate results of QuantiFERON-TB test.

Characteristics	Multivariate	
	p value	OR (95% C.I.)
Age, per 1 year increment	0.205	
Gender, male vs. female	0.075	
Smoking, current vs. none	0.130	
Dialysis duration, per 1 year increment	0.023	1.113 (1.015–1.221)
Prior TB history	0.424	
Dialysis mode, HD vs. PD	0.025	10.535 (1.336–83.093)
Anemia, presence vs. absence	0.049	8.760 (1.014–75.651)
Serum albumin, per 1 g/dL increment	0.008	0.244 (0.086–0.693)
Symptoms at examination*	0.052	
Any lesion by chest radiograph	0.135	
Diabetes mellitus	0.388	
Malignancy	0.635	

*Presence of chronic cough, dyspnea, or constitutional symptoms.

observation suggests that transmission of TB to HD patients within crowded dialysis facilities may be similar to PD patients at home [36]. This suggests that the study institute has an effective TB infection control policy on early detection, prompt treatment, and rapid isolation.

Although 71.4% of QFT-indeterminate patients have definite

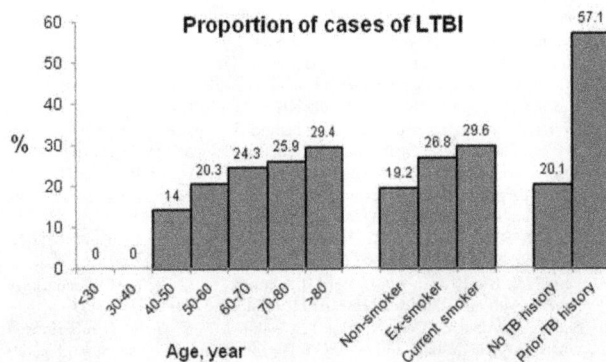

Figure 1. The proportion of latent tuberculosis infection (LTBI) cases defined by QuantiFERON-TB test was plotted according to age, smoking status, and history of TB.

Table 4. Multivariate logistic regression for latent tuberculosis (TB) infection diagnosed by QuantiFERON-TB test.

Characteristics	Multivariate	
	p value	OR (95% C.I.)
Age, per 1 year increment	0.001	1.034 (1.013–1.056)
Gender, male vs. female	0.677	
Smoking status, current vs. none	0.037	2.675 (1.061–6.747)
Dialysis duration, per 1 year increment	0.142	
Prior TB history, presence vs. absence	0.002	6.467 (1.985–21.066)
Serum albumin, per 1 g/dL increment	0.077	
Symptoms at examination*	0.769	
Any lesion by chest radiograph	0.225	
Diabetes mellitus	0.894	
Malignancy	0.228	

*Presence of chronic cough, dyspnea, or constitutional symptoms.

results after repeat testing, 4.7% of the initial QFT tests with an indeterminate result are associated with hypoalbuminemia, anemia, HD, and longer dialysis duration. The association between anemia and indeterminate status has been shown before [37]. Along with hypoalbuminemia, these predictors suggest that malnutrition attenuates immune response and compromises the performance of IGRA [38]. The current finding that HD, but not PD, is associated with QFT-indeterminate is interesting and worth discussing further. A previous study reveals that while both HD and PD patients have lower but insignificant HLD-DR expression on peripheral blood monocytes compared to healthy controls, HLA-DR expression is significantly higher in PD than in HD patients [39]. This implies that continuous dialysis like PD can attenuate immune dysfunction compared to intermittent modes like HD. Moreover, longer duration of dialysis in dialysis patients has been correlated with worse cellular immunity [40]. This may

explain how a much higher percentage (95%) of QFT-indeterminate results in the present study may come from low mitogen responses, compared to 51% in a public health clinic setting [24]. For diagnosing LTBI in such patients, IGRA should be meticulously applied. Repeating IGRA or using alternative tests may be necessary.

In contrast to a previous report [24], female gender is not an independent factor of QFT-indeterminate results in the present study. This may be due to different patient characteristics, such as age, race, and prevalence of HIV infection, between studies. Further large-scale investigations are necessary to confirm this finding and investigate possible reasons.

The present study has several limitations. First, this study was conducted in a tertiary referral center and its branch, so patients had more underlying co-morbidities and the LTBI prevalence might be higher. Second, without detailed contact investigation, the epidemiologic link and biological implication of QFT-positivity cannot be confirmed. Lastly, this is a cross-sectional study. Further prospective studies with long-term follow-up on the development of active TB are needed.

In conclusion, patients receiving PD have a similar prevalence of LTBI as those receiving HD (19% and 22%, respectively). The prevalence of LTBI in long-term dialysis patients is even higher in the elderly, current smokers, and those with prior TB history. These risk factors can be used to select a target group for cost-effective LTBI screening. Patients receiving HD or long duration of dialysis, and those with anemia or lower albumin level are likely to have a QFT-indeterminate result. For such patients, repeat IGRA or alternative test may be necessary to detect LTBI.

Disclosures

Parts of the study results have been presented as a poster in the 2011 Congress of the Asia Pacific Society of Respirology and the 2012 International Conference of the American Thoracic Society.

Author Contributions

Conceived and designed the experiments: LNL JYW CCS. Performed the experiments: CCS FJY SCP TSL JTW VCW. Analyzed the data: JYW CCS. Wrote the paper: JYW VCW CCS.

References

1. Rose DN (2000) Benefits of screening for latent Mycobacterium tuberculosis infection. Arch Intern Med 160: 1513–1521.
2. Christopoulos AI, Diamantopoulos AA, Dimopoulos PA, Gumenos DS, Barbalias GA (2006) Risk of tuberculosis in dialysis patients: association of tuberculin and 2,4-dinitrochlorobenzene reactivity with risk of tuberculosis. Int Urol Nephrol 38: 745–751.
3. Dobler CC, McDonald SP, Marks GB (2011) Risk of tuberculosis in dialysis patients: a nationwide cohort study. PLoS One 6: e29563.
4. Lundin AP, Adler AJ, Berlyne GM, Friedman EA (1979) Tuberculosis in patients undergoing maintenance hemodialysis. Am J Med 67: 597–602.
5. Smirnoff M, Patt C, Seckler B, Adler JJ (1998) Tuberculin and anergy skin testing of patients receiving long-term hemodialysis. Chest 113: 25–27.
6. Jick SS, Lieberman ES, Rahman MU, Choi HK (2006) Glucocorticoid use, other associated factors, and the risk of tuberculosis. Arthritis Rheum 55: 19–26.
7. (2000) Targeted tuberculin testing and treatment of latent tuberculosis infection. American Thoracic Society. MMWR Recomm Rep 49: 1–51.
8. Venkata RK, Kumar S, Krishna RP, Kumar SB, Padmanabhan S (2007) Tuberculosis in chronic kidney disease. Clin Nephrol 67: 217–220.
9. Fang HC, Lee PT, Chen CL, Wu MJ, Chou KJ, et al. (2004) Tuberculosis in patients with end-stage renal disease. Int J Tuberc Lung Dis 8: 92–97.
10. Simsek H, Alpar S, Ucar N, Aksu F, Ceyhan I, et al. (2010) Comparison of tuberculin skin testing and T-SPOT.TB for diagnosis of latent and active tuberculosis. Jpn J Infect Dis 63: 99–102.
11. Brock I, Weldingh K, Lillebaek T, Follmann F, Andersen P (2004) Comparison of tuberculin skin test and new specific blood test in tuberculosis contacts. Am J Respir Crit Care Med 170: 65–69.
12. Diel R, Loddenkemper R, Meywald-Walter K, Niemann S, Nienhaus A (2008) Predictive value of a whole blood IFN-gamma assay for the development of

active tuberculosis disease after recent infection with Mycobacterium tuberculosis. Am J Respir Crit Care Med 177: 1164–1170.
13. Triverio PA, Bridevaux PO, Roux-Lombard P, Niksic L, Rochat T, et al. (2009) Interferon-gamma release assays versus tuberculin skin testing for detection of latent tuberculosis in chronic haemodialysis patients. Nephrol Dial Transplant 24: 1952–1956.
14. Lee SS, Chou KJ, Su IJ, Chen YS, Fang HC, et al. (2009) High prevalence of latent tuberculosis infection in patients in end-stage renal disease on hemodialysis: Comparison of QuantiFERON-TB GOLD, ELISPOT, and tuberculin skin test. Infection 37: 96–102.
15. Lee SS, Chou KJ, Dou HY, Huang TS, Ni YY, et al. (2010) High prevalence of latent tuberculosis infection in dialysis patients using the interferon-gamma release assay and tuberculin skin test. Clin J Am Soc Nephrol 5: 1451–1457.
16. Chung WK, Zheng ZL, Sung JY, Kim S, Lee HH, et al. (2010) Validity of interferon-gamma-release assays for the diagnosis of latent tuberculosis in haemodialysis patients. Clin Microbiol Infect 16: 960–965.
17. Sester M, Sester U, Clauer P, Heine G, Mack U, et al. (2004) Tuberculin skin testing underestimates a high prevalence of latent tuberculosis infection in hemodialysis patients. Kidney Int 65: 1826–1834.
18. Stevens LA, Viswanathan G, Weiner DE (2010) Chronic kidney disease and end-stage renal disease in the elderly population: current prevalence, future projections, and clinical significance. Adv Chronic Kidney Dis 17: 293–301.
19. Hill CJ, Fogarty DG (2012) Changing trends in end-stage renal disease due to diabetes in the United kingdom. J Ren Care 38 Suppl 1: 12–22.
20. Shu CC, Wang JT, Lee CH, Wang JY, Lee LN, et al. (2010) Predicting results of mycobacterial culture on sputum smear reversion after anti-tuberculous treatment: a case control study. BMC Infect Dis 10: 48.

21. Pugh RN, Murray-Lyon IM, Dawson JL, Pietroni MC, Williams R (1973) Transection of the oesophagus for bleeding oesophageal varices. Br J Surg 60: 646–649.
22. Lalvani A, Pathan AA, McShane H, Wilkinson RJ, Latif M, et al. (2001) Rapid detection of *Mycobacterium tuberculosis* infection by enumeration of antigen-specific T cells. Am J Respir Crit Care Med 163: 824–828.
23. Dyrhol-Riise AM, Gran G, Wentzel-Larsen T, Blomberg B, Haanshuus CG, et al. (2010) Diagnosis and follow-up of treatment of latent tuberculosis; the utility of the QuantiFERON-TB Gold In-tube assay in outpatients from a tuberculosis low-endemic country. BMC Infect Dis 10: 57.
24. Banach DB, Harris TG (2011) Indeterminate QuantiFERON(R)-TB Gold results in a public health clinic setting. Int J Tuberc Lung Dis 15: 1623–1630.
25. (1997) NKF-DOQI clinical practice guidelines for hemodialysis adequacy. National Kidney Foundation. Am J Kidney Dis 30: S15–66.
26. Lukowsky LR, Kheifets L, Arah OA, Nissenson AR, Kalantar-Zadeh K (2012) Patterns and Predictors of Early Mortality in Incident Hemodialysis Patients: New Insights. Am J Nephrol 35: 548–558.
27. Lin HH, Ezzati M, Chang HY, Murray M (2009) Association between tobacco smoking and active tuberculosis in Taiwan: prospective cohort study. Am J Respir Crit Care Med 180: 475–480.
28. Jasmer RM, Snyder DC, Chin DP, Hopewell PC, Cuthbert SS, et al. (2000) Twelve months of isoniazid compared with four months of isoniazid and rifampin for persons with radiographic evidence of previous tuberculosis: an outcome and cost-effectiveness analysis. Am J Respir Crit Care Med 162: 1648–1652.
29. Yu MC, Suo J, Huang C, Bai KJ, Lin TP, et al. (1999) Annual risk of tuberculous infection in Taiwan, 1996–1998. J Formos Med Assoc 98: 496–499.
30. Lai CC, Tan CK, Chou CH, Hsu HL, Liao CH, et al. (2010) Increasing incidence of nontuberculous mycobacteria, Taiwan, 2000–2008. Emerg Infect Dis 16: 294–296.
31. Centers of Disease Control DoH, R.O.C. (Taiwan) (2010) CDC Annual Report 2011. Taipei: Centers of Disease Control, Department of Health, R.O.C. (Taiwan).
32. Wang JY, Shu CC, Lee CH, Yu CJ, Lee LN, et al. (2012) Interferon-gamma release assay and Rifampicin therapy for household contacts of tuberculosis. J Infect 64: 291–298.
33. Shu CC, Wu HD, Yu MC, Wang JT, Lee CH, et al. (2010) Use of high-dose inhaled corticosteroids is associated with pulmonary tuberculosis in patients with chronic obstructive pulmonary disease. Medicine (Baltimore) 89: 53–61.
34. Bates MN, Khalakdina A, Pai M, Chang L, Lessa F, et al. (2007) Risk of tuberculosis from exposure to tobacco smoke: a systematic review and meta-analysis. Arch Intern Med 167: 335–342.
35. Palomar R, Arias Guillen M, Robledo C, Aguero R, Aguero J, et al. (2011) Detection of latent tuberculosis infection in peritoneal dialysis patients: new methods. Nefrologia 31: 169–173.
36. Chavers BM, Solid CA, Gilbertson DT, Collins AJ (2007) Infection-related hospitalization rates in pediatric versus adult patients with end-stage renal disease in the United States. J Am Soc Nephrol 18: 952–959.
37. Lange B, Vavra M, Kern WV, Wagner D (2010) Indeterminate results of a tuberculosis-specific interferon-gamma release assay in immunocompromised patients. Eur Respir J 35: 1179–1182.
38. Fabrizi F, Dixit V, Martin P, Jadoul M, Messa P (2011) Meta-Analysis: The Impact of Nutritional Status on the Immune Response to Hepatitis B Virus Vaccine in Chronic Kidney Disease. Dig Dis Sci 2012; 57:1366–1372.
39. de Cal M, Cruz DN, Corradi V, Nalesso F, Polanco N, et al. (2008) HLA-DR expression and apoptosis: a cross-sectional controlled study in hemodialysis and peritoneal dialysis patients. Blood Purif 26: 249–254.
40. Vacher-Coponat H, Brunet C, Lyonnet L, Bonnet E, Loundou A, et al. (2008) Natural killer cell alterations correlate with loss of renal function and dialysis duration in uraemic patients. Nephrol Dial Transplant 23: 1406–1414.

Safety Issues of Long-Term Glucose Load in Patients on Peritoneal Dialysis

Hon-Yen Wu[1,2,5], Kuan-Yu Hung[2,3*⊕], Tao-Min Huang[2,5], Fu-Chang Hu[4,6], Yu-Sen Peng[1,2], Jenq-Wen Huang[2*⊕], Shuei-Liong Lin[2], Yung-Ming Chen[2,5], Tzong-Shinn Chu[2], Tun-Jun Tsai[2], Kwan-Dun Wu[2]

1 Department of Internal Medicine, Far Eastern Memorial Hospital, New Taipei City, Taiwan, 2 Department of Internal Medicine, National Taiwan University Hospital, Taipei, Taiwan, 3 Center of Quality Management, National Taiwan University Hospital, Taipei, Taiwan, 4 National Center of Excellence for General Clinical Trial and Research, National Taiwan University Hospital, Taipei, Taiwan, 5 Department of Internal Medicine, Yun-Lin Branch, National Taiwan University Hospital, Yun-Lin, Taiwan, 6 International Harvard Statistical Consulting Company, Taipei, Taiwan

Abstract

Background: Effects of long-term glucose load on peritoneal dialysis (PD) patient safety and outcomes have seldom been reported. This study demonstrates the influence of long-term glucose load on patient and technique survival.

Methods: We surveyed 173 incident PD patients. Long-term glucose load was evaluated by calculating the average dialysate glucose concentration since initiation of PD. Risk factors were assessed by fitting Cox's models with repeatedly measured time-dependent covariates.

Results: We noted that older age, higher glucose concentration, and lower residual renal function (RRF) were significantly associated with a worse patient survival. We found that female gender, absence of diabetes, lower glucose concentration, use of icodextrin, higher serum high density lipoprotein cholesterol, and higher RRF were significantly associated with a better technique survival.

Conclusions: Long-term glucose load predicted mortality and technique failure in chronic PD patients. These findings emphasize the importance of minimizing glucose load in PD patients.

Editor: Paolo Fiorina, Children's Hospital Boston/Harvard Medical School, United States of America

Funding: This work was supported by grants from the National Science Council of Taiwan (to Kuan-Yu Hung; NSC-95-2314-B-002-238-MY2), the Ta-Tung Kidney Foundation, and the Mrs. Hsiu-Chin Lee Kidney Research Foundation (Taipei, Taiwan), and grants from the Yun-Lin Branch, National Taiwan University Hospital (to Hon-Yen Wu; NTUHYL.97.S007 and NTUHYL.98.S010, Yun-Lin, Taiwan). The funders had no role in study design, data collection and analysis, decision to publish, or preparation of the manuscript.

Competing Interests: The authors have declared that no competing interests exist.

* E-mail: kyhung@ntu.edu.tw (K-YH); 007378@ntuh.gov.tw (J-WH)

⊕ These authors contributed equally to this work.

Introduction

Glucose is the main osmotic agents providing ultrafiltration (UF) to peritoneal dialysis (PD) patients [1], however, a high glucose load may cause peritoneal damage, hyperglycemia, hyperinsulinemia, dyslipidemia, oxidative stress, and increased incidences of metabolic syndrome, as well as cardiovascular diseases (CVD) [2,3,4]. We recently reported that higher initial glucose load, defined as the average dialysate glucose concentration prescribed in the first 6 months of PD therapy, predicted a worse PD technique survival [1]. In addition, we also identified that patients with diabetes mellitus (DM), high body mass index (BMI), and low residual renal function (RRF) tend to have a high dialysate glucose load during long-term PD therapy [5]. Regarding long-term patient safety, the accumulative effects from glucose load have rarely been reported. In this retrospective 7-year cohort study of chronic PD patients, we analyze the accumulative effects of long-term glucose load on patient outcomes by applying repeatedly measured time-dependent covariates in survival analysis.

Methods

Ethics Statement

The Institutional Review Board of National Taiwan University Hospital approved the retrospective cohort study. Written informed consent was not needed because the study retrospectively collected available medical records in the hospital. The Institutional Review Board specifically granted a waiver for the "no consent needed".

Study participants: inclusion and exclusion criteria

202 patients initiated PD therapy at our PD center between September 2001 and January 2006. We excluded those who were younger than 18 years old (n = 4) or had active malignancy (n = 3). Patients who had a PD technique survival shorter than 6 months (n = 10) or had undergone PD previously (n = 12) were also excluded. A total of 173 end-stage renal disease (ESRD) patients were enrolled in our study and were followed until February 2008. The mean follow-up period was 42.0 ± 17.2 (range 6–78) months.

We reviewed clinical data of each patient, including age, gender, and annual data of comorbid diseases, body height, body weight, RRF, peritoneal transport characteristics and solute clearance, cardiothoracic ratio (CTR), and blood laboratory exams. Comorbid diseases included DM, CVD, and chronic hepatic diseases. Patients with a history of stroke, coronary or peripheral artery diseases, or left ventricular ejection fraction less than 30% were considered to have CVD [5,6]. Chronic hepatic diseases included liver cirrhosis and chronic viral hepatitis [7].

Definitions of patient survival and PD technique survival

The primary outcome of this study was actuarial patient survival and the secondary outcome was PD technique survival. In the analysis of patient survival, the causes of drop-out were classified as death, renal transplantation, and hospital transfer. Because long-term survival is much better for renal transplant recipients than patients who remain on dialysis [8], renal transplantation, as well as hospital transfer, were considered as censoring events in the analysis of patient survival. In the analysis of PD technique survival, the reasons for terminating PD were categorized as hospital transfer, renal transplantation, death, and switching to hemodialysis (HD). Among them, events of switching to HD were recognized as PD technique failure, while the others were regarded as censoring events.

PD regimens and calculation of glucose load

The PD regimen and modality for each patient were evaluated and prescribed in our PD unit during monthly follow-up. We reviewed the detailed PD regimen of each patient. Our evaluations for glucose exposure included glucose weight and glucose load. Glucose weight was defined as the sum of the products of glucose concentration and the volume for each exchange of glucose solution (Dianeal®; Baxter Healthcare Corporation, Deerfield, IL, U.S.A.) over a time period [9], whereas glucose load was calculated as the average dialysate glucose concentration (i.e., [total glucose weight]/[total volume of glucose solution]) over a time period [10,11]. The administered volume of icodextrin solution (Extraneal®; Baxter Healthcare) and amino acid solution (Nutrineal®; Baxter Healthcare) for each patient was also evaluated.

Laboratory examinations and peritoneal dialysis assessments

The blood for laboratory exams was drawn after patients had fasted for at least 8 hours. We evaluated dialysate-to-plasma ratio of creatinine (D/P Cre) and UF volume by the peritoneal equilibration test (PET) [12]. We measured peritoneal solute clearance by weekly peritoneal Kt/V, evaluated RRF based on weekly renal Kt/V, and estimated protein intake by normalized protein nitrogen appearance (nPNA) [13]. All biochemical and hematological tests were performed with automatic analyzers.

Statistical analyses

Data are expressed as mean ± standard deviation (SD) or frequency and percentage, unless otherwise indicated. As descriptive analysis, univariate analyses were performed by using two-sample t tests, one-way analysis of variance (ANOVA), Pearson's chi-square test, or Fisher's exact test, as appropriate. In multivariate analysis, the risk factors of mortality and PD technique failure were assessed by fitting two different Cox's models with repeatedly measured time-dependent covariates using the counting process approach. The repeatedly measured time-dependent covariates included body weight, comorbidity status, dialysate prescription, PD modality, laboratory blood exams, peritoneal transport, estimated protein intake, and solute clearance by the peritoneum and kidneys. Among them, each subject's dialysate prescription was represented by (1) the accumulative glucose exposure and (2) the accumulative volumes of icodextrin solution and amino acid solution, from the time of PD initiation to each time at which a PD technique failure or death occurred in the Cox's models for PD technique failure or mortality.

Next, the predictors of each year's annual average dialysate glucose concentration over the 6-year follow-up period were examined. Since the missing data in the repeated-measurements of glucose concentration at later times was most likely due to PD technique failure, 6 separate multiple linear regression models were fitted to the data of the subjects who were still at risk in the beginning of each year.

To assure the quality of the analysis results, we applied basic model-fitting techniques, including stepwise variable selection, goodness-of-fit assessment, and regression diagnostics (e.g., residual analysis, detection of influential cases, and checks for multicollinearity), in our regression analysis. The stepwise variable selection procedure (with iterations between the forward and backward steps) was applied to obtain the candidate final regression model. All the univariate significant and non-significant relevant covariates and some of their interactions were put on the variable list to be selected. The significance levels for entry and for stay were set to 0.15 or larger. Since the statistical testing at each step of the stepwise variable selection procedure was conditioning on the other covariates in the regression model, the concern about multiple analyses is minor. We used the variance inflation factor to detect the potential multicollinearity problem. A grid search method was applied to discover appropriate cut-off points for representing nonlinear effects of some continuous covariates. A two-sided P value ≤0.05 was considered statistically significant. The statistical analyses were conducted using SAS software, version 9.1.3 (SAS Institute Inc., Cary, NC, USA).

Results

Patient characteristics

There were 87 men and 86 women enrolled in our study with a mean age of 54.6±15.6 years at PD initiation. Patients with longer technique survivals had higher BMI, higher serum levels of total cholesterol, triglyceride (TG), albumin, and creatinine (Table 1). We noted a trend of a decrease in RRF with increasing peritoneal Kt/V among patients who had more prolonged PD therapy. Moreover, these patients were prescribed with higher doses of icodextrin solution and showed a higher UF volume in later years (Table 1). Patients with longer overall survivals had higher BMI and higher serum levels of total cholesterol, TG, albumin, and creatinine (Table 2). During the study period, 4 cases of new-onset DM were diagnosed, and we considered the change in DM status as a repeatedly measured time-dependent covariate in the regression analysis.

Patient survival analysis

By the end of the follow-up, there were 60 dropouts, including 31 deaths, 20 renal transplantations, and 9 patients transferred to other hospitals. The major causes of death included infectious diseases (64.5%) and CVD (12.9%). The annual patient survival rates by using the Kaplan-Meier method were 94.7%, 90.5%, 85.5%, 78.0%, and 75.5% at the beginning of year-2, year-3, year-4, year-5, and year-6, respectively. Kaplan-Meier survival curves showed a significant worse patient survival in the subjects with higher glucose load (Figure 1A, $P=0.03$). The mean patient

Table 1. Demographic and clinical data of patients who remained on PD at the beginning of each year.

Variable	Treatment Year											
	First year		Second year		Third year		Fourth year		Fifth year		Sixth year	
Patient number	173		151		133		86		49		13	
Gender(M:F)	87 :	86	75 :	76	64 :	69	37 :	49	22 :	27	5 :	8
Baseline age (years)	54.6 ±	15.6	53.3 ±	14.7	53.2 ±	14.0	51.0 ±	12.0	50.8 ±	9.2	52.0 ±	8.6
Glucose concentration (%)*	1.81 ±	0.26	1.79 ±	0.33	1.80 ±	0.39	1.81 ±	0.42	1.76 ±	0.71	1.90 ±	0.68
Glucose weight (Kg/month)**	4.9 ±	1.5	4.9 ±	1.7	5.0 ±	1.7	5.1 ±	1.9	4.8 ±	2.3	4.3 ±	1.9
Icodextrin solution (L/month)**, §	3.6 ±	14.1	7.2 ±	18.9	12.5 ±	24.9	9.8 ±	21.4	11.5 ±	21.1	25.5 ±	25.8
Amino acid solution (L/month)**	1.3 ±	5.4	2.2 ±	8.0	2.0 ±	8.7	0.7 ±	3.2	0.8 ±	2.7	0.0 ±	0.0
Body mass index (Kg/m²)§	21.6 ±	3.2	22.8 ±	3.4	23.0 ±	3.3	22.9 ±	2.8	23.0 ±	2.4	22.6 ±	2.8
Comorbid diseases												
Diabetes mellitus	37	(21.4)	29	(19.2)	22	(16.5)	10	(11.6)	5	(10.2)	3	(23.1)
Cardiovascular diseases	64	(37.0)	52	(34.4)	41	(30.8)	24	(27.9)	10	(20.4)	5	(38.5)
D/P Cre	0.63 ±	0.10	0.62 ±	0.10	0.61 ±	0.10	0.61 ±	0.10	0.62 ±	0.10	0.65 ±	0.07
Ultrafiltration volume (ml)***, §	278 ±	187	333 ±	173	376 ±	332	347 ±	221	441 ±	265	456 ±	154
PD modality (CAPD:APD)	144 :	29	121 :	30	97 :	36	61 :	25	36 :	13	12 :	1
Weekly peritoneal Kt/V§	1.71 ±	0.36	1.85 ±	0.33	1.94 ±	0.27	1.96 ±	0.28	2.09 ±	0.29	2.09 ±	0.33
Weekly renal Kt/V§	0.60 ±	0.44	0.37 ±	0.36	0.25 ±	0.31	0.21 ±	0.30	0.10 ±	0.19	0.04 ±	0.15
Daily urine output (ml)§	742 ±	558	580 ±	555	440 ±	568	365 ±	514	190 ±	346	130 ±	413
nPNA (g/Kg/d)	1.10 ±	0.25	1.09 ±	0.23	1.08 ±	0.23	1.05 ±	0.22	1.04 ±	0.20	0.98 ±	0.24
Cardiothoracic ratio (%)	51.4 ±	7.5	50.1 ±	6.7	49.9 ±	6.7	49.6 ±	6.6	50.5 ±	6.2	49.5 ±	10.8
Hemoglobin (g/dL)	9.9 ±	1.6	9.8 ±	1.3	9.8 ±	1.4	9.9 ±	1.3	9.8 ±	1.8	10.0 ±	1.5
Blood biochemistry												
Total cholesterol (mg/dL)§	201 ±	52	222 ±	52	217 ±	52	214 ±	47	204 ±	60	218 ±	83
Triglyceride (mg/dL)§	156 ±	111	213 ±	151	218 ±	171	221 ±	166	214 ±	155	313 ±	431
HDL (mg/dL)	44.0 ±	13.6	41.7 ±	11.5	41.5 ±	15.6	40.3 ±	8.9	40.5 ±	9.3	40.8 ±	9.2
Fasting glucose (mg/dL)	111 ±	43	111 ±	39	103 ±	43	100 ±	29	107 ±	28	99 ±	18
Albumin (g/dL)§	3.8 ±	0.5	4.0 ±	0.4	4.0 ±	0.4	4.0 ±	0.3	4.1 ±	0.4	4.0 ±	0.2
Urea nitrogen (mg/dL)	65.5 ±	22.2	62.8 ±	16.0	63.3 ±	16.4	62.9 ±	15.1	64.1 ±	16.9	63.1 ±	10.8
Creatinine (mg/dL)§	9.2 ±	3.0	11.0 ±	2.9	11.6 ±	2.9	11.5 ±	3.3	12.3 ±	2.5	11.3 ±	2.3

NOTE. Data are expressed as mean ± SD. Conversion factors for units: hemoglobin in g/dL to g/L, ×10; cholesterol and HDL in mg/dL to mmol/L, ×0.02586; triglyceride in mg/dL to mmol/L, ×0.01129; glucose in mg/dL to mmol/L, ×0.05551; albumin in g/dL to to g/L, ×10; urea nitrogen in mg/dL to mmol/L, ×0.357; creatinine in mg/dL to μmol/L, ×88.4.

Abbreviations: D/P, dialysate-to-plasma; CAPD, continuous ambulatory peritoneal dialysis; APD, automated peritoneal dialysis; nPNA, normalized protein nitrogen appearance; HDL, high-density lipoprotein cholesterol.

*The annual average dialysate glucose concentration prescribed within each year.

**Obtained from all the PD solution prescribed within each year.

***Obtained from the peritoneal equilibration test.

§$P<0.05$ for the statistical testing between years.

survival time was 65.5 ± 1.9 months. By fitting Cox's models with repeatedly measured time-dependent covariates, we found that older age, higher glucose load, lower RRF, higher blood urea nitrogen (BUN), and lower serum creatinine were significantly associated with a worse patient survival (Table 3). The presence of CVD had a borderline significant influence on patient survival (Table 3), and the positive association between the presence of CVD and DM was highly significant (odds ratio = 7.224, $P<0.001$). This could explain why only the presence of CVD, but not also DM, was significant in patient survival analysis.

PD technique survival analysis

By the end of the follow-up, there were 42 PD technique failures, including peritonitis (42.9%), UF failure (21.4%), exit site infection (19.0%), and inadequate solute clearance (14.3%). Events of random censorings included 20 renal transplantations, 3 hospital transfers, and 19 deaths (mainly due to infectious diseases and CVD). The annual PD technique survival rates by using the Kaplan-Meier method were 95.7%, 88.5%, 79.8%, 71.6%, and 56.4% at the beginning of year-2, year-3, year-4, year-5, and year-6, respectively. Kaplan-Meier survival curves showed a borderline significant worse technique survival in the subjects with higher glucose load (Figure 1B, $P=0.057$). The mean technique survival time was 58.8 ± 2.1 months. By fitting Cox's models with repeatedly measured time-dependent covariates, we found that male gender, the presence of DM, higher glucose load, lower RRF, and lower serum high-density lipoprotein (HDL) were significantly associated with a worse technique survival (Table 3).

Table 2. Demographic and clinical data of patients who remained alive at the beginning of each year.

Variable	First year		Second year		Third year		Fourth year		Fifth year		Sixth year	
	Treatment Year											
Patient number	173		159		147		99		58		21	
Gender(M:F)	87 :	86	81 :	78	75 :	72	46 :	53	29 :	29	9 :	12
Baseline age (years)	54.6 ±	15.6	53.9 ±	15.2	53.3 ±	14.2	51.0 ±	12.7	49.9 ±	11.9	49.3 ±	9.1
Glucose concentration (%)*, ξ	1.81 ±	0.26	1.70 ±	0.51	1.63 ±	0.65	1.57 ±	0.73	1.48 ±	0.91	1.17 ±	1.08
Glucose weight (Kg/month)**, ξ	4.9 ±	1.5	4.7 ±	2.0	4.5 ±	2.2	4.5 ±	2.5	4.1 ±	2.8	2.7 ±	2.6
Icodextrin solution (L/month)**, ξ	3.6 ±	14.1	6.8 ±	18.5	11.5 ±	23.9	8.5 ±	20.2	9.7 ±	19.8	15.8 ±	23.7
Body mass index (Kg/m²)ξ	21.6 ±	3.2	22.7 ±	3.4	23.1 ±	3.4	22.9 ±	2.9	22.8 ±	2.5	23.2 ±	3.3
Comorbid diseases												
Diabetes mellitus	37	(21.4)	32	(20.1)	29	(19.7)	13	(13.1)	6	(10.3)	4	(19.0)
Cardiovascular diseases	64	(37.0)	56	(35.2)	47	(32.0)	26	(26.3)	11	(19.0)	6	(28.6)
Weekly renal Kt/Vξ	0.60 ±	0.44	0.37 ±	0.37	0.25 ±	0.30	0.21 ±	0.29	0.10 ±	0.19	0.03 ±	0.13
Hemoglobin (g/dL)	9.9 ±	1.6	9.75 ±	1.29	9.86 ±	1.42	9.88 ±	1.51	9.82 ±	2.00	10.38 ±	1.94
Blood biochemistry												
Total cholesterol (mg/dL)ξ	201 ±	52	221 ±	52	215 ±	52	211 ±	48	200 ±	59	212 ±	80
Triglyceride (mg/dL)ξ	156 ±	111	213 ±	149	212 ±	166	218 ±	166	206 ±	149	282 ±	372
Fasting glucose (mg/dL)	111 ±	43	113 ±	42	104 ±	43	100 ±	29	106 ±	27	101 ±	20
Albumin (g/dL)ξ	3.8 ±	0.5	3.9 ±	0.4	4.0 ±	0.4	4.0 ±	0.4	4.1 ±	0.4	4.0 ±	0.4
Urea nitrogen (mg/dL)	65.5 ±	22.2	62.8 ±	16.1	63.8 ±	17.3	62.6 ±	15.7	63.6 ±	17.6	60.6 ±	13.4
Creatinine (mg/dL)ξ	9.2 ±	3.0	10.9 ±	3.0	11.5 ±	2.9	11.5 ±	3.3	12.2 ±	2.5	10.5 ±	3.0

NOTE. Data are expressed as mean ± S.D. Conversion factors for units: hemoglobin in g/dL to g/L, ×10; cholesterol in mg/dL to mmol/L, ×0.02586; triglyceride in mg/dL to mmol/L, ×0.01129; glucose in mg/dL to mmol/L, ×0.05551; albumin in g/dL to to g/L, ×10; urea nitrogen in mg/dL to mmol/L, ×0.357; creatinine in mg/dL to μmol/L, ×88.4.
*The annual average dialysate glucose concentration prescribed within each year.
**Obtained from all the PD solution prescribed within each year.
ξP<0.05 for the statistical testing between years.

Higher glucose weight and the use of icodextrin solution were significantly associated with a better technique survival (Table 3). By Pearson's correlation analysis, a higher dialysate glucose weight was significantly correlated with a higher volume of glucose solution ($r = 0.861$, $P<0.001$), and the correlation between the volume of glucose solution and average dialysate glucose concentration was much lower ($r = 0.274$, $P<0.001$). Higher peritoneal Kt/V (without adding weekly renal Kt/V) was not persistently associated with a better technique survival. Further analysis of discretized weekly peritoneal Kt/V (without adding weekly renal Kt/V) with different cut-off values revealed that the range between 1.4 and 1.7 was associated with the best technique survival (Table 3).

Factors determining annual glucose load

Figure 2 shows the distributions of glucose load in our study population. Considering the gradual increase in the number of dropouts due to technique failure, we performed multiple linear regressions to analyze the predictors for annual glucose load (average dialysate glucose concentration) among patients who remained on PD at the beginning of that year. We applied PD year-specific multiple linear regression models, using the stepwise variable selection method, to analyze the effect of gender, age, BMI, comorbid diseases, PD modality, icodextrin solution, amino acid solution, peritoneal characteristics and solute clearance, RRF, CTR, and results of blood tests. As shown in Table 4, the presence of DM, higher BMI, lower weekly renal Kt/V, younger age, and the use of icodextrin solution were significantly correlated with

higher glucose load during most of the years of the study period. We also observed that the modality of automated PD (APD), higher CTR, lower peritoneal UF volume, lower serum albumin, and lower BUN were significantly correlated with higher glucose load in some years during the study period (Table 4).

Discussion

This is the first detailed survival analysis describing the long-term effects of glucose load on PD outcomes by applying the repeatedly measured time-dependent method. In this 7-year cohort, patients with higher long-term glucose load were significantly associated with worse actuarial patient survival and PD technique survival (Table 3). In addition, the prescription of icodextrin solution was significantly associated with a better PD technique survival (Table 3). Furthermore, younger age was one of the main risk factors for high glucose load in long-term PD (Table 4).

Previous studies on PD patients have shown that the actual glucose absorption by the peritoneum can be precisely predicted from the average glucose concentration in the dialysate inflow, which offers an easy way to evaluate glucose uptake in long-term PD patients [11]. In the present study, we demonstrated further that a higher chronic glucose load was significantly associated with a worse patient survival, as well as a worse technique survival (Table 3). This result is compatible with our previous report regarding the harmful effects of the average dialysate glucose concentration in the initial 6 months after PD commencement [1].

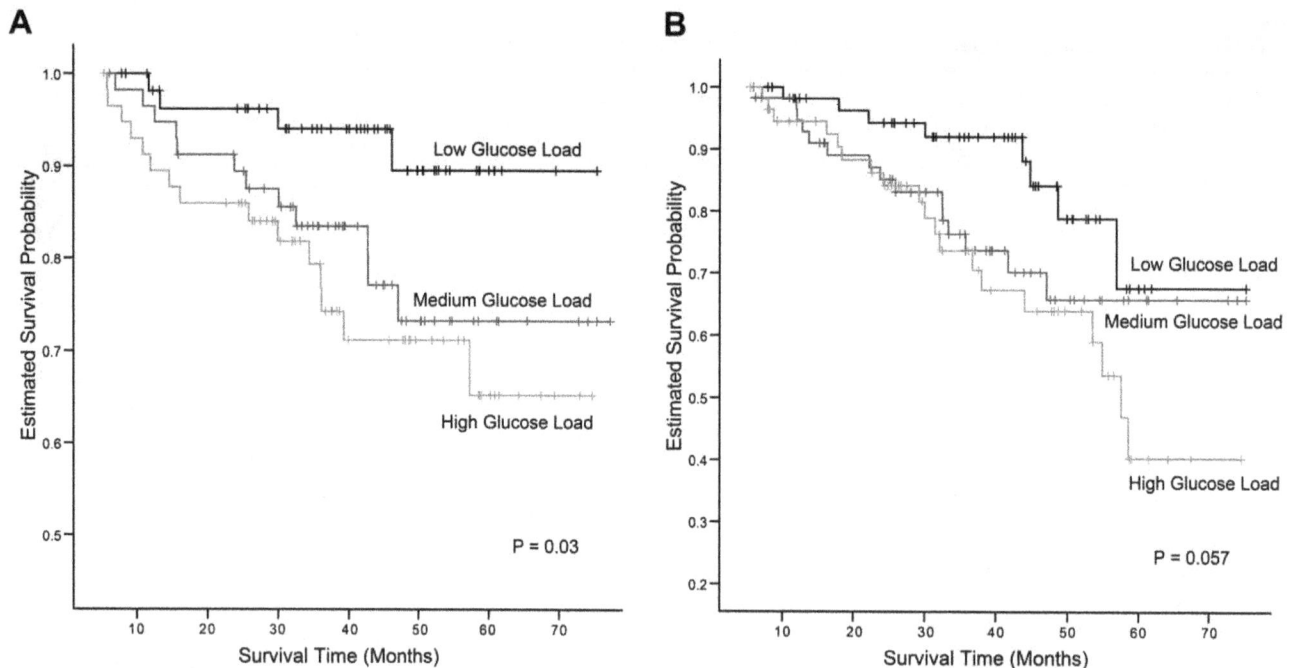

Figure 1. Cumulative survival curves for (A) patient survival and (B) technique survival. All subjects were divided into tertiles (low, medium, or high glucose load group) according to the average dialysate glucose concentration administered since PD initiation. Survival curves are constructed by the Kaplan-Meier method and compared by the log-rank test. Subjects with higher glucose load showed worse patient and technique survivals.

Table 3. Multivariate analyses of the risk factors for patient and technique survival using Cox's models with repeatedly measured time-dependent covariates.

Covariate	Parameter Estimate (B)	Standard Error	P Value	Hazard Ratio	95% Confidence Interval	
Patient Survival[1]:						
Baseline age (years)	0.07	0.02	< 0.001	1.07	1.03	- 1.11
Cardiovascular diseases	0.99	0.54	0.07	2.68	0.92	- 7.76
Glucose concentration (%)*	1.83	0.81	0.02	6.23	1.26	- 30.74
Weekly renal Kt/V	- 3.18	1.04	0.002	0.04	0.01	- 0.32
Blood urea nitrogen (mg/dL)	0.02	0.01	0.01	1.02	1.004	- 1.04
Creatinine (mg/dL)	- 0.40	0.09	< 0.001	0.67	0.56	- 0.80
Technique Survival[2]:						
Male gender	1.39	0.40	< 0.001	4.03	1.85	- 8.75
Diabetes mellitus	1.53	0.41	< 0.001	4.64	2.07	- 10.38
Glucose concentration (%)*	2.25	0.90	0.01	9.46	1.62	- 55.35
Glucose weight (Kg/month)*	- 0.64	0.17	< 0.001	0.53	0.38	- 0.73
Icodextrin solution (L/month)*	- 0.02	0.01	0.03	0.98	0.96	- 0.997
Weekly renal Kt/V	- 2.03	0.72	< 0.01	0.13	0.03	- 0.53
1.4 ≤ Weekly peritoneal Kt/V <1.7	- 1.53	0.63	0.02	0.22	0.06	- 0.74
HDL (mg/dL)	- 0.05	0.02	0.02	0.95	0.92	- 0.99

NOTES. Conversion factors for units: HDL in mg/dL to mmol/L, ×0.02586; urea nitrogen in mg/dL to mmol/L, ×0.357; creatinine in mg/dL to μmol/L, ×88.4.
Abbreviations: HDL, high-density lipoprotein cholesterol.
[1]Cox's model with 4 repeatedly measured time-dependent covariates (glucose concentration, weekly renal Kt/V, blood urea nitrogen, and creatinine), adjusted generalized $R^2 = 0.58$.
[2]Cox's model with 7 repeatedly measured time-dependent covariates (diabetes mellitus, glucose concentration, glucose weight, icodextrin solution, weekly renal Kt/V, weekly peritoneal Kt/V, and HDL), adjusted generalized $R^2 = 0.31$.
*Each subject's dialysate prescription was represented by (1) the accumulative glucose exposure and (2) the accumulative volumes of icodextrin solution, from the time of PD initiation to each time at which a PD technique failure or death occurred in the Cox's models for PD technique failure or mortality.

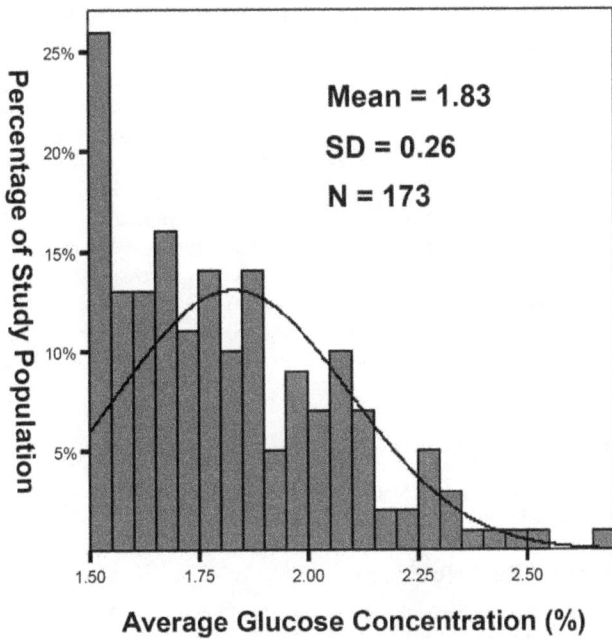

Mean = 1.83

SD = 0.26

N = 173

Figure 2. Frequency distribution of average dialysate glucose concentration in the study population. Average dialysate glucose concentration of each subject was calculated as: [total glucose weight]/ [total volume of glucose solution] administered since initiation of PD.

A higher average dialysate glucose concentration is more directly related with the consumption of high glucose-containing PD solution, implying more glucose uptake, poor fluid control, and

more peritoneal damage [3,5,11]. In contrast, prescription of icodextrin solution is associated with a better PD technique survival, which may result from the beneficial effects of icodextrin in improving fluid control and metabolic abnormalities [2,3,14].

Because of the regulations of the health insurance system in Taiwan, icodextrin solution is prescribed to patients who require 2.5% or 4.25% dextrose solution in more than half of their daily dialysate volume. This leads to the association between the use of icodextrin solution and higher average dialysate glucose concentration (Table 4). PD patients require dialysate with higher glucose concentration if their fluid control is inadequate, thus higher CTR and lower peritoneal UF volume have some associations with higher glucose load (Table 4). Daily oral intake in elderly PD patients may decrease due to diminished appetite, dental problems, constipation, and increased intra-abdominal pressure by the dialysate [15]. This may result in less use of PD solution with high glucose concentration in elderly patients (Table 4).

PD patients with lower levels of serum creatinine or higher levels of BUN were significantly associated with higher mortality (Table 3). Serum creatinine is highly correlated with lean body mass and nutritional condition in patients on chronic dialysis therapy, and the association between low serum creatinine and high mortality has been reported in previous studies [16]. A "U"-shaped pattern of the influence of BUN on dialysis patients has been reported, with higher mortality in patients with BUN over 110 mg/dL or below 60 mg/dL. This phenomenon might result from malnutrition in low BUN groups and under dialysis in high BUN groups [16,17]. This explains the association between higher mortality and lower levels of serum creatinine or higher levels of BUN (Table 3).

There is a significant correlation between high glucose weight and high dialysate volume ($r = 0.861$), hence, the beneficial effect

Table 4. Multiple linear regression analyses of predictors associated with annual average dialysate glucose concentration administered within each year[a].

| Covariate | Treatment Year | | | | | |
	First year[1]	Second year[2]	Third year[3]	Fourth year[4]	Fifth year[5]	Sixth year[6]
Baseline age (years)	—	−0.004 ± 0.002*	−0.003 ± 0.002*	−0.011 ± 0.003**	−0.022 ± 0.005**	−0.020 ± 0.007**
Diabetes mellitus	0.226 ± 0.040**	0.177 ± 0.056**	0.266 ± 0.064**	0.186 ± 0.093*	0.599 ± 0.136**	0.288 ± 0.160[§]
Body mass index (Kg/m²)	0.020 ± 0.005**	0.028 ± 0.006**	0.028 ± 0.007**	0.036 ± 0.012**	—	—
Cardiothoracic ratio (%)	—	0.783 ± 0.336*	—	1.328 ± 0.493**	—	—
Weekly renal Kt/V	−0.090 ± 0.036**	−0.174 ± 0.055**	−0.355 ± 0.071**	−0.232 ± 0.096*	—	—
Icodextrin solution (kl/month)[b]	0.033 ± 0.008**	0.025 ± 0.008**	—	—	0.055 ± 0.026*	0.107 ± 0.019**
Ultrafiltration volume (L)[c]	—	—	−0.418 ± 0.128**	−0.479 ± 0.139**	—	—
Automated peritoneal dialysis	0.081 ± 0.041*	—	—	—	—	—
Albumin (g/dL)	−0.079 ± 0.031**	—	—	—	—	—
Blood urea nitrogen (mg/dL)	—	—	—	−0.004 ± 0.002*	—	—

NOTE. Conversion factors for units: albumin in g/dL to to g/L, ×10; urea nitrogen in mg/dL to mmol/L, ×0.357.
[a]The numbers listed in the table are the least squares estimates of regression coefficients ± estimates of the corresponding standard errors.
[b]Obtained from all the PD solution prescribed within each year.
[c]Obtained from the peritoneal equilibration test.
*$p \leq 0.05$.
**$p \leq 0.01$.
[§]$0.05 < P < 0.1$.
[1]Linear regression model: n = 173, $R^2 = 0.4101$.
[2]Linear regression model: n = 150, $R^2 = 0.3751$.
[3]Linear regression model: n = 129, $R^2 = 0.4534$.
[4]Linear regression model: n = 84, $R^2 = 0.4466$.
[5]Linear regression model: n = 44, $R^2 = 0.5664$.
[6]Linear regression model: n = 22, $R^2 = 0.7284$.

of total glucose weight (Table 3) might reflect a better peritoneal solute clearance. We noted that patients with weekly peritoneal Kt/V (without adding weekly renal Kt/V) between 1.4 and 1.7 had significantly better technique survivals (Table 3). Similar results were also reported by Lo et al. They noted a "V" shaped curve of mortality risk in female anuric PD patients, with the best survival rates among those with weekly peritoneal Kt/V between 1.67 and 1.86 [18]. According to the guidelines for solute removal in chronic PD, the weekly total Kt/V (peritoneal Kt/V plus renal Kt/V) should be at least 1.7 or above [19]. However, there are no additional beneficial effects on patient outcomes when increasing the weekly total Kt/V further, and potential adverse effects of increasing PD dose include increased intraperitoneal pressure, failure to increase clearance of middle molecules, and increased exposure to glucose [18].

This study certainly has a few limitations. First, this is a retrospective cohort analysis, and the causal relationships between variables and outcomes could be influenced by confounding factors. Even though we have controlled for several important covariates, the possibility of residual confounding still remains. Second, the patient number of our study cohort is slightly limited; however, the statistical power for testing important hypotheses should be enough in Cox's models using repeatedly measured time-dependent covariates. Third, it is difficult to clearly distinguish the study population into either continuous ambulatory PD (CAPD) or APD groups. Patients initiated PD with the modality of CAPD, and may have shifted between APD and CAPD according to medical advice and individual family facilities or convenience. We tried to minimize this limitation by applying PD modality as a repeatedly measured time-dependent covariate in the regression analysis. Fourth, although our PD center belongs to a tertiary referral university hospital with patients from the whole country, this is a single-center study and the applicability of our findings to general PD population is still limited. To resolve these limitations, a prospective, large scale, multi-center randomized trial comparing different PD regimens is necessary.

In conclusion, our study demonstrates that long-term glucose load predicts mortality and technique failure in chronic PD patients, and the use of icodextrin is associated with a better technique survival.

Acknowledgments

We thank Ms. Ling-Chu Wu and Ms. Chia-Chi Cheng for their assistance in statistical computing.

Author Contributions

Conceived and designed the experiments: H-YW K-YH J-WH. Performed the experiments: H-YW T-MH F-CH. Analyzed the data: H-YW Y-SP S-LL Y-MC. Contributed reagents/materials/analysis tools: F-CH. Wrote the paper: H-YW K-YH J-WH. Reviewed and edited the manuscript: T-SC T-JT K-DW.

References

1. Wu HY, Hung KY, Huang JW, Chen YM, Tsai TJ, et al. (2008) Initial glucose load predicts technique survival in patients on chronic peritoneal dialysis. Am J Nephrol 28: 765–771.
2. Li PK, Kwan BC, Ko GT, Chow KM, Leung CB, et al. (2009) Treatment of metabolic syndrome in peritoneal dialysis patients. Perit Dial Int 29 Suppl 2: S149–152.
3. Holmes C, Mujais S (2006) Glucose sparing in peritoneal dialysis: implications and metrics. Kidney Int Suppl. pp S104–109.
4. Liu J, Rosner MH (2006) Lipid abnormalities associated with end-stage renal disease. Semin Dial 19: 32–40.
5. Wu HY, Hung KY, Hu FC, Chen YM, Chu TS, et al. (2010) Risk factors for high dialysate glucose use in PD patients–A retrospective 5-year cohort study. Perit Dial Int 30: 448–455.
6. Peng YS, Chiang CK, Hung KY, Chiang SS, Lu CS, et al. (2007) The association of higher depressive symptoms and sexual dysfunction in male haemodialysis patients. Nephrol Dial Transplant 22: 857–861.
7. Chaudhary K, Khanna R (2008) Renal replacement therapy in end-stage renal disease patients with chronic liver disease and ascites: role of peritoneal dialysis. Perit Dial Int 28: 113–117.
8. Wolfe RA, Ashby VB, Milford EL, Ojo AO, Ettenger RE, et al. (1999) Comparison of mortality in all patients on dialysis, patients on dialysis awaiting transplantation, and recipients of a first cadaveric transplant. N Engl J Med 341: 1725–1730.
9. Davies SJ, Phillips L, Naish PF, Russell GI (2001) Peritoneal glucose exposure and changes in membrane solute transport with time on peritoneal dialysis. J Am Soc Nephrol 12: 1046–1051.
10. Davies SJ, Brown EA, Frandsen NE, Rodrigues AS, Rodriguez-Carmona A, et al. (2005) Longitudinal membrane function in functionally anuric patients treated with APD: data from EAPOS on the effects of glucose and icodextrin prescription. Kidney Int 67: 1609–1615.
11. Grodstein GP, Blumenkrantz MJ, Kopple JD, Moran JK, Coburn JW (1981) Glucose absorption during continuous ambulatory peritoneal dialysis. Kidney Int 19: 564–567.
12. Twardowski ZJ, Nolph KD, Khanna R, Prowant BF, Ryan LP, et al. (1987) Peritoneal equilibration test. Perit Dial Bull 7: 138–147.
13. Bergstrom J, Heimburger O, Lindholm B (1998) Calculation of the protein equivalent of total nitrogen appearance from urea appearance. Which formulas should be used? Perit Dial Int 18: 467–473.
14. Adachi Y, Nakagawa Y, Nishio A (2006) Icodextrin preserves residual renal function in patients treated with automated peritoneal dialysis. Perit Dial Int 26: 405–407.
15. Ho-dac-Pannekeet MM (2006) PD in the elderly–a challenge for the (pre)dialysis team. Nephrol Dial Transplant 21 Suppl 2: ii60–62.
16. Lowrie EG, Lew NL (1990) Death risk in hemodialysis patients: the predictive value of commonly measured variables and an evaluation of death rate differences between facilities. Am J Kidney Dis 15: 458–482.
17. Laird NM, Berkey CS, Lowrie EG (1983) Modeling success or failure of dialysis therapy: the National Cooperative Dialysis Study. Kidney Int Suppl: S101–106.
18. Lo WK, Lui SL, Chan TM, Li FK, Lam MF, et al. (2005) Minimal and optimal peritoneal Kt/V targets: results of an anuric peritoneal dialysis patient's survival analysis. Kidney Int 67: 2032–2038.
19. Peritoneal Dialysis Adequacy Work Group. (2006) Clinical practice guidelines for peritoneal dialysis adequacy. Am J Kidney Dis 48 Suppl 1: S98–129.

The Spectrum of Podoplanin Expression in Encapsulating Peritoneal Sclerosis

Niko Braun[1], M. Dominik Alscher[1,2], Peter Fritz[2,3], Joerg Latus[1], Ilka Edenhofer[4,5], Fabian Reimold[1,6], Seth L. Alper[6], Martin Kimmel[1], Dagmar Biegger[7], Maja Lindenmeyer[4,8], Clemens D. Cohen[4,8], Rudolf P. Wüthrich[4], Stephan Segerer[4,5]*

1 Department of Internal Medicine, Division of General Internal Medicine and Nephrology, Robert-Bosch-Hospital, Stuttgart, Germany, 2 Institute of Digital Medicine, Stuttgart, Germany, 3 Department of Diagnostic Medicine, Division of Pathology, Robert-Bosch-Hospital, Stuttgart, Germany, 4 Division of Nephrology, University Hospital, Zurich, Switzerland, 5 Institute of Anatomy, University of Zurich, Zurich, Switzerland, 6 Division of Nephrology, Beth Israel Deaconess Medical Center, Department of Medicine, Harvard Medical School, Boston, United States of America, 7 Margarete Fischer-Bosch Institute of Clinical Pharmacology, University of Tuebingen, Stuttgart, Germany, 8 Institute of Physiology, University of Zurich, Zurich, Switzerland

Abstract

Encapsulating peritoneal sclerosis (EPS) is a life threatening complication of peritoneal dialysis (PD). Podoplanin is a glycoprotein expressed by mesothelial cells, lymphatic endothelial cells, and myofibroblasts in peritoneal biopsies from patients with EPS. To evaluate podoplanin as a marker of EPS we measured podoplanin mRNA and described the morphological patterns of podoplanin-positive cells in EPS. Included were 20 peritoneal biopsies from patients with the diagnosis of EPS (n = 5), patients on PD without signs of EPS (n = 5), and control patients (uremic patients not on PD, n = 5, non-uremic patients n = 5). EPS patient biopsies revealed significantly elevated levels of podoplanin mRNA (p<0.05). In 24 peritoneal biopsies from patients with EPS, podoplanin and smooth muscle actin (SMA) were localized by immunohistochemistry. Four patterns of podoplanin distribution were distinguishable. The most common pattern (8 of 24) consisted of organized, longitudinal layers of podoplanin-positive cells and vessels in the fibrotic zone ("organized" pattern). 7 of 24 biopsies demonstrated a diffuse distribution of podoplanin-positive cells, accompanied by occasional, dense clusters of podoplanin-positive cells. Five biopsies exhibited a mixed pattern, with some diffuse areas and some organized areas ("mixed"). These contained cuboidal podoplanin-positive cells within SMA-negative epithelial structures embedded in extracellular matrix. Less frequently observed was the complete absence of, or only focal accumulations of podoplanin-positive fibroblasts outside of lymphatic vessels (podoplanin "low", 4 of 24 biopsies). Patients in this group exhibited a lower index of systemic inflammation and a longer symptomatic period than in EPS patients with biopsies of the "mixed" type (p<0.05). In summary we confirm the increased expression of podoplanin in EPS, and distinguish EPS biopsies according to different podoplanin expression patterns which are associated with clinical parameters. Podoplanin might serve as a useful adjunct to the morphological workup of peritoneal biopsies.

Editor: Mitsunobu R. Kano, Okayama University, Japan

Funding: SS is supported by a grant by Baxter and a grant by the Swiss National Science Foundation (SNF 32003B_129710); NB by the Robert-Bosch Foundation and a grant by Baxter, FR by the Robert-Bosch Foundation; CDC by SNF (32-122439/1); SLA by the Harvard Digestive Diseases Center (DK34854). The funders had no role in study design, data collection and analysis, decision to publish, or preparation of the manuscript.

Competing Interests: The study was supported by a Grant from Baxter. Stephan Segerer receives benefits from ROCHE as a consultant. Otherwise the authors do not declare competing interests. This does not alter the authors' adherence to all the PLOS ONE policies on sharing data and materials.

* E-mail: Stephan.segerer@usz.ch

Introduction

Encapsulating peritoneal sclerosis (EPS) is a rare, but life-threatening complication of long-term PD [1,2,3]. Recent PD registries described rates of 0.7–3.3%, an incidence of 4.9 per 1000 person-years, and a mortality of 42% one year post diagnosis [4]. The diagnosis is based on the combination of clinical symptoms (bowel obstruction), radiological findings (suggesting extensive thickening of the peritoneal membrane as the cause of bowel obstruction), and/or the histo-morphological picture [1]. Peritoneal thickening, bowel tethering, peritoneal calcification, peritoneal enhancement and loculated fluid collections can be visualized by computed tomography [1]. Peritoneal biopsy histo-morphological features pathognomonic for EPS have not been defined, and the importance of peritoneal biopsy in the clinical diagnosis of EPS remains poorly established. Morphological signs such as mesothelial denudation, extreme fibrotic thickening, peritoneal fibroblast swelling, interstitial fibrosis, angiogenesis with increased capillary density, and mononuclear cell infiltration are all typical for EPS, but not specific [5,6,7]. Fibrin deposits may lead to adhesions and permanent scarring, eventually resulting in bowel obstruction.

Podoplanin, a member of a type-1 transmembrane sialomucin-like glycoprotein family, serves as a marker of lymphatic endothelial cells but is also expressed by mesothelial cells [8,9]. In a previous study we described podoplanin expression in 69 peritoneal biopsies including 18 patients with EPS. 15 of these biopsies demonstrated a diffuse infiltration with podoplanin-positive cells [10]. These cells were identified as SMA-positive myofibroblasts, which did not express endothelial or other

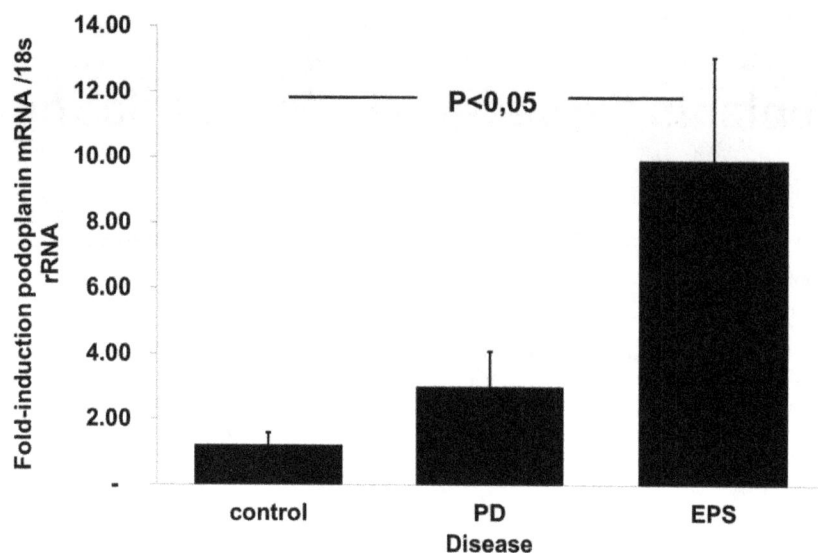

Figure 1. Podoplanin mRNA levels are increased in EPS. RNA samples from patients on PD without signs of EPS (n = 5), and with EPS (n = 5), as well as control biopsies from patients with uremia (n = 5) and normal peritoneum taken during laparatomy (n = 5). The two groups were pooled as "control" samples. Podoplanin mRNA levels were analyzed by real-time RT-PCR. The mean fold induction of podoplanin mRNA was normalized to normal control samples.

Table 1. Clinical information and laboratory values of patients from whom originated biopsy specimens studied by RT-PCR.

Variable	Uremic patients (not on PD)	PD	EPS	Normal biopsies
n =	5	5	5	5
Gender (male:female)	3:2	4:1	4:1	1:4
Age (years;mean ±SD)	54.4 (±16.2)	64.4 (±11.8)	51.6 (±11.0)	56.2 (±12.3)
PD-duration in months		35.2 (±38.2), n.s.	72.6 (±24.3)	
Peritonitis		1:22 months	1:46 months	
PDF: Neutral		4	2	
Acidic		0	2	
N.D.		1	1	
Transporter status				
High/high average		2	3	
Low/low average		1	0	
N.D.		1	2	
Icodextrin		2/5	4/5	
Diabetes	4/5	2/5	0/5	0/5
Smoker	2/5	1/5	2/5	0/5
Hypertension	3/5	3/5	5/5	2/5
Hb (g/dl ± SD [13–18])	10.7 (±1.0)	12.2 (±1.9)	9.7 (±1.8)	12.4 (±2.6)
Leukocytes (G/L ± SD [4.0–11.3])	8.5 (±1.5)	6.4 (±1.4)	6.7 (±3.5)	5.4 (±1.3)
CRP (mg/dl ± SD [<0.1])	1.1 (±2.4)	1.9 (±2.4)	6.4 (±7.5)	0.1 (±0.1)
Phosphate (mmol/l [0.68–1.68])	1.7 (±0.25)	1.3 (±0.3)	1.2 (±2.2)	
Calcium (mmol/l [1.90–2.70])	2.05 (±0.12)	2.2 (±0.1)	2.1 (±0.3)	2.28 (±0.1)
PTH (pmol/l [1.1–7.3])	34.3 (±6.8)	31.1 (±26)	46 (±49.4)	
Urea-N (mg/dl [10–25])	62.2 (±22.9)	42.5 (±22.2)	35.4 (±14.2)	
Creatinine (mg/dl [0.5–1.4])	5.1 (±0.94)	5.1 (±2.3)	6.4 (±2.9)	0.8 (±0.14)

PD, peritoneal dialysis; EPS, encapsulating peritoneal sclerosis; n.s. not significant compared to EPS. PDF, peritoneal dialysis fluid; Hb, haemoglobin; PTH, parathyroid hormone; CRP, C-reactive protein.

Table 2. Clinical information and laboratory values of patients with EPS.

Variable	EPS
n =	24
Gender (male:female)	21/3
Age (years; mean ±SD)	55.1 (±11.0)
PD-duration (months)	80 (±35)
Peritonitis episodes	60 in 1919 months (1:32)
PDF	
Neutral	9/24
Acidic	8/24
Both or N.D.	7/24
Transporter status	11
High/high average	5
Low/low average	8
N.D. last 6 months	
Icodextrin	18/24
Diabetes	17/24
Smoker	9/24
Hypertension	22/24
Hb (g/dl, 13–18)	10.6 (±2.9)
Leukocytes (G/L, 4.0–11.3)	8.7 (±3.4)
Phosphate (mmol/l, 0.68–1.68)	1.3 (±0.5)
Calcium (mmol/l, 1.9–2.7)	2.3 (±0.3)
PTH (pmol/l, 1.1–7.3)	25.6 (±25.1)
Urea-N (mg/dl, 10–25)	41.2 (±15.6)
Creatinine (mg/dl, 0.5–1.4)	6.9 (±2.2)
Time of onset of complaints to Surgery (months)	7.1 (±5.5)
CRP (mg/dl, <0.1)	9.0 (±10.7)

Hb, haemoglobin; EPS, encapsulating peritoneal sclerosis; PD, peritoneal dialysis;
PDF, peritoneal dialysis fluid; PTH, parathyroid hormone; CRP, C-reactive protein; SD, standard deviation.

mesothelial markers [10]. This cell type was focally present in only 3 out of 16 specimens from PD patients without signs of EPS, and in none of 35 controls [10]. The accumulation of podoplanin-positive myofibroblasts in EPS was confirmed by Yaginuma and colleagues using immunoelectron microscopy [11].

Here we confirm the prominent expression of podoplanin using quantitative real-time RT-PCR, and describe four histological patterns of podoplanin-positive cells in EPS biopsies which, we propose, will facilitate morphologic diagnosis of EPS.

Results

Podoplanin mRNA Expression in Peritoneal Biopsies

To evaluate podoplanin expression on transcript level we performed real-time RT-PCR on peritoneal biopsies (Table 1) taken from uremic patients not on PD (n = 5), patients on PD (n = 5), and from PD patients with clinical signs of EPS (n = 5). An additional set of control biopsies were taken from normal peritoneum during abdominal surgery (see material and methods). Both control groups were pooled in this analysis (Figure 1). A prominent and statistically significant induction of podoplanin mRNA was demonstrated. Therefore the previously described accumulation of podoplanin-positive myofibroblasts in EPS was associated with significant induction of podoplanin mRNA expression [10,11].

Podoplanin Patterns by Immunohistochemistry

The clinical and laboratory data of the 24 patients with EPS included in the morphological analysis are presented in Table 2. Podoplanin staining was first analyzed without knowledge of the clinical information. This analysis led to segregation into four groups of podoplanin patterns. Podoplanin-positive lymphatic vessels were present in all four groups, whereas the groups differed in the appearance of podoplanin-positive cells with the morphology of myofibroblasts.

The most common pattern of podoplanin-positive cells was a prominent staining of the superficial fibrotic layer, with longitudinal alignment of podoplanin-positive cells and vessels (Figure 2 A). These longitudinal layers appeared well organized (Figure 2 A, E) with podoplanin-positive cells and vessels arrayed in parallel orientation ("organized" pattern, 8 out 24 biopsies). The corresponding distribution of SMA-positive cells was similar to the pattern of podoplanin (Figure 2 B, D). In the podoplanin-stained sections, prominent lymphatic vessels present in the fibrotic layer (Figure 2 A, B arrowheads) were negative for SMA expression on consecutive sections (Figure 2 D). In some fibrotic zones the superficial layer contained fewer podoplanin- and SMA-

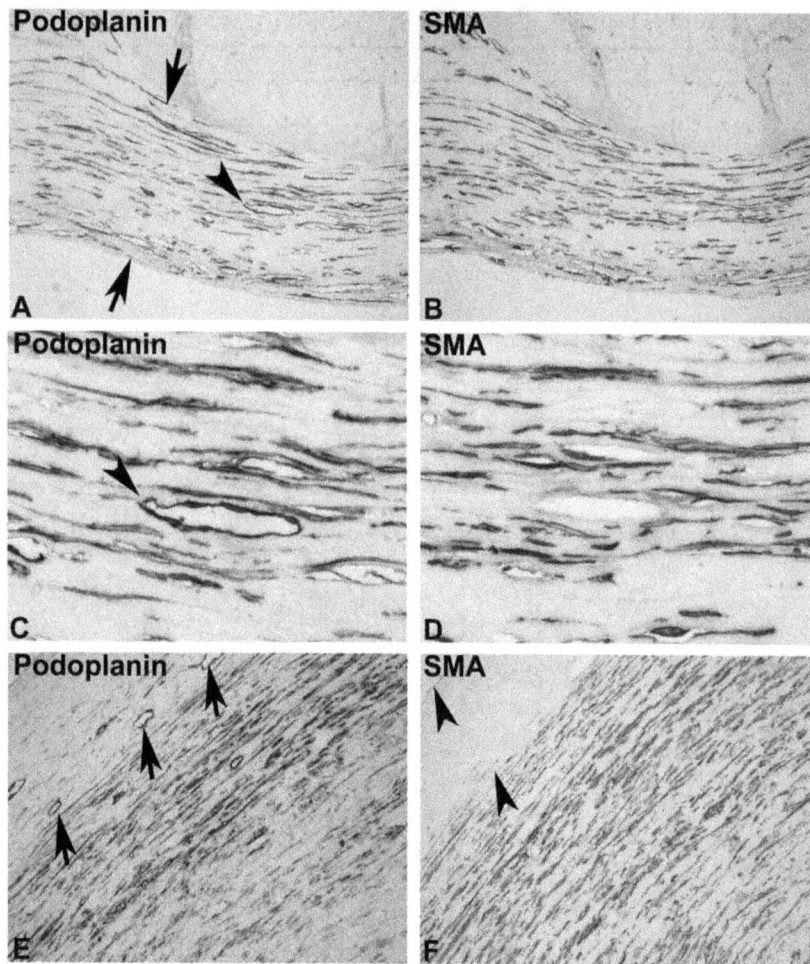

Figure 2. Examples of the "organized" pattern of podoplanin in EPS. Peritoneal biopsies from patients with EPS were stained with monoclonal antibodies against podoplanin (A, C, E). Consecutive section stained with monoclonal antibody against SMA (B, D, F) showed that many cells appeared to express both proteins. In the fibrotic zone (between arrows in A) longitudinal layers of podoplanin-positive cells and vessels (A, C arrowhead) are present, and on consecutive sections SMA-positive cells are detected. These "organized" longitudinal layers led to the description as an "organized" pattern. The superficial layer illustrated in E (upper left corner) contains only some podoplanin-positive vessels, but few SMA-positive cells. Below this superficial layer a prominent zone with podoplanin- and SMA-positive cells is present, as in panels A and B. Panels A-D are from a single individual, panels E and F are from a different individual. (Original magnification, 200X in A, B, E, F; 630X in C, D.).

positive cells (Figure 2 F left upper corner, between arrowheads). Podoplanin-positive lymphatic vessels were detectable in this superficial layer (arrows in Figure 2 E).

The second most common appearance of podoplanin (7 out of 24 biopsies) was in a diffuse pattern with an irregular, random distribution of podoplanin-positive cells ("diffuse" pattern, Figure 3). The cells seemed to be randomly distributed and oriented within the fibrotic zones (Figure 3 A), in contrast to the longitudinal orientation in the "organized" pattern (Figure 2 A). Podoplanin-positive cells occupied a larger proportion of the visual fields in biopsies of "diffuse" pattern (Figure 3 E). The individual podoplanin-positive cells were embedded in extracellular matrix (Figure 3 A). Other areas demonstrated dense accumulations of podoplanin-positive cells with correspondingly less prominent extracellular matrix (Figure 3 E). The SMA expression pattern was very similar to the podoplanin staining (Figure 3 B, D, F), but SMA-positive smooth muscle cells in vessel walls were podoplanin-negative (Figure 3 C, D).

In 5 out of 24 biopsies areas of both "organized" (Figure 4 A, B) and "diffuse" pattern (Figure 4 C, D) were observed, which we

referred to as "mixed" pattern. These biopsies demonstrated the most variable appearance of podoplanin-positive cells. Interestingly, these biopsies contained areas of cuboidal podoplanin-positive cells, which were embedded in extracellular matrix (Figure 4 E, F). Consecutive sections revealed that these cells (arrowhead in 4 E) were SMA-negative (Figure 4 F). It is important to note that this podoplanin-positive, SMA-negative cell type differs in morphology (cuboidal rather than fibroblastic) and in SMA expression from the majority of podoplanin-positive cells. Clusters of podoplanin-positive, SMA-negative cuboidal cells were completely surrounded by dense extracellular matrix. Some podoplanin positive cells were separated from these structures. Also these cells were completely surrounded by extracellular matrix on consecutive sections a major part (but not all) demonstrated expression of calretinin (indicating an mesothelial origin/and or mesothelial differentiation, not illustrated).

In four out of 24 biopsies the expression of podoplanin was mainly restricted to lymphatic endothelial cells (Figure 5). Particularly in the fibrotic zones, where a prominent accumulation of podoplanin-positive cells was present in the biopsies with the other

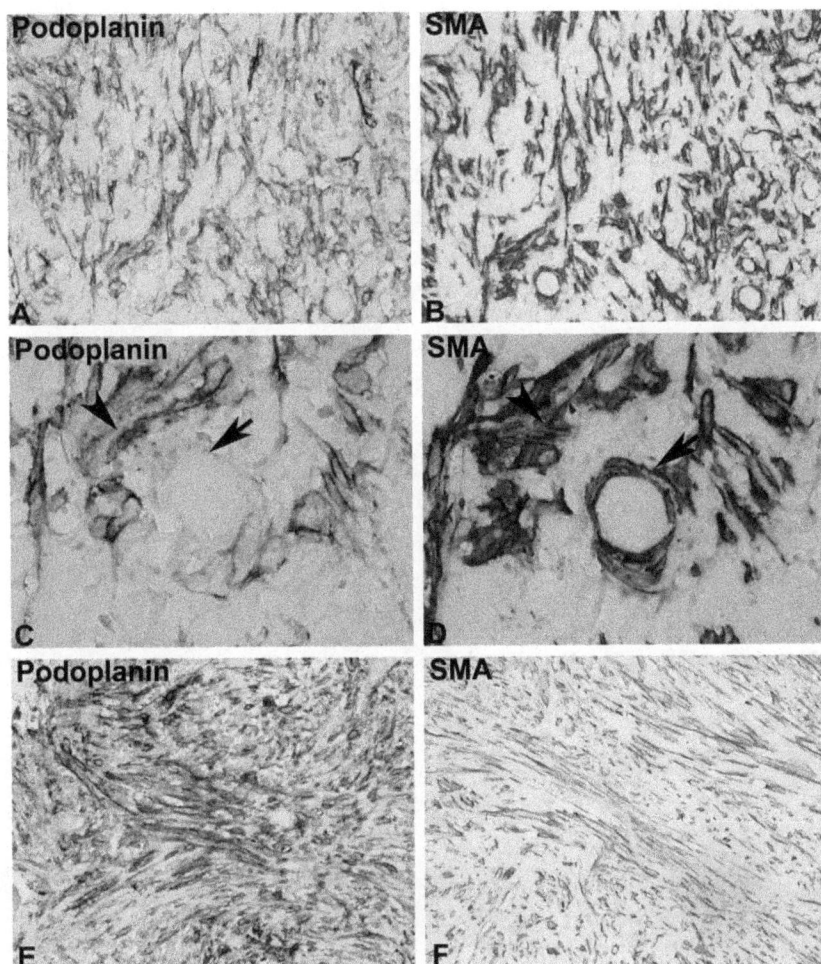

Figure 3. Examples of the "diffuse" pattern. Peritoneal biopsies from patients with EPS were stained with monoclonal antibodies against podoplanin (A, C, E). Consecutive sections were stained with a monoclonal antibody against SMA (B, D, F). The diffusely distributed and randomly oriented pattern of individual podoplanin-positive cells separated by matrix is illustrated in A, and at higher magnification in C. In E the same pattern is illustrated with more densely distributed podoplanin-positive cells. At a higher magnification (C, D) the SMA-positive cells of arteries (arrow) were podoplanin-negative, but the SMA-positive myofibroblasts (arrowhead) were podoplanin-positive. Panels A-D are from a single individual, panels E and F are from a different individual. (Original magnification, 200X in A, B, E, F; 630X in C, D.).

patterns, no podoplanin-positive myofibroblasts were detectable (podoplanin "low" pattern. Figure 5 A, B). In some biopsies focal accumulations of podoplanin-positive fibroblastic cells were detected (Figure 5 C, D). In this histological class of biopsies, location and detection of these scarce, focal areas of podoplanin-positive cells may require analysis of several biopsy specimens from one individual.

Importantly, patients with biopsies with the podoplanin "low" pattern had a significantly lower level of systemic inflammation (as reflected by serum C-reactive protein concentrations, Figure 6 A), but the longest time with symptoms (Figure 6 B). The groups did not differ in mean age, time on PD, or number or frequency of peritonitis episodes (Table 3). The number of CD20 positive B cells, CD3 T cells and CD68 positive macrophages/DCs were scored semi-quantitatively. Most biopsies demonstrated either a mild (score 1) or severe (score 2) diffuse infiltration of CD3 and more prominent CD68 positive cells. CD20 positive B cells were rare within the fibrotic membranes. A single biopsy contained two nodular accumulations on the abluminal side of the fibrotic membrane. Larger accumualtions of infiltrating cells (score 3) were rare. The mean scores of CD3 and CD68 positive infiltrating cells in the biopsies were similarly distributed as the C-reactive protein, with the highest scores in biopsies with a diffuse or mixed pattern (Figure 6 C, D). B cells demonstrated low scores and no differences between the groups.

Discussion

In a previous study we described a podoplanin-positive, SMA positive cell population in 15 of 18 biopsies from patients with EPS, whereas only focal accumulations of podoplanin-positive cells were present in biopsies from 3 of 16 patients on PD without signs of EPS [10]. We thus suggested that podoplanin staining might be suitable as an adjunct to the morphological diagnosis of EPS. The current study had two goals. The first was to examine podoplanin expression in EPS with a different technique (i.e. mRNA measurement by quantitative real-time RT-PCR). The second goal was to further describe the pattern of podoplanin-positive cells, particularly in those biopsies without the typical accumulation of podoplanin-positive myofibroblasts.

Using quantitative real-time RT-PCR we were able to confirm increased levels of podoplanin mRNA in peritoneal biopsies from

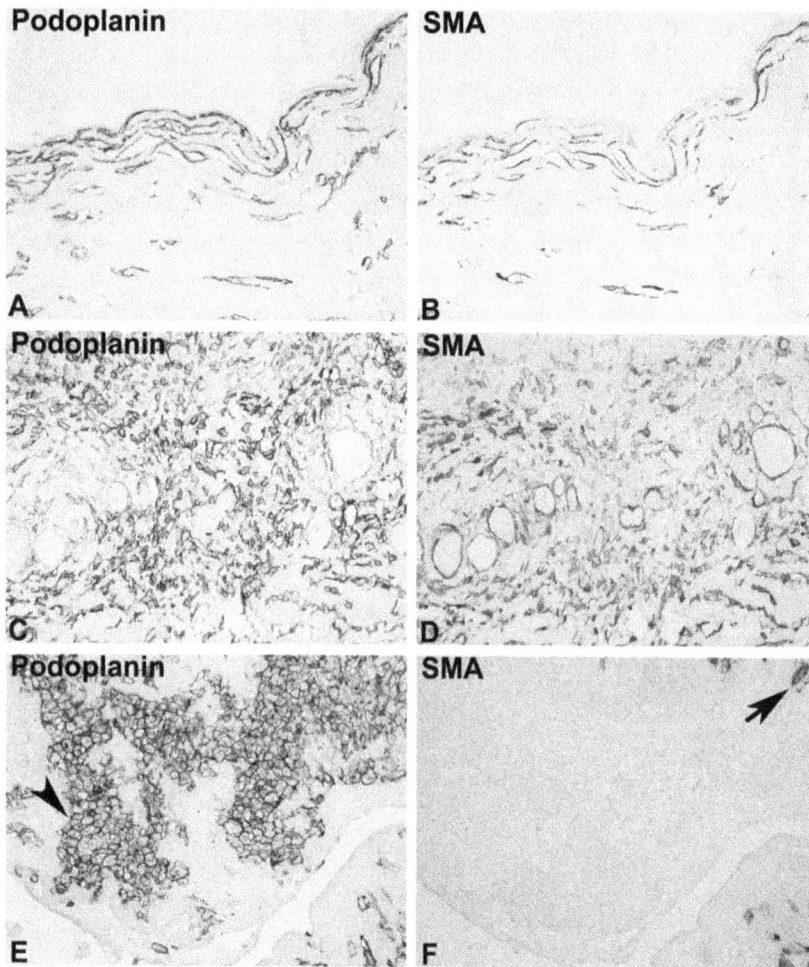

Figure 4. Illustration of the "mixed" pattern. Peritoneal biopsies from patients with EPS were stained with monoclonal antibodies against podoplanin (A, C, E). Consecutive sections were stained with monoclonal antibody against SMA (B, D, F). Examples of "organized" (A, B) and "diffuse" (C, D) patterns are illustrated from the same tissue specimen. An area of podoplanin-positive, cuboidal cells embedded in matrix is illustrated in E (arrowhead), but these cells were SMA negative on consecutive sections (F). An SMA-positive myofibroblast is illustrated by the arrow (F, upper right). Panels A-D are from a single individual, panels E and F are from a different individual. (Original magnification, 200X.).

patients with EPS on PD. Furthermore, a recent study confirmed the existence of these podoplanin-positive fibroblastic cells by both immunohistochemistry and by immunoelectron microscopy [11]. Thus, the first goal of the paper was achieved, as another technique demonstrated increased podoplanin expression in a different group of EPS patients.

The second part of the work aimed to extend the histological description and pattern(s) of podoplanin-positive cells in peritoneal biopsies. We found that the biopsies could be separated into four morphological groups. From the diagnostic point of view, the group with rare podoplanin-positive cells ("podoplanin low") is an important one, as this category might generate false negative results for EPS. Four of 24 patients demonstrated podoplanin-positive vessels (lymphatics), but only small and focal sites of accumulation of podoplanin-positive cells. In our previous study, the proportion of patients with this pattern was similar (with 3 of 16). Therefore, between 15 and 20% of biopsies from patients with EPS exhibit a "low" podoplanin pattern. Patients with this histological pattern had the lowest level of systemic inflammation (as judged by serum levels of C-reactive protein), and the longest history of symptoms. Therefore, this pattern could reflect a late (and/or slowly progressive) disease state (fibrotic, or "burnt out").

It is important to note that these small clusters of podoplanin-positive cells can usually be detected when sufficient material is available and thoroughly examined, but these areas can easily be missed on smaller biopsies.

Two additional, distinct patterns and a mixed pattern could be identified. The "organized" pattern and the "diffuse" pattern were observed with equal frequency, and were together most commonly found. The "organized" pattern was characterized by a longitudinal organization of podoplanin-positive cells throughout the fibrotic layer or the basal part of the fibrotic zone. In contrast, the "diffuse" pattern was distinguished by a random accumulation of podoplanin-positive cells across a larger area of biopsy. Five of 24 biopsies demonstrated a "mixed" pattern (with features of both "organized" and "diffuse" patterns). The "mixed" pattern group exhibited the highest level of inflammation and the shortest history of symptoms prior to surgery. The "mixed" and the "diffuse" types likely reflect the most active and aggressive phases of EPS, with sites of very prominent podoplanin- and SMA-positive cell accumulation. Furthermore the "mixed" and the "diffuse" type demonstrated the strongest infiltration by T cells and CD68 positive macrophages/DCs.

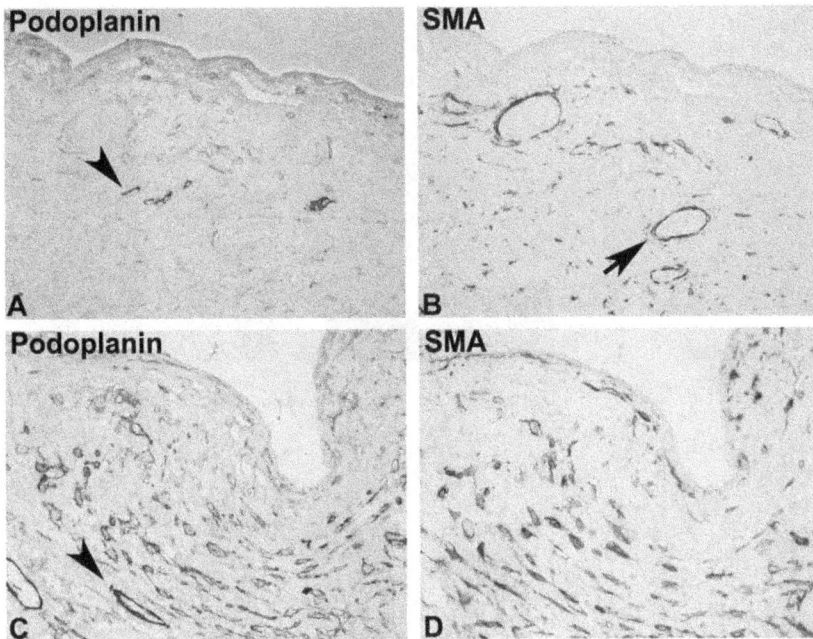

Figure 5. Example of the podoplanin "low" pattern. A peritoneal biopsy from an EPS patient was stained with monoclonal antibodies against podoplanin (A, C), and consecutive sections were stained with a monoclonal antibody against SMA (B, D, orig. X200). Panel A illustrates an area in which the fibrotic zone does not demonstrate a significant accumulation of podoplanin-positive cells (the arrowhead show some positive small vessels). In small areas of the biopsy the typical presence of podoplanin-positive myofibroblast was detectable The arrowhead in B marks a podoplanin-positive lymphatic vessel, not stained by SMA on the consecutive section (D).

The morphological patterns were not associated with the number of peritonitis episodes and the groups did not differ in age, time on PD, Icodextrin exposure, parathyroid hormon, and calcium. Also not quite significant, patients with mixed pattern demonstrated a trend towards higher leukocytes, lower urea and lower phosphate (likely reflecting poorer nutritional status).

It is currently unclear whether the different morphological podoplanin patterns are related to differences in the quantitative podoplanin mRNA expression. Particularly, the podoplanin "low" pattern is likely associated with a decreased podoplanin mRNA expression. Currently, the materials available for matched podoplanin staining and mRNA quantification were not sufficient to answer this question, but it will be evaluated in a future study.

The fibroblastic podoplanin- and SMA-positive cell type typical for EPS was found to be negative for calretinin (a marker of mesothelial cells [10]. Podoplanin positive stromal cells (called lymphoid stromal cells,) have been described as follicular reticular cells (also positive for SMA) in T cell zones of secondary lymphatic organs, in thymic medulla, in intestinal lamina propria, and in tertiary lymphoid organs formed during chronic infiltration [17,18,19]. During development of secondary lymphoid organs the lymphoid tissue inducer cells activate podoplanin positive stromal cells via lymphotoxin to release chemokines and upregulate adhesion molecules [18]. Some forms of Inflammation recapitulate the formation of lymphoid stromal cells as the accumulation of podoplanin positive stromal cells was demonstrated in different inflammatory models in the mouse (e.g. models of autoimmunity, inflammation of mouse ears induced by adjuvant) [18]. During inflammation the lymphoid stromal cells resulted from local proliferation of non-epithelial precursor cells [18]. The development of these cells seems to be dependent on the injury process. Studies in chronically inflamed kidneys did not demonstrate the accumulation of podoplanin positive myofibro-

blasts, whereas SMA positive cells form a prominent part of the interstitial fibroblasts in chronic renal injury [16]. Furthermore, in patients on PD with simple peritoneal fibrosis, diffuse accumulation of podoplanin positive myofibroblasts was rarely detected. Therefore the podoplanin positive cells in EPS reflect features of lymphoid stromal cells. As nodular infiltrates were rarely present full tertiary lymphoid organs were not present, these cells do not seem to promote the formation of lymphoid tissue in the EPS membranes. Future studies will need to further describe these cells with other markers of lymphoid stromal cells. The question remains whether these cells are the consequence of the injury process of EPS or a driving force.

Another podoplanin positive cell type has been described in mice. During zymosan peritonitis a F4/80 positive cell expressing podoplanin has been described and called fibroblastic macrophages [20]. In our study the overall pattern of CD68 (a marker of human monocyte/macrophages/DCs) did not match the podoplanin staining, but further studies using double labelling need to evaluate whether similar fibroblastic macrophages are present in human EPS.

In the biopsies with a "mixed" pattern clusters of podoplanin-positive cuboidal cells were found embedded in extracellular-matrix (illustrated in Figure 4E). As these cells cells were SMA negative, these might reflect mesothelial cells [21]. In parallel staining for calretinin (as a marker of mesothelial cells) a major part of these cells demonstrated calretinin expression, but a smaller part did not. Therefore these cells do not seem to be typical mesothelial cells but the differentiation of these cells need further description. In Figure 4C the excess of podoplanin-positive cells over SMA-positive cells (in Figure 4 D) may reflect the presence of this cell type. These areas might reflect sites of early epithelial-to-mesenchymal cell transition or a cell on the way towards a mesothelial phenotype.

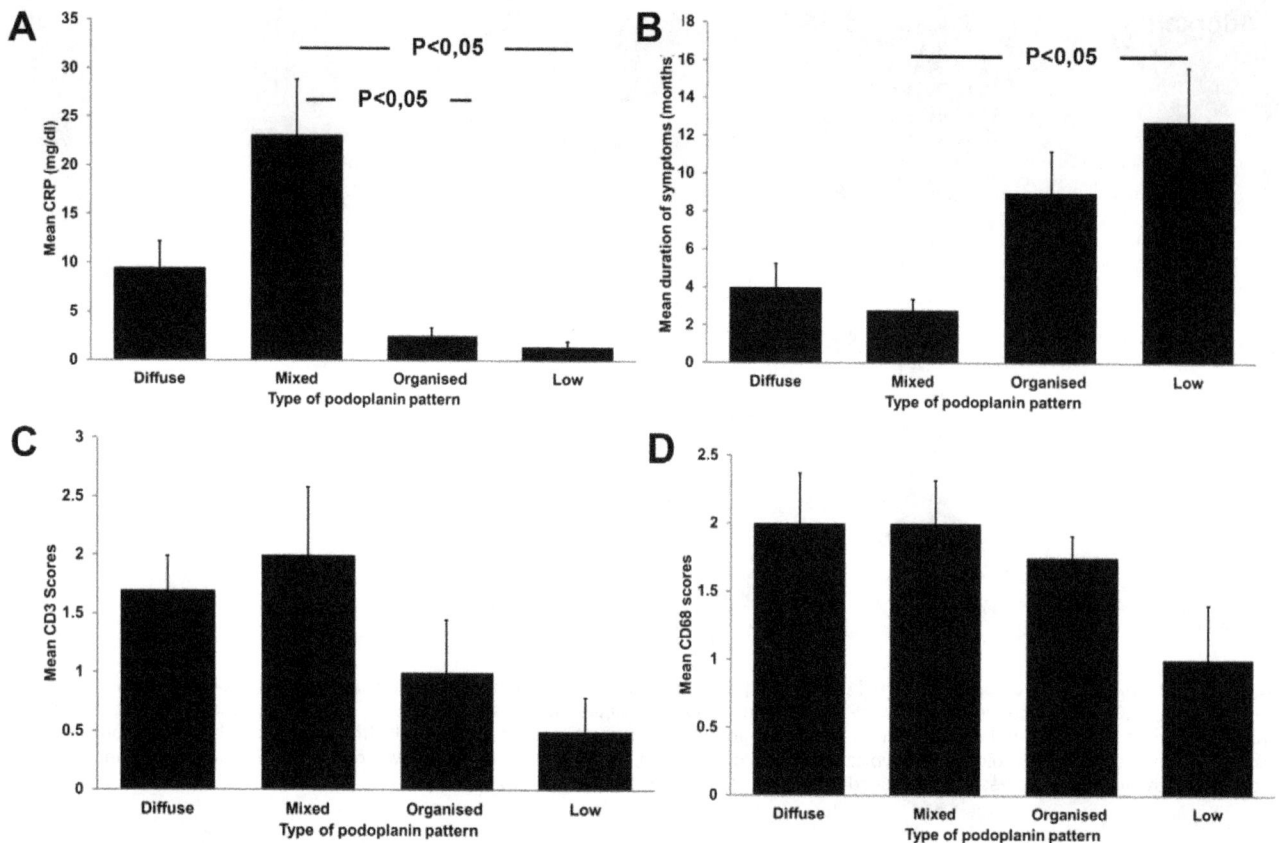

Figure 6. Association between podoplanin pattern and clinical parameters and morphological scores of inflammatory cells. Illustrated are the mean C reactive protein (CRP) levels (A), the mean duration of symptoms (in months, B), the mean scores for CD3 positive T cells (C) and the mean scores for CD68 positive cells (D) for the four histological groups of podoplanin patterns. The infiltrating cells were scored semi-quantitatively as described in materials and methods.

The question remains whether the patterns illustrated reflect a continuum (likely from "mixed/diffuse" pattern via "organized" towards "low" pattern) or different disease entities. The clinical data suggest that the "mixed/diffuse" pattern reflects earlier (active) phases, whereas the "organized" and, particularly, the podoplanin "low" pattern are rather later stages. If true, then the "low" pattern might not be susceptible to anti-inflammatory treatment, a hypothesis that could be tested. This novel stratification of EPS patients into groups exhibiting distinct podoplanin expression patterns could be of significant diagnostic and prognostic impact, if it can be confirmed in other EPS biopsy registries.

Methods

All peritoneal biopsies were obtained from the peritoneal biopsy registry at the Robert-Bosch-Hospital, Stuttgart, Germany. The human peritoneal tissue, blood and peritoneal dialysate for research purposes were collected after written consent of the patient was given. The study was approved by the local ethics committee (#322/2009BO1, Eberhard-Karls University Tuebingen, Germany).

Additionally, shortly after tissue excision, 20 samples from patients on PD without EPS (n = 5), patients with EPS (n = 5), uremic patients not on PD (n = 5), and normal tissue taken during cholecystectomy (n = 3), hemicolectomy (n = 1) and closure of loop-colostomy (n = 1), all without signs of systemic and local inflammation, were washed in 0.9% saline solution, placed in RNAlater (Qiagen, Hilden, Germany), then stored at −80°C for subsequent RNA extraction.

Clinical data collection included demographic data, cause of primary renal disease, comorbidities (diabetes, hypertension and smoking status), PD details and the date of dialysis initiation. Body mass index, peritonitis rate, medications, and time of onset of symptoms were also recorded. The diagnosis of EPS was made according to the clinical criteria of Nakamoto et al. [12], the radiological criteria of Vlijm et al. [13] and the histological criteria of Honda et al. [5]. Biopsies of the parietal peritoneum were taken, formalin-fixed and embedded in paraffin following routine protocols. All patients were on hemodialysis after surgery.

Quantitative Real-time RT-PCR

RNA was isolated from tissues frozen and immersed in RNAlater (Qiagen), using the miRNeasy Mini-Kit (Qiagen) according to the description of the manufacturer. 50–100 mg tissue samples were incubated in 0.7 ml Qiazol reagent and homogenized using a rotor-stator homogenizer (Ultra-Turrax T8, IKA-Werke Staufen, Germany) for 1 minute. The homogenate was extracted with 0.14 ml chloroform, and phase separation of the solution was achieved by centrifugation. The clear, aqueous supernatant containing total RNA was removed, and total RNA was twice precipitated with 75% ethanol, and re-suspended in nuclease-free water.

Table 3. Clinical information and laboratory values according to the morphological pattern of podoplanin.

	Diffuse	Mixed	Organised	Low
n =	7	5	8	4
Gender (male:female)	7/0	4/1	7/1	4/0
Age (years;mean ±SD)	51.7 (±15.9)	46.4 (±7.3)	55.5 (±12.2)	47.3 (±17.2)
PD-duration in months	71 (±37)	99 (±33)	86 (±29)	59 (±39)
Peritonitis	1:26	1:37	1:33	1:26
PDF				
Neutral	3	1	4	1
Acidic	2	1	3	2
Both or N.D.	2	3	1	1
Transporter status				
High/high average	2	3	5	1
Low/low average	1	1	1	2
N.D.	4	1	2	1
Icodextrin	4	5	6	3
Diabetes	2	1	2	1
Smoker	3	2	2	2
Hypertension	6	4	8	4
Hb (g/dl ± SD [13–18])	84 (±31.1)	115 (±29.3)	116 (±21.0)	113 (±26.4)
Leukocytes (G/L ±SD [4.0–11.3])	8.4 (±2.3)	11.2 (±5.2)	8.6 (±3)	6.5 (±2.2)
Phosphate (mmol/l [0.68–1.68])	1.7 (±0.6)	1.0 (±0.5)	1.3 (±0.5)	1.4 (±0.6)
Calcium (mmol/l [1.90–2.70])	2.1 (±0.2)	2.3 (±0.3)	2.4 (±0.3)	2.3 (±0.4)
PTH (pmol/l [1.1–7.3])	28.5 (±17.6)	12.9 (±8.8)	21 (±30.5)	43 (±30.8)
Urea-N (mg/dl [10–25])	92.1 (±32)	69.8 (±27.5)	87.4 (±27.8)	105.8 (±52.3)
Creatinine (mg/dl [0.5–1.4])	6.8 (±2.4)	6.8 (±2.1)	7 (±2.2)	6.7 (±3.1)

PD, peritoneal dialysis; EPS, encapsulating peritoneal sclerosis; PDF, peritoneal dialysis fluid; Hb, haemoglobin; PTH, parathyroid hormone.

RNA was measured using a NanoDrop Spectrophotometer 2000c (Peqlab Biotechnologie GmbH, Erlangen, Germany). RNA integrity was assessed using the Agilent 2100 Bioanalyzer (Agilent Technologies, Santa Clara, CA). First-strand cDNA was synthesized with TaqMan RT reagents (Applied Biosystems, Darmstadt, Germany). Pre-developed TaqMan reagents were used for human podoplanin and housekeeping genes GAPDH and 18SrRNA (Applied Biosystems, Darmstadt, Germany). The mRNA expression was analyzed by the delta delta Ct method as previously described [14].

Immunohistochemistry

Immunohistochemistry was performed as previously described [10,15]. In brief, paraffin-embedded tissue sections were deparaffinized in xylene, rehydrated in a graded series of ethanols, and incubated in 3% hydrogen peroxide (to block endogenous peroxidases). Antigen retrieval was performed in an autoclave oven, using antigen retrieval solution (Vector, Burlingame, CA). The primary antibodies were applied for 1 hour. Incubation with biotinylated secondary reagents (Vector) was performed for 30 minutes, followed by washing, then exposure to ABC reagent (Vector). 3'3'diaminobenzidine (DAB, Sigma, Taufkirchen, Germany) with metal enhancement (resulting in a black colour product) was used as a detection system. Nuclei were counterstained with methyl green.

A monoclonal mouse anti-human podoplanin antibody (D2–40, Signet Laboratories, Dedham, MA) was used on all biopsies [15,16]. As control tissues we used sections of human renal allograft nephrectomies, including the replacement of the primary antibody by isotype-matched control immunoglobulins (Figure S1). These controls did not demonstrate positive staining (Figure S1 B). For detection of SMA a monoclonal mouse antibody was used (1A4, DakoCytomation, Glostrup, Denmark), which stains smooth muscle cells in arterial walls and in myofibroblasts (Figure S1 C, D). Additional sections were stained with a monoclonal antibody against CD68 (Clone PG-M1, DAKO Germany, Hamburg), with a monoclonal antibody against CD3 (clone: CD3–12, rat anti-human, Serotec, Oxford, UK), and with a monoclonal antibody against CD20 (clone L26; DakoCytomation, Dako Deutschland, Hamburg, Germany) [16]. Selected biopsies were stained with calretinin (Dak Calret 1, DakoCytomation, Glostrup, Denmark) a marker of mesothelial cells. The extent of inflammatory infiltrates were semi-quantitatively scored from 0 (no or scattered cells), 1 (milde diffuse infiltrates), 2 (severe diffuse infiltrates) to 3 (severe diffuse infiltrates with larger cell accumulations) by an observer blinded to the morphological podoplanin pattern and the clinical information.

Statistical Analysis

Statistical analysis was performed using InStat® software (Version 3.05, Intuitive Software for Science, San Diego, CA). For comparison of means, the non-parametric Kruskal-Wallis test and Dunn's multiple comparisons test were applied. A $p < 0.05$ was considered to be significant. Error bars demonstrate standard error of the mean (SEM).

Conclusions

The current study confirms elevated podoplanin expression in EPS peritoneal biopsies. The morphological evaluation of podoplanin can separate histological groups with different clinical features, and in the future might guide both diagnosis and treatment of EPS. The similarity of these podoplanin positive cells with lymphoid stromal cells needs further evaluation.

Supporting Information

Figure S1 Illustration of podoplanin and SMA in control tissue. Immunohistochemistry was performed on tissue sections from an allograft nephrectomy (A, C), with monoclonal antibodies against podoplanin (A) and smooth muscle actin (C). Consecutive sections of the renal allograft were stained with the isotype

immunoglobulin control (as negative control B, D). Note the staining of periarterial lymphatic vessels (arrowhead in A) and the absence of staining in B. Panel C shows SMA-positive cells in the walls of an artery (arrowhead) and an arteriole (arrow). No staining is present in the isotype immunoglobulin control (D). (Original magnification, 200X)

Acknowledgments

Microscopes were provided by the Center of Microscopy and Image Analysis (University of Zurich).

Author Contributions

Conceived and designed the experiments: NB MDA SLA ML CDC SS. Performed the experiments: SS IE DB. Analyzed the data: NB MDA SLA ML CDC SS PF JL FR MK. Contributed reagents/materials/analysis tools: NB MK DB ML CDC. Wrote the paper: NB SS RW.

References

1. Augustine T, Brown PW, Davies SD, Summers AM, Wilkie ME (2009) Encapsulating peritoneal sclerosis: clinical significance and implications. Nephron Clin Pract 111: c149–154; discussion c154.
2. Braun N, Alscher MD, Kimmel M, Amann K, Buttner M (2011) Encapsulating peritoneal sclerosis - an overview. Nephrol Ther 7: 162–171.
3. Korte MR, Sampimon DE, Betjes MG, Krediet RT (2011) Encapsulating peritoneal sclerosis: the state of affairs. Nat Rev Nephrol 7: 528–538.
4. Brown MC, Simpson K, Kerssens JJ, Mactier RA (2009) Encapsulating Peritoneal Sclerosis in the New Millennium: A National Cohort Study. Clin J Am Soc Nephrol.
5. Honda K, Nitta K, Horita S, Tsukada M, Itabashi M, et al. (2003) Histologic criteria for diagnosing encapsulating peritoneal sclerosis in continuous ambulatory peritoneal dialysis patients. Adv Perit Dial 19: 169–175.
6. Alscher DM, Braun N, Biegger D, Fritz P (2007) Peritoneal mast cells in peritoneal dialysis patients, particularly in encapsulating peritoneal sclerosis patients. Am J Kidney Dis 49: 452–461.
7. Garosi G, Di Paolo N (2001) Morphological aspects of peritoneal sclerosis. J Nephrol 14 Suppl 4: S30–38.
8. Raica M, Cimpean AM, Ribatti D (2008) The role of podoplanin in tumor progression and metastasis. Anticancer Res 28: 2997–3006.
9. Kalof AN, Cooper K (2009) D2-40 immunohistochemistry-so far! Adv Anat Pathol 16: 62–64.
10. Braun N, Alscher DM, Fritz P, Edenhofer I, Kimmel M, et al. (2011) Podoplanin-positive cells are a hallmark of encapsulating peritoneal sclerosis. Nephrol Dial Transplant 26: 1033–1041.
11. Yaginuma T, Yamamoto I, Yamamoto H, Mitome J, Tanno Y, et al. (2012) Increased Lymphatic Vessels in Patients with Encapsulatingperitoneal Sclerosis. Perit Dial Int.
12. Nakamoto H (2005) Encapsulating peritoneal sclerosis-a clinician's approach to diagnosis and medical treatment. Perit Dial Int 25 Suppl 4: S30–38.
13. Vlijm A, Stoker J, Bipat S, Spijkerboer AM, Phoa SS, et al. (2009) Computed tomographic findings characteristic for encapsulating peritoneal sclerosis: a case-control study. Perit Dial Int 29: 517–522.
14. Cohen CD, Frach K, Schlondorff D, Kretzler M (2002) Quantitative gene expression analysis in renal biopsies: a novel protocol for a high-throughput multicenter application. Kidney Int 61: 133–140.
15. Neusser MA, Kraus AK, Regele H, Cohen CD, Fehr T, et al. (2010) The chemokine receptor CXCR7 is expressed on lymphatic endothelial cells during renal allograft rejection. Kidney Int 77: 801–808.
16. Heller F, Lindenmeyer MT, Cohen CD, Brandt U, Draganovici D, et al. (2007) The contribution of B cells to renal interstitial inflammation. Am J Pathol 170: 457–468.
17. Link A, Hardie DL, Favre S, Britschgi MR, Adams DH, et al. (2011) Association of T-zone reticular networks and conduits with ectopic lymphoid tissues in mice and humans. Am J Pathol 178: 1662–1675.
18. Peduto L, Dulauroy S, Lochner M, Spath GF, Morales MA, et al. (2009) Inflammation recapitulates the ontogeny of lymphoid stromal cells. J Immunol 182: 5789–5799.
19. Link A, Vogt TK, Favre S, Britschgi MR, Acha-Orbea H, et al. (2007) Fibroblastic reticular cells in lymph nodes regulate the homeostasis of naive T cells. Nat Immunol 8: 1255–1265.
20. Hou TZ, Bystrom J, Sherlock JP, Qureshi O, Parnell SM, et al. (2010) A distinct subset of podoplanin (gp38) expressing F4/80+ macrophages mediate phagocytosis and are induced following zymosan peritonitis. FEBS letters 584: 3955–3961.
21. Kimura N, Kimura I (2005) Podoplanin as a marker for mesothelioma. Pathol Int 55: 83–86.

Peritoneal Dialysis-Related Peritonitis due to *Staphylococcus aureus*: A Single-Center Experience over 15 Years

Pasqual Barretti[1], Taíse M. C. Moraes[1,2], Carlos H. Camargo[1,2], Jacqueline C. T. Caramori[1], Alessandro L. Mondelli[1], Augusto C. Montelli[1,2], Maria de Lourdes R. S. da Cunha[2]*

1 Departamento de Clínica Médica, Faculdade de Medicina, UNESP - Universidade Estadual Paulista, Botucatu, São Paulo, Brazil, 2 Departamento de Microbiologia e Imunologia, Instituto de Biociências, UNESP - Universidade Estadual Paulista, Botucatu, São Paulo, Brazil

Abstract

Peritonitis caused by *Staphylococcus aureus* is a serious complication of peritoneal dialysis (PD), which is associated with poor outcome and high PD failure rates. We reviewed the records of 62 *S. aureus* peritonitis episodes that occurred between 1996 and 2010 in the dialysis unit of a single university hospital and evaluated the host and bacterial factors influencing peritonitis outcome. Peritonitis incidence was calculated for three subsequent 5-year periods and compared using a Poisson regression model. The production of biofilm, enzymes, and toxins was evaluated. Oxacillin resistance was evaluated based on minimum inhibitory concentration and presence of the *mec*A gene. Logistic regression was used for the analysis of demographic, clinical, and microbiological factors influencing peritonitis outcome. Resolution and death rates were compared with 117 contemporary coagulase-negative staphylococcus (CoNS) episodes. The incidence of *S. aureus* peritonitis declined significantly over time from 0.13 in 1996–2000 to 0.04 episodes/patient/year in 2006–2010 ($p = 0.03$). The oxacillin resistance rate was 11.3%. Toxin and enzyme production was expressive, except for enterotoxin D. Biofilm production was positive in 88.7% of strains. The presence of the *mec*A gene was associated with a higher frequency of fever and abdominal pain. The logistic regression model showed that diabetes mellitus ($p = 0.009$) and β-hemolysin production ($p = 0.006$) were independent predictors of non-resolution of infection. The probability of resolution was higher among patients aged 41 to 60 years than among those >60 years ($p = 0.02$). A trend to higher death rate was observed for *S. aureus* episodes (9.7%) compared to CoNS episodes (2.5%), ($p = 0.08$), whereas resolution rates were similar. Despite the decline in incidence, *S. aureus* peritonitis remains a serious complication of PD that is associated with a high death rate. The outcome of this infection is negatively influenced by host factors such as age and diabetes mellitus. In addition, β-hemolysin production is predictive of non-resolution of infection, suggesting a pathogenic role of this factor in PD-related *S. aureus* peritonitis.

Editor: Michael Otto, National Institutes of Health, United States of America

Funding: This work was supported by a grant from the São Paulo state funding agency Fundação de Amparo à Pesquisa do Estado de São Paulo (FAPESP). The funding agency played no role in the study design, data collection and analysis, decision to publish, or preparation of the manuscript

Competing Interests: The authors have declared that no competing interests exist.

* E-mail: cunhamlr@ibb.unesp.br

Introduction

Peritonitis is a serious complication of peritoneal dialysis (PD) and is responsible for a high rate of technique failure and death in PD patients [1]. Gram-positive cocci are the main etiological agents of peritonitis in the world, with coagulase-negative staphylococci (CoNS) being the most common microbial agents, whereas *Staphylococcus aureus* is associated with more severe episodes, a higher risk of hospitalization, catheter removal, and death [1,2]. Although *S. aureus* is responsible for a small proportion of peritonitis episodes in most countries, it continues to be the leading cause of this infection in some Latin American countries, particularly in Brazil [3].

A poor prognosis of PD-related *S. aureus* peritonitis has been frequently reported [2,4,5], but there are only two reports [6,7] that specifically describe the clinical outcome and predictors of treatment response in this infection. In the largest series,

Govindarajulu et al. [6] showed that methicillin-resistant *S. aureus* (MRSA) peritonitis was independently predictive of an increased risk of permanent hemodialysis transfer and tended to be associated with a high risk of hospitalization. Szeto et al. [7] reported a lower primary response rate and complete cure rate for episodes caused by MRSA compared to episodes due to other *S. aureus*. In both cases the clinical outcome of *S. aureus* peritonitis was not encouraging. The rates of relapse, catheter removal and hospitalization were 20%, 23% and 67%, respectively, in the study of Govindarajulu et al. [6]. In the series of Szeto et al. [7], only 51% of patients with methicillin-susceptible *S. aureus* peritonitis and 46% with MRSA peritonitis presented complete cure without relapse, recurrent or repeat episodes, or need for catheter removal.

In addition to antibiotic resistance, the severity of *S. aureus* infections is associated with virulence factors produced by this bacterium, such as enzymes (coagulase, lipase, and nucleases) and multiple toxins with diverse activities. One family of protein toxins are the staphylococcal enterotoxins and the related toxic shock syndrome toxin-1 (TSST-1) that act as superantigens [8]. The biofilm produced by most *S. aureus* strains facilitates bacterial adhesion to catheters and colonization and simultaneously worsens the response to infection, protecting bacterial cells from the host's natural defense mechanisms and from the action of antibiotics [8,9]. Although these products may influence clinical outcome, their role in PD-related *S. aureus* peritonitis is still not fully defined. Data published by Haslinger-Löffler et al. [10] suggest that α-hemolysin plays a specific role in the pathogenesis of peritonitis. Using cultured human peritoneal mesothelial cells, these authors showed that α-hemolysin produced by *S. aureus* was able to induce caspase-independent cell death. In a recent study, our group demonstrated that biofilm and α-hemolysin production were the only independent predictors of non-resolution of staphylococcal peritonitis [11]. However, the small number of *S. aureus* episodes analyzed was an important limitation of that study.

For the last 15 years we have monitored clinical and microbiological characteristics of *S. aureus* peritonitis in PD patients, including virulence factors produced by this pathogen and presence of the *mec*A gene that confers resistance to methicillin/oxacillin. The objective of the present study was to describe the experience of a single Brazilian center with PD-related *S. aureus* peritonitis, focusing on host and bacterial factors that influence peritonitis outcome.

Results

A total of 682 peritonitis episodes were diagnosed in our unit between 1996 and 2010. The overall peritonitis rate was 0.96 episodes per patient per year. Seventy-three (10.7%) episodes were caused by S. *aureus*. After application of the exclusion criteria, 62 episodes that occurred in 56 patients were analyzed. The demographic and baseline clinical data of the patients are summarized in Table 1. The clinical findings in peritonitis

Table 1. Summary of Patient Characteristics at Baseline (*n* = 56).

	Frequency	%
Age (years)		
≤20	4	7.2
21–40	12	21.4
41–60	20	35.7
>60	20	35.7
Male gender	23	41.1
Presence of diabetes	28	50
Educational Level		
Elementary	30	53.6
Secondary	8	14.3
Higher	6	10.7
Illiterate	7	12.5
Unknown	5	8.9
PD modality		
APD	9	16.6
CAPD	47	83.3

PD, peritoneal dialysis; APD, automated peritoneal dialysis; CAPD, continuous ambulatory peritoneal dialysis.

episodes were expressed in Table 2. The incidence of *S. aureus* peritonitis declined significantly over time and was 0.13 episodes per patient per year in 1996–2000, 0.10 in 2001–2005, and 0.04 in 2006–2010 (*p* = 0.03). The annual *S. aureus* peritonitis rate is presented in figure 1; a strong decline of the incidence was observed after 2003. Vancomycin was used in 35 (56.5%) episodes. Overall, 32 (51.6%) episodes were resolved; among cases that were not resolved one (0.16%) relapsed, 18 (29%) required removal of the catheter due to refractory peritonitis, five (8%) were resolved with a second antibiotic regimen, and six (9.7%) progressed to death. Of 117 contemporary CoNS peritonitis episodes, 63 (53.8%) were resolved and three (2.5%) progressed to death. The death rate tended to be lower among episodes caused by CoNS than among *S. aureus* episodes (*p* = 0.08), whereas resolution rates were similar (*p* = 0.16).

All strains were susceptible to vancomycin (MIC≤3 µg/ml) and seven (11.3%) were resistant to oxacillin (MIC≥4 µg/ml). The vancomycin MIC or proportion of oxacillin-resistant isolates did not change significantly over time (Figure 2). The *mec*A gene was detected in seven (11.3%) strains.

The rates of toxin and enzyme production by *S. aureus* are shown in Table 3. No associations were observed between the production of virulence factors and the frequency of initial clinical findings. However, fever was observed in 83.3% of episodes caused by bacteria expressing the *mec*A gene, whereas this clinical symptom was present in only 24% of episodes due to *mec*A gene-negative strains (*p* = 0.03). In addition, there was a trend towards a higher rate of abdominal pain (100%) among strains expressing the *mec*A gene compared to *mec*A gene-negative isolates (64.8%) (*p* = 0.08). The production of virulence factors and presence of the *mec*A gene were not associated with catheter removal, hospitalization, or death rate.

Gender, age, vancomycin use, presence of diabetes, production of virulence factors (β-hemolysin, lecithinase, deoxyribonuclease, SEC, and TSST-1), presence of the *mec*A gene, and dialysis vintage were associated with a higher chance of non-resolution in univariate analysis (Table 4), and were therefore included in the multivariate logistic regression model. Multivariate analysis showed that the presence of diabetes and β-hemolysin production were factors independently associated with a higher odds ratio of non-resolution of peritonitis episodes. In contrast, age of 41–60 years was associated with a lower chance of non-resolution when compared to age >60 years. No significant association with peritonitis outcome was observed for the other variables (Table 4).

Discussion

The present results showed a marked decline in the incidence and proportion of peritonitis episodes caused by *S. aureus* over the past 15 years, in agreement with other studies [3,12]. The introduction of safer connection systems and the routine use of

Table 2. Clinical findings in *S. aureus* peritonitis episodes.

Sign or symptom	N	%
Cloudy Dialysis Effluent	60	96.8
Abdominal pain	42	67.7
Nausea or vomiting	26	41.9
Fever	18	29.0
Hypotension	12	19.3

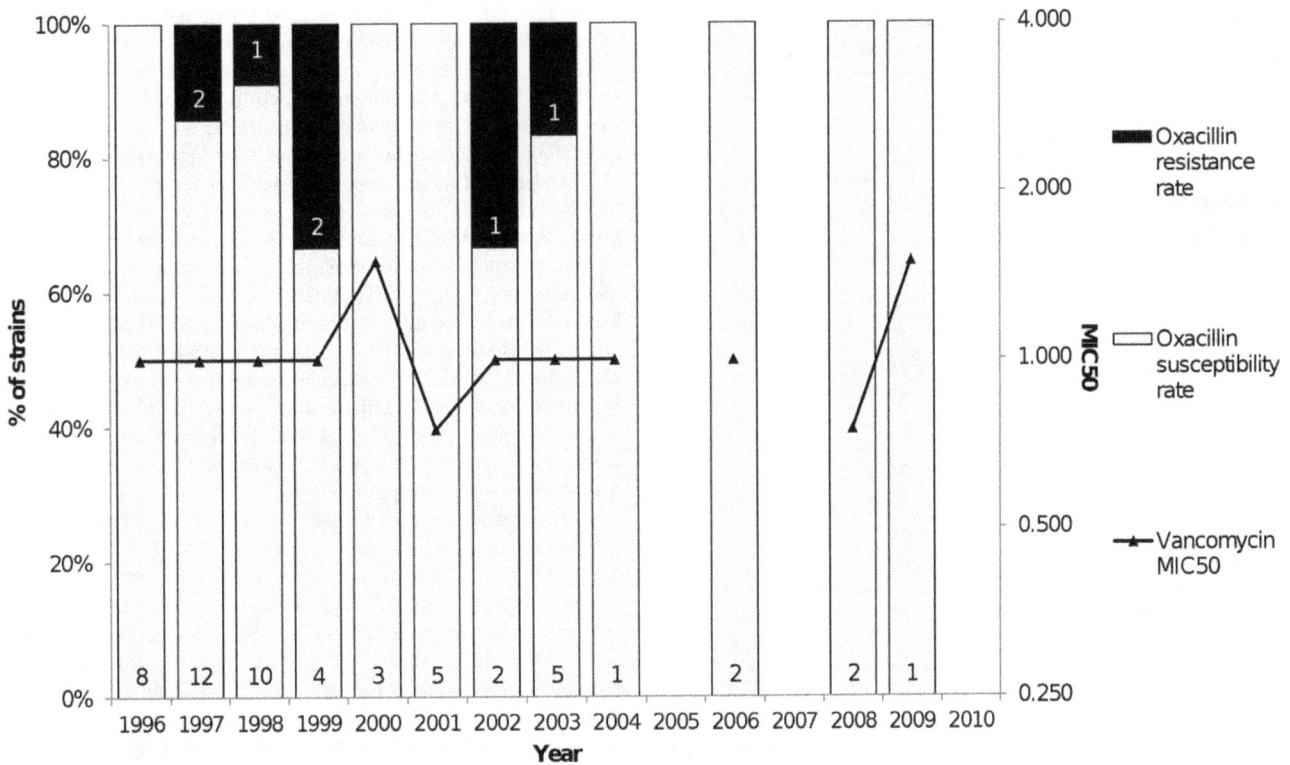

Figure 1. Annual Rate (episodes/patient/year) of *Staphylococcus aureus* Peritonitis from January 1996 to December 2010.

prophylactic antibiotics at the catheter exit site possibly contributed to the reduction of the incidence of *S. aureus* peritonitis; however the strong decline in the incidence observed after the introduction of the prophylaxis with mupirocin reinforces the role of this strategy on *S. aureus* peritonitis prevention. In addition, in the present series we observed a higher death rate among *S. aureus* episodes compared to episodes caused by CoNS as previously reported [1].

There are few studies reporting the influence of demographic and clinical factors on the prognosis of *S. aureus* peritonitis episodes. Szeto et al. [7] observed an association between adjuvant rifampicin treatment and a significantly lower risk of relapse,

whereas the complete cure rate was similar for cephalosporin and vancomycin empiric treatment protocols. Govindarajulu et al. [6] found that the presence of peripheral vascular disease and the use of vancomycin compared to cephalosporins were significantly associated with an increased risk of relapse of *S. aureus* peritonitis. According to these authors, female gender and middle tertile of age were independent predictors of a lower risk of relapse. Similarly, we observed that patient age of 41 to 60 years was associated with a higher chance of peritonitis resolution when compared to older patients. In addition, the presence of diabetes was an independent predictor of non-resolution of peritonitis. It is known that the immune response is dysregulated in diabetic

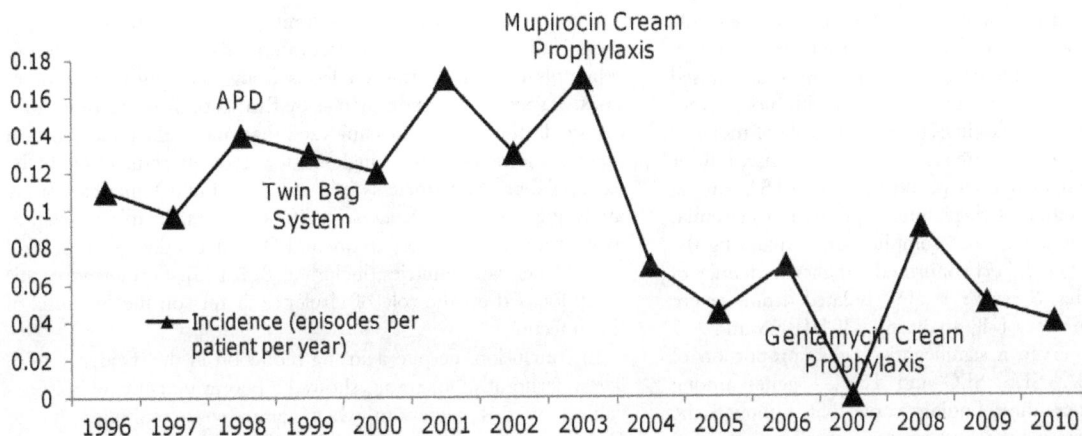

Figure 2. Vancomycin Minimum Inhibitory Concentration (MIC50) and Proportion of Oxacillin-Resistant *Staphylococcus aureus* Strains Isolated from Peritoneal Dialysis Patients with Peritonitis between 1996 and 2010.

Table 3. Production Rates of Pathogenic Factors by *S. aureus* strains Isolated from 62 Peritonitis Episodes.

	N	%
Enzymes		
α-Hemolysin	27	43.5
β-Hemolysin	24	38.7
Lipase	52	83.9
Lecithinase	57	91.9
Deoxyribonuclease	58	93.5
Thermonuclease	56	90.3
Toxins		
SEA	7	11.3
SEB	17	27.4
SEC	12	19.4
TSST-1	17	27.4
Biofilm	55	88.7

SEA, SEB, SEC, enterotoxins A, B and C, respectively; TSST-1, toxic shock syndrome toxin-1.

patients, increasing the risk of developing infection. In addition, advanced glycation end-products act on peritoneal mesothelial cells, with a potentially negative impact on the local immune response [13]. Although diabetes has been reported to be a risk factor for peritonitis [14], to our knowledge, there are no studies showing diabetes to be a predictor of poor outcome after a peritonitis episode. In the present series, vancomycin use was not an independent predictor of outcome, in agreement with the study of Szeto et al. [7]. We observed no influence of other demographic or clinical factors on resolution rate. Similar results have been reported by Krishnan et al. [15] in a retrospective series of peritonitis episodes of different causes.

Little is known about the influence of specific virulence factors on peritonitis caused by *S. aureus*. MRSA peritonitis has been associated with poor outcome in the two largest series of *S. aureus* peritonitis [6,7]. In the present series, we found a low oxacillin resistance rate, which was confirmed by determination of the *mecA* gene. On the other hand, the *S. aureus* strains studied presented expressive enzyme, toxin, and biofilm production. In contrast to previous studies we found no association between oxacillin resistance and resolution rate; however, in the present series only seven peritonitis episodes were caused by oxacillin-resistant *S. aureus*, a fact that may have influenced the results. Episodes caused by *mecA*-positive *S. aureus* isolates were associated with more severe initial clinical symptoms. Studies investigating the role of the *mecA* gene in the virulence of *S. aureus* are scarce in the literature. Fowler Jr et al. [16] found an increasing proportion of MRSA among strains isolated from nasal carriage, uncomplicated bacteremia, and bacteremia with hematogenous complications. Analyzing the same sample later, Gill et al. [17] confirmed a higher frequency of the *mecA* gene among *S. aureus* strains isolated from severe infections. In our laboratory [18] analyzing 336 MRSA and 107 MSSA strains, we observed a significantly higher proportion of strains expressing SEA, SEB, SEC and TSST-1 genes among MRSA. Taken together, these findings show that, although the number of strains expressing the *mecA* gene was small in this series, a role of the *mecA* gene in *S. aureus* virulence cannot be ruled out.

Among bacterial factors studied, β-hemolysin production was significantly and independently associated with lower resolution

odds. The role of β-hemolysin in the pathogenesis of *S. aureus* infections has not been previously reported in PD-related peritonitis. Nevertheless, some pathways may be suggested based on the findings of experimental models. β-Hemolysin is one of the toxins produced by *S. aureus* which acts as a sphingomyelinase, degrading sphingomyelin in the outer layer of cell membranes [19]. Deletion of the catalase and β-toxin genes in *S. aureus* strains has been shown to cause strong attenuation of virulence in intramammary and subcutaneous experimental infections of ewes and lambs and in a murine skin abscess model [19]. Using a mouse model of lung injury, Hayashida et al. [20] found that animals infected with β-hemolysin-deficient *S. aureus* presented significantly attenuated lesions compared to those infected with *S. aureus* expressing this toxin. This experimental disease was characterized by intense neutrophilic inflammation and reduced expression of syndecan-1 in alveolar epithelial cells and could be reproduced by administration of recombinant β-hemolysin, but not of mutant β-hemolysin deficient in sphingomyelinase activity.

Extracellular DNA is a major structural component in the biofilms of pathogenic *S. aureus*. Huseby et al. [21] showed that β-hemolysin forms covalent cross-links to itself in the presence of DNA, irrespective of sphingomyelinase activity, producing an insoluble nucleoprotein matrix in vitro. Using an infectious endocarditis rabbit model, the authors observed that this toxin stimulates biofilm formation in vivo. β-Hemolysin does not lyse most types of host cells but leaves them vulnerable to a number of other lytic agents, such as α-hemolysin and Panton-Valentine leukocidin [20]. We recently demonstrated that α-hemolysin production predicts poor outcome in peritonitis episodes caused by *S. aureus* and CoNS [11].

A reservoir of phospholipids exists on the peritoneal surface and the main constituents of peritoneal phospholipids are phosphatidylcholine and sphingomyelin [22]. Indeed, evidence suggests that the phospholipids present on the peritoneal surface are derived from peritoneal mesothelial cells. In this respect, β-hemolysin, a sphingomyelinase, may participate directly in biofilm formation, contributing to a poorer outcome of peritonitis episodes, or may render host peritoneal cells susceptible to other pathogenic factors.

Surprisingly, biofilm production was not a predictor of peritonitis resolution. However, the percentages of non-producers was low, a fact impairing the comparison with biofilm producers; therefore, a role of biofilm production in peritonitis outcome cannot be ruled out. Finally, other *S. aureus* virulence factors that act in a synergistic and coordinated fashion may play a pathogenic role.

The present study has several limitations, the most important of them is the absence of more accurate tests to assess production of β-hemolysin such as mRNA levels using quantitative real time-PCR or specific detection such as by ELISA or Western Blot. Also, the small number of cases analyzed that may reduce its statistical power, and since it is a single-center study its results cannot be extrapolated. Nevertheless, it is the first Latin American study analyzing a series of *S. aureus* peritonitis cases. In this respect, *S. aureus* remains the most frequent PD-related etiology in several Latin American countries, including Brazil [3]. Furthermore, this study focused on the role of virulence factors on the outcome of this infection.

In conclusion, despite a strong reduction in the incidence of *S. aureus* peritonitis, our results showed a poorer outcome of episodes caused by this bacterium when compared to episodes due to CoNS, particularly a higher death rate. Among demographic factors, older age and diabetes were predictors of a lower resolution rate. These findings highlight the importance of peritonitis as a serious complication of PD, particularly among

Table 4. Odds Comparison of Peritonitis Resolution by Logistic Regression Analysis.

Factor	p value (univariate)	p value (multivariate)	OR	95% CI
Gender (female)	0.109	0.143	4.551	0.599–34.611
Caucasian race	0.642			
Age (years)	0.042			
≤20		0.999	Exp(3.849)	0.000–
21–40		0.871	0.845	0.111–6.466
41–60		0.020	0.091	0.012–0.684
>60 (reference)				
Educational level	0.934			
Elementary				
Secondary				
Higher				
Illiteracy				
Vancomycin use	0.037	0.242	0.325	0.049–2.140
Presence of diabetes	0.042	0.009	14.682	1.960–112.676
Enzyme production				
α-Hemolysin	0.632			
β-Hemolysin	0.077	0.006	16.597	2.246–122.615
Lipase	0.204			
Lecithinase	0.185	0.697	2.248	0.038–131.697
Deoxyribonuclease	0.033	0.999	Exp(6.296)	0.000–
Thermonuclease	0.934			
Presence of mecA gene	0.195	0.838	1.430	0.046–44.342
Biofilm production	0.623			
Toxin production				
SEA	0.265			
SEB	0.312			
SEC	0.071	0.217	5.621	0.363–87.052
TSST-1	0.205	0.399	0.365	0.035–3.805
Dialysis vintage (months)	0.07	0.092	0.943	0.880–1.010
Dialysis modality (APD vs CAPD)	0.477			

SEA, SEB, SEC, enterotoxins A, B and C, respectively; TSST-1: toxic shock syndrome toxin-1; APD, automated peritoneal dialysis; CAPD, continuous ambulatory peritoneal dialysis.

elderly and diabetic patients. β-Hemolysin production was the only virulence factor that negatively influenced peritonitis outcome; however further studies using specific tests to detect the presence of β-hemolysin are necessary to confirm this result.

Materials and Methods

All episodes of ambulatory PD-related peritonitis caused by *Staphylococcus aureus* between January 1996 and December 2010 were reviewed. The diagnosis of peritonitis was made when at least two of the following criteria were present: 1) presence of a cloudy peritoneal effluent; 2) abdominal pain; 3) dialysate containing more than 100 white blood cells per μl (at least 50% polymorphonuclear cells), and 4) positive culture of peritoneal effluent [23,24]. Exclusion criteria were episodes of relapsing *S. aureus* peritonitis, presence of concomitant exit site or tunnel infections, and incomplete clinical data. Resolution was defined as the disappearance of signs and symptoms within 96 h after the beginning of antibiotic therapy and

a negative peritoneal fluid culture at least 28 days after treatment completion [23,24]. Relapse was defined as an episode due to the same organism, or a negative culture result that occurs within 28 days of completion of antibiotic therapy for a prior *S. aureus* episode [23,24]. Death related to peritonitis was defined as death of a patient with active peritonitis, or admitted with peritonitis, or within 2 weeks of a peritonitis episode [23,24]. Non-resolution was the term used for cases presenting initial non-resolution, relapse, peritoneal catheter removal due to refractory peritonitis, need for a second antibiotic regimen, or death.

The following information was recorded for each case: 1) episode: date, clinical findings, treatment, and outcome (resolution, relapse, catheter removal, or death); 2) presence of diabetes mellitus; 3) demographic data: age, gender and race (Caucasian, non-Caucasian), and dialysis treatment time; 4) dialysis modality (continuous ambulatory peritoneal dialysis or automated peritoneal dialysis); 5) educational level (illiterate, elementary, secondary, and higher).

The study was approved by the Research Ethics Committee of the Faculty of Medicine of Botucatu, Brazil (OF. 028/08-CEP). This study was exempted from the requirement to obtain written informed consent from the participants and/or their legal guardians because the *Staphylococcus* strains included in the study had already been isolated and stored in the Culture Collection of the Department of Microbiology and Immunology, UNESP, Botucatu, São Paulo, Brazil.

Patients were treated within 24 h of the onset of the first clinical signs or symptoms using contemporary empiric antibiotic recommendations [23–25]. From 1996 to 2000 (period 1) empiric antibiotic therapy consisted of intraperitoneal (i.p.) cefazolin plus amikacin. Two protocols were used from 2000 to 2005 (period 2): the first consisted of i.p. cefazolin plus amikacin and the second of i.p. cefazolin plus ceftazidime. After 2005 (period 3) all episodes were first treated with i.p. vancomycin plus amikacin. Therapy was evaluated and adjusted as soon as the culture results were available. The duration of antibiotic therapy was 21 days.

In the period 1 no antibiotic prophylaxis at exit site was prescribed and two connection systems were used: the Y set system and the twin bag system, which was introduced in 1999; automated PD (APD) was used from 1998. In the period 2 no antibiotic prophylaxis at exit site was prescribed until 2003, when daily mupirocin cream application at exit site began to be recommended; the twin bag system or APD were prescribed for all patients. In the period 3 until December 2006 all patients were oriented to daily mupirocin cream application, and from January 2007 daily gentamicin cream application at exit site was prescribed to all incident patients; the twin bag system or APD were prescribed for all patients.

The incidence of *S. aureus* peritonitis was calculated for the three subsequent periods of 5 years and is expressed as episodes per patient per year.

The initial cultures were performed with the Bactec® Automated System (Becton Dickinson Company, Sparks, Maryland, USA) and then seeded onto blood agar. The isolates were Gram stained to confirm purity and to determine morphology and specific color. After confirmation of these characteristics, tests for identification of the isolates were performed as recommended by Koneman et al. [26]. The isolates were stored in a culture collection.

The in vitro susceptibility of *S. aureus* to oxacillin and vancomycin was evaluated based on the minimum inhibitory concentration determined by the E-test (AB Biodisk, Solna, Sweden). This quantitative method uses a transparent strip of inert plastic that contains drug concentrations ranging from 0.002 to 256 µg/ml. The proportion of strains susceptible to each drug was defined based on the 2011 CLSI breakpoints [27]. Strains presenting intermediate values were considered to be resistant.

Whole nucleic acids were extracted from *S. aureus* strains cultured on blood agar, individually inoculated into brain heart infusion (BHI) broth, and incubated at 37°C for 24 h. Nucleic acids were extracted using the illustra blood genomic Prep Mini Spin kit (GE Healthcare, Little Chalfont, Buckinghamshire, UK) according to manufacturer instructions. Staphylococcal cells were first digested with lysozyme (10 mg/ml) and proteinase K (20 mg/ml). Next, 500 µl extraction solution was added to the mixture. After centrifugation at 5000 g for 1 min, the supernatant was transferred to a GFX column and centrifuged at 5000 g for 1 min. The supernatant was discarded and 500 µl extraction solution was added to the column. After centrifugation and disposal of the supernatant, 500 µl wash solution was added to the column. The column was then centrifuged at 14,000 rpm for 3 min and transferred to a 1.5-ml tube. Milli-Q water (200 µl) preheated to 70°C was used for elution. The isolates were centrifuged at 5000 g

for 1 min and the GFX column was discarded. Extracted DNA was stored under refrigeration at 4°C.

PCR amplification was performed in 0.5-ml microcentrifuge tubes containing 10 pmol of each primer, 2.0 U Taq DNA polymerase, 100 µM deoxyribonucleotide triphosphates, 10 mM Tris-HCl (pH 8.4), 0.75 mM MgCl$_2$, and 3 µl nucleic acid in a total volume of 25 µl. Gene *mec*A amplification was carried out in an appropriate thermal cycler using the mecA1 (AAA ATC GAT GGT AAA GGT TGG) and mecA2 (AGT TCT GCA GTA CCG GAT TTG) primers as described by Murakami et al. [28]: 40 cycles of denaturation at 94°C for 30 s, annealing of primers at 55.5°C for 30 s, and extension at 72°C for 1 min. After completion of the 40 cycles, the tubes were incubated at 72°C for 5 min and then cooled to 4°C. The *S. aureus* ATCC 33591 and ATCC 25923 references strains were included in all reactions as positive and negative controls, respectively.

The efficiency of amplification was monitored by electrophoresis on 1.5% agarose gel prepared in 1× TBE buffer and stained with ethidium bromide. The size of the amplified products was compared with a 100-bp standard and the gels were photographed under UV transillumination.

Biofilm production was evaluated according to Christensen et al. [29]. Colonies isolated on blood agar were inoculated into tubes measuring 12.0×75.0 mm and containing 2.0 ml trypticase soy broth and incubated at 37°C for 48 h. Next, 1.0 ml 0.4% trypan blue or Toluidine blue O solution was added to the tubes. After gentle shaking to guarantee staining of the material adhered to the inner surface of the tubes, the dye was discarded. A positive result was defined as the presence of a layer of stained material adhered to the inner wall of the tube. The presence of a colored ring only at the liquid-air surface was classified as a negative result.

Production of α- and β-hemolysin were determined on plates containing blood agar supplemented with 5% rabbit blood and 5% sheep blood, respectively. The plates were incubated at 37°C for 24 h. The formation of hemolysis zones around the isolated colonies indicated a positive result.

Lipolytic activity was evaluated on plates containing blood agar enriched with 0.01% CaCl$_2$:2H$_2$O and 1% Tween 80. A positive result was defined as the formation of opacity around the colony after incubation at 37°C for 18 h, followed by incubation at room temperature for 24 h [30]. The production of lecithinase was evaluated using Baird-Parker medium. The formation of an opaque halo around the colony indicated a positive result [31].

Nuclease (DNAse) and thermonuclease (TNAse) were determined by the metachromatic Toluidine blue O agar diffusion-DNA technique according to Lachica et al. [32]. Supernatants obtained by the sac culture method of Donnelly et al. [33] as described below were transferred to the wells of plates containing metachromatic Toluidine blue O agar. The culture supernatant was first heated in a water bath for 20 min for the detection of TNAse. Nuclease (DNAse and TNAse) activity was evaluated by measuring the diameter of pink halos (mm) formed on the medium. Positive results were interpreted by comparing the halos with those obtained for a standard DNAse- and TNAse-positive *S. aureus* strain (ATCC 25923).

For the evaluation of the production of enterotoxins and TSST-1, the sac culture method [33] was used to determine the toxigenic profile of the strains. Dialysis sacs filled with 50 ml double-concentrated BHI broth were placed in U-shaped Erlenmeyer flasks and autoclaved at 121°C for 15 min. A loopful of organisms was added to 18 ml sterile 0.2 M phosphate buffer in 0.9% NaCl, pH 7.4. After incubation at 37°C for 24 h on a shaker at 200 rpm, the cultures were centrifuged at 8000 g for 10 min at 4°C and the supernatants obtained were stored at −20°C until the time of use.

The extracellular products were detected by reverse passive latex agglutination (RPLA) using the SET-RPLA-T900 and TST-RPLA-TD940 kits (Oxoid Diagnostic Reagents, Cambridge, UK) for the detection of enterotoxins A (SEA), B (SEB), C (SEC) and D (SED) and TSST-1, respectively, according to manufacturer instructions. Samples that presented nonspecific reactions after this treatment were filtered through a Millipore membrane (0.22 μm) and, if necessary, diluted 1:10 with 0.02 M phosphate buffer in 0.9% NaCl, pH 7.4. A positive reaction was classified as (+), (++) and (+++) according to the agglutination pattern described by the manufacturer of the kit. The formation of a rose button was interpreted as a negative result.

Statistical analysis

Peritonitis incidences were compared using the Poisson regression model. The association between microbiological characteristics (oxacillin resistance, presence of *mec*A gene and production of pathogenic factors) and the frequency of clinical findings at initial presentation (abdominal pain, fever, nausea or vomiting, and arterial hypotension) was analyzed by the chi-square or Fisher's exact test. These tests were also used to compare resolution and death rates between *S. aureus* peritonitis episodes and 117 contemporary CoNS cases. Multivariate analysis by logistic regression was used to test baseline demographic, clinical, and microbiological factors that independently predicted the outcome of a peritonitis episode. Outcome was classified as two mutually exhausted and exclusive results (resolution or non-resolution). For this purpose, univariate analysis using the chi-square or Fisher's exact test (binary variables) or logistic regression (continuous variables) was first performed to select the variables that would enter the final model, with $p>0.20$ being used as an elimination criterion. A p value less than 0.05 was considered to be significant. All statistical analyses were performed using the SPSS 16.0 software (SPSS®, Inc.).

Author Contributions

Conceived and designed the experiments: PB JCTC ACM MLRSC. Performed the experiments: TMCM CHC ALM ACM. Analyzed the data: PB CHC MLRSC. Contributed reagents/materials/analysis tools: PB MLRSC. Wrote the paper: PB CHC MLRSC. Collection of the clinical data: PB JCTC.

References

1. Pérez Fontan M, Rodríguez-Carmona A, García-Naveiro R, Rosales M, Villaverde P, et al. (2005) Peritonitis-related mortality in patients undergoing chronic peritoneal dialysis. Perit Dial Int 25: 274–284.
2. Cunha MLRS, Montelli AC, Fioravante AM, Neves Batalha JE, Teixeira Caramori JC, et al. (2005) Predictive factors of outcome following staphylococcal peritonitis in continuous ambulatory peritoneal dialysis. Clin Nephrol 64: 378–382.
3. Barretti P, Bastos KA, Dominguez J, Caramori JC (2007) Peritonitis in Latin America. Perit Dial Int 27: 332–339.
4. Bunke CM, Brier ME, Golper TA (1997) Outcomes of single organism peritonitis in peritoneal dialysis: gram negatives versus gram positives in the Network 9 Peritonitis Study. Kidney Int 52: 524–529.
5. Peacock SJ, Howe PA, Day NP, Crook DW, Winearls CG, et al. (2000) Outcome following staphylococcal peritonitis. Perit Dial Int 20: 215–219.
6. Govindarajulu S, Hawley CM, McDonald SP, Brown FG, Rosman JB, et al. (2010) *Staphylococcus aureus* peritonitis in Australian peritoneal dialysis patients: predictors, treatment, and outcomes in 503 cases. Perit Dial Int 30: 311–319.
7. Szeto CC, Chow KM, Kwan BC, Law MC, Chung KY, et al. (2007) *Staphylococcus aureus* peritonitis complicates peritoneal dialysis: review of 245 consecutive cases. Clin J Am Soc Nephrol 2: 245–251.
8. DeLeo FR, Diep BA, Otto M (2009) Host defense and pathogenesis in *Staphylococcus aureus* infections. Infect Dis Clin North Am 23: 17–34.
9. Alexander W, Rimland D (1987) Lack of correlation of slime production with pathogenicity in continuous ambulatory peritoneal dialysis peritonitis caused by coagulase negative staphylococci. Diagn Microbiol Infect Dis 8: 215–220.
10. Haslinger-Löffler B, Wagner B, Brück M, Strangfeld K, Grundmeier M, et al. (2006) *Staphylococcus aureus* induces caspase-independent cell death in human peritoneal mesothelial cells. Kidney Int 70: 1089–1098.
11. Barretti P, Montelli AC, Batalha JE, Caramori JC, Cunha MLRS (2009) The role of virulence factors in the outcome of staphylococcal peritonitis in CAPD patients. BMC Infect Dis 9: 212.
12. Moraes TP, Pecoits-Filho R, Ribeiro SC, Rigo M, Silva MM, et al. (2009) Peritoneal dialysis in Brazil: twenty-five years of experience in a single center. Perit Dial Int 29: 492–498.
13. Ortiz A, Wieslander A, Linden T, Santamaria B, Sanz A, et al. (2006) 3,4-DGE is important for side effects in peritoneal dialysis what about its role in diabetes. Curr Med Chem 13: 2695–2702.
14. Han SH, Lee JE, Ahn SV, Lee JE, Kim DK, et al. (2007) Reduced residual renal function is a risk of peritonitis in continuous ambulatory peritoneal dialysis patients. Nephrol Dial Transplant 22: 2653–2658.
15. Krishnan M, Thodis E, Ikonomopoulos D, Vidgen E, Chu M, et al. (2002) Predictors of outcome following bacterial peritonitis in peritoneal dialysis. Perit Dial Int 22: 573–581.
16. Fowler VG, Nelson CL, McIntyre LM, Kreiswirth BN, Monk A, et al. (2007) Potential associations between hematogenous complications and bacterial genotype in *Staphylococcus aureus* infection. J Infect Dis 196: 738–747.
17. Gill SR, McIntyre LM, Nelson CL, Remortel B, Rude T, et al. (2011) Potential associations between severity of infection and the presence of virulence-associated genes in clinical strains of *Staphylococcus aureus*. PLoS One 6: e18673.
18. Pimenta-Rodrigues MV (2011) Epidemiologia molecular e fatores de risco para aquisição de clones endêmicos de *Staphylococcus aureus* resistente à meticilina (MRSA) em um hospital de ensino. [Tese]. Botucatu: Univ Estadual Paulista.
19. Martínez-Pulgarín S, Domínguez-Bernal G, Orden JA, de la Fuente R (2009) Simultaneous lack of catalase and beta-toxin in *Staphylococcus aureus* leads to increased intracellular survival in macrophages and epithelial cells and to attenuated virulence in murine and ovine models. Microbiology 155: 1505–1515.
20. Hayashida A, Bartlett AH, Foster TJ, Park PW (2009) *Staphylococcus aureus* beta-toxin induces lung injury through syndecan-1. Am J Pathol 174: 509–518.
21. Huseby MJ, Kruse AC, Digre J, Kohler PL, Vocke JA, et al. (2010) Beta toxin catalyzes formation of nucleoprotein matrix in staphylococcal biofilms. Proc Natl Acad Sci U S A 107: 14407–14412.
22. Zhong JH, Guo QY, Ye RG, Lindholm B, Wang T (2000) Phospholipids in dialysate and the peritoneal surface layer. Adv Perit Dial 16: 36–41.
23. Li PK, Szeto CC, Piraino B, Bernardini J, Figueiredo AE, et al. (2010) Peritoneal dialysis-related infections recommendations: 2010 update. Perit Dial Int 30: 393–423.
24. Piraino B, Bailie GR, Bernardini J, Boeschoten E, Gupta A, et al. (2005) Peritoneal dialysis-related infections recommendations: 2005 update. Perit Dial Int 25: 107–131.
25. Keane WF, Bailie GR, Boeschoten E, Gokal R, Golper TA, et al. (2000) Adult peritoneal dialysis-related peritonitis treatment recommendations: 2000 update. Perit Dial Int 20: 396–411.
26. Koneman EW, Allen SD, Janda WM, Scheckenberger PC, Winn WC (1992) Color Atlas and text book of Diagnostic Microbiology. Philadelphia: J. B. Lippincott Company.
27. Clinical and Laboratory Standards Institute (2008) Performance standards for antimicrobial susceptibility testing: eighteenth informational supplement M100-S18. 18th ed. Wayne PA: CLSI.
28. Murakami K, Minamide W, Wada K, Nakamura E, Teraoka H, et al. (1991) Identification of methicillin-resistant strains of staphylococci by polymerase chain reaction. J Clin Microbiol 29: 2240–2244.
29. Christensen GD, Simpson WA, Bisno AL, Beachey EH (1982) Adherence of slime-producing strains of *Staphylococcus epidermidis* to smooth surfaces. Infect Immun 37: 318–326.
30. Jessen O, Faber V, Rosendal K, Eriksen KR (1959) Some properties of *Staphylococcus aureus*, possibly related to pathogenicity. Part 1. A study of 446 strains from different types of human infection. Acta Pathol Microbiol Scand 47: 316–326.
31. Matos JE, Harmon RJ, Langlois BE (1995) Lecithinase reaction of *Staphylococcus aureus* strains of different origin on Baird-Parker medium. Lett Appl Microbiol 21: 334–335.
32. Lachica RV, Genigeorgis C, Hoeprich PD (1971) Metachromatic agar-diffusion methods for detecting staphylococcal nuclease activity. Appl Microbiol 21: 585–587.
33. Donnelly CB, Leslie JE, Black LA, Lewis KH (1967) Serological identification of enterotoxigenic staphylococci from cheese. Appl Microbiol 15: 1382–1387.

Transcriptional Patterns in Peritoneal Tissue of Encapsulating Peritoneal Sclerosis, a Complication of Chronic Peritoneal Dialysis

Fabian R. Reimold[1,2,3], **Niko Braun**[3,4], **Zsuzsanna K. Zsengellér**[5], **Isaac E. Stillman**[1,5], **S. Ananth Karumanchi**[1,2,6], **Hakan R. Toka**[1,7], **Joerg Latus**[3,4], **Peter Fritz**[8], **Dagmar Biegger**[8,9], **Stephan Segerer**[10], **M. Dominik Alscher**[3,4], **Manoj K. Bhasin**[2,11ᗋ], **Seth L. Alper**[1,2,6]*ᗋ

1 Renal Division, Beth Israel Deaconess Medical Center, Harvard Medical School, Boston, Massachusetts, United States of America, 2 Department of Medicine, Harvard Medical School, Boston, Massachusetts, United States of America, 3 Department of General Internal Medicine and Nephrology, Robert-Bosch Hospital, Stuttgart, Germany, 4 Institute of Digital Medicine, Stuttgart, Germany, 5 Department of Pathology, Beth Israel Deaconess Medical Center and Harvard Medical School, Boston, Massachusetts, United States of America, 6 Center for Vascular Biology Research, Beth Israel Deaconess Medical Center and Harvard Medical School, Boston, Massachusetts, United States of America, 7 Division of Nephrology and Department of Medicine, Brigham and Women's Hospital and Harvard Medical School, Boston, Massachusetts, United States of America, 8 Division of Pathology, Department of Diagnostic Medicine, Robert-Bosch Hospital, Stuttgart, Germany, 9 Margarete Fischer-Bosch Institute of Clinical Pharmacology, Stuttgart, Germany, 10 Division of Nephrology, University Hospital Zurich, Zurich, Switzerland, 11 Division of Interdisciplinary Medicine and Biotechnology and Department of Medicine, Beth Israel Deaconess Medical Center and Harvard Medical School, Boston, Massachusetts, United States of America

Abstract

Encapsulating peritoneal sclerosis (EPS) is a devastating complication of peritoneal dialysis (PD), characterized by marked inflammation and severe fibrosis of the peritoneum, and associated with high morbidity and mortality. EPS can occur years after termination of PD and, in severe cases, leads to intestinal obstruction and ileus requiring surgical intervention. Despite ongoing research, the pathogenesis of EPS remains unclear. We performed a global transcriptome analysis of peritoneal tissue specimens from EPS patients, PD patients without EPS, and uremic patients without history of PD or EPS (Uremic). Unsupervised and supervised bioinformatics analysis revealed distinct transcriptional patterns that discriminated these three clinical groups. The analysis identified a signature of 219 genes expressed differentially in EPS as compared to PD and Uremic groups. Canonical pathway analysis of differentially expressed genes showed enrichment in several pathways, including antigen presentation, dendritic cell maturation, B cell development, chemokine signaling and humoral and cellular immunity (P value<0.05). Further interactive network analysis depicted effects of EPS-associated genes on networks linked to inflammation, immunological response, and cell proliferation. Gene expression changes were confirmed by qRT-PCR for a subset of the differentially expressed genes. EPS patient tissues exhibited elevated expression of genes encoding sulfatase1, thrombospondin 1, fibronectin 1 and alpha smooth muscle actin, among many others, while in EPS and PD tissues mRNAs encoding leptin and retinol-binding protein 4 were markedly down-regulated, compared to Uremic group patients. Immunolocalization of Collagen 1 alpha 1 revealed that Col1a1 protein was predominantly expressed in the submesothelial compact zone of EPS patient peritoneal samples, whereas PD patient peritoneal samples exhibited homogenous Col1a1 staining throughout the tissue samples. The results are compatible with the hypothesis that encapsulating peritoneal sclerosis is a distinct pathological process from the simple peritoneal fibrosis that accompanies all PD treatment.

Editor: Andre Van Wijnen, University of Massachusetts Medical, United States of America

Funding: This work was supported by Baxter International, Inc. (NB, SS and MDA), the Howard Hughes Medical Institute (SAK) and NIH DK34854 (Harvard Digestive Diseases Center to SLA). FRR was supported by a Fellowship of the Robert Bosch Foundation. SS is supported by the Swiss National Science Foundation (32003B-129710). The funders had no role in study design, data collection and analysis, decision to publish, or preparation of the manuscript.

Competing Interests: The authors have the following interests. This study was partly funded by Baxter International, Inc. There are no patents, products in development or marketed products to declare. This does not alter the authors' adherence to all the PLOS ONE policies on sharing data and materials, as detailed online in the guide for authors.

* E-mail: salper@bidmc.harvard.edu

ᗋ These authors contributed equally to this work.

Introduction

Renal replacement therapy is currently restricted to renal transplantation, hemodialysis (HD), and peritoneal dialysis (PD). Peritoneal dialysis constitutes <10% of current renal replacement therapy in the US and in much of Europe, but up to 80% in Mexico and Taiwan [1]. However, reimbursement changes expected to accompany health care reform in the US will promote renewed interest in and increased use of PD.

Encapsulating peritoneal sclerosis (EPS) is a rare but dangerous complication of peritoneal dialysis (PD). Mortality rates as high as 57% [2,3] have been reduced at centers specializing in the medical and surgical treatment of EPS, even in late stage disease characterized by severe intestinal obstruction [3,4,5]. Although sporadic idiopathic EPS has been reported [6,7,8], prior duration of PD remains the most important risk factor identified to date [2,9]. EPS epidemiology has been complicated by regional differences in PD use and in reported EPS incidence, likely exacerbated by non-uniform diagnostic criteria. EPS rates among 7000 patients from Australia and New Zealand were 0.3% after 3 years on PD, 0.8% after 5 years, and 3.9% after 8 years [9], but 8.1% of UK patients treated with PD for 5 years developed EPS [10]. In a Japanese cohort of PD patients with overall EPS incidence of 2.5%, EPS was diagnosed in 17–70% of patients with PD duration >15 years [11,12,13]. 72% of EPS is recognized only after discontinuation of PD due to ultrafiltration failure, switch to hemodialysis, or transplantation [9]. Among transplanted PD patients in the Dutch multicenter EPS study, EPS was the fourth most common cause of death after infection, cardiovascular disease, and malignancy [14].

The pathogenesis of EPS remains incompletely understood. Simple peritoneal fibrosis accompanies nearly all PD treatment, resulting in gradual impairment of ultrafiltration that can necessitate transition to HD [15]. Risk factors and signaling pathway abnormalities distinguishing the malignant fibrotic process of EPS from simple peritoneal fibrosis are poorly defined. The current two-hit model envisions as a first hit the long-term exposure to advanced glycation end products (AGEs) in peritoneal dialysate [16,17], leading to increased expression of profibrotic factors such as transforming growth factor β (TGF-β) and of angiogenic mediators such as vascular endothelial growth factor (VEGF). In addition, declining numbers of pro-fibrinolytic mast cells promote enhanced fibrin deposition [18]. A contributing role has also been proposed for the turbulent fluid shear stress intrinsic to the process of PD [19,20]. The second hit remains unknown, but may be a clinically obvious or occult inflammatory or ischemic stimulus. Peritoneal mesothelial cells are believed to undergo epithelial-to-mesenchymal transition (EMT), leading in EPS to complete mesothelial denudation that accompanies the severe fibrosis [21,22]. However, the high rates of EPS among patients treated with PD over lengthy periods also suggest an alternate hypothesis. EPS may instead represent the natural evolution of PD-associated peritoneal fibrosis, influenced by patient-specific risk modifier gene profiles that determine the kinetics of progression from simple fibrosis to EPS.

The absence of blood tests specific for EPS requires diagnosis based on clinical presentation, radiologic and histologic findings [2]. The clinical presentation of EPS is characterized by varied and nonspecific symptoms, including bowel obstruction, loss of appetite, fever, nausea and vomiting, ascites, constipation, diarrhea and weight loss. The diagnosis of EPS is most commonly made by CT scan, but the radiological picture can be nonspecific [23]. Diagnosis also can be made by peritoneoscopy or laparotomy, classically revealing abdominal cocooning (bands or layers of fibrotic tissue surrounding and constricting bowel loops), sometimes accompanied by a fibrotic "sugar coating" appearance. Histologically, EPS peritoneal tissues often contain myofibroblast-like cells expressing smooth muscle actin-1 and podoplanin [22]. Braun et al. have recently proposed additional novel histological criteria for the diagnosis of EPS, including mesothelial denudation, fibrin deposits, and presence of fibroblast-like cells [24].

Non-surgical therapeutic options for EPS are few, and randomized controlled trials non-existent [12]. Glucocorticoids have been used, especially in settings of marked inflammation [12,25,26,27]. Clinical responses to azathioprine or mycophenolate have been reported [28], but the increased post-transplant prevalence of EPS suggests possible deleterious, profibrotic actions of calcineurin inhibitors [29]. Anecdotal reports of beneficial

treatment with tamoxifen have been attributed to inhibition of profibrotic TGF-β [30,31]. Inhibitors of the renin angiotensin aldosterone system (RAAS), widely used in PD patients and including angiotensin converting enzyme inhibitors (ACEi) and angiotensin receptor blockers (ARB), have been proposed to deter development of EPS in PD patients [32]. Indeed, RAAS inhibition in rat models has reduced angiogenesis and peritoneal thickening [32], and retarded or reduced progression from simple fibrosis to a condition resembling EPS [33]. However, severe EPS cases characterized by enteral obstruction or ileus usually require urgent surgical enterolysis and debridement. Although the outcomes of acute surgical intervention are often favorable, EPS recurs in up to 23% of these post-surgical patients [12,34].

Models of peritoneal fibrosis in rats and mice [35] have been generated by peritoneal insertion of foreign bodies [36], by peritoneal instillation of peritoneal dialysate containing glucose oxidation products for periods up to 3 weeks [37], by peritoneal instillation of inflammatory agents such as chlorhexidine gluconate [38], and by adenovirus-driven overexpression of TGF-β1 [39]. These models have offered opportunities for unbiased examinations of changes in global gene expression [36,37,38] that might shed light on the pathogenesis of peritoneal fibrosis. However the relationships between these short-term rodent models and the human conditions of PD-associated slowly progressive peritoneal fibrosis or the more serious and aggressive EPS remain unclear.

Therefore, we have performed a pilot study to compare transcriptomes of fresh-frozen peritoneal biopsy samples from EPS patients with those of PD patients without EPS, and with those of uremic patients (Uremic) prior to initiation of dialysis. We employed systems biology and interactive network analyses to identify pathways and interactive networks enriched with EPS-dysregulated genes, to establish the feasibility of using this approach to unravel pathophysiological mechanisms of EPS development in PD patients. This pilot study lays an empiric foundation for future investigations to understand biological mechanisms of EPS and to identify novel prognostic and therapeutic biomarkers.

Methods

Sample accrual

All samples were obtained from the peritoneal biopsy registry at Robert-Bosch Hospital, Stuttgart, Germany. Human peritoneal tissue, blood and peritoneal dialysate was collected at time of surgery at Robert-Bosch Hospital. Written informed consent was obtained from Patients according to an approved protocol (#322/2009BO1, Ethik-Kommission, Eberhard-Karls-Universität Tbingen, Germany). The approved protocol included a patient information sheet explaining the purpose of the study and the envisioned use of the tissue specimen. All patients agreeing to participate in the study signed, in the presence of an authorized clinical investigator, a detailed written consent form previously approved by the "Ethik-Kommission" of Eberhard-Karls-Universität Tbingen, Germany. Patients were provided one day during which to reconsider their written consent. Surgeries included implantation or reimplantation of peritoneal dialysis (PD) catheters or, for EPS patients, enterolyses or peritonectomies. The diagnosis of EPS was based on clinical and radiological findings and on histological criteria that included fibrosis, fibroblast-like cells, exudation, cellularity and its variability, vessel density and its variability, acute or chronic inflammation, hemorrhage, mesothelial hyperplasia, fibrin deposits, presence of vasculopathy, mesothelial denudation, presence of acellular areas, presence of iron and/or calcium deposits, and osseous metaplasia

[23,25,40]. Shortly after excision, tissue samples were washed in 0.9% saline solution, placed in RNAlater (Ambion, Woodlands, TX) for 12 hours at room temperature, then stored at −80°C. Clinical and laboratory data were recorded for all patients. Clinical data included peritoneal transporter status, peritoneal dialysis efficiency, and number of peritonitis episodes.

RNA isolation from fresh-frozen (FF) tissue

RNA was isolated from fresh-frozen tissues using Trizol reagent (Invitrogen, Carlsbad, CA). Frozen tissue samples were homogenized in 1 ml Trizol reagent using a rotor-stator homogenizer (Tissue Tearor, BioSpec Products, Bartlesville, OK) for 1 minute. After chloroform extraction of the homogenate, the aqueous RNA-containing supernatant was twice ethanol-precipitated and resuspended in nuclease-free water. RNA concentration was measured by UV spectrophotometry (NanoDrop ND-1000, NanoDrop Technologies, Wilmington, DE). RNA integrity was assessed using the Agilent 2100 Bioanalyzer (Agilent Technologies, Santa Clara, CA).

cDNA synthesis

Tissue RNA samples were DNAse-treated (DNA-free kit, Applied Biosystems, Carlsbad, CA, Foster City, CA), and 250 ng total RNA from each specimen was reverse-transcribed using the High Capacity cDNA Reverse Transcription Kit (Applied Biosystems) for 10 min at 25°C, 120 min at 37°C, and 5 min at 85°C in a GeneAmp PCR System 2700 thermal cycler (Applied Biosystems). Resultant cDNA samples were diluted 10-fold.

Quantitative reverse transcriptase polymerase chain reaction (qRT-PCR) for individual gene expression assays

qRT-PCR was performed in duplicate with TaqMan gene expression kits and TaqMan Fast Universal PCR master mix (2x) using the "fast protocol" performed on the 7500 Fast Real-Time PCR System (Applied Biosystems) in bar-coded MicroAmp 96-well plates (Applied Biosystems), per manufacturer's instructions. The gene products analyzed included Thrombospondin 1 (THBS1), Matrix Metalloproteinase 2 (MMP2), Leptin (LEP), Retinol-Binding Protein 4 (RBP4), Runt-Related Transcription Factor 2 (RUNX2), Intercellular Adhesion Molecule 1 (ICAM-1), α Smooth Muscle Actin (ACTA2), Fibronectin 1 (FN1), Collagen 1α1 (Col1a1), and Sulfatase 1 (SULF1). β-actin (ACTB) was used as an endogenous control.

DNA microarrays

Total RNA was reverse transcribed into cDNA using the Ovation Pico WTA System (NuGen Technologies, San Carlos, CA). cDNA samples were cleaved and 3′-biotinylated using the Encore Biotin Module (NuGen Technologies, San Carlos, CA), yielding biotinylated single-stranded cDNA probes of 50–100 nt in length. The probe mix was hybridized with the GeneChip Human Genome HT U133 Plus PM Array plate (Affymetrix, Santa Clara, CA), presenting >54,000 target probe sets representing 47,000 transcripts encoding >33,000 well characterized human genes. Microarray analysis was conducted by the Beth Israel Deaconess Medical Center Genomics and Proteomics Center according to standard Affymetrix protocol, using a high throughput hybridization and scanning system. The quality of hybridized chips was assessed using Affymetrix guidelines based on PM mean, 3′ to 5′ ratios for beta-actin and GAPDH, and values for spike-in control transcripts. We also monitored sample reproducibility by chip-to-chip correlation and signal-to-noise ratio (SNR) methods for replicate arrays using the bioconductor package, arrayQuality-

Table 1. Patient characteristics.

Clinical data	EPS (4)	PD (2)	Uremic (2)
Age [a]	60.75±12.42	68.50	56.50
Sex	2 m, 2 f	1 m, 1 f	2 m
Time on PD [months]	74.00±33.52	23	-
Kt/V	1.96±0.32	2.41	-
Bacterial peritonitis [# of episodes]	2.25±2.63	0.50	-
24 h urine output [mL]	275.00±246.64	440.00	2000.00
Nicotine abuse	2/4	0/2	2/2
Arterial hypertension	4/4	1/2	2/2
Diabetes of any kind	1/4	2/2	2/2
PD fluids	2 neutral/2 acidic	both neutral	-
Icodextrin use	4/4	2/2	-
Laboratory values			
Hemoglobin [g/L]	111.75±7.63	100.00	131.50
Leucocytes [×10⁹/L]	8.79±3.41	4.70	6.40
CRP [mg/dL]	2.97±3.35	1.35	0.30
Creatinine [mg/dL]	3.55±1.84	4.00	5.80
BUN [mg/dL]	86.58±36.40	61.00	173.00
Calcium [mM/L]	2.35±0.10	2.09	2.51
Phosphate [mM/L]	1.45±0.34	1.51	1.45

Clinical data and laboratory values of (n) patients, collected before the surgeries that allowed collection of peritoneal biopsy samples. Values are shown as means ± s.e.m. for the EPS group and as means for the smaller PD and Uremic groups. Smoking history was not stratified by duration. Uremic group 24 h urine output was higher than that of the combined PD and EPS groups (p<0.001). Arterial hypertension was defined as resting arterial blood pressure ≥140/90 mmHg. Acidic PD solutions were lactate-buffered with pH 5.0–5.5. Neutral (multicomponent) solutions were of pH 6.5. Icodextrin status was listed as positive if used at any time during the course of PD.
EPS, Encapsulating peritoneal sclerosis; PD, Peritoneal dialysis; CrP, C reactive protein; BUN, blood urea nitrogen.

Metrics [41]. All high quality arrays were included for unsupervised and supervised bioinformatics analysis.

To obtain signal values, chips were further analyzed using the Robust Multichip Average (RMA) method in R using Bioconductor and associated packages. RMA performed background adjustment, quantile normalization and final summarization of 11 oligonucleotides per transcript using the median polish algorithm [42]. Unsupervised analysis was performed using Principal Component Analysis (PCA), which projects multivariate data objects onto a lower dimensional space while retaining as much of the original variance as possible [43,44]. Before PCA, transcripts were filtered to include only those with absolute expression ≥10 in at least 10% of samples. When comparing two groups of samples to identify genes enriched in a given phenotype, i.e. enriched in Uremic vs. both EPS and PD, differentially expressed genes were defined as those with LCB>2, serving as a stringent estimate of the FC [45]. (LCB is defined as the 90% Lower Confidence Bound of the fold change (FC) between the two groups, providing 90% confidence that the actual FC exceeds the threshold LCB).

Self Organizing Maps (SOM)

Identification of functionally related genes differentially expressed in the profiles of EPS, or in the profiles of both EPS and

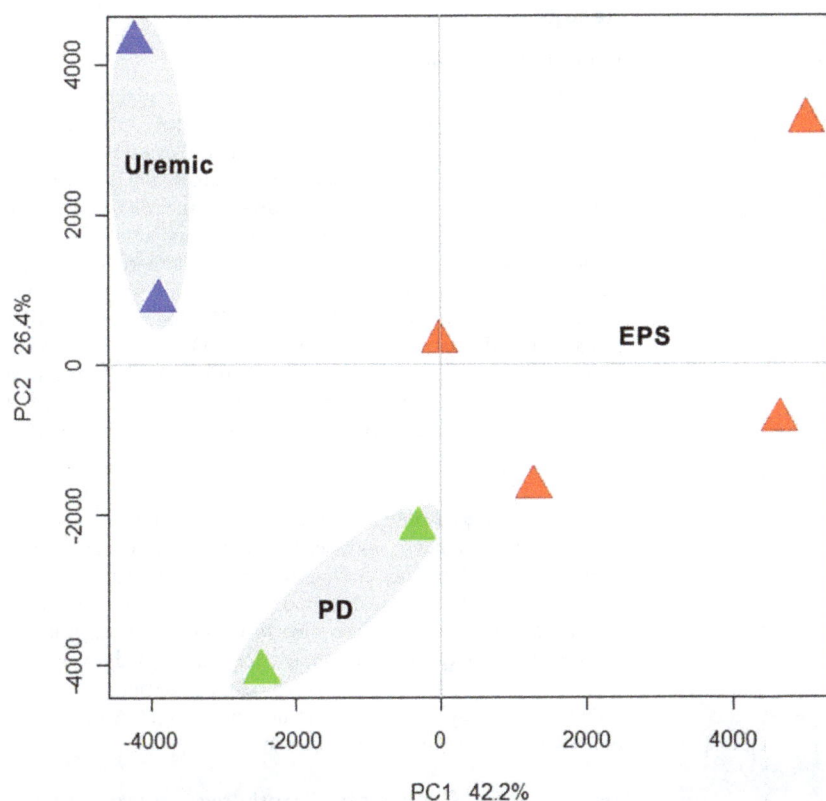

Figure 1. Principal Component Analysis (PCA) of normalized expression data obtained from Uremic, PD and EPS samples. The first component with highest variance (42.2%) is on the X-axis separating Uremic and PD from EPS samples. The second highest (26.4%) is on the Y-axis depicting maximum variation between PD and Uremic samples. The Uremic, PD and EPS samples formed three separate clusters on the PCA plot.

PD as compared to Uremic, was by self-organizing map (SOM) analysis of the differentially expressed genes. We performed SOM clustering on transcript expression values using Pearson correlation coefficient-based distance metrics and a target of 40 groups. SOM allowed grouping of gene expression patterns into an imposed structure in which adjacent clusters are related, thereby identifying sets of genes that follow common expression patterns (transcription signatures) across different conditions [45,46].

Pathways and interactive network analysis

Ingenuity Pathway Analysis (IPA 7.0, Ingenuity Systems, Inc., Redwood City, CA) was used to identify pathways and interaction networks significantly affected by genes with expression changes specifically associated with EPS or with both EPS and PD. The knowledge base of this software consists of functions, pathways and network models derived by systematic exploration of the peer-reviewed scientific literature. IPA analysis calculates a P-value for each pathway according to the fit of user data to the IPA database, using a one-tailed Fisher exact test (http//www.ingenuity.com). Pathways with multiple test-corrected P-values<0.05 were considered significantly affected.

An IPA score [(−log(P value)]>2 indicates a probability >99% that the affected network was not generated at random, but reflects statistically (and biologically) meaningful relationships among a set of genes with specifically altered expression. The ability to rank networks based on relevance to the queried data sets allows network prioritization according to highest predicted impact on the disease process.

Immunohistochemistry

Deparaffinized, rehydrated tissue sections were incubated in Peroxidase Blocking Solution (S 2023, DAKO, Hamburg, Germany). Immunostaining was performed with a TechMate 500 Plus (DAKO), using a dextran-coated peroxidase-coupled polymer system (Dako REAL^{TM} EnVision^{TM} Detection Kit, Peroxidase/DAB+, Rabbit/Mouse, K 5007, DAKO). The primary antibody was rabbit monoclonal anti-human collagen 1 α 1 (AB292, Abcam, Cambridge, MA) diluted 1:100 in DAKO S 2022 diluent. Skin tissue from a human non-diabetic leg served as a positive tissue control. Omission of primary antibody served as negative control. Adjacent tissue sections were stained with Hematoxylin and Eosin (H&E).

Semiquantitative analysis of Collagen 1 α 1 immunostaining was performed within defined areas from 0–100 μm and from 100–200 μm inward from the mesothelial tissue edges towards the adventitia, using ImageJ 1.46 (NIH). Color images recorded by an Olympus BX41 microscope equipped with an Olympus DP71 camera were converted to 32-bit black and white. Immunostaining detection threshold was zeroed at background staining intensity, and ranged from 0–255 arbitrary units. Measurements were recorded at three or more discreet locations within each specimen. Scaled intensity values in the region 0–100 μm from the mesothelial edge were divided by the intensity values in the adjacent region 100–200 μm from the edge. The mean intensity ratios for each group were normalized to that of the Uremic group, to which was assigned a relative intensity ratio value of 1.0.

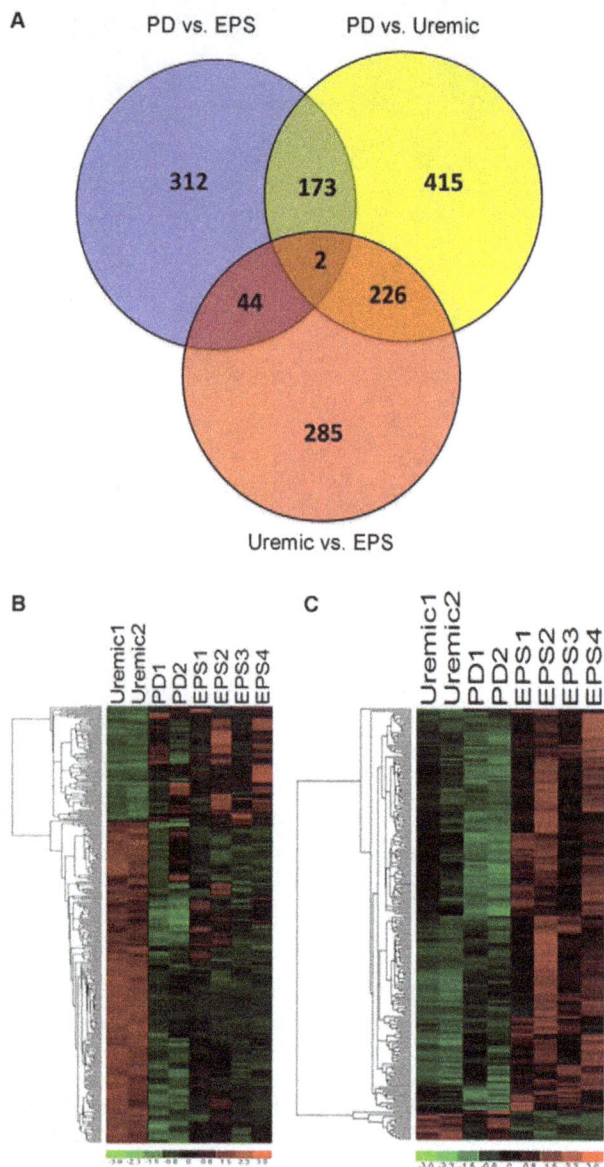

Figure 2. Differentially expressed genes identified from supervised analyses. A. Venn diagram comparing significantly differentially expressed genes identified from the pairwise comparisons Uremic vs. PD (yellow), PD vs. EPS (blue), and Uremic vs. EPS (red). The genes were selected using supervised analysis on the basis of the 90% lower confidence bound (LCB) of the fold change (FC) by pairwise comparison of the groups. The analysis was performed on preprocessed data by filtering out low-expressing probes on the basis of absolute intensity (Intensity <10 in 90% of samples). **B.** Heatmap of genes differentially expressed in both EPS and PD groups as compared to Uremic group (P<0.05). **C.** Heatmap of genes differentially expressed only in EPS as compared to both PD and Uremic groups (P<0.05). Columns represent the samples, with rows representing genes. Gene expression levels are presented in pseudocolor (scale −3 to 3), with red and green respectively denoting high and low expression levels.

Statistical Analysis

Clinical data and laboratory values were compared by ANOVA (Sigmaplot 11.0, Systat Software Inc., San Jose, CA). Differences in results were considered statistically significant for P<0.05.

Results

Patient characteristics

Tissue samples were available from 8 patients: 4 with encapsulating peritoneal sclerosis (EPS, 2 males and 2 females, of mean age 60.8 yrs and mean PD duration 74±34 months), 2 chronic peritoneal dialysis patients (PD, 1 male and 1 female, of mean age 68.5 yrs and mean PD duration 23 months), and 2 male Uremic patients of mean age 56.5 yrs, as yet undialyzed (Table 1, Table S1). Uremic patients had an estimated glomerular filtration rate (eGFR)<15 mL/min/1,73 m^2 body surface area. Residual renal function (urine output, RRF) was 275±246 mL in the EPS group, 440 mL for the PD group, and 2000 mL in the Uremic group (p<0.01 Uremic vs. both groups). Additional clinical characteristics are summarized in Table 1 and (for individual patients) Tables S2a and S2b. Serum chemistries are presented in Table S1.

DNA microarray analysis - unsupervised analysis

Unsupervised analysis was performed on ~11,500 transcripts after preprocessing and normalization of high quality DNA expression data. By principal component analysis, we demonstrated that samples separated according to EPS status along primary component (PC) 1, which accounted for 42.2% of the variation between samples. The analysis revealed three distinct clusters of gene expression by principal component analysis (PCA) (Figure 1), consistent with the three clinical groups.

Identification of genes significantly dysregulated only with EPS or both EPS and PD

Supervised analysis applying a 90% lower confidence bound of the fold change (LCB of FC), and expressed as corrected fold-change >2.0, revealed 531 genes differentially expressed between EPS and PD groups, 557 genes differentially expressed between EPS and Uremic groups, and 816 genes differentially expressed between PD and Uremic groups (Figure 2A). Tables S2, S3, S4 present the 50 genes most highly differentially expressed in pairwise comparisons of the three clinical groups. The group of genes upregulated in EPS compared to PD is dominated by genes involved in immunological processes (e.g. MHC class II and associated proteins). The comparison of EPS to the Uremic group featured upregulation of genes encoding collagens and other matrix proteins, and downregulation of lipid metabolism genes such as glycerol-3-phosphate acyltransferase (~20-fold). In contrast, comparison of PD with Uremic reveals significant upregulation of lipid metabolism genes (20-fold increased glycerol-3-phosphate acyltransferase) and downregulation of matrix metabolism genes, including integrins and collagens.

The Venn diagram of Figure 2A shows that 228 transcripts are differentially expressed in both the comparisons between EPS and the Uremic control group and between PD and Uremic groups, and these represent a candidate transcription signature for peritoneal fibrosis. The Venn diagram also depicts a set of 641 transcripts that are differentially expressed uniquely in EPS as compared to PD or Uremic, and so might include candidate genes linked to the pathological progression from uremic changes, through the simple peritoneal fibrosis of PD, and on to EPS.

When using gene clustering and self-organizing maps (SOM) to detect groups of differentially expressed genes with similar expression patterns, we arbitrarily drew 40 separate maps according to Pearson correlation coefficient-based distance metrics (Figure S1). Evaluation of the maps revealed groups of similarly structured expression patterns, allowing selective merger of patterns depicting specific dysregulation in EPS vs. both PD and

A

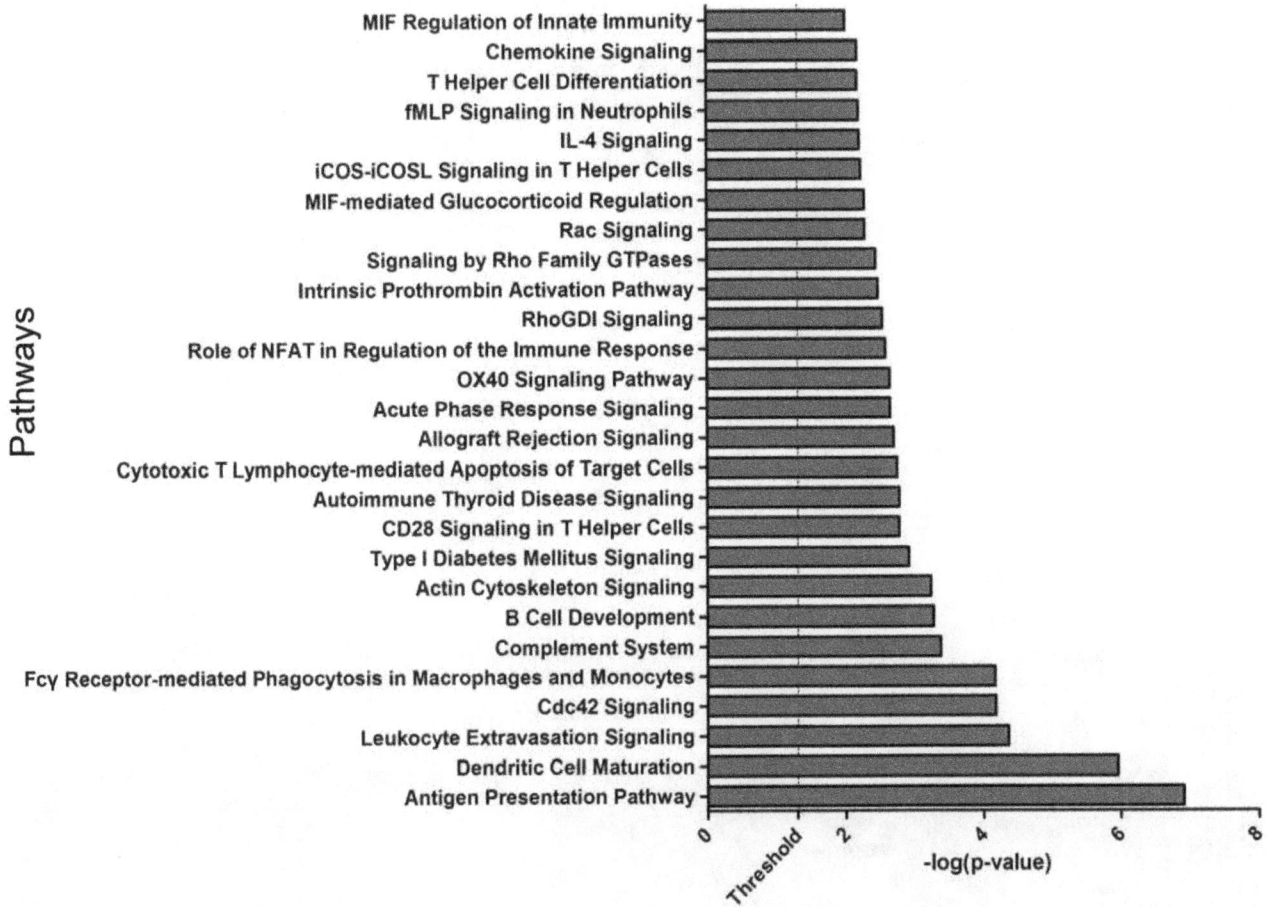

B

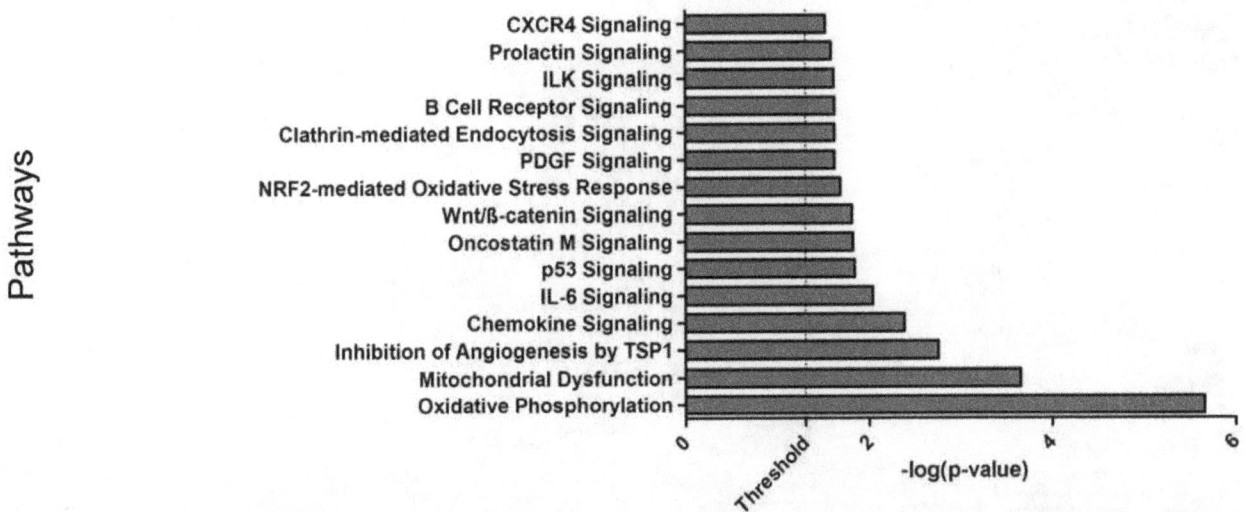

Figure 3. Pathway enrichment analysis of differentially expressed genes. A. Genes differentially expressed only in EPS as compared to PD and Uremic groups. **B.** Genes differentially expressed in both EPS and PD groups as compared to the Uremic group. Each bar represents a significantly enriched pathway as determined by Fisher's Exact Test P value [depicted on the X-axis as −log10(P value)]. The analysis for canonical pathways was performed using Ingenuity Systems software (www.ingenuity.com).

A

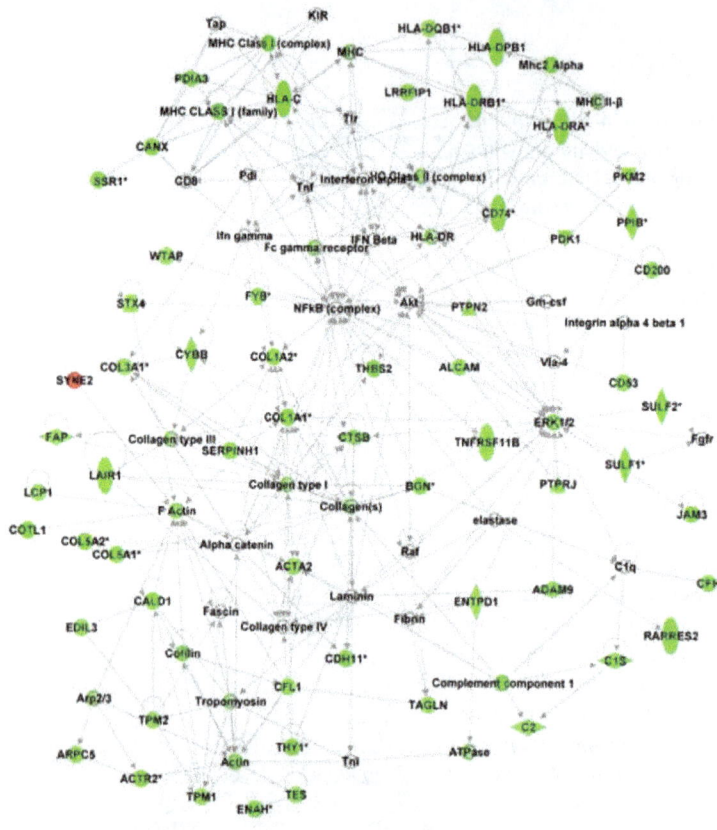

B

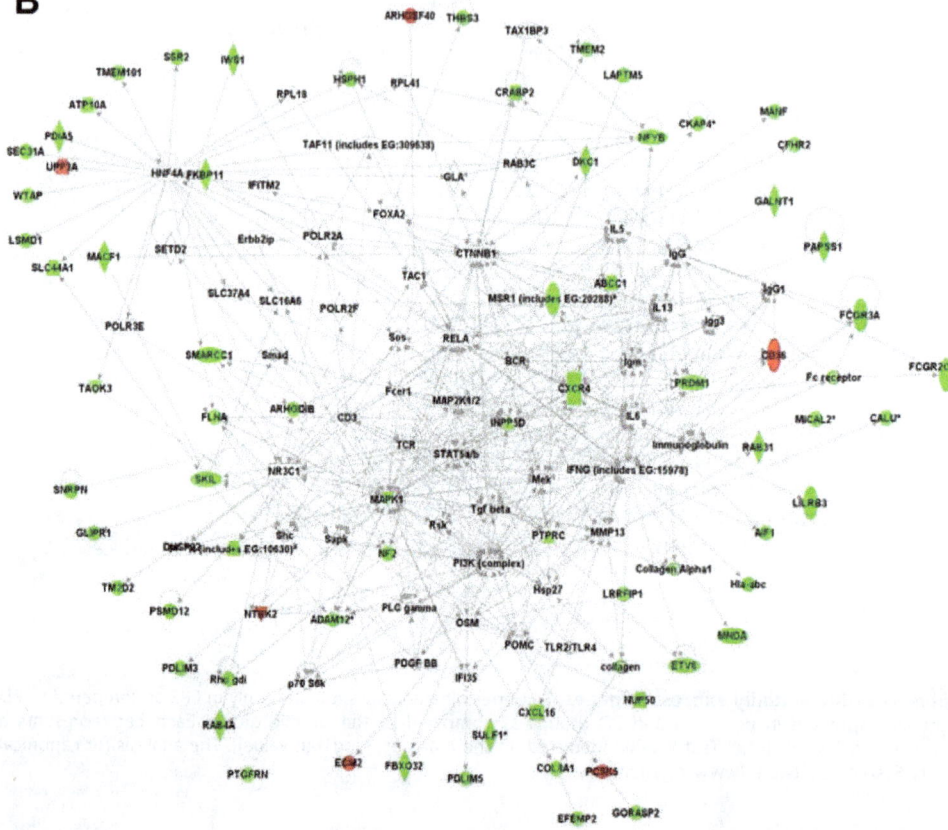

Figure 4. Network representation of cellular functions differentially expressed specifically in EPS but not in PD or Uremic groups.
A. Network related to cell assembly and organization as well as to connective tissue and skeletal muscle tissue disorders. This network has NF-κB, collagen, and ERK1/2 genes as primary regulatory focus nodes. **B.** Network enriched with genes involved in cellular growth and proliferation, carbohydrate metabolism, and gastrointestinal and immunological diseases. This network has PI3K, IFNγ and MAPK1 genes as primary regulatory focus nodes. Ingenuity Pathways Analysis software was used to generate comprehensive gene networks that merged affected networks of related function. Downregulated genes are shown in green, upregulated genes in red. All networks shown were significantly affected in EPS with a score >15 (−log 10[Fisher's Exact Test]).

Uremic, or dysregulation in both EPS and PD as compared to Uremic. The analysis identified a set of 316 transcripts differentially expressed in both EPS and PD as compared to Uremic (fibrosis signature) (Figure 2B). This analysis also identified another set of 219 transcripts specifically differentially expressed in EPS vs. PD as well as in EPS vs. Uremic (EPS Signature) (Figure 2C).

Canonical pathways analysis of EPS and Disease Signatures

We performed canonical pathways enrichment analysis (IPA 7.0) to gain further insight into the functional pathways associated with genes dysregulated only in EPS (EPS signature), and with those dysregulated in both EPS and PD (Disease signature). EPS-associated genes were significantly over-represented (P value<0.05) in pathways related to immune response, inflammation and cytoskeleton signaling, including *"antigen presentation"*, *"Dendritic cell maturation"*, *"B cell development"*, *"complement system"*, *"chemokine signaling"* and *"humoral and cellular immunity"* (Figure 3A). Most of the genes in these pathways were upregulated in EPS, suggesting enhanced activity of innate immune and inflammation pathways.

Pathway analysis of the genes differentially expressed in both the EPS vs. Uremic and the PD vs. Uremic comparisons showed significant association with pathways involved in cell signaling, immune response and metabolism, including *"Oxidative Phosphorylation"*, *"Mitochondrial Dysfunction"*, *"Oncostatin M-"*, *"ILK-"*, *"CXCR4-"* and *"PDGF -"* signaling (Figure 3B).

EPS impacts critical molecules and networks linked to inflammation, immunological response, and cell proliferation

To integrate a functional view of critical regulatory molecules associated with EPS, we performed interactive network analysis on the 228 genes specifically dysregulated in EPS tissue specimens (Figure 2C). The *Ingenuity Pathways Analysis* tool was applied to generate interaction networks based on known functional interactions such as protein-protein interactions or gene regulation interactions (Figure 4). The analysis identified 8 different networks that were significantly affected in EPS with a score >20 (−log 10 [Fisher's Exact Test]). Networks of related function were merged to generate more comprehensive networks. Three different networks related to cell assembly and organization and connective tissue and skeletal muscle tissue disorders were merged to generate an integrated view of cell cycle-related dysregulation in EPS tissue (Figure 4A), featuring the NF-κB, collagen, and ERK1/2 genes as major critical regulatory nodes. Another EPS-associated comprehensive network merging subnetworks linked to cell growth and proliferation and to carbohydrate metabolism (as in gastrointestinal and immunological diseases) features the PI3K, IFNγ and MAPK1 genes as major regulatory focus nodes. These regulatory focus nodes are likely critical to network function, such that therapeutic (or pathologic) alteration of expression of these genes predicts perturbation of the entire network.

EPS and PD both impact critical molecules and networks associated with inflammatory disease, metabolism, cell motility, and cell signaling

To gain further insight into functional consequences of genes that are altered both in both EPS and PD as compared to the Uremic group, we again performed IPA interactive network analysis, identifying 8 different networks significantly affected in both EPS and PD compared to the Uremic control group with a significance score >20. Three networks related to inflammatory and immunological diseases were merged to identify critical regulatory genes (Figure 5A). The resulting merged network highlighted NFKB, JUN, SP1 as critical regulatory molecules. The independent merged network in Figure 5B is enriched in genes involved in lipid metabolism, cellular assembly and movement, and cell death, and reveals the PI3K, AKT and TP53 genes as major regulatory focus nodes.

qRT-PCR Validation of DNA array data

Selected cases of differential gene expression were validated by qRT-PCR assays. β-actin was used as an endogenous "control" transcript. The data were analyzed using the $2^{-\Delta CT}$ calculation, and then normalized to the Uremic group, for which relative gene expression = 1.0. The results of the DNA chip array are presented as mean raw signal intensities. Col1a1 showed >20-fold upregulation in EPS over Uremic and a 2.5-fold increase in gene expression over PD as judged by qRT-PCR, while the DNA chip array showed >5-fold transcript induction in EPS over Uremic and ~1.5-fold upregulation over PD (Figure 6). α-Smooth muscle actin (ACTA2), Sulfatase 1 (SULF1) and Intracellular adhesion molecule 1 (ICAM1) exhibited similar expression patterns (Figure S2), with EPS showing the highest levels of transcript induction. Fibronectin 1 (FN1) and Thrombospondin 1 (THBS1) showed yet greater upregulation in EPS compared to EPS and Uremic control groups (Figure 6), whereas Retinol-binding protein 4 (RBP4) (Figure 6) and Leptin (LEP) (Figure S3) were substantially downregulated in both EPS and PD groups compared to the Uremic control group (figure 6). The DNA array results generally correlated well with the qRT-PCR data. However, whereas array data indicated highest expression of Runt-related transcription factor 2 (RUNX2) and Matrix metalloproteinase 2 (MMP2) in the EPS group, qRT-PCR indicated highest expression in the PD group (Figure S4).

Immunostaining for Collagen 1 α 1 (Col1a1)

To determine protein expression of Col1a1, one of the more highly upregulated genes in EPS, we performed anti-Col1a1 immunohistochemical staining of formalin-fixed, paraffin-embedded tissue sections corresponding to the fresh frozen specimens from which RNA was isolated. EPS and PD tissues showed marked immunostaining for Col1a1, indicating fibrosis. In most of the EPS and PD samples the mesothelium was not detectable. PD sections were strongly and homogeneously stained with Col1a1 throughout the entire specimen. In contrast, EPS samples exhibited pronounced Col1a1 immunostaining predominantly in the area of the (most superficial) submesothelial zone. We

A

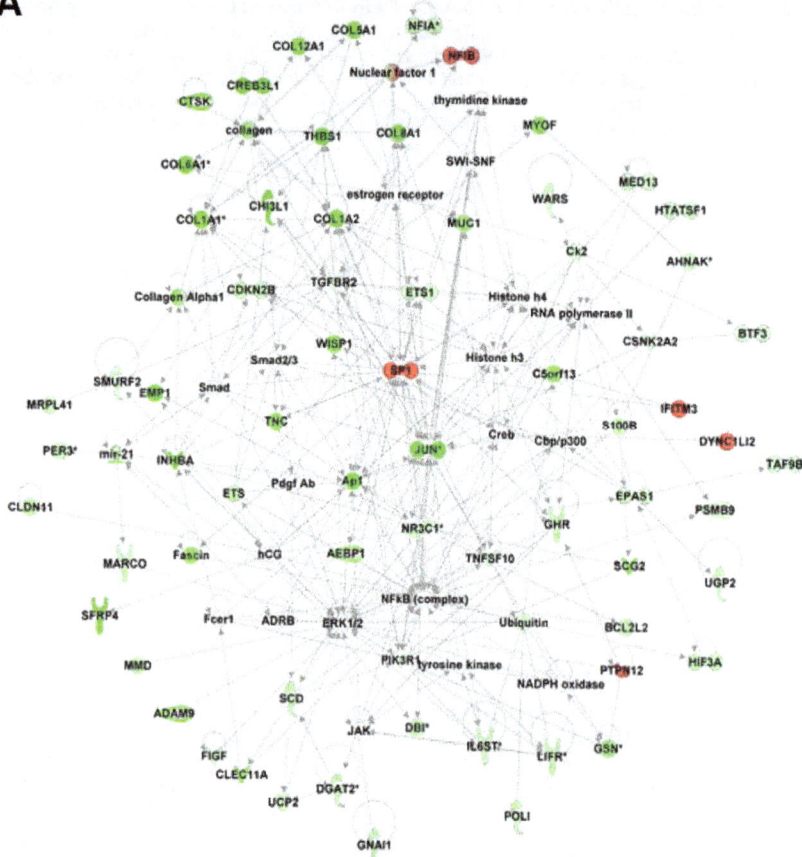

B

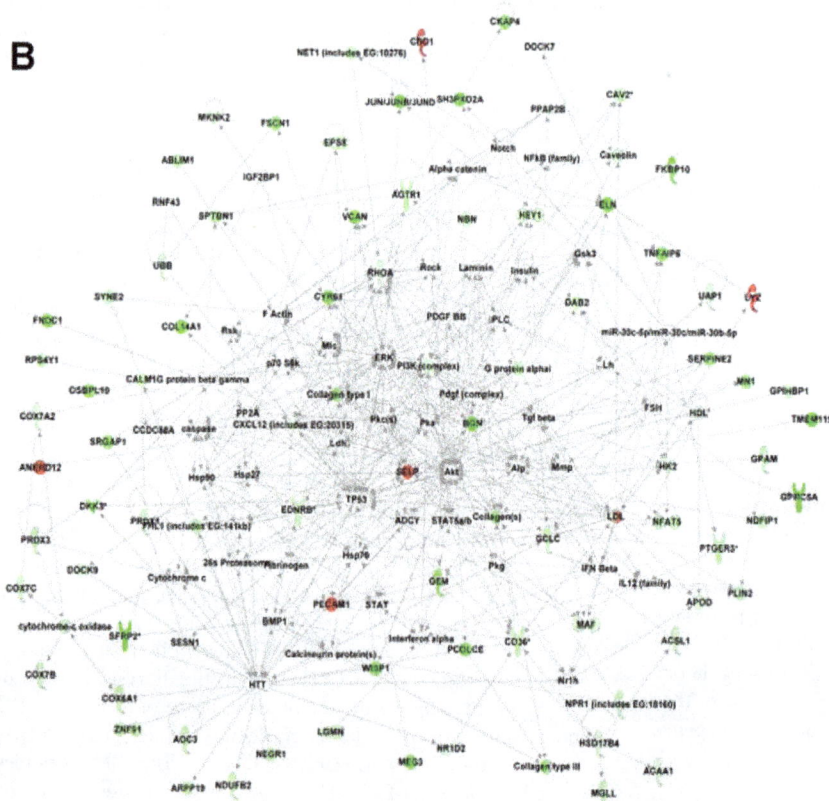

Figure 5. Network representation of the cellular functions affected specifically in both EPS and PD groups, but not in the Uremic group. A. Network related to inflammatory and immunological diseases, including NF-κB, JUN, and SP1 genes as primary regulatory focus nodes. **B.** Network enriched with genes involved in lipid metabolism, cellular assembly and movement, and cell death, including PI3K, AKT and TP53 genes as primary regulatory focus nodes. The Ingenuity Pathways Analysis tool was used to generate comprehensive gene networks that merged with affected networks of related function. Downregulated genes are shown in green, upregulated genes in red. Geometric shapes are associated with individual gene products according to Ingenuity definitions. All networks shown were significantly affected in EPS with a score >20 (−log 10[Fisher's Exact Test]).

quantified the extent of the latter staining pattern by making staining intensity measurements in the submesothelial zone (0–100 μm) and the adjacent, deeper zone (100–200 μm from the surface of the tissue block zone moving towards the adventitial layer). The normalized submesothelial staining intensity of the 0–100 μm zone relative to the deeper 100–200 μm zone was 7-fold higher in the EPS group than in the PD or Uremic groups (Figure 7). Similar zonal analyses with zone thicknesses of 200 and or 500 μm yielded the same result.

Discussion

EPS is among the most serious complications of chronic PD. Although PD duration seems to be a major risk factor, spontaneous EPS has been reported, and the causes of EPS remain obscure. The factors that govern progression from the common PD-associated condition of simple peritoneal fibrosis to the rare but aggressive condition of EPS are poorly understood. The pilot study presented here is the first comparison of transcriptomes of human peritoneal tissues taken from patients with EPS, PD patients without EPS, and predialytic uremic patients. The three groups show distinct gene expression patterns that allow their separation by principal component and heat map analyses. The results constitute proof-of-principle for a larger-scale study that could generate hypotheses for future EPS research, leading to more rigorous biochemical or cell biologic diagnostic criteria for EPS, and to definition of prognostic markers. Correlation of these and future transcriptome data with proteomics studies from peritoneal tissue and fluid would add further insight into EPS disease pathways and could improve early diagnosis and prevention.

Patients and tissue samples

The samples examined in this study were the first fresh-frozen tissue samples collected by the Peritoneal Biobank at the Robert-Bosch Hospital in Stuttgart, Germany, as part of a comprehensive database of tissues, serum, whole-blood and peritoneal effluent samples from PD patients, PD patients with EPS, and control patients without and with uremia. Collection of formalin-fixed, paraffin-embedded peritoneal tissue blocks had been initiated previously. The early stage of fresh tissue collection is reflected in the small sample sizes of the current study and the imperfect clinical matching of specimens in terms of PD duration, number of peritonitis episodes, Kt/V, systemic baseline inflammatory state, and use of acidic dialysate likely containing glucose oxidation products [47,48,49,50]. Consistent with their predialytic status, patients of the Uremic control group exhibited higher values of residual urine excretion, blood hemoglobin, serum creatinine, BUN, and calcium than did PD patients (p<0.05 for BUN and calcium) or EPS patients (Table 1).

The limited number and mass of patient samples available for this pilot study also prevented uniformity of dominant tissue histological features of the RNA source tissues within and among clinical groups. Later studies might employ laser capture microdissection to facilitate comparison of histologically similar regions within and among groups.

Transcriptome patterns and pathways

Transcriptome results exhibited good inter-individual agreement. Unsupervised analysis identified three distinct gene expression patterns consistent with the samples' clinical groupings (Figure 1). Several hundred genes were identified by a moderately stringent criterion as differentially expressed in each pairwise comparison (Figure 2A). Subsets of these genes predictably differentiated the Uremic group from both EPS and PD groups (Figure 2B). However, another subset served to differentiate EPS from both PD and the Uremic group (Figure 2C).

The differentially expressed genes could be organized into canonical pathways that distinguished EPS as a separate group from both the PD and the Uremic groups (Figure 3A), and into pathways that distinguished the Uremic control group from both EPS and PD groups (Figure 3B). The pathways uniting genes upregulated uniquely in EPS are dominated by pathways involved in cellular and humoral defense, including those controlling antigen presentation, dendritic cell maturation, phagocytic function, and leukocyte degranulation. The EPS-upregulated degranulation product, lysozyme, is a component of renal amyloid, but histological evidence of amyloid has not been observed in EPS. Additional serological, immunocyte-related, and innate immune response pathways are also regulated preferentially in EPS (Figure 3A). These results are consistent with the reported contribution of peritoneal complement activation to peritoneal fibrin deposition and early peritoneal fibrosis in a murine model [50,51]. They are likewise consistent with the reported local proliferation of alternatively activated Mφ2 macrophages without macrophage recruitment from distant sites [52]. These macrophages can secrete proinflammatory mediators during episodes of infectious peritonitis [53], associated with increased risk of EPS. In addition, macrophages express the EPS-upregulated scavenger receptor A (SRA/MSR1), previously associated with fibrotic processes [54]. The elevation in EPS tissue of genes encoding neurotropin receptors and their ligands GDNF, BDNF, neurotrophin-3 and MANF (not shown) is also consistent with increased macrophage activation or function. Coincident upregulation of matrix protease inhibitors such as TIMP1 and SERPINH1 and proteases such as ADAM9 and MM2 is also apparent (not shown).

The pathways shared by EPS and PD groups that differentiate them both from the Uremic group (Figure 3B) feature oxidative mitochondrial metabolism and dysfunction, and a variety of cell signaling pathways. PD is known to promote malnutrition and excessive loss of free amino acids, essential fatty acids [55], and albumin [56], leading to muscle wasting [57]. The downregulation of leptin mRNA in peritoneal tissues from both EPS and PD patients (Figure S2) may reflect malnourishment in chronic PD patients, as serum leptin levels fall during long-term fasting [58]. In contrast, elevated serum and dialysate leptin have been reported during chronic PD [59,60]. Moreover, treatment of hyperacutely uremic rats with high glucose PD solutions produced hyperleptinemia, and acute exposure of 3T3-L1 adipocytes to high-glucose PD solution increased leptin mRNA levels [61,62]. The striking downregulation of retinol-binding protein 4 (RBP4) mRNA to <10% of Uremic group levels in both PD and EPS groups has

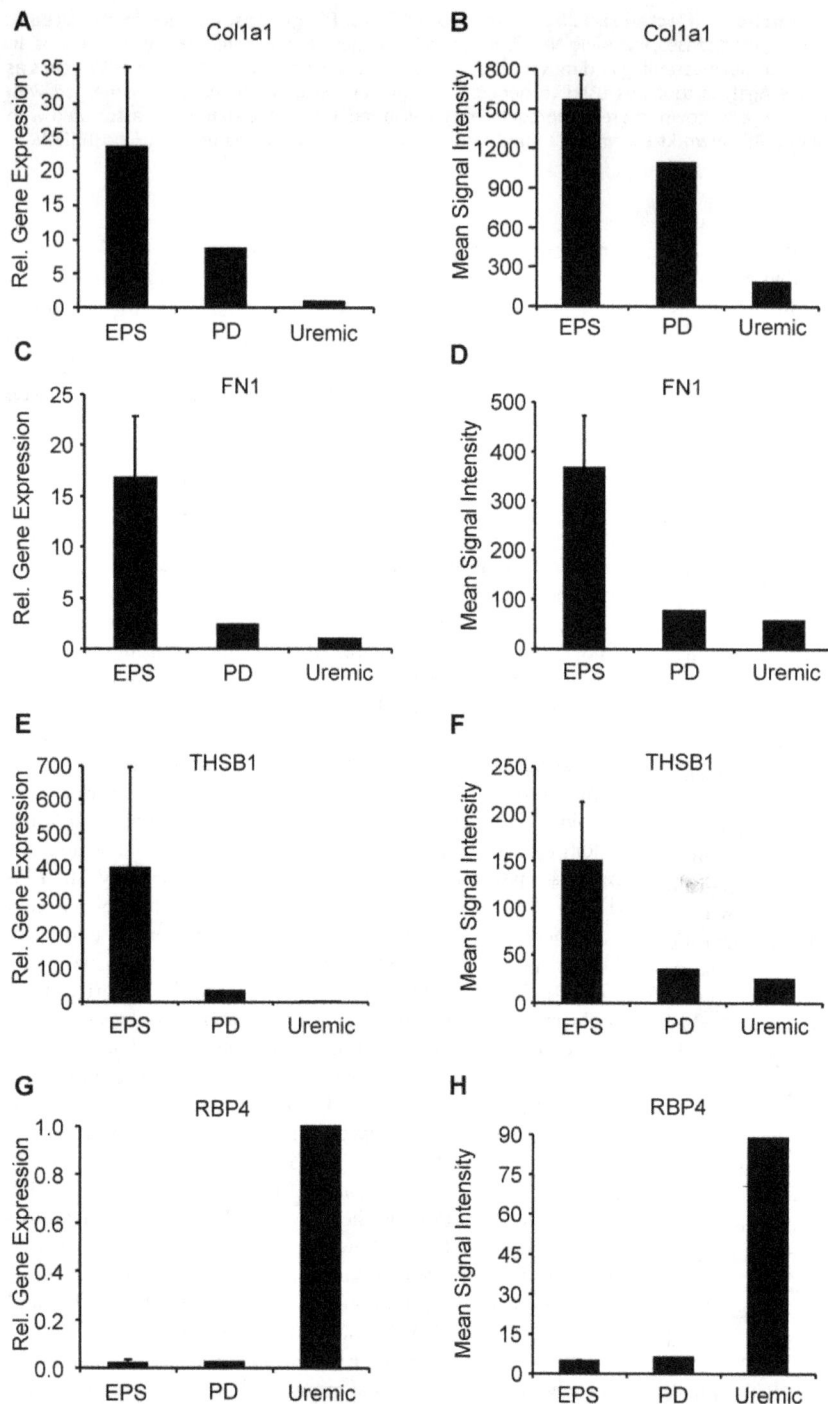

Figure 6. mRNA expression levels of selected gene products determined through qRT-PCR correlate well with corresponding data from the DNA chip array. Collagen 1 α 1 (Col1a1), Fibronectin 1 (FN1), and thrombospondin 1 (THBS1) were highly upregulated in EPS compared to PD and Uremic groups, while retinol-binding protein 4 (RBP4) was highly downregulated in EPS and PD groups compared to the Uremic group. **A.,** **C., E.,** and **G.** Normalized mRNA expression levels determined through qRT-PCR of indicated gene products. Individual gene expression levels were calculated using the equation $2^{-\Delta CT}$ with β-actin (ACTB) as endogenous control. Mean gene expression levels of biological groups were normalized to the Uremic group, defining the relative gene expression in this group as 1.0. **B., D., F.,** and **H.** Mean raw signal intensity of indicated gene products calculated from DNA array probe signals.

been associated with lean body mass [63] and with ovarian cancer [64], but impaired glucose tolerance and obesity were associated with elevated serum RBP4. RBP4 has not been studied in peritoneal dialysis patients.

Networks of differentially expressed genes

Figures 4 and 5 provide network views of the interactions of differentially expressed gene products. Figure 4A highlights the importance of multiple collagen isoforms, consistent with the

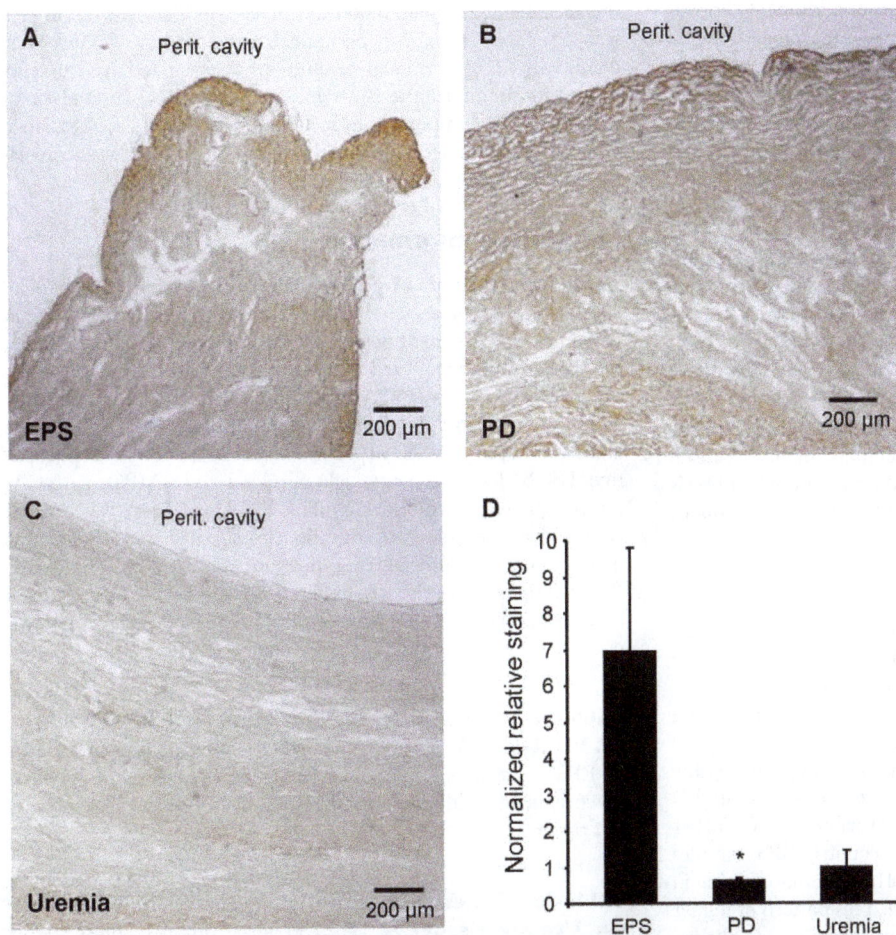

Figure 7. Immunohistochemical expression patterns of collagen 1 α 1 (Col1a1) polypeptide in peritoneal biopsy samples. Peritoneal biopsy sections from (**A.**) EPS, (**B.**) PD, and (**C.**) Uremic groups were analyzed for Col1a1 immunolocalization. Each panel indicates location of peritoneal cavity adjacent to the tissue surface. **D.** Normalized ratios of staining intensities measured in rectangular areas of thickness depth 0–100 μm and 100–200 μm from the peritoneal cavity tissue surface. P<0.05 for EPS vs. PD (One Way ANOVA with Dunn's Multiple Comparison post-test).

exacerbated fibrotic processes underlying EPS. COL1a1 mRNA showed the highest proportional increase in the EPS group (Figure 6 and Table S3). Col1a1 is not only a major component of fibrotic peritoneal tissue (Figure 6), but has also been reported as a marker of peritoneal fibrocytes together with CD45/PTPRC [65], another gene product upregulated in EPS (Table S2). Also upregulated were matrix proteases and protease inhibitors, and thrombospondin 1 (THBS1), activated through a NF-κB signaling pathway which acts as one of the major regulatory nodes in the presented networks [66]. THBS1 is involved in physiological tissue repair and extracellular matrix remodeling as a regulator of TGF-β-mediated fibrosis [67], and as a proinflammatory and profibrotic factor in chronic kidney disease and kidney fibrosis [68]. Also markedly upregulated was sulfatase 1 (SULF1) mRNA (Figure 6), which like SULF2 modulates the sonic hedgehog (Shh), wingless (Wnt), fibroblast growth factor (FGF), and vascular endothelial growth factor (VEGF) signaling pathways. The highly upregulated Fibronectin 1 transcript (Figure 6) encodes a ubiquitously expressed extracellular matrix protein involved in wound healing [69,70] and is overexpressed in fibrotic tissues [71,72], induced in fibroblasts and myofibroblasts, and implicated in glomerular and interstitial renal fibrosis [73].

The myofibroblast marker α-smooth muscle actin (ACTA2) mRNA was also upregulated (Figure S2). ACTA2 has been implicated in TGF-β-induced epithelial-to-mesenchymal transition (EMT) in bronchial cells in a cellular model of asthma [74], and in numerous other models of tissue fibrosis. EMT is believed to play an important role in EPS, especially in postulated mesothelial cell transformation into myofibroblasts [75]. One of the important pathways through which EMT is induced is the ERK1/2 pathway [76], another central regulatory node in the EPS-related networks (Figure 4A). The transcription factor TWIST, upregulated 5-fold in PD and 2.5-fold in EPS (not shown), has been widely implicated as a driver of EMT, most recently in a mouse model of peritoneal fibrosis [77]. Lysyl oxidase, best known for its post-translational lysine hydroxylation of collagen, was recently identified as a transcriptional activator of TWIST and TWIST-mediated EMT [78]. Interestingly, expression of the closely related LOXL2 transcript was 4.2-fold higher in the EPS group than in the PD group (Table S2). LOXL2 transcription can be increased by VEGF and by high glucose [79]. LOXL2 can deaminate Lys4 in histone H3 [80], but at least some of its effects as an inhibitor of differentiation are independent of its enzymatic activity [81].

Several transcriptome studies of rodent peritoneal fibrosis models have recently appeared. Yokoi et al [38] suggested that pleiotrophin plays an important role in both inflammation and fibrosis following acute chlorhexidine gluconate-induced peritoneal injury in mice. Pleiotrophin upregulation was not observed in tissue from our EPS patients compared to chronic PD or Uremic groups. However, observations of elevated procollagen, CCl5, Cxcl16, and Adam12 in that mouse model [38] were also noted in our human EPS specimens. Imai et al described a rat model in which intraperitoneal instillation of high-dose glucose-degradation products led to peritoneal fibrotic changes consistent with a role for EMT in development of peritoneal fibrosis [37]. Le et al induced peritoneal fibrosis in rats via foreign body insertion [36]. As in our observations with human tissue, they observed upregulation of α-smooth muscle actin and other myofibroblast markers, as well as overexpression of profibrotic agents such as TGF-β and CTGF. However, interpretation of mechanistic comparisons between animal models of induced peritoneal fibrosis and PD-associated peritoneal fibrosis and EPS in humans remains difficult.

Col1a1 IHC Immunohistochemistry

Histochemical expression of collagen I was compared to the increased Col1a1 mRNA levels in EPS tissue. The increased Col1a1 mRNA level in EPS tissue was not paralleled by higher total Col1a1 polypeptide levels, as judged by immunostaining intensity across entire fields of view. Although EPS tissue showed greater Col1a1 expression than did Uremic group tissue, the highest levels of Col1a1 immunostaining were observed in PD tissues. In contrast to the homogeneous distribution of Col1a1 immunostaining across entire PD tissue sections, EPS samples exhibited pronounced intensification of Col1a1 immunostaining in the submesothelial compact zone (Figure 7). This pattern of higher density of fibrous tissue and pronounced accumulation of collagen 1 α 1 protein was also noted in the peritoneal submesothelial compact zone in rats after 4 weeks exposure to PD fluid [82].

Conclusion

Although EPS remains a poorly understood disease, we have demonstrated a distinct transcriptional pattern of peritoneal tissue from EPS patients that differed from those of PD patients and predialytic uremic patients. The distinct transcriptional patterns of EPS and PD tissues presented here are consistent with the hypothesis that EPS constitutes a separate disease entity, possibly requiring a "second hit", and not merely an exacerbation of the simple peritoneal sclerosis believed present in all PD patients. However, the data also are consistent with EPS representing a malignant acceleration of PD-associated peritoneal fibrosis influenced by patient-specific risk modifier genes and, possibly, by transplant and/or immunosuppression therapy.

Although our small study does not point to a principal pathogenic mechanism in EPS distinct from that of the simple peritoneal fibrosis of chronic PD, the study does serve as proof-of-principle for future array studies with peritoneal tissue from larger groups of patients. Preliminary data (not shown) indicates that the spectrum and abundance of mRNA isolated from formalin-fixed paraffin-embedded tissues from the same patients studied in this paper were very similar to those of mRNA isolated from fresh-frozen tissue (correlation coefficient >0.91). This suggests the reliability of transcriptome analysis applied to archived paraffin blocks of tissues from EPS and PD patients, especially when combined with laser capture microdissection for comparison of histologically similar regions of tissue. Similar transcriptome studies should be conducted with peritoneal dialysate fluid and cell specimens, and with blood specimens, since accrual of samples will be easier than for peritoneal tissue samples. Moreover, definition of transcriptional signatures may prove to have value for diagnostic monitoring and prognosis. Comprehensive analysis of miRNAs will be important to include in these future studies, since they (or their antagomirs) can be easily envisioned as intraperitoneal therapeutic agents.

Supporting Information

Table S1 Individual patient characteristics. The clinical features and laboratory values represent those of each individual patient's last assessment before the surgical procedure that yielded the tissue samples analyzed in this study. Underlying renal diseases are abbreviated as: IgA, IgA nephropathy; GN, chronic glomerulonephritis; PaI-RPGN, pauci-immune rapid progressive glomerulonephritis; NS, nephrosclerosis; DN, diabetic nephropathy; FSGS, focal segmental glomerulosclerosis; MPO, pANCA-positive (myeloperoxidase) vasculitis. Smoking history was defined as positive regardless of duration. Arterial hypertension was defined as resting arterial blood pressure ≥140/90 mmHg. Acidic PD solutions were lactate-buffered with pH 5.0–5.5. Neutral (multicomponent) solutions were of pH 6.5. Icodextrin status was positive if used at any time during course of PD.

Table S2 Genes differentially expressed in EPS tissue vs. PD tissue. A. The 50 gene products most highly upregulated in EPS tissue as compared to PD tissue. **B.** All gene products downregulated with corrected FC>2.0 in EPS tissue compared to PD tissue.

Table S3 Genes differentially expressed in EPS tissue vs. Uremic tissue. A. The 50 gene products most highly upregulated in EPS tissue as compared to Uremic tissue. **B.** The 50 most downregulated gene products in EPS tissue as compared to Uremic tissue.

Table S4 Genes differentially expressed in PD tissue vs. Uremic tissue. A. The 50 gene products most highly upregulated in PD tissue as compared to Uremic tissue. **B.** All gene products downregulated with corrected FC>2.0 in PD tissue compared to Uremic tissue.

Figure S1 Selected genomic expression patterns depicting progression from uremia to EPS. Genes differentially expressed in any group comparison (e.g. Uremic vs. PD, Uremic vs. EPS, PD vs. EPS) were used as the seed set for Self-Organizing Map (SOM) analysis of gene expression. These differentially expressed genes were partitioned to 40 separate maps according to Pearson correlation coefficient-based distance metrics. Selected, biologically interesting SOM maps were manually clustered into 2 biologically relevant categories, each representative of at least two similar SOM patterns: EPS-specific [I, EPS vs. (PD+Uremic), left], and fibrosis-specific [II, (EPS+PD) vs. Uremic, right]. The X-axis arrays individual biological samples, and the Y-axis represents changes in gene expression on a scale from −3 to +3.

Figure S2 Upregulated gene expression in EPS determined by qRT-PCR correlates well with that measured by DNA microarray. α-smooth muscle actin (ACTA2) (A,B), sulfatase 1 (SULF1) (C,D), and intra-cellular adhesion molecule 1 (ICAM1) (E,F) are highly upregulated in EPS compared to PD and

Uremic groups, as judged both by qRT-PCR data (A,C,E) and by DNA microarray data (B,D,F). Uremic group qRT-PCR expression values were normalized to a value of 1.0, and β-actin mRNA served as endogenous control. DNA array signal intensities are raw probe values.

Figure S3 Down-regulated gene expression in EPS determined by qRT-PCR correlates well with that measured by DNA microarray. Leptin (LEP) mRNA levels are greatly downregulated in tissues from EPS and PD patients compared to Uremic group tissues, as judged by normalized qRT-PCR data (A) and by DNA microarray data (B). Uremic group qRT-PCR expression values were normalized to a value of 1.0, and β-actin mRNA served as endogenous control. DNA array signal intensities are raw probe values.

Figure S4 Two examples of lower correlation between gene expression measured by qRT-PCR and by DNA microarray. Normalized Runt-related transcription factor 2 (Runx2) mRNA levels measured by qRT-PCR did not significantly differ (A), although DNA microarray suggested that

expression in EPS tissue exceeded that in Uremic group tissue (B). Normalized MMP2 mRNA levels measured by qRT-PCR suggested higher levels in EPS and PD tissues than in Uremic group tissues (C), whereas MMP2 levels detected by DNA microarray appeared higher in EPS than in PD or Uremic group tissues (D). Uremic group qRT-PCR expression values were normalized to a value of 1.0, and β-actin mRNA served as endogenous control. DNA array signal intensities are raw probe values.

Acknowledgments

We thank Boris E. Shmukler, Augustine Rajakumar, Dongsheng Zhang, and Jack Lawler for helpful discussion and sharing reagents.

Author Contributions

Conceived and designed the experiments: FRR SLA MKB IES ZKZ NB MDA. Performed the experiments: FRR ZKZ NB DB PF. Analyzed the data: FRR SLA MKB IES ZKZ NB DB PF SAK HRT. Contributed reagents/materials/analysis tools: SLA MKB IES ZKZ NB DB PF JL. Wrote the paper: FRR SLA MKB NB SS.

References

1. Lameire N, Van Biesen W (2010) Epidemiology of peritoneal dialysis: a story of believers and nonbelievers. Nat Rev Nephrol 6: 75–82.
2. Braun N, Alscher MD, Kimmel M, Amann K, Buttner M (2011) Encapsulating peritoneal sclerosis - an overview. Nephrol Ther 7: 162–171.
3. Kawanishi H, Shintaku S, Moriishi M, Dohi K, Tsuchiya S (2011) Seventeen years' experience of surgical options for encapsulating peritoneal sclerosis. Adv Perit Dial 27: 53–58.
4. Ulmer C, Braun N, Rieber F, Latus J, Hirschburger S, et al. (2012) Efficacy and morbidity of surgical therapy in late-stage encapsulating peritoneal sclerosis. Surgery.
5. Latus J, Ulmer C, Fritz P, Rettenmaier B, Biegger D, et al. (2012) Encapsulating peritoneal sclerosis: a rare, serious but potentially curable complication of peritoneal dialysis-experience of a referral centre in Germany. Nephrol Dial Transplant.
6. Da Luz MM, Barral SM, Barral CM, Bechara Cde S, Lacerda-Filho A (2011) Idiopathic encapsulating peritonitis: report of two cases. Surg Today 41: 1644–1648.
7. Koak Y, Gertner D, Forbes A, Ribeiro BF (2008) Idiopathic sclerosing peritonitis. Eur J Gastroenterol Hepatol 20: 148–150.
8. Minutolo V, Gagliano G, Angirillo G, Minutolo O, Morello A, et al. (2008) Intestinal obstruction due to idiopathic sclerosing encapsulating peritonitis. Clinical report and review of literature. G Chir 29: 173–176.
9. Johnson DW, Cho Y, Livingston BE, Hawley CM, McDonald SP, et al. (2010) Encapsulating peritoneal sclerosis: incidence, predictors, and outcomes. Kidney Int 77: 904–912.
10. Brown MC, Simpson K, Kerssens JJ, Mactier RA (2009) Encapsulating peritoneal sclerosis in the new millennium: a national cohort study. Clin J Am Soc Nephrol 4: 1222–1229.
11. Toyohara T, Ubara Y, Higa Y, Suwabe T, Hoshino J, et al. (2011) Prognosis of patients on continuous ambulatory peritoneal dialysis (CAPD) for over 10 years. Intern Med 50: 2519–2523.
12. Kawanishi H, Kawaguchi Y, Fukui H, Hara S, Imada A, et al. (2004) Encapsulating peritoneal sclerosis in Japan: a prospective, controlled, multicenter study. Am J Kidney Dis 44: 729–737.
13. Kawanishi H, Moriishi M (2005) Epidemiology of encapsulating peritoneal sclerosis in Japan. Perit Dial Int 25 Suppl 4: S14–18.
14. Korte MR, Habib SM, Lingsma H, Weimar W, Betjes MG (2011) Posttransplantation encapsulating peritoneal sclerosis contributes significantly to mortality after kidney transplantation. Am J Transplant 11: 599–605.
15. Braun N, Alscher DM, Schwenger V, Amann K, Büttner M (2010) Deutsches Peritonealdialyseregister (DPR). Der Nephrologe 5: 531–534.
16. Nakamura S, Niwa T (2004) Advanced glycation end-products and peritoneal sclerosis. Semin Nephrol 24: 502–505.
17. Schwenger V, Morath C, Salava A, Amann K, Seregin Y, et al. (2006) Damage to the peritoneal membrane by glucose degradation products is mediated by the receptor for advanced glycation end-products. J Am Soc Nephrol 17: 199–207.
18. Alscher DM, Braun N, Biegger D, Fritz P (2007) Peritoneal mast cells in peritoneal dialysis patients, particularly in encapsulating peritoneal sclerosis patients. Am J Kidney Dis 49: 452–461.
19. Aoki S, Ikeda S, Takezawa T, Kishi T, Makino J, et al. (2011) Prolonged effect of fluid flow stress on the proliferative activity of mesothelial cells after abrupt

discontinuation of fluid streaming. Biochem Biophys Res Commun 416: 391–396.
20. Aoki S, Makino J, Nagashima A, Takezawa T, Nomoto N, et al. (2011) Fluid flow stress affects peritoneal cell kinetics: possible pathogenesis of peritoneal fibrosis. Perit Dial Int 31: 466–476.
21. Augustine T, Brown PW, Davies SD, Summers AM, Wilkie ME (2009) Encapsulating peritoneal sclerosis: clinical significance and implications. Nephron Clin Pract 111: c149–154; discussion c154.
22. Braun N, Alscher DM, Fritz P, Edenhofer I, Kimmel M, et al. (2011) Podoplanin-positive cells are a hallmark of encapsulating peritoneal sclerosis. Nephrol Dial Transplant 26: 1033–1041.
23. Vlijm A, Stoker J, Bipat S, Spijkerboer AM, Phoa SS, et al. (2009) Computed tomographic findings characteristic for encapsulating peritoneal sclerosis: a case-control study. Perit Dial Int 29: 517–522.
24. Braun N, Fritz P, Ulmer C, Kimmel M, Biegger D, et al. (2012) The Definition of Histological Criteria for Encapsulating Peritoneal Sclerosis – A Standardized Approach [Abstract]. PLoS One In press.
25. Nakamoto H (2005) Encapsulating peritoneal sclerosis–a clinician's approach to diagnosis and medical treatment. Perit Dial Int 25 Suppl 4: S30–38.
26. Kawanishi H, Harada Y, Noriyuki T, Kawai T, Takahashi S, et al. (2001) Treatment options for encapsulating peritoneal sclerosis based on progressive stage. Adv Perit Dial 17: 200–204.
27. Yamamoto H, Nakayama M, yamamoto R, Otsuka Y, Takahashi H, et al. (2002) Fifteen cases of encapsulating peritoneal sclerosis related to peritoneal dialysis: a single-center experience in Japan. Adv Perit Dial 18: 135–138.
28. Wong CF, Beshir S, Khalil A, Pai P, Ahmad R (2005) Successful treatment of encapsulating peritoneal sclerosis with azathioprine and prednisolone. Perit Dial Int 25: 285–287.
29. Fieren MW, Betjes MG, Korte MR, Boer WH (2007) Posttransplant encapsulating peritoneal sclerosis: a worrying new trend? Perit Dial Int 27: 619–624.
30. Korte MR, Fieren MW, Sampimon DE, Lingsma HF, Weimar W, et al. (2011) Tamoxifen is associated with lower mortality of encapsulating peritoneal sclerosis: results of the Dutch Multicentre EPS Study. Nephrol Dial Transplant 26: 691–697.
31. Braun N, Fritz P, Biegger D, Kimmel M, Reimold F, et al. (2011) Difference in the expression of hormone receptors and fibrotic markers in the human peritoneum–implications for therapeutic targets to prevent encapsulating peritoneal sclerosis. Perit Dial Int 31: 291–300.
32. Bhasin M, Yuan L, Keskin DB, Otu HH, Libermann TA, et al. (2010) Bioinformatic identification and characterization of human endothelial cell-restricted genes. BMC Genomics 11: 342.
33. Nakamoto H, Imai H, Fukushima R, Ishida Y, Yamanouchi Y, et al. (2008) Role of the renin-angiotensin system in the pathogenesis of peritoneal fibrosis. Perit Dial Int 28 Suppl 3: S83–87.
34. Kawanishi H, Ide K, Yamashita M, Shimomura M, Moriishi M, et al. (2008) Surgical techniques for prevention of recurrence after total enterolysis in encapsulating peritoneal sclerosis. Adv Perit Dial 24: 51–55.
35. Park SH, Kim YL, Lindholm B (2008) Experimental encapsulating peritoneal sclerosis models: pathogenesis and treatment. Perit Dial Int 28 Suppl 5: S21–28.

36. Le SJ, Gongora M, Zhang B, Grimmond S, Campbell GR, et al. (2010) Gene expression profile of the fibrotic response in the peritoneal cavity. Differentiation 79: 232–243.
37. Imai T, Hirahara I, Morishita Y, Onishi A, Inoue M, et al. (2011) DNA microarray analysis of the epithelial-mesenchymal transition of mesothelial cells in a rat model of peritoneal dialysis. Adv Perit Dial 27: 11–15.
38. Yokoi H, Kasahara M, Mori K, Ogawa Y, Kuwabara T, et al. (2012) Pleiotrophin triggers inflammation and increased peritoneal permeability leading to peritoneal fibrosis. Kidney Int 81: 160–169.
39. Margetts PJ, Bonniaud P, Liu L, Hoff CM, Holmes CJ, et al. (2005) Transient overexpression of TGF-β1 induces epithelial mesenchymal transition in the rodent peritoneum. J Am Soc Nephrol 16: 425–436.
40. Honda K, Nitta K, Horita S, Tsukada M, Itabashi M, et al. (2003) Histologic criteria for diagnosing encapsulating peritoneal sclerosis in continuous ambulatory peritoneal dialysis patients. Adv Perit Dial 19: 169–175.
41. Kauffmann A, Gentleman R, Huber W (2009) arrayQualityMetrics–a bioconductor package for quality assessment of microarray data. Bioinformatics 25: 415–416.
42. Irizarry RA, Hobbs B, Collin F, Beazer-Barclay YD, Antonellis KJ, et al. (2003) Exploration, normalization, and summaries of high density oligonucleotide array probe level data. Biostatistics 4: 249–264.
43. Wang C, Rao N, Wang Y (2007) [Principal component analysis for exploring gene expression patterns]. Sheng wu yi xue gong cheng xue za zhi = Journal of biomedical engineering = Shengwu yixue gongchengxue zazhi 24: 736–741.
44. Yeung KY, Ruzzo WL (2001) Principal component analysis for clustering gene expression data. Bioinformatics 17: 763–774.
45. Li C, Wong WH (2001) Model-based analysis of oligonucleotide arrays: expression index computation and outlier detection. Proceedings of the National Academy of Sciences of the United States of America 98: 31–36.
46. Tamayo P, Slonim D, Mesirov J, Zhu Q, Kitareewan S, et al. (1999) Interpreting patterns of gene expression with self-organizing maps: methods and application to hematopoietic differentiation. Proc Natl Acad Sci U S A 96: 2907–2912.
47. Ayuzawa N, Ishibashi Y, Takazawa Y, Kume H, Fujita T (2012) Peritoneal morphology after long-term peritoneal dialysis with biocompatible fluid: recent clinical practice in Japan. Perit Dial Int 32: 159–167.
48. Garcia-Lopez E, Lindholm B, Davies S (2012) An update on peritoneal dialysis solutions. Nat Rev Nephrol 8: 224–233.
49. Baroni G, Schuinski A, de Moraes TP, Meyer F, Pecoits-Filho R (2012) Inflammation and the peritoneal membrane: causes and impact on structure and function during peritoneal dialysis. Mediators Inflamm 2012: 912595.
50. Mizuno M, Ito Y, Mizuno T, Harris CL, Suzuki Y, et al. (2012) Membrane complement regulators protect against fibrin exudation increases in a severe peritoneal inflammation model in rats. Am J Physiol Renal Physiol 302: F1245–1251.
51. Mizuno T, Mizuno M, Morgan BP, Noda Y, Yamada K, et al. (2011) Specific collaboration between rat membrane complement regulators Crry and CD59 protects peritoneum from damage by autologous complement activation. Nephrol Dial Transplant 26: 1821–1830.
52. Jenkins SJ, Ruckerl D, Cook PC, Jones LH, Finkelman FD, et al. (2011) Local macrophage proliferation, rather than recruitment from the blood, is a signature of TH2 inflammation. Science 332: 1284–1288.
53. Fieren MW (2012) The local inflammatory responses to infection of the peritoneal cavity in humans: their regulation by cytokines, macrophages, and other leukocytes. Mediators Inflamm 2012: 976241.
54. Wang W, Wang H, Shi W, Liang X, Ma J, et al. (2012) Deletion of scavenger receptor A protects mice from progressive nephropathy independent of lipid control during diet-induced hyperlipidemia. Kidney Int 81: 1002–1014.
55. Yerlikaya FH, Mehmetoglu I, Kurban S, Tonbul Z (2011) Plasma fatty acid composition in continuous ambulatory peritoneal dialysis patients: an increased omega-6/omega-3 ratio and deficiency of essential fatty acids. Ren Fail 33: 819–823.
56. Mehrotra R, Duong U, Jiwakanon S, Kovesdy CP, Moran J, et al. (2011) Serum albumin as a predictor of mortality in peritoneal dialysis: comparisons with hemodialysis. Am J Kidney Dis 58: 418–428.
57. Garibotto G, Sofia A, Saffioti S, Bonanni A, Mannucci I, et al. (2012) Effects of peritoneal dialysis on protein metabolism. Nutr Metab Cardiovasc Dis.
58. Weigle DS, Duell PB, Connor WE, Steiner RA, Soules MR, et al. (1997) Effect of fasting, refeeding, and dietary fat restriction on plasma leptin levels. J Clin Endocrinol Metab 82: 561–565.
59. Lai KN, Lam MF, Leung JC, Chan LY, Lam CW, et al. (2012) A study of the clinical and biochemical profile of peritoneal dialysis fluid low in glucose degradation products. Perit Dial Int 32: 280–291.
60. Wojcik K, Stompor T, Krzanowski M, Miarka P, Zdzienicka A, et al. (2007) The relationships between activation of non-specific inflammatory process and malnutrition in patients on peritoneal dialysis. Med Pregl 60 Suppl 2: 114–116.
61. Matsubara K, Kiyomoto H, Moriwaki K, Hara T, Kondo N, et al. (2004) Leptin kinetics during peritoneal dialysis in acutely uraemic rats. Nephrology (Carlton) 9: 256–261.
62. Teta D, Tedjani A, Burnier M, Bevington A, Brown J, et al. (2005) Glucose-containing peritoneal dialysis fluids regulate leptin secretion from 3T3-L1 adipocytes. Nephrol Dial Transplant 20: 1329–1335.
63. Graham TE, Yang Q, Bluher M, Hammarstedt A, Ciaraldi TP, et al. (2006) Retinol-binding protein 4 and insulin resistance in lean, obese, and diabetic subjects. N Engl J Med 354: 2552–2563.
64. Lorkova L, Pospisilova J, Lacheta J, Leahomschi S, Zivny J, et al. (2012) Decreased concentrations of retinol-binding protein 4 in sera of epithelial ovarian cancer patients: a potential biomarker identified by proteomics. Oncol Rep 27: 318–324.
65. Sagara A, Sakai N, Shinozaki Y, Kitajima S, Toyama T, et al. (2011) Histone Acetyltransferase Activity Is Involved in the Pathogenesis of Experimental Peritoneal Fibrosis [Abstract]. J Am Soc Nephrol: 36A.
66. Wang HR, Chen DL, Zhao M, Shu SW, Xiong SX, et al. (2012) C-reactive protein induces interleukin-6 and thrombospondin-1 protein and mRNA expression through activation of nuclear factor-kB in HK-2 cells. Kidney Blood Press Res 35: 211–219.
67. Sweetwyne MT, Murphy-Ullrich JE (2012) Thrombospondin1 in tissue repair and fibrosis: TGF-beta-dependent and independent mechanisms. Matrix Biol 31: 178–186.
68. Bige N, Shweke N, Benhassine S, Jouanneau C, Vandermeersch S, et al. (2012) Thrombospondin-1 plays a profibrotic and pro-inflammatory role during ureteric obstruction. Kidney Int 81: 1226–1238.
69. Grinnell F (1984) Fibronectin and wound healing. J Cell Biochem 26: 107–116.
70. Valenick LV, Hsia HC, Schwarzbauer JE (2005) Fibronectin fragmentation promotes alpha4beta1 integrin-mediated contraction of a fibrin-fibronectin provisional matrix. Exp Cell Res 309: 48–55.
71. Muro AF, Moretti FA, Moore BB, Yan M, Atrasz RG, et al. (2008) An essential role for fibronectin extra type III domain A in pulmonary fibrosis. Am J Respir Crit Care Med 177: 638–645.
72. Leask A, Abraham DJ (2004) TGF-beta signaling and the fibrotic response. FASEB J 18: 816–827.
73. Van Vliet A, Baelde HJ, Vleming IJ, de Heer E, Bruijn JA (2001) Distribution of fibronectin isoforms in human renal disease. J Pathol 193: 256–262.
74. Doerner AM, Zuraw BL (2009) TGF-beta1 induced epithelial to mesenchymal transition (EMT) in human bronchial epithelial cells is enhanced by IL-1beta but not abrogated by corticosteroids. Respir Res 10: 100.
75. Yanez-Mo M, Lara-Pezzi E, Selgas R, Ramirez-Huesca M, Dominguez-Jimenez C, et al. (2003) Peritoneal dialysis and epithelial-to-mesenchymal transition of mesothelial cells. N Engl J Med 348: 403–413.
76. Han M, Liu M, Wang Y, Chen X, Xu J, et al. (2012) Antagonism of miR-21 Reverses Epithelial-Mesenchymal Transition and Cancer Stem Cell Phenotype through AKT/ERK1/2 Inactivation by Targeting PTEN. PLoS One 7: e39520.
77. Margetts PJ (2012) Twist: a new player in the epithelial-mesenchymal transition of the peritoneal mesothelial cells. Nephrol Dial Transplant.
78. El-Haibi CP, Bell GW, Zhang J, Collmann AY, Wood D, et al. (2012) Critical role for lysyl oxidase in mesenchymal stem cell-driven breast cancer malignancy. Proc Natl Acad Sci U S A.
79. Coral K, Madhavan J, Pukhraj R, Angayarkanni N (2012) High Glucose Induced Differential Expression of Lysyl Oxidase and Its Isoform in ARPE-19 Cells. Curr Eye Res.
80. Herranz N, Dave N, Millanes-Romero A, Morey L, Diaz VM, et al. (2012) Lysyl oxidase-like 2 deaminates lysine 4 in histone H3. Mol Cell 46: 369–376.
81. Lugassy J, Zaffryar-Eilot S, Soueid S, Mordoviz A, Smith V, et al. (2012) The enzymatic activity of lysyl oxidase-like-2 (LOXL2) is not required for LOXL2-induced inhibition of keratinocyte differentiation. J Biol Chem 287: 3541–3549.
82. Guo H, Leung JC, Lam MF, Chan LY, Tsang AW, et al. (2007) Smad7 transgene attenuates peritoneal fibrosis in uremic rats treated with peritoneal dialysis. J Am Soc Nephrol 18: 2689–2703.

The Associations between the Family Education and Mortality of Patients on Peritoneal Dialysis

Zhi-Kai Yang[1], Qing-Feng Han[2], Tong-Ying Zhu[3], Ye-Ping Ren[4], Jiang-Hua Chen[5], Hui-Ping Zhao[6], Meng-Hua Chen[7], Jie Dong[1]*, Yue Wang[2], Chuan- Ming Hao[3], Rui Zhang[4], Xiao-Hui Zhang[5], Mei Wang[6], Na Tian[7], Hai-Yan Wang[1]

1 Renal Division, Department of Medicine, Peking University First Hospital, Institute of Nephrology, Peking University, Key Laboratory of Renal Disease, Ministry of Health, Key Laboratory of Renal Disease, Ministry of Education, Beijing, China, 2 Department of Nephrology, Peking University Third Hospital, Beijing, China, 3 Department of Nephrology, Huashan Hospital of Fudan University, Shanghai, China, 4 Department of Nephrology, Second Affiliated Hospital of Harbin Medical University, Heilongjiang, China, 5 Kidney Disease Center, The First Affiliated Hospital, College of Medicine, Zhejiang University, Hangzhou, China, 6 Department of Nephrology, Peking University People's Hospital, Beijing, China, 7 Department of Nephrology, General Hospital of Ningxia Medical University, Ningxia, China

Abstract

Aims: To investigate whether education level of family members predicts all-cause and cardiovascular death and initial-episode peritonitis in patients on peritoneal dialysis (PD).

Methods: A total of 2264 patients on chronic PD were collected from seven centers affiliated with the Socioeconomic Status on the Outcome of Peritoneal Dialysis (SSOP) Study. All demographic, socioeconomic and laboratory data of patients and the education level of all family members were recorded at baseline. Multivariate Cox regression was used to calculate the hazard ratio (HR) of all-cause and cardiovascular mortality, and initial-episode peritonitis with adjustments for recognized traditional factors.

Results: There were no significant differences in baseline characteristics between patients with (n = 1752) and without (n = 512) complete education information. According to the highest education level of patients' family, included 1752 patients were divided into four groups, i.e. elementary or lower (15%), middle (27%), high (24%) and more than high school (34%). The family highest education (using elementary school or lower group as reference, hazard ratio and 95% confidence interval of middle school group, high school group and more than high school group was 0.68[0.48–0.96], 0.64[0.45–0.91], 0.66[0.48–0.91], respectively) rather than their average education level or patients' or spouse's education was significantly associated with the higher mortality. Neither patients' nor family education level did correlate to the risk for cardiovascular death or initial-episode peritonitis.

Conclusions: Family members' education level was found to be a novel predictor of PD outcome. Family, as the main source of health care providers, should be paid more attention in our practice.

Editor: Hamid Reza Baradaran, Iran University of Medical Sciences, Iran (Islamic Republic Of)

Funding: This study is in part supported by New Century Excellent Talents from Education Department, China, Baxer Clinical Research Award from Baxter Corp, China and ISN Research Award from ISN GO R&P Committee. The funders had no role in study design, data collection and analysis, decision to publish, or preparation of the manuscript.

Competing Interests: This study is in part supported by New Century Excellent Talents from Education Department, China, Baxer Clinical Research Award from Baxter Corp, China and ISN Research Award from ISN GO R&P Committee. The funders had no role in study design, data collection and analysis, decision to publish, or preparation of the manuscript. The authors confirm that this does not alter their adherence to PLOS ONE policies on sharing data and materials.

* E-mail: dongjie@medmail.com.cn

Introduction

Peritoneal dialysis (PD) has been utilized as one of the main renal replacement therapies since the 1980s. Although the number of PD patients has markedly increased in both developing and developed countries[1], PD outcomes, such as mortality, technique failure, and hospitalization, have not markedly improved. Potential risk factors for poor outcome have been continuously explored in recent years. Among these, socioeconomic status (SES) has been indicated as a key predictor through multi-center PD cohort studies from various countries. These studies indicate that SES evaluated by individual education[2] and income[3], housing

status[4], remote location[5,6], or social support[7–11] play the critical role in the outcomes of dialysis patients. Based on the inverse relationship between individual SES and mortality from our large-scale multi-center retrospective PD cohort study[3], we would further explore the association of social support and PD outcome.

Social support is the intricate network in which patients with various chronic illnesses may give and receive information and aid and have emotional needs met[12], which is mainly sourced from family members including a spouse, children and relatives, friends, and colleagues. For patients who receive long-term home care therapy, family members are the most important healthcare providers. At the start of dialysis, family members the main drivers for choosing PD or hemodialysis (HD) as a treatment[13,14]. Family members are also involved in the accommodation of lifestyle and living environment changes, and helping patients to improve their compliance to a therapy regime. For elderly or disabled patients, family members are more likely to take more responsibility for PD-associated care, such as performing the PD exchange and exit-site care, monitoring symptoms and signs daily, and contributing to food preparation and nutrition provision. All of the above are dependent on a strong education base[15]. Hence, it is hypothesized that the education level of family members may play a key role in the quality of therapy and PD outcome. To date, social support as a general index of SES rather than family members' education status has been investigated with respect to its impact on dialysis outcome in previous studies[7–11].

Therefore, we aimed to investigate associations between education level of PD patients' family members and outcome events, including all-cause and cardiovascular death and first-episode peritonitis through a large-scale multi-center retrospective cohort study, which will be helpful for unpacking the black box of the family education-outcome puzzle for PD population.

Methods

This is an affiliated study with the Socioeconomic Status on the Outcome of Peritoneal Dialysis (SSOP) study, which is a retrospective multi-center cohort study as described in detail in our previous paper[3]. The ethics committee of Peking University First Hospitl, China approved this study. Written consent was given by the patients for their information to be stored in the hospital database and used for research.

Center Enrollment

Centers with professional PD doctors and nurses and well-developed databases maintained for least 3 years, recording baseline characteristics and follow-up data every 1 to 3 months, participated in this study voluntarily. Nine centers were qualified, and seven of these, accounting for about 70% of all incident patients attending the nine centers, agreed to participate. The included PD centers were located in five different provinces and four geographical regions (north, northeast, northwest, and east) of China. Data from each center were collected within a strict quality control framework and further inspected and optimized to ensure the integrity and accuracy of the database. All study investigators and staff members completed a training program that taught them the methods and processes of the study. A manual of detailed instructions for data collection was distributed.

Subject Selection

All incident patients receiving chronic PD between the date of intact database creation and August 2011 were enrolled into this study. After starting PD, each patient signed informed consent agreeing to the use of their demographic and laboratory data in future studies. Those without information of education levels of family members were excluded. All subjects began the PD program within 1 month after catheter implantation and were given lactate-buffered glucose dialysate with a twin-bag connection system (Baxter Healthcare, Guangzhou, China).

Data collection

Demographic and clinical data including age, gender, body mass index (BMI), primary renal disease, history of cardiovascular disease (CVD), and presence of diabetes mellitus (DM) were collected at baseline. CVD was recorded if one of the following conditions was present: angina, class III/IV congestive heart failure (New York Heart Association), transient ischemic attack, history of myocardial infarction or cerebro-vascular accident, or peripheral arterial disease[16]. Baseline biochemistry data including hemoglobin, serum albumin, calcium, phosphate and intact parathyroid hormone (iPTH) were examined using an automatic Hitachi chemistry analyzer and then calculated as the mean of measurements made during the first 3 months. Dialysis adequacy and residual renal function (RRF) were measured during the first 6 months. RRF was defined as the mean of residual creatinine clearance and residual urea clearance. Dialysis adequacy was determined from the total Kt/V and total creatinine clearance (Ccr). Center size was also recorded according to the number of enrolled patients from each center.

The education level of patients and each family member, including spouses of those who are married was recorded from 1 to 4 as ordinal categorical variables according to diploma obtained based on school level: elementary school or lower $= 1$; middle school $= 2$; high school $= 3$; and more than high school $= 4$. Average education of a whole family except for the patient was calculated as the arithmetic mean of the education levels of all family members. The highest education of any one family member was recorded as the maximum education level of family members.

Family income was defined as the yearly household income per person and was divided into low (<¥20,000, <$3160,), medium (¥20,000–40,000, $3160–6320) and high (>¥40,000, >$6320) according to average income for urban information in 2011 from the bureau of statistics (http://www.bjstats.gov.cn/nj/main/2011-tjnj/index.htm) since most subjects were from urban. Information of reimbursement type and family residence was also collected. The frequent visitor was defined as someone visiting doctors at least one time every 3 months. Whether medical expenses are covered by national health care system was also recorded

Definition of Outcome Events

The Primary outcome was defined as all-cause death and cardiovascular death. Cardiovascular death was defined as death due to myocardial infarction, congestive heart failure, cerebral bleeding, cerebral infarction, arrhythmia, peripheral arterial disease, and sudden death. The secondary outcome was initial peritonitis, which was diagnosed according to International Society for Peritoneal Dialysis 2010 guidelines[17]. In all analyses, data of transferring to hemodialysis (HD), loss to follow-up, renal transplantation or till the end of the study (November 1, 2011) were censored.

Statistical Analysis

Continuous data were presented as mean with standard deviation except that RRF was presented as the median (interquartile range) because of high skew. Categorical variables were presented as proportions. Relevant characteristics were compared between different education groups, respectively. Patient data were compared using the one-way ANOVA for normally distributed continuous variables, or the Kruskall–Wallis H test for skewed continuous variables, and the Chi-square test for categorical variables. Spearman correlations were explored to identify correlation among various indices of education level and family income. To determine predictive effect of education level of the patient and family (couple education, average education and the highest education) on the outcome events, stratified multivariable Cox regression models were explored, adjusted by age, gender, BMI, presence of DM, CVD history, baseline albumin, hemoglobin, RRF, and family income, and center size was as the stratified factor to adjust for center effects. The center effect was reflected not only in disparity of center size (ranging from 78 patients to 815 patients), which has been demonstrated to be an independent predictor of PD outcome[18–20], but also in differences in practice patterns and biochemical assays between centers. We reported the multivariable adjusted hazard ratios (HRs) with 95% confidence interval (CI). All probabilities were two- tailed, and the level of significance was set at 0.05. Statistical analyses were performed using SPSS for Windows software version 15.0 (SPSS Inc., Chicago, IL).

Results

Baseline characteristics

Data from 2,264 patients were collected. Five hundred and twelve patients were excluded due to missing family education data. In the final cohort, the included 1,752 patients had a mean age of 57.93±15.30 years, with male patients accounting for 49.9%. Overall, 38.8% were diabetic and cerebrovascular disease (CVD) was present in 43.4% of subjects at baseline. The total follow-up duration was 27.6 (14.3–45.4) months. Chronic glomerulonephritis (CGN) was the most common cause of end-stage renal disease (ESRD) (34.4%), followed by diabetic nephropathy (29.7%) and hypertensive nephropathy (16.4%). There were no significant differences in age, gender, body mass index (BMI), or distribution of education level of patients and their family members between the included and excluded subjects (P> 0.05).

Education levels of PD patients and their family members

The constitutions of education levels of the patients and their partners were nearly equivalent; e.g. elementary school 26.7% and 25.9%, middle school 30.0% and 34.5%, high school 23.3% and 22.2%, and more than high school 20.0% and 17.4%, respectively. As for the highest education level of the family members, 33.7% had more than high school level (**Figure 1**).

Comparing patients according to their family's highest level of education showed significant differences in age (over 65 years or not), gender, education and income level, reimbursement type (healthcare or not), or the percentage of rural residence (P<0.001 or 0.05; **Table 1**). Patients whose family's highest education was elementary or lower were more likely to be the eldest male patients from a rural area. They were also less likely to be covered by national healthcare, and had lower family income and lower education level. These patients also had the lowest plasma albumin at baseline. There were no significant differences in the presence of diabetes mellitus (DM), CVD history, percentage of frequent visitor, total Kt/V and Ccr, RRF, BMI, or hemoglobin (P>0.05).

Education levels of patients, their spouses, and the average and highest level of education of their family members, had positive correlations (r = 0.241~0.695; P<0.001 for all). Likewise, each education level was correlated with yearly personal income (r = 0.241~0.265; P<0.001 for all; **Table 2**).

Follow-up and outcomes

Among the 497 patients who died, 190 deaths (38.2%) were due to CVD and 120 (24.1%) infection; other causes were malignancy, gastrointestinal bleeding, malnutrition, miscellaneous, and undefined. One hundred and forty-eight patients were transferred to HD, most due to PD-associated infection (67 cases, 45.3%).

The time to first-episode peritonitis was 20.88 (9.73–35.23) months. Among 392 episodes of initial peritonitis during the study period, there were 139 episodes (35.5%) due to Gram-positive organisms, while 84 (21.4%) were due to Gram-negative organisms and 7 (1.8%) fungi.

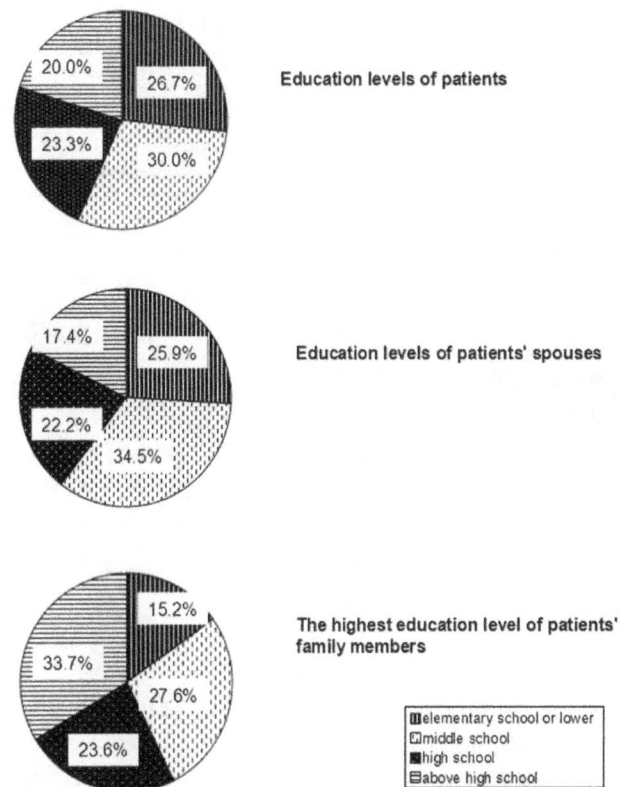

Figure 1. Education levels of PD patients and their family members.

Associations of education levels with outcome

By multivariable Cox regression analysis (**Table 3**), similar to our previous report[3], patient education level did not predict patient survival after adjusting for age, gender, BMI, presence of DM, CVD history, baseline albumin, hemoglobin, RRF, and family income, and using center size as a stratified factor to adjust for center effects. However, the highest education of family members was significantly associated with higher mortality. As compared to the family's highest education of elementary school or lower group, middle, high and more than high school education decreased the risk of death by 32%, 36%, and 34%, respectively. There also a trend that each increase of 1 in average education level decreased mortality by 11% (P = 0.05). As for spouse's education, middle education rather than high school or more than high school also predicted a lower mortality. For cardiovascular death and initial-episode peritonitis, neither PD patients nor their family members' education level were associated with the higher risk after adjusting for the abovementioned covariates. No interactions between education level and age, gender, DM, or CVD history were found for predicting all-cause mortality, CV death, or initial-episode peritonitis.

Discussion

In this large-scale multi-center retrospective study, the highest education of family members were identified as independent predictive factors of PD outcome; however, no such effects were detected for CV death or occurrence of the first episode of peritonitis after adjustment for well-recognized confounders. The education level of a PD patient was not found to contribute to any outcome events, similar to our previous reports[3]. To our

Table 1. The baseline characteristics and clinical data of PD patients according to their family's highest education level.

	The highest education level of patients' family members				
	elementary school or lower	middle school	high school	above high school	P
Age>65 yrs (%)	50.38	38.30	29.30	38.47	<0.001
Male(%)	55.26	52.80	47.22	46.95	0.048
BMI (Kg/m2)	22.63±3.88	22.93±3.51	23.05±3.59	22.81±3.39	0.47
DM (%)	39.02	40.22	36.39	39.18	0.70
CVD (%)	43.68	39.28	41.83	47.20	0.06
Family income					<0.001
Low (%)	61.89	53.11	48.54	34.92	
Medium (%)	30.57	38.59	39.08	34.92	
High (%)	7.55	8.30	12.38	30.15	
Education levels of patients					<0.001
Elementary school or lower (%)	53.01	27.44	21.31	18.00	
Middle school (%)	27.82	41.37	28.33	22.75	
High school (%)	12.03	22.25	32.93	22.54	
Above high school (%)	7.14	8.94	17.43	36.67	
Education levels of patients' spouse					NA
Elementary school or lower (%)	100.00	14.14	12.39	12.03	
Middle school (%)	0.00	85.86	18.13	17.15	
High school (%)	0.00	0.00	69.49	17.15	
Above high school (%)	0.00	0.00	0.00	53.67	
Average education level	1.00±0.00	1.88±0.22	2.65±0.44	3.38±0.63	<0.001
Rural residence (%)	34.2	23.8	21.1	8.6	<0.001
Health care (%)[#]	59.4	68.7	73.5	84.1	<0.001
Frequent visitors (%)[□]	85.71	88.54	86.68	90.15	0.19
Hemoglobin (g/L)	98.76±18.16	101.82±19.39	101.45±17.51	101.52±17.16	0.07
Serum albumin (g/L)	34.32±5.76	34.80±5.21	35.45±5.25	35.29±5.13	0.023
Calcium(mmol/L)	2.16±0.25	2.17±0.23	2.19±0.25	2.20±0.24	0.08
Phosphate(mmol/L)	1.53±0.47	1.58±0.50	1.54±0.46	1.56±0.42	0.36
iPTH (pg/ml)	179.2(78~343)	180.9(93.05~327.15)	192(87.7~338.5)	148(64.57~313.15)	0.07
Total Kt/V	2.03±0.66	2.05±0.63	2.12±0.67	2.02±.64	0.13
Total Ccr (L/w/1.73 m²)	77.25±41.43	77.9±47.99	76.9±30.9	74.78±29.9	0.64
RRF (ml/min)	3.02(1.30–5.62)	3.30(1.76–5.40)	3.72(1.94–5.57)	3.51(1.93–5.50)	0.26

Abbreviations: BMI, body mass index; DM, diabetes mellitus; CVD, cardiovascular disease; iPTH, intact parathyroid hormone; Kt/V, urea clearance; Ccr, creatinine clearance; RRF, residual renal function.
[#]Healthcare % represents the percentage of patients whose medical expenses are covered more than 90% by the national healthcare system.
[□]Frequent visitor was defined as someone visiting doctors at least once every 3 months.

Table 2. Coefficient correlations between the education levels of PD patients and their family members and family income[#].

	Patients' education	Spouse's education	The highest education	Average education	Family income
Patients' education	NA				
Spouse's education	0.566	NA			
The highest education	0.335	0.695	NA		
Average education	0.428	0.825	0.874	NA	
Family income	0.265	0.281	0.241	0.262	NA

Abbreviation: NA, non analysis.
[#]All P values for the correlation analyses were <0.001.

Table 3. The predictive role of education level of patients and their family members by multivariable Cox regression analysis.

	Death			Cardiovascular death			Initial- episode peritonitis		
	HR	95% CI	P	HR	95% CI	P	HR	95% CI	P
Patients' education									
Low	ref		0.47	ref		0.95	ref		0.85
Middle	0.81	0.61 1.09	0.17	0.93	0.57 1.50	0.77	0.93	0.69 1.25	0.63
High	0.87	0.63 1.21	0.40	0.88	0.52 1.49	0.64	0.91	0.66 1.27	0.59
>high	1.00	0.71 1.41	0.99	0.85	0.48 1.52	0.59	0.86	0.60 1.24	0.86
The highest education									
Low	ref		0.04	ref		0.49	ref		0.26
middle	0.68	0.48 0.96	0.03	0.74	0.42 1.33	0.31	0.85	0.58 1.26	0.43
High	0.64	0.45 0.91	0.01	0.62	0.34 1.13	0.12	1.08	0.74 1.59	0.67
>high	0.66	0.48 0.91	0.01	0.75	0.44 1.29	0.30	1.14	0.79 1.64	0.49
Spouse's education									
Low	ref		0.07	ref		0.18	ref		0.06
middle	0.69	0.49 0.97	0.03	0.69	0.41 1.17	0.17	0.90	0.62 1.29	0.56
High	0.72	0.49 1.07	0.10	0.62	0.33 1.17	0.14	1.39	0.95 2.05	0.09
>high	0.98	0.67 1.43	0.92	1.08	0.60 1.97	0.79	1.19	0.79 1.81	0.41
Average education	0.89	0.78 1.00	0.05	0.94	0.77 1.14	0.52	1.07	0.95 1.22	0.28

Notes:All models are adjusted for age, gender, BMI, presence of DM, CVD history, baseline albumin, hemoglobin, RRF and family income, and center size was used as a stratified factor to adjust for center effects. The HRs and 95%CI for all-cause death, cardiovascular death, and initial-episode peritonitis are shown respectively using low level (elementary school or lower) as the reference. The HR and 95% of average education level as a continuous variable is also shown.

knowledge, this is the first study to offer insight into the impact of family members' education status on PD patient outcomes.

Most patients with chronic kidney disease will develop ESRD and sooner or later require renal replacement therapy. This is unpleasant and has a great impact on both the patients and their family members. Undoubtedly, the patients' illness affects the physical and mental health of families in this population[21–23]. On the other hand, family members as a primary source of social support can make great contributions to patients' disease management. To date, only a few studies have shown that spouse's behavior and attitude can affect patient management of diabetes[24,25], stroke[26], and osteoarthritis[27] rehabilitation therapy. For the dialysis population, although previous studies have indicated the significant impact of social support on satisfaction, psychological status, quality of life, hospitalization, and mortality for PD and HD patients[7–11], the association between a specific aspect of family members, such as education status and PD outcome has rarely been explored.

Our novel findings presented here revealed a close relationship between education level of family members and poor PD outcome. There are several reasons for these results. Firstly, for patients with ESRD, medical decisions are largely dependent on consultation with family members. Family members with high education backgrounds are more likely to get access to healthcare and offer better information sharing and advice. Such good social support from family probably leads to early referral to nephrologists, appropriate choice of dialysis modality, and timely preparation with dialysis access[28]. Secondly, once a dialysis program starts, the whole family has to strive to adapt to the changes in their daily lives, including dietary, complex medication regimens, some social isolation, frequent clinic visits, and hospitalization. Care giving activities, including appraising, advocating, and coaching, provided by family members is dependent on a strong knowledge base[15]. Family members with higher education levels can understand all the changes easily and are apt to adjust patients' lifestyles as suggested. As shown in a previous study, there is a very strong correlation between coherence and functionality of the non-chronically-ill spouse, social support, and compliance to chronic illness to his or her situation[29]. Besides the family-unit therapy nature of PD, according to our practice, deep-rooted family conception of Chinese patients may reveal the unnegligible affection from the whole family to the patient, hence patients' own education levels seemed less important. However, there was not such a linear trend that the family highest education level of middle school and above would be more benefit for patients' mortality. Though educated family would be expected to have better adherence to treatment and adaptation to daily life change, they also bear heavier mental pressure and endure more fierce decision conflict when accidents happen. Leadership, the role most likely played by person with the highest family education, might be important at such a difficult point to decision making, which would affect patients' outcomes.In addition, although close relationships among family's education level, income level, rural residence, and less healthcare were found, multivariate analysis could not validate that the predicting role of family's education level is confounded by these factors. Future studies should focus on the effect of improved social support from family members on the physical or psychosocial well-being of patients[30].

It is interesting that higher education level of the spouse did not decrease the death risk for PD patients despite the fact that the spouse has the closest relationship with patients acting as a caregiver, confidant, and primary source of emotional support. The cause for this phenomenon is not clear. However, recent studies have suggested that the quality of marriage rather than the presence of a marriage significantly influences the outcome for dialysis patients. Low patient marital satisfaction evaluated by the Dyadic Adjustment Scale is found to be associated with poorer psychological status of the partners and higher mortality[31]. Whether or how the education level of a spouse correlates to the quality of marriage and family support needs to be explored.

Based on our data, the education level of patients and their family members has no impact on initial-episode peritonitis. One possible explanation for this is that selected centers were equipped with professional PD clinicians and well-developed training programs[32]. In most centers, patients and their homecare helpers were often and repeatedly trained and examined for proper techniques with respect to bag exchange. Under these circumstances, it is likely that biological factors leading to the occurrence of peritonitis may outweigh the effects of education level of patients and their family members.

This study has several strengths. First, this is the only study to disclose the impact of education levels of both PD patients and their family members on PD outcomes with large sample sizes. The detailed information on the education status offers us a valuable chance to reveal a family education-outcome relationship. Our results alert clinicians to highlight the importance of family factors on the therapeutic effects of family-based treatment, such as in PD. In addition, the baseline education level is a fixed variable for the majority adult patients and their family. As compared to social support, a variable index during long-term follow up, baseline education status as a potential prognostic factor is more appropriate to be explored.

There are some limitations to this study. First, potential mechanisms for the association of family members' education and PD outcome are not clear since we did not evaluate a patient's satisfaction with care providers, perception of accessibility of care or to therapy for patients from less-educated families. Until such research is conducted, a determination of whether and how family members' education directly affects quality of therapy and PD outcome is difficult to make. Secondly, we should be aware of the possibility of residual confounding and recall bias because of the retrospective nature of this study. However, if confounding occurred, it would result in underestimation of the association but not change our main findings at all. In addition, we should be aware of the possibilities of ascertainment bias (totally 22.6% eligible patients were not included). Finally, as an observational study, a cause-effect relationship could not be established.

In conclusion, PD patients with well-educated family members have a lower death risk. This novel finding is helpful for us to understand the key role that family support plays in the quality of PD therapy, such a home-based therapy. Further research focusing on family-unit therapy and individualized care based on family education background should be designed to investigate their potential benefits for PD patients. The issues raised by the present study also highlight some challenges for caring practices in home-based therapy for conditions like PD.

Acknowledgments

The authors express their appreciation to the patients, doctors, and nursing staff of the peritoneal dialysis center of Peking University First Hospital, Division of Nephrology of Peking University Third Hospital, Division of Nephrology of Huashan Hospital, Fudan University, Division of Nephrology of the second affiliated hospital of Harbin Medical University, Division of Nephrology of Peking University People's Hospital, Division of Nephrology of the first affiliated hospital of Zhejiang University School of Medicine, Division of Nephrology of General Hospital of NingXia Medical University, for their participation in this study.

Author Contributions

Conceived and designed the experiments: JD HYW. Performed the

experiments: QFH TYZ YPR JHC HPZ MHC JD YW CMH RZ XHZ MW NT. Analyzed the data: ZKY JD. Wrote the paper: ZKY JD.

References

1. Jain AK, Blake P, Cordy P, Garg AX (2012) Global trends in rates of peritoneal dialysis. J Am Soc Nephrol 23: 533–544.
2. Martin LC, Caramori JC, Fernandes N, Divino-Filho JC, Pecoits-Filho R, et al. (2011) Geographic and educational factors and risk of the first peritonitis episode in Brazilian Peritoneal Dialysis study (BRAZPD) patients. Clin J Am Soc Nephrol 6: 1944–1951.
3. Xu R, Han QF, Zhu TY, Ren YP, Chen JH, et al. (2012) Impact of individual and environmental socioeconomic status on peritoneal dialysis outcomes: a retrospective multicenter cohort study. PLoS One 7: e50766.
4. Farias MG, Soucie JM, McClellan W, Mitch WE (1994) Race and the risk of peritonitis: an analysis of factors associated with the initial episode. Kidney Int 46: 1392–1396.
5. Tonelli M, Hemmelgarn B, Culleton B, Klarenbach S, Gill JS, et al. (2007) Mortality of Canadians treated by peritoneal dialysis in remote locations. Kidney Int 72: 1023–1028.
6. Mehrotra R, Story K, Guest S, Fedunyszyn M (2012) Neighborhood location, rurality, geography, and outcomes of peritoneal dialysis patients in the United States. Perit Dial Int 32: 322–331.
7. Thong MS, Kaptein AA, Krediet RT, Boeschoten EW, Dekker FW (2007) Social support predicts survival in dialysis patients. Nephrol Dial Transplant 22: 845–850.
8. Szeto CC, Chow KM, Kwan BC, Law MC, Chung KY, et al. (2008) The impact of social support on the survival of Chinese peritoneal dialysis patients. Perit Dial Int 28: 252–258.
9. Plantinga LC, Fink NE, Harrington-Levey R, Finkelstein FO, Hebah N, et al. (2010) Association of social support with outcomes in incident dialysis patients. Clin J Am Soc Nephrol 5: 1480–1488.
10. Untas A, Thumma J, Rascle N, Rayner H, Mapes D, et al. (2011) The associations of social support and other psychosocial factors with mortality and quality of life in the dialysis outcomes and practice patterns study. Clin J Am Soc Nephrol 6: 142–152.
11. Ye XQ, Chen WQ, Lin JX, Wang RP, Zhang ZH, et al. (2008) Effect of social support on psychological-stress-induced anxiety and depressive symptoms in patients receiving peritoneal dialysis. J Psychosom Res 65: 157–164.
12. Patel SS, Peterson RA, Kimmel PL (2005) The impact of social support on end-stage renal disease. Semin Dial 18: 98–102.
13. Oliver MJ, Garg AX, Blake PG, Johnson JF, Verrelli M, et al. (2010) Impact of contraindications, barriers to self-care and support on incident peritoneal dialysis utilization. Nephrol Dial Transplant 25: 2737–2744.
14. Griva K, Li ZH, Lai AY, Choong MC, Foo MW (2013) Perspectives of patients, families, and health care professionals on decision-making about dialysis modality—the good, the bad, and the misunderstandings! Perit Dial Int 33: 280–289.
15. Beanlands H, Horsburgh ME, Fox S, Howe A, Locking-Cusolito H, et al. (2005) Caregiving by family and friends of adults receiving dialysis. Nephrol Nurs J 32: 621–631.
16. Smith SC, Jr., Jackson R, Pearson TA, Fuster V, Yusuf S, et al. (2004) Principles for national and regional guidelines on cardiovascular disease prevention: a scientific statement from the World Heart and Stroke Forum. Circulation 109: 3112–3121.
17. Li PK, Szeto CC, Piraino B, Bernardini J, Figueiredo AE, et al. (2010) Peritoneal dialysis-related infections recommendations: 2010 update. Perit Dial Int 30: 393–423.
18. Afolalu B, Troidle L, Osayimwen O, Bhargava J, Kitsen J, et al. (2009) Technique failure and center size in a large cohort of peritoneal dialysis patients in a defined geographic area. Perit Dial Int 29: 292–296.
19. Mujais S, Story K (2006) Peritoneal dialysis in the US: evaluation of outcomes in contemporary cohorts. Kidney Int Suppl: S21–26.
20. Schaubel DE, Blake PG, Fenton SS (2001) Effect of renal center characteristics on mortality and technique failure on peritoneal dialysis. Kidney Int 60: 1517–1524.
21. Sezer S, Uyar ME, Bal Z, Tutal E, Ozdemir Acar FN (2013) The influence of socioeconomic factors on depression in maintenance hemodialysis patients and their caregivers. Clin Nephrol 80: 342–348.
22. Schipper K, Abma TA (2011) Coping, family and mastery: top priorities for social science research by patients with chronic kidney disease. Nephrol Dial Transplant 26: 3189–3195.
23. Tsai TC, Liu SI, Tsai JD, Chou LH (2006) Psychosocial effects on caregivers for children on chronic peritoneal dialysis. Kidney Int 70: 1983–1987.
24. Stephens MA, Franks MM, Rook KS, Iida M, Hemphill RC, et al. (2013) Spouses' attempts to regulate day-to-day dietary adherence among patients with type 2 diabetes. Health Psychol 32: 1029–1037.
25. Khan CM, Stephens MA, Franks MM, Rook KS, Salem JK (2013) Influences of spousal support and control on diabetes management through physical activity. Health Psychol 32: 739–747.
26. Molloy GJ, Johnston M, Johnston DW, Pollard B, Morrison V, et al. (2008) Spousal caregiver confidence and recovery from ambulatory activity limitations in stroke survivors. Health Psychol 27: 286–290.
27. Stephens MA, Fekete EM, Franks MM, Rook KS, Druley JA, et al. (2009) Spouses' use of pressure and persuasion to promote osteoarthritis patients' medical adherence after orthopedic surgery. Health Psychol 28: 48–55.
28. Cohen SD, Sharma T, Acquaviva K, Peterson RA, Patel SS, et al. (2007) Social support and chronic kidney disease: an update. Adv Chronic Kidney Dis 14: 335–344.
29. Horsburgh ME, Rice VH, Matuk L (1998) Sense of coherence and life satisfaction: patient and spousal adaptation to home dialysis. ANNA J 25: 219–228; discussion 229–230.
30. Tong A, Sainsbury P, Craig JC (2008) Support interventions for caregivers of people with chronic kidney disease: a systematic review. Nephrol Dial Transplant 23: 3960–3965.
31. Kimmel PL, Peterson RA, Weihs KL, Shidler N, Simmens SJ, et al. (2000) Dyadic relationship conflict, gender, and mortality in urban hemodialysis patients. J Am Soc Nephrol 11: 1518–1525.
32. Xu R, Zhuo M, Yang Z, Dong J (2012) Experiences with assisted peritoneal dialysis in China. Perit Dial Int 32: 94–101.

Pneumonia and Mortality Risk in Continuous Ambulatory Peritoneal Dialysis Patients with Diabetic Nephropathy

Feng He*[9], Xianfeng Wu[9], Xi Xia, Fenfen Peng, Fengxian Huang, Xueqing Yu*

Department of Nephrology, The First Affiliated Hospital, Sun Yat-sen University, Guangzhou, China

Abstract

Background: Although clinical experience suggests that patients with diabetes mellitus are more susceptible to several types of infections, the overall scope of pneumonia in continuous ambulatory peritoneal dialysis (CAPD) patients with diabetic nephropathy (DN) has received little attention.

Methods: This was a prospective observational cohort study in CAPD patients in which prognostic risks of pneumonia were evaluated in DN and non-DN patients by Cox regression analysis. Hazard ratios of pneumonia events, all-cause and pneumonia-related mortality were calculated by Kaplan-Meier curves and the Cox proportional hazards model for DN versus non-DN patients.

Results: A total of 1148 patients (58.6% male, 48.34±15.78 years) had a median follow-up of 23.8 months and a maximum follow-up of 72.0 months. The pneumonia incidence rate of 62.3/1,000 patient-years in CAPD patients with DN was significantly higher than that of 28.5/1,000 patient-years in non-DN patients. On multivariate analysis, independent predictors of pneumonia occurrence in CAPD patients with DN were high body mass index (hazard ratio [HR], 1.15; 95% confidence interval [CI], 1.01–1.31; P = 0.037) and low serum albumin level (HR, 0.87; 95% CI, 0.78–0.98; P = 0.014). Older age (HR, 1.63; 95% CI, 1.35–1.96; P<0.001) was an independent risk factor for the presence of pneumonia in non-DN patients. CAPD patients with DN had higher pneumonia-related mortality (HR, 4.424; 95% CI, 1.871–10.461; P<0.001) and all-cause mortality (HR, 2.608; 95% CI, 1.890–3.599; P<0.001) hazards than their non-DN counterparts, even when extensive demographics, comorbidities, and lab adjustments were made.

Conclusions: The pneumonia and all-cause mortality risks were strikingly higher in CAPD patients with DN than in non-DN counterparts, which may warrant further investigation and therapeutic care intensification.

Editor: Emmanuel A. Burdmann, University of Sao Paulo Medical School, Brazil

Funding: This study was supported by the grants from the National Key Basic Research Program of China (grant number 2011CB504005), the National Key Technology Research and Development Program of the Ministry of Science and Technology of China (grant number 2011BAI10B05), the National Natural Science Foundation of China (grant number 81170765), and the Guangdong Natural Science Foundation (grant number S2011020002359). The funders had no role in study design, data collection and analysis, decision to publish, or preparation of the manuscript.

Competing Interests: The authors have declared that no competing interests exist.

* E-mail: hfxyl@163.net (F. He); yuxq@mail.sysu.edu.cn (XY)

[9] These authors contributed equally to this work.

Introduction

Registry studies typically rank infection second to cardiovascular disease as a cause of death in dialysis patients, and approximately one in every five infection-related deaths is attributed to pulmonary causes [1]. Regarding pneumonia, the mortality rate of pulmonary infection in hemodialysis (HD) patients has been reported to be 14- to 16-fold higher than in the general population [2]. In another study, the cumulative probability of pneumonia hospitalizations at 5 years was 36% in hemodialysis patients [3]. Although hemodialysis patients have an increased risk of pulmonary infection, which contributes to sizeable morbidity and mortality, the overall scope of pneumonia in continuous ambulatory peritoneal dialysis patients has received little attention.

Patients with diabetes mellitus (DM) are considered to be more susceptible to several types of infections, including pneumonia, urinary tract infection, and skin infection [4,5]. Diabetic patients may have increased susceptibility to pneumonia due to hyperglycemia, increased risk of aspiration, decreased immunity, pulmonary microangiopathy, impaired lung function, and coexisting morbidity [6]. Moreover, diabetic nephropathy (DN) may occur in approximately 40% of patients with DM and has become the leading cause of end-stage renal disease (ESRD), which may further impair patient ability to combat pneumonia due to a chronic uremic milieu, older age, and the presence of comorbidities [3,7,8]. To the best of our knowledge, few if any studies have attempted to estimate the incidence, risk factors, and prognosis of pneumonia in CAPD patients with diabetic nephropathy.

Therefore, the objective of the current study was to define the clinical features and outcomes of pneumonia in CAPD patients. Specifically, we wished to define: (1) the incidence rate of pneumonia, (2) the prognostic risks of pneumonia events, and (3) the association with mortality in CAPD patients with DN.

Materials and Methods

Study design and participants

This was a prospective, observational cohort study of patients recruited from a single peritoneal dialysis (PD) center of the First Affiliated Hospital of Sun Yat-sen University. Enrollment occurred from February 1, 2006 to February 1, 2011 and follow-up extended to February 1, 2012, including a total of 1148 patients older than 18 years who had received CAPD for >3 months. Patients were followed every 3 months after the start of CAPD until death or censoring, which occurred because of a transfer to a non-participating dialysis center, withdrawal from the study, kidney transplantation, at the end of the follow-up period on February 1, 2012, or at a maximum follow-up of 6 years. We divided patients into DN and non-DN group according to diabetic nephropathy. For all participants, the total number of episodes of pneumonia infection and the date of the first episode were recorded. The occurrence of pneumonia was determined from Part A Medicare in-patient claims, using the following International Classification of Diseases, Ninth Revision, Clinical Modification codes: (1) viral pneumonia, 480.x. and 484.1; (2) pneumococcal pneumonia 481; (3) other bacterial pneumonia 482.xx and 483.x; (4) fungal pneumonia 112.4, 114.0, 115.xx, 484.6, 484.7; (5) pneumonia caused by other or unspecified organisms 482.89, 482.9, 483.8, 484.3, 484.5, 484.8, 485, and 486 [3]. We defined our main outcome of pneumonia as presence of one of these diagnostic codes and exhibiting signs of infection on chest x-rays. The endpoint of follow-up was pneumonia-related mortality or all-cause mortality. The study design was approved by the Clinical Research Ethics Committee of the First Affiliated Hospital of Sun Yat-sen University. All participants provided their written informed consent before inclusion.

Data collection and laboratory measurements

Baseline demographic data and clinical data such as age, gender, diabetes, diabetic nephropathy (with proven biopsy, or an urinary albumin: creatinine ratio (ACR)>30 mg/g), hypertension, history of cardiovascular disease (myocardial infarction, ischemic stroke, or limb amputation due to peripheral arterial disease), and history of stroke were collected at the start of CAPD treatment. Diabetes was defined on the basis of diabetes mellitus registered as a primary kidney disease or as a comorbid condition [9]. Hypertension was recorded if the patient was taking antihypertensive drugs or had two separated measured blood pressures ≥140/90 mmHg. Stroke was defined as evidence of an acute disturbance of focal neurological function with symptoms lasting>24 hours and considered to be due to intracerebral hemorrhage or ischemia [10].

Baseline biochemical parameters were collected 3 months after the start of CAPD and included blood pressure, hemoglobin, serum albumin, C-reactive protein, total triglycerides, total cholesterol, HDL-C, LDL-C, plasma urea, and plasma creatinine. All parameters were measured in the biochemical laboratory of the First Affiliated Hospital of Sun Yat-sen University. Renal function was calculated using the mean creatinine and urea clearance, adjusted for body surface area (mL/min/1.73 m^2), and renal function was calculated every 3 months. All PD patients selected peritoneal dialysis as the initial dialysis, and no patient was anuric when initiating the study. Patients were interviewed by trial nurses for general condition and concomitant medication information monthly in person or by telephone.

Statistical analysis

Variables are presented in this study as mean ± SD, median (interquartile range), or number (proportion) where appropriate. Differences in variables between the DN and non-diabetic nephropathy (non-DN) group were tested using the Student's t-test, the non-parametric Mann-Whitney test, or the chi-square test where appropriate. Timeline incidence data were analyzed using a Poisson model. Life tables were used to calculate cumulative proportions surviving during follow-up. Cox regression analysis was used to evaluate the prognostic risks of the presence of pneumonia in the DN and non-DN group at baseline. Two different approaches were applied: (1) univariate Cox regression analysis was selected from the following variables: age, body mass index, hypertension, cardiovascular disease, stroke, diastolic blood pressure (DBP), mean artery pressure (MAP), estimated glomerular filtration rate (eGFR), C-reactive protein, and serum albumin for the presence of pneumonia, which were statistically different in baseline parameters comparison between two groups, and (2) the multivariate Cox regression analysis model using covariates by a backward stepwise selection procedure (entry: P≤0.05; removal: P>0.1, the selection criterion was from acquiesce in SPSS software system as well as the importance of clinical concern). Time-to-event analysis of pneumonia events, all-cause mortality and pneumonia-related mortality was performed using Kaplan-Meier survival curves, the Log-Rank test and the Cox proportional hazards model for the DN group compared with non-DN group. Multivariate models were constructed sequentially using only the group, then adding demographic characteristics (age at enrollment, gender, and BMI), then adding comorbidities (hypertension, cardiovascular disease, and stroke), then adding eGFR, and finally adding laboratory values (serum albumin, HDL-C, and LDL-C), in addition, other parameters exclusion by collinearity. Statistical significance was defined as P<0.05 using two-tailed tests. Statistical analyses were performed using SPSS 13.0 for Windows (SPSS, Chicago, IL, USA).

Results

Patient characteristics at baseline

The demographic and clinical characteristics of CAPD patients are summarized in Table 1, and categorized according to diabetic nephropathy. A total of 1148 patients were enrolled in this study (age 48.34±15.78 years, male 58.6%), with a median follow-up of 23.8 months and a maximum follow-up of 72.0 months, including 190 (16.6%) patients with DN (DN group: age 60.13±11.12 years, male 56.3%), and 958 (83.4%) patients without DN (non-DN group: age 46.02±15.53 years, male 59.1%). Reasons for exclusion were lost to follow-up (n = 25), transfer to hemodialysis (n = 60), renal transplantation (n = 151), transfer to other centers (n = 35), and poor compliance (n = 8). Compared with non-DN patients, DN patients more frequently had hypertension, cardiovascular disease, and stroke, as well as presented with a higher BMI, eGFR, and CRP, but a lower DBP, MAP, and serum albumin. However, no significant differences in baseline parameters were found between diabetic nephropathy patients with (n = 103) and without biopsy (n = 87).

Characteristics of pneumonia patients

The characteristics of pneumonia patients are shown in Table 2. During the study period, a total of 78 pneumonia events occurred in all patients, including 24 events in the DN group and 54 events in the non-DN group. Pneumonia incidence rates were 12.63% higher in the DN group than that of 5.63% in the non-DN group (P = 0.001). The overall incidence rate of pneumonia was 34.3/

Table 1. Baseline characteristics of 1148 CAPD patients.

Characteristics	Total	DN	Non-DN	P value
Demographics				
All, n(%)	1148(100.0)	190(16.6)	958(83.4)	
Age (years)	48.34±15.78	60.13±11.12	46.02±15.53	<0.001
Male, n(%)	673(58.6)	107(56.3)	566(59.1)	0.531
Body mass index (kg/m²)	21.20±3.42	22.32±3.84	20.99±3.33	<0.001
Comorbidities, n(%)				
Diabetes mellitus	262(22.8)	190(100)	72(7.5)	<0.001
Hypertension	753(65.6)	144(75.8)	609(63.6)	0.002
Cardiovascular disease	79(6.9)	38(20.0)	41(4.3)	<0.001
Stroke	89(7.8)	28(14.7)	61(6.4)	<0.001
Blood Pressure				
SBP (mmHg)	130.94±20.38	137.93±22.86	136.93±19.85	0.563
DBP (mmHg)	84.70±14.55	75.48±12.61	88.55±14.21	<0.001
MAP (mmHg)	101.14±17.84	96.30±14.48	102.11±18.28	<0.001
eGFR (mL/min per 1.73m²)	7.97±3.42	9.23±3.64	7.73±3.40	<0.001
Laboratory data				
Hemoglobin (g/L)	95.01±22.85	97.20±20.67	94.57±23.24	0.119
Serum albumin (g/L)	36.80±5.69	34.28±4.75	37.31±5.73	<0.001
C-reactive protein (mg/L)[a]	1.94 (0.76–7.18)	2.98 (1.00–10.47)	1.70 (0.73–6.53)	<0.001
Total triglycerides (mmol/L)	1.79 ± 1.38	1.82 ± 1.16	1.73 ± 1.42	0.335
Total cholesterol (mmol/L)	5.08±2.60	5.28±1.50	5.04±2.77	0.096
HDL-C (mmol/L)	1.26±0.58	1.22±0.52	1.27±0.59	0.317
LDL-C (mmol/L)	2.93±1.33	2.99±1.06	2.92±1.38	0.516

Data expressed with a plus/minus sign are the mean±SD.
[a]Median (interquartile range).
Abbreviations: CAPD, continuous ambulatory peritoneal dialysis; SBP, systolic blood pressure; DBP, diastolic blood pressure; MAP, mean artery pressure; eGFR, estimated glomerular filtration rate; HDL, high-density lipoprotein-C; LDL-C, low-density lipoprotein.

1,000 patient-years (62.3/1,000 patient-years in the DN group and 28.5/1,000 patient-years in the non-DN group, P<0.001). Obviously, the cumulative hazard of developing pneumonia was significantly higher in the DN group than that in the non-DN group (HR, 2.176; 95% CI, 1.344–3.522; P = 0.003) (Figure 1). Additionally, The cumulative pneumonia survival was 87%, 82%, and 68% at 1, 3, and 5 years, respectively, in the DN group compared with 96%, 88%, and 83% at 1, 3, and 5 years, respectively, in the non-DN group. Furthermore, patients with DN had a higher BMI (23.60±1.80 vs. 20.99±2.99; P=0.001), a stroke more frequently (12.5% vs. 11.1%; P=0.049), decreased DBP (71.91±8.56 vs. 82.00±13.15; P=0.001), decreased MAP (92.42±8.95 vs. 99.71±14.70; P=0.009), decreased eGFR (7.29±2.96 vs. 9.69±5.13; P=0.013), and decreased serum albumin (33.03±4.54 vs. 37.60±4.99; P<0.001) than patients without DN. However, there was no difference with regard to age or C-reactive protein level between the two groups.

Independent predictors of pneumonia

Clinical and laboratory variables that were statistically different in Table 1 were included in the Cox regression analysis. Table 3 shows the predictors of pneumonia for CAPD patients with DN. There were no significant variables using univariate Cox regression analysis, however, the multivariate analysis model identified higher BMI and lower serum albumin as independent predictors of pneumonia occurrence after adjusting for age,

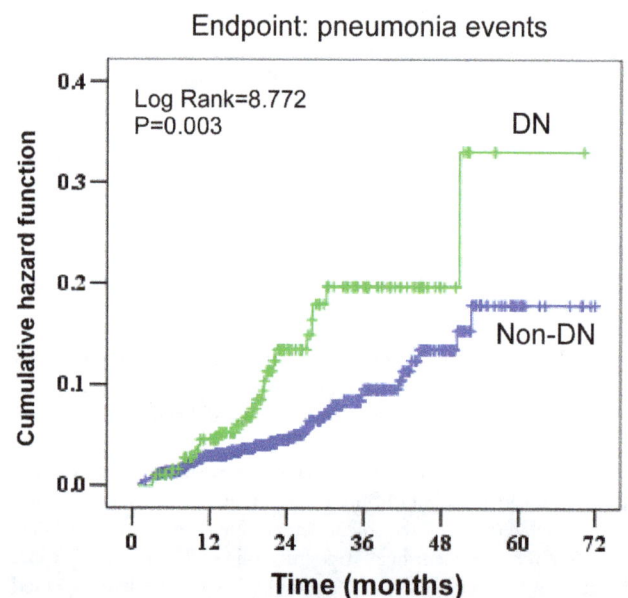

Figure 1. Cumulative incidence of pneumonia events according to diabetic nephropathy.

Table 2. Characteristics of pneumonia patients with and without diabetic nephropathy.

Characteristics	DN	Non-DN	P value
Demographics			
All, n(%)	24 (30.8)	54 (69.2)	
Age (years)	60.13±11.12	46.02±15.53	0.074
Male, n(%)	16 (66.7)	25 (46.3)	0.156
Body mass index (kg/m²)	23.60±1.80	20.99±2.99	0.001
Comorbidities, n(%)			
Diabetes mellitus	24(100)	7(13.0)	<0.001
Hypertension	19(79.2)	40(74.1)	0.843
Cardiovascular disease	3(12.5)	1(1.9)	0.158
Stroke	3(12.5)	6(11.1)	0.049
Blood Pressure			
SBP (mmHg)	133.46±15.11	135.13±21.99	0.743
DBP (mmHg)	71.91±8.56	82.00±13.15	0.001
MAP (mmHg)	92.42±8.95	99.71±14.70	0.009
eGFR (mL/min per 1.73m²)	7.29±2.96	9.69±5.13	0.013
Laboratory data			
Hemoglobin (g/L)	94.51±14.43	99.57±24.37	0.257
Serum albumin (g/L)	33.03±4.54	37.60±4.99	<0.001
C-reactive protein (mg/L)[a]	1.76(0.69–11.42)	3.02(1.28–8.40)	0.432
Total triglycerides (mmol/L)	1.90±1.38	1.84±1.12	0.216
Total cholesterol (mmol/L)	4.73±1.04	5.25±1.12	0.079
HDL-C (mmol/L)	1.29±0.35	1.33±0.55	0.116
LDL-C (mmol/L)	2.70±0.69	2.99±1.01	0.158

Data expressed with a plus/minus sign are the mean±SD.
[a]Median (interquartile range).
Abbreviations: SBP, systolic blood pressure; DBP, diastolic blood pressure; MAP, mean artery pressure; eGFR, estimated glomerular filtration rate; HDL-C, high-density lipoprotein; LDL-C, low-density lipoprotein.

Table 3. Predictor variables and multivariate model for pneumonia events in patients with diabetic nephropathy.

Predictors	Hazard ratio	95% CI	P value
Predictor variables			
Age (per 10-year age increase)	1.27	0.87–1.87	0.215
Body mass index (per 1 kg/m² increase)	1.08	0.96–1.22	0.185
Hypertension (yes/no)	1.45	0.54–3.90	0.459
Cardiovascular disease (yes/no)	0.60	0.18–2.01	0.407
Stroke (yes/no)	0.77	0.23–2.60	0.674
DBP (per 1 mmHg increase)	0.98	0.95–1.01	0.133
MAP (per 1 mmHg increase)	0.98	0.91–1.01	0.182
eGFR (per 1mL/min per 1.73m² increase)	1.00	0.90–1.13	0.883
C-reactive protein(per 1 mg/L increase)	0.98	0.91–1.05	0.539
Serum albumin (per 1g/L increase)	0.93	0.86–1.01	0.066
Multivariate model[a]			
Body mass index (per 1 kg/m² increase)	1.15	1.01–1.31	0.037
Serum albumin (per 1g/L increase)	0.87	0.78–0.98	0.014

Abbreviations: DBP, diastolic blood pressure; MAP, mean artery pressure; eGFR, estimated glomerular filtration rate; CI, confidence interval.
[a]Adjusted for variables from the above predictor variables using a backward stepwise cox proportional hazards model with a stay criterion of 0.10. P<0.05 represents statistical significant.

Table 4. Predictor variables and multivariate model for pneumonia events in patients without diabetic nephropathy.

Predictors	Hazard ratio	95% CI	P value
Predictor variables			
Age (per 10-year age increase)	1.51	1.27–1.80	<0.001
Body mass index (per 1 kg/m² increase)	1.00	0.92–1.09	0.938
Hypertension (yes/no)	1.72	0.94–3.17	0.081
Cardiovascular disease (yes/no)	0.35	0.05–2.54	0.300
Stroke (yes/no)	1.75	0.75–4.10	0.195
DBP (per 1 mmHg increase)	0.97	0.95–0.99	0.003
MAP (per 1 mmHg increase)	0.99	0.98–1.00	0.071
eGFR (per 1mL/min per 1.73m² increase)	0.93	0.85–1.03	0.146
C-reactive protein(per 1 mg/L increase)	1.00	0.98–1.03	0.852
Serum albumin (per 1g/L increase)	1.00	0.95–1.05	0.937
Multivariate model[a]			
Age (per 10-year age increase)	1.63	1.35–1.96	<0.001

Abbreviations: DBP, diastolic blood pressure; MAP, mean artery pressure; eGFR, estimated glomerular filtration rate; CI, confidence interval.
[a]Adjusted for variables from the above predictor variables using a backward stepwise cox proportional hazards model with a stay criterion of 0.10. P<0.05 represents statistical significant.

hypertension, cardiovascular disease, stroke, DBP, MAP, and eGFR. The predictors of pneumonia for the non-DN group are summarized in Table 4. Significant variables included age and DBP by univariate Cox regression analysis. Only older age remained significant in the multivariate model after adjusting for BMI, hypertension, cardiovascular disease, stroke, DBP, MAP, eGFR, CRP, and serum albumin, which showed that every 10-year increase in age increased the risk of a pneumonia event by 63% (HR, 1.63; 95% CI, 1.35–1.96; P<0.001).

Pneumonia and survival

Fatal events were registered during follow-up. A total of 164 patients died and 21 deaths were pneumonia related. In terms of all-cause death, 57 occurred in the DN group and 107 in the non-DN group. In terms of pneumonia-related deaths, 10 occurred in the DN group and 11 in the non-DN group. Furthermore, the cumulative pneumonia-related mortality was 4%, 10%, and 23% at 1, 3, and 5 years, respectively, in the DN group compared with 1%, 4%, and 6% at 1, 3, and 5 years, respectively, in the non-DN group. Meanwhile, the cumulative overall mortality at 1, 3, and 5 years was 25%, 50%, and 58%, respectively, in the DN group compared with 9%, 24%, and 33%, respectively, in the non-DN group.

Mortality analyses

Compared with non-DN patients, DN patients were at increased risk of all-cause and pneumonia-related mortality based on Kaplan-Meier curves and Cox regression analysis (Figure 2). In univariate analysis risk of diabetic nephropathy, the cumulative hazard was significantly higher in the DN group. Specifically, it was 2.608 (95% CI, 1.890–3.599; P<0.001) for all-cause mortality and 4.424 (95% CI, 1.871–10.461; P<0.001) for pneumonia-related mortality. Furthermore, the association between DN and all-cause or pneumonia-related mortality was studied by multivariate Cox analysis (Figure 3). Similar to the univariate analysis of model 1, this elevated risk of all-cause mortality persisted after adjustment for various potential confounders, whereas adjustments for age, gender, and BMI in model 2 slightly decreased the strength (HR,1.581; 95% CI, 1.082–2.226; P = 0.017). There was still a statistically significant association found between DN and the risk of pneumonia-related mortality by additional adjustment for various confounders. In a full model including demographics, comorbidities, and labs, the adjusted HR was 4.831 (95% CI, 1.927–12.109; P = 0.001).

Discussion

This prospective study of a single peritoneal dialysis center offers a detailed evaluation of the epidemiology, clinical features, and outcomes of pneumonia in CAPD patients. The main findings are that (i) CAPD patients with DN had a higher incidence of developing pneumonia than non-DN patients; (ii) risk factors for pneumonia occurrence were higher BMI and lower serum albumin in DN patients during CAPD, whereas older age was an independent predictor of the incidence of pneumonia in non-DN patients; and (iii) all-cause and pneumonia-related mortality rates were significantly higher in CAPD patients with DN.

The clinical epidemiology of pneumonia in dialysis patients has received comparatively little attention to date. The United States Renal Data System shows that in dialysis patients pulmonary infections account for about 115 hospital admissions per 1000 patient-years of risk [1]. Other observational studies suggest that

nosocomial infections, including pneumonia, are much more common in hospitalized dialysis patients than in their non-dialyzed counterparts [11]. Guo et al. reported a pneumonia rate of 29.0 episodes per 100 patient-years in hemodialysis patients [12], which was higher than the rate of hospitalization for pneumonia as the primary diagnosis (18.2 per 100 patient-years) in peritoneal dialysis patients. For comparison with our population, we collected all pneumonia incidences (diagnosed by chest x-rays exhibiting signs of infection in the lungs), including hospital and community-acquired pneumonia. We found the overall pneumonia rates were 34.3/1,000 patient-years, and pneumonia rates in the DN patients were 62.3/1,000 patient-years, as well as 28.5/1,000 patient-years in the non-DN patients. There may be several explanations for the lower prevalence of pneumonia in our population than in the data reported previously in dialysis patients. On the one hand, we applied a uniform and relatively strict standard in diagnosing pneumonia by chest x-rays, which may have lead to us missing some cases. On the other hand, our participants were mainly from Guangdong province located in southern China where the climate is so mild that the occurrence of pneumonia is not very prevalent. Interestingly, we found that the CAPD patients with DN were more susceptible to develop pneumonia. Importantly, we found the hazard of developing pneumonia for CAPD patients with DN was significantly higher than the patients without DN.

Diabetes is frequently associated with multiple complications, such as hypertension, ischemic heart disease, left ventricular hypertrophy, arrhythmia, diabetic nephropathy, arteriosclerosis obliterans, diabetic retinopathy, hyperglycemia, and dyslipidemia, which exist even before the pre-dialysis stage [13]. In the present study, CAPD patients with DN were older, and more commonly had comorbidities of hypertension, a cardiovascular condition (chronic heart or cerebrovascular disease), and stroke. Moreover, we found that pneumonia patients with DN were significantly associated with higher BMI and lower serum albumin, which also were independent predictors of pneumonia occurrence even when extensive demographics, comorbidities, and lab adjustments were made. Our results agree with the report which showed that low levels of serum albumin associated with greater pneumonia risk in

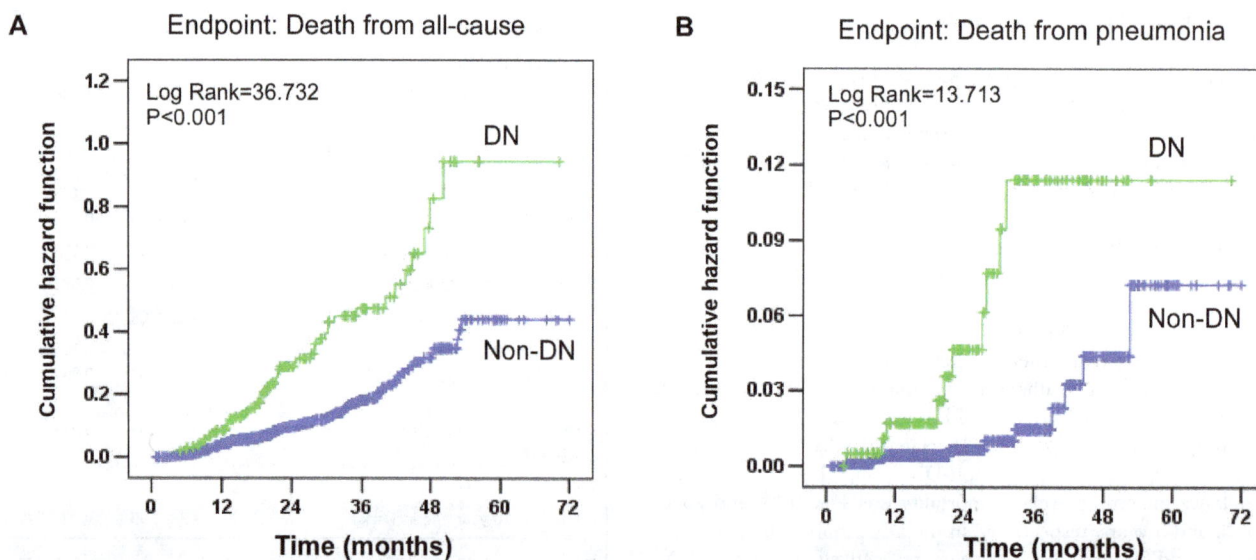

Figure 2. Cumulative incidences of all-cause and pneumonia-related death according to diabetic nephropathy. (A) Cumulative hazard of all-cause death. The HR in the DN, as compared with non-DN, was 2.608 (95% CI, 1.890–3.599). (B) Cumulative hazard of pneumonia death, for which the HR in the DN group was 4.424 (95% CI, 1.871–10.461).

A   Hazard Ratio (95% CI)

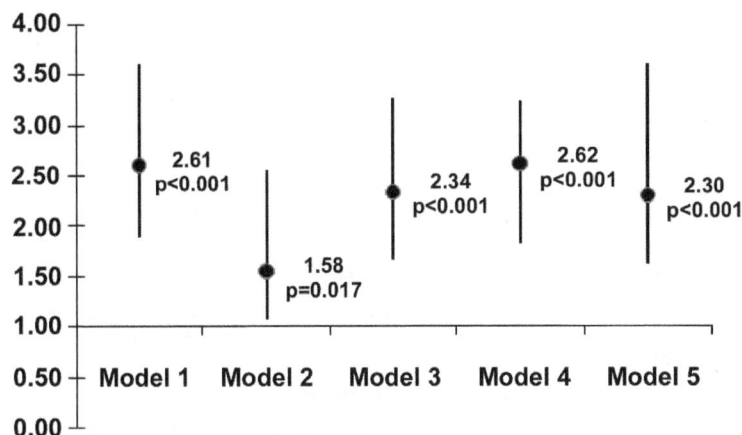

B   Hazard Ratio (95% CI)

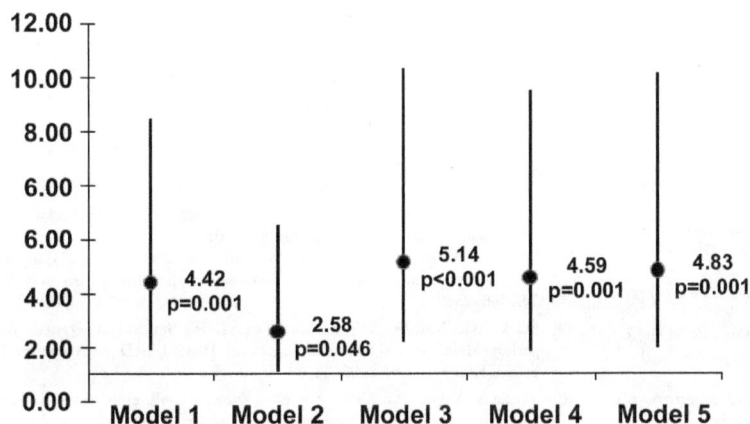

Model 1: Univariate analysis risk of diabetic nephropathy
Model 2: 1+ age, sex, BMI
Model 3: 2+ hypertension, cardiovascular disease, stroke
Model 4: 3+ eGFR
Model 5: 4+ serum albumin, HDL-C, LDL-C

Figure 3. The hazard ratios of diabetic nephropathy on CAPD for the prediction of all-cause and pneumonia-related mortality. (A) All-cause mortality and (B) pneumonia-related mortality by diabetic nephropathy. BMI, body mass index; eGFR, estimated glomerular filtration rate; MAP, mean artery pressure; CRP, C-reactive protein; HDL-C, high-density lipoprotein; LDL-C, low-density lipoprotein; HR, hazard ratio; CI, confidence interval.

dialysis patients [12]. Obviously, obesity (measured as a BMI) increases the risk for diabetes and is also an independent risk factor for ESRD [14–16]. Likewise, our findings are partially consistent with large studies (of >1000 participants) among incident dialysis patients with a long-term follow-up (5–10 years) which showed that high BMI was associated with worse dialysis outcomes and increased mortality risk among peritoneal dialysis and hemodialysis patients [17–19]. Therefore, intensive management of risk factors (high BMI and low albumin) and prompt recognition of infection is therefore recommended for CAPD patients with DN to improve quality of life. In addition, an independent risk factor in our study for the presence of pneumonia in non-DN patients was older age. A similar observation was previously made among older patients [20,21].

Sarnak and Jaber reported that pulmonary infection mortality rates are 14–16 times higher in dialysis patients than in the general population [2]. In our study, the pulmonary mortality of 5.3% found in CAPD patients with DN, was five times higher than in non-DN patients. Meanwhile, the cumulative hazard was 4.831 (95% CI, 1.927–12.109; P = 0.001) for pneumonia-related mortality when adjustments were made for extensive demographics, comorbidities, and labs in DN patients after an episode of pneumonia. A similar trend was observed for all-cause mortality. According to the report, patients with diabetes mellitus are considered to be immunocompromised and therefore more susceptible to infections [22]. ESRD is widely understood to be a state of inflammatory, endothelial, and redox dysfunction [23–25]. Micro-inflammation is a pivotal contributor to the pathogenesis of cardiovascular disease [26]. Therefore, DN patients on CAPD may be chronically immunosuppressed, by virtue of the uremic internal milieu and the very frequent coexistence of serious comorbid medical conditions. Pneumonia typically leads to 'macro'-inflammation. Standard indices of inflammatory activity were not available in this study. Thus, our hypothesis that pneumonia and subsequent mortality reflect sudden increases in inflammatory activity remains speculative.

This study was limited in that it was a prospective observational study and pneumonia was identified based on results of a chest x-ray test, which might miss some pneumonia patients. A substantial number of pneumonia cases likely occurred after admission to the hospital with another serious illness. In this scenario, an association between pneumonia and mortality could reflect the occurrence of this other serious illness, without a direct causal link between pneumonia and death. Our study involved a prevalent cohort of CAPD patients; therefore, patients were not studied at a uniform phase of their chronic kidney disease. Smoking and microbiologic test data were not used because of incomplete information.

Despite its limitations, our study may have practical implications. We found that higher BMI and lower serum albumin are independent predictors for pneumonia in CAPD patients with DN, which suggests that these patients should pay attention to weight control but avoid malnutrition. Furthermore, both the burden of disease and mortality associations were noteworthy. These findings might encourage the use of preventive measures, timely diagnosis of pneumonia, and prompt initiation of appropriate treatment. Prospective mechanistic, observational, and therapeutic research is greatly needed in this population.

Acknowledgments

We thank the trial nurses in our peritoneal dialysis center. We express our gratitude to all patients who participated in the study.

Author Contributions

Conceived and designed the experiments: F. Huang XY. Performed the experiments: F. He XW XX FP. Analyzed the data: F. He XW. Contributed reagents/materials/analysis tools: F. Huang. Wrote the paper: F. He.

References

1. Bethesda (2006) US Renal Data System. USRDS 2006 Annual Data Report. National Institutes of Health, National Institute of Diabetes and Digestive and Kidney Diseases.
2. Sarnak MJ, Jaber BL (2001) Pulmonary infectious mortality among patients with end-stage renal disease. Chest 120: 1883–1887.
3. Slinin Y, Foley RN, Collins AJ (2006) Clinical epidemiology of pneumonia in hemodialysis patients: the USRDS waves 1, 3, and 4 study. Kidney Int 70:1135–1141.
4. Benfield T, Jensen JS, Nordestgaard BG (2007) Influence of diabetes and hyperglycaemia on infectious disease hospitalisation and outcome. Diabetologia 50:549–554.
5. Shah BR, Hux JE (2003) Quantifying the risk of infectious diseases for people with diabetes. Diabetes Care 26:510–513.
6. Kaparianos A, Argyropoulou E, Sampsonas F, Karkoulias K, Tsiamita M, et al. (2008) Pulmonary complications in diabetes mellitus. Chron Respir Dis 5:101–108.
7. Remuzzi G, Macia M, Ruggenenti P (2006) Prevention and treatment of diabetic renal disease in type 2 diabetes: the BENEDICT study. J Am Soc Nephrol 17(4 Suppl 2):S90–S97.
8. Xie Y, Chen X (2008) Epidemiology, major outcomes, risk factors, prevention and management of chronic kidney disease in China. Am J Nephrol 28: 1–7.
9. Hoogeveen EK, Halbesma N, Rothman KJ, Stijnen T, van Dijk S, et al. (2012) Obesity and mortality risk among younger dialysis patients. Clin J Am Soc Nephrol 7:280–288.
10. (1989) Recommendations on stroke prevention, diagnosis, and therapy. Report of the WHO Task Force on Stroke and other Cerebrovascular Disorders. Stroke 20:1407–1431.
11. D'Agata EM, Mount DB, Thayer V, Schaffner W (2000) Hospital-acquired infections among chronic hemodialysis patients. Am J Kidney Dis 35:1083–1088.
12. Guo H, Liu J, Collins AJ, Foley RN (2008) Pneumonia in incident dialysis patients-the United States Renal Data System. Nephrol Dial Transplant 23:680–686.
13. Kuriyama S (2007) Peritoneal dialysis in patients with diabetes: are the benefits greater than the disadvantages? Perit Dial Int 27:S190–S195.
14. Adams KF, Schatzkin A, Harris TB, Kipnis V, Mouw T, et al. (2006) Overweight, obesity, and mortality in a large prospective cohort of persons 50 to 71 years old. N Engl J Med 355:763–78.
15. de Mutsert R, Snijder MB, van der Sman-de Beer F, Seidell JC, Boeschoten EW, et al. (2007) Association between body mass index and mortality is similar in the hemodialysis population and the general population at high age and equal duration of follow-up. J Am Soc Nephrol 18:967–974.
16. Praga M (2002) Obesity-a neglected culprit in renal disease. Nephrol Dial Transplant 17:1157–1159.
17. McDonald SP, Collins JF, Johnson DW (2003) Obesity is associated with worse peritoneal dialysis outcomes in the Australia and New Zealand patient populations. J Am Soc Nephrol 14:2894–901.
18. Beddhu S, Pappas LM, Ramkumar N, Samore M (2003) Effects of body size and body composition on survival in hemodialysis patients. J Am Soc Nephrol 14:2366–2372.
19. Stack AG, Murthy BV, Molony DA (2004) Survival differences between peritoneal dialysis and hemodialysis among "large" ESRD patients in the United States. Kidney Int 65:2398–2408.
20. Yende S, Angus DC, Ali IS, Somes G, Newman AB, et al. (2007) Influence of comorbid conditions on long-term mortality after pneumonia in older people. J Am Geriatr Soc 55:518–525.
21. O'Meara ES, White M, Siscovick DS, Lyles MF, Kuller LH (2005) Hospitalization for pneumonia in the Cardiovascular Health Study: incidence, mortality, and influence on longer-term survival. J Am Geriatr Soc 53:1108–1116.
22. Vardakas KZ, Siempos II, Falagas ME (2007) Diabetes mellitus as a risk factor for nosocomial pneumonia and associated mortality. Diabet Med 24:1168–1171.
23. Stenvinkel P, Heimbürger O, Paultre F, Diczfalusy U, Wang T, et al. (1999) Strong association between malnutrition, inflammation, and atherosclerosis in chronic renal failure. Kidney Int 55:1899–1911.
24. Miyamoto T, Carrero JJ, Stenvinkel P (2011) Inflammation as a risk factor and target for therapy in chronic kidney disease. Curr Opin Nephrol Hypertens 20:662–8.
25. Piroddi M, Depunzio I, Calabrese V, Mancuso C, Aisa CM, et al. (2007) Oxidatively-modified and glycated proteins as candidate pro-inflammatory toxins in uremia and dialysis patients. Amino Acids 32:573–592.
26. Navab KD, Elboudwarej O, Gharif M, Yu J, Hama SY, et al. (2011) Chronic inflammatory disorders and accelerated atherosclerosis: chronic kidney disease. Curr Pharm Des 17:17–20.

The Associations of Uric Acid, Cardiovascular and All-Cause Mortality in Peritoneal Dialysis Patients

Jie Dong[1]*, Qing-Feng Han[2], Tong-Ying Zhu[3], Ye-Ping Ren[4], Jiang-Hua Chen[5], Hui-Ping Zhao[6], Meng-Hua Chen[7], Rong Xu[1], Yue Wang[2], Chuan-Ming Hao[3], Rui Zhang[4], Xiao-Hui Zhang[5], Mei Wang[6], Na Tian[7], Hai-Yan Wang[1]

1 Renal Division, Department of Medicine, Peking University First Hospital; Institute of Nephrology, Peking University; Key Laboratory of Renal Disease, Ministry of Health; Key Laboratory of Renal Disease, Ministry of Education; Beijing, China, 2 Department of Nephrology, Peking University Third Hospital, Beijing, China, 3 Department of Nephrology, Huashan Hospital of Fudan University, Shanghai, China, 4 Department of Nephrology, Second Affiliated Hospital of Harbin Medical University, Heilongjiang, China, 5 Kidney Disease Center, The First Affiliated Hospital, College of Medicine, Zhejiang University, Hangzhou, China, 6 Department of Nephrology, Peking University People's Hospital, Beijing, China, 7 Department of Nephrology, General Hospital of Ningxia Medical University, Ningxia, China

Abstract

Aims: To investigate whether uric acid (UA) is an independent predictor of cardiovascular (CV) and all-cause mortality in peritoneal dialysis (PD) patients after controlling for recognized CV risk factors.

Methods: A total of 2264 patients on chronic PD were collected from seven centers affiliated with the Socioeconomic Status on the Outcome of Peritoneal Dialysis (SSOP) Study. All demographic and laboratory data were recorded at baseline. Multivariate Cox regression was used to calculate the hazard ratio (HR) of CV and all-cause mortality with adjustments for recognized traditional and uremia-related CV factors.

Results: There were no significant differences in baseline characteristics between patients with (n = 2193) and without (n = 71) UA measured. Each 1 mg/dL of increase in UA was associated with higher all-cause mortality with 1.05(1.00~1.10) of HR and higher CV mortality with 1.12 (1.05~1.20) of HR after adjusting for age, gender and center size. The highest gender-specific tertile of UA predicted higher all-cause mortality with 1.23(1.00~1.52) of HR and higher CV mortality with 1.69 (1.21~2.38) of HR after adjusting for age, gender and center size. The predictive value of UA was stronger in patients younger than 65 years without CV disease or diabetes at baseline. The prognostic value of UA as both continuous and categorical variable weakened or disappeared after further adjusted for uremia-related and traditional CV risk factors.

Conclusions: The prognostic value of UA in CV and all-cause mortality was weak in PD patients generally, which was confounded by uremia-related and traditional CV risk factors.

Editor: Yan Li, Shanghai Institute of Hypertension, China

Funding: This study is supported in part by New Century Excellent Talents from The Education Department, China, Baxer Clinical Research Award from Baxter Corp, China, and an ISN Research Award from the ISN GO R&P Committee. The funders had no role in study design, data collection and analysis, decision to publish, or preparation of the manuscript.

Competing Interests: This study was partly funded by Baxter Corp and there are no patents, products in development or marketed products to declare. This does not alter adherence to all the PLOS ONE policies on sharing data and materials, as detailed online in the guide for authors.

* E-mail: dongjie@medmail.com.cn

Introduction

Increased cardiovascular (CV) events have been extensively documented in patients with end-stage renal disease (ESRD) including peritoneal dialysis (PD) and hemodialysis(HD) population [1,2]. CV events still accounts for approximately 40% of the annual mortality in dialysis patients [3]. Although numerous risk factors, categorized into traditional, uremic-related and non-traditional factors, have been recognized in recent years [4,5], series of meta-analysis have not been able to demonstrate significant effect of targeting some of factors such as hyperlipidemia [6], hyperhomocystinemia [7], oxidative stress [8] and hyperphosphatemia [9] on outcomes in this high-risk patient group. Exploring novel and potentially modifiable risk factors for CV and all-cause mortality is therefore urgent.

Uric acid (UA), as one of novel risk factors, has been paid more attention in recent years. In general population, previous studies have shown that UA is closely associated with hypertension, coronary heart disease and chronic kidney disease (CKD) [10–12]. High UA also could independently predict CV events and mortality for ones with chronic diseases including CKD [13–15]. For dialysis population, a few studies from HD population indicated inconsistent relationship between UA and outcomes, that is, UA is negatively or 'J-shaped' related to all-cause or CV mortality [16–19]. There is no specific data on UA and outcomes for PD population yet.

In the present study, we aimed to explore associations of UA, all-cause and CV mortality in a large-scale multi-center PD cohort. The prognostic value of UA would be compared between patients≥65 years and <65years, with or without CV disease

(CVD), diabetes and non-diabetes at baseline respectively. In addition, we determined whether associations of UA and outcomes would be changed after controlling for uremic-related factors(albumin, hemoglobin, residual renal function, phosphate etc) and traditional CV risk factors (hypertension, hyperlipidemia, obesity, diabetes, etc).

Methods

This is an affiliated study with the Socioeconomic Status on the Outcome of Peritoneal Dialysis (SSOP) Study, which is a retrospective multi-center cohort study as described in detail in our previous paper [20]. The ethics committee of Peking University First Hospital approved this study.

Centers enrollment

Centers which have professional PD doctors and PD nurses, and have well-developed databases of at least 3-years duration, recording baseline characteristics and follow-up data every 1~3 months for each patient in our country participated this study voluntarily. Totally 9 centers were qualified, and 7 of them agreed to participate providing about 70 percent of all incident patients from 9 centers. Enrolled centers were from 5 provinces and located at 4 geographical regions (north, northeast, northwest, or east) in China. Data from each center have been collected within the strict quality control framework and further inspected and optimized to keep integrity and accuracy of the database. All study investigators and staff members completed a training program that taught them the methods and processes of the study. A manual of detailed instructions for data collection was distributed.

Subjects selection

All the incident patients on chronic PD between the date of intact database creation and August 2011 were enrolled into this study. Each patient signed informed consent to agree their demographic and lab data to be used in future studies since they started PD therapy. All subjects began the PD program within one month after catheter implantation and were given lactate-buffered glucose dialysate with a twin-bag connection system (Baxter Healthcare, Guangzhou, China).

Data collection

Demographic and clinical data including age, gender, body mass index (BMI), socioeconomic status (income and education level, living condition, etc), primary renal disease, the presence of cardiovascular disease (CVD) and diabetes mellitus (DM) were collected at baseline. Center size was also recorded according to number of enrolled patients of each center. CVD was recorded if one of the following conditions was present: angina, class III–IV congestive heart failure (NYHA), trandient ischemic attack, history of myocardial infarction or cerebrovascular accident and peripheral arterial disease [21].

Blood pressures were measured according to the guidelines presented in the Seventh Report of the Joint National Committee on Prevention, Detection, Evaluation and Treatment of High Blood pressure [22]. Patients took antihypertensive medications and performed the bag exchange as usual at their home on the morning of each clinic visit. A skilled nurse using a mercury sphygmomanometer measured brachial blood pressure in sitting position after they had rested for at least 10 minutes in a quiet and peaceful room. Systolic and diastolic blood pressure, and calculated mean arterial pressure during the first 3 months were averaged for at least three times of readings.

Biochemistry data including hemoglobin, serum albumin, UA, lipids spectrum, glucose, calcium, phosphate and intact parathyroid hormone (iPTH) were examined using an automatic Hitachi chemistry analyzer. The first testing was completed within one month of PD at the first visit, and then repeatedly once a month. The mean values in the first 3 months were calculated. The coefficient of variation of UA from multiple measurements was 5.3% for subjects from Peking University First Hospital but not recorded for those from other hospitals. Serum UA was measured by the uricase method using the same autoanalyzer. Serum high sensitive C-reactive protein (CRP) was measured by immune rate nephelometric analysis. Dialysis adequacy and residual renal function (RRF) were measured after one month of dialysis therapy. RRF was defined as the mean of residual creatinine clearance and residual urea clearance. Dialysis adequacy was defined as total Kt/V and total creatinine clearance. Corrected calcium was calculated by standard equation: Corrected calcium = serum total calcium+0.02*(40-serum albumin in g/L).

Definition of outcome event

The outcomes were defined as cardiovascular and all-cause death. The cardiovascular death was defined as death due to myocardial infarction, congestive heart failure, cerebral bleeding, cerebral infarction, arrhythmia, peripheral arterial disease, and sudden death. In all analysis, we censored follow-up at trandferring to HD, loss to follow-up, renal trandplantation, or the end of the study (November 1, 2011).

Statistical analysis

Continuous data were presented as mean with SDs except for CRP and RRF, which were presented as median (interquartile range) because of a high skew. Categorical variables were presented as proportions. Patients' data were compared by using the t-test or ANOVA F-test for normally distributed continuous variables, chi-square test for categorical variables, and Mann-Whitney U test for skewed continuous variables. UA was trandformed into categorical variable by gender-specific tertiles or quartiles.

For determining associations of UA, CV and all-cause mortality, UA as continuous variable was first examined in Cox regression models after adjusting for age, gender and center size (model 1) for all participants, and then in subgroups such as patients≥65 years or <65 years, with or without CVD, with or without DM respectively. Next, we explored whether associations of UA and CV/all-cause mortality in all participants were confounded by traditional and uremia-related CVD factors. Uremia-related factors such as serum albumin, hemoglobin, phosphate, RRF and CRP (model 2), and additional traditional CV factors such as BMI, the history of diabetes or CVD, mean arterial pressure and LDL cholesterol(model 3) were constructed respectively. For these examinations, UA was also considered as categorical variable by gender-specific tertiles or quartiles respectively but only gender-specific tertiles of UA was shown in the context since similar linear trends were indicated. Gender was not included as the adjusted variable if UA is examined as the gender-specific variable.

We reported the multivariable adjusted hazards ratios (HRs) with 95% CIs. All probabilities were two-tailed, and the level of significance was set at 0.05. Statistical analysis was performed by SPSS for Windows software version 13.0 (SPSS Inc., Chicago, IL).

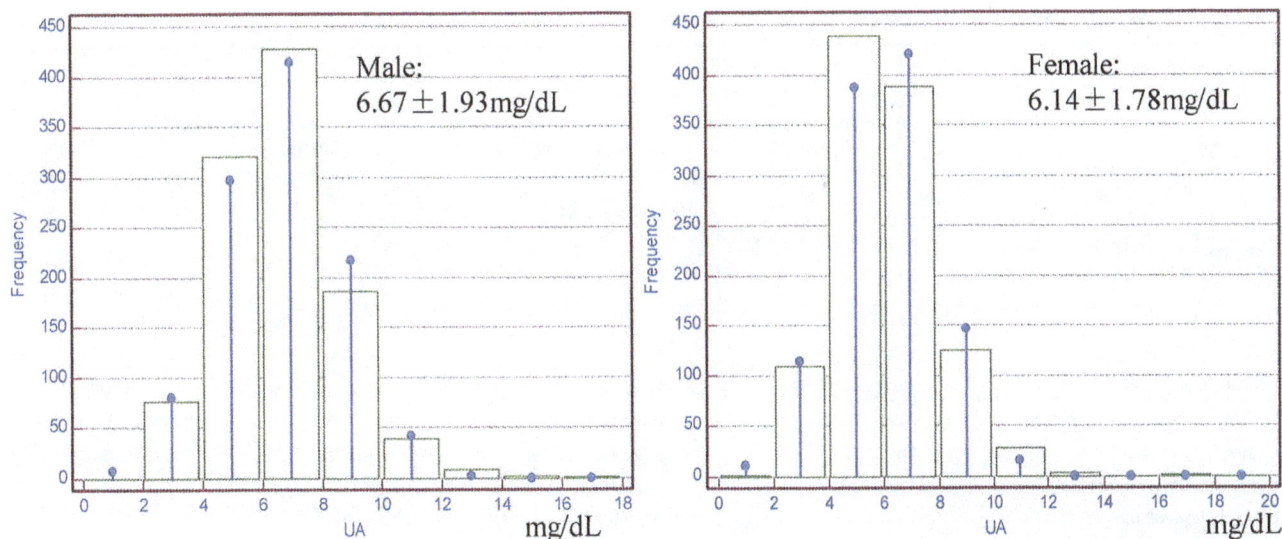

n=1078 for male, 1115 for female

Figure 1. The distribution chart of serum uric acid.

Results

Baseline characteristics and follow-up

A total of 2264 PD patients were collected, with a mean age of 58.1 ± 15.5 years, BMI of 22.9 ± 3.6 kg/m^2; 37.7% were diabetic and CVD was present in 41.5% of subjects at baseline. Chronic glomerulonephritis was the most common cause of ESRD (34.4%), followed by diabetic nephropathy (29.3%) and hypertensive nephropathy (15.5%). There were 71 of 2264 patients without UA values at baseline. The mean age, BMI, MBP, serum lipids, distribution of primary renal disease, CVD history, prevalence of DM were not significantly different between those who had measured UA and those who did not (2193 patients) ($P > 0.05$). A total of 80 patients with inactive solid organ tumors at baseline were not excluded since their UA values were comparable to the remainders, and linear trends of UA and outcomes were not changed when they were excluded. Thereafter, 2193 patients were included in the final analysis.

The median follow-up time was 26.5(13.6~43.6) months. At the end of study, of 586 (26.7% of 2193) patients who died, 231 cases (39.4%) were due to CVD, 140 cases (23.8%) were due to infection, and other causes of death included malignancy (11.9%), gastrointestinal bleeding (4.3%), severe malnutrition (4.8%), miscellaneous (5.1%), and undefined (10.6%). Of 231 patients who died from CVD, the leading cause was myocardial infarction (52 cases, 22.5%), followed by congestive heart failure (19.0%), cerebral bleeding (14.3%), cerebral infarction (12.9%), sudden death (9.5%), arrhythmia (4.8%), peripheral arterial disease (1.3%), and undefined causes (15.1%).

UA and clinic characteristics

The mean values of UA were 6.41 ± 1.87 mg/dL for the whole cohort. The normal distribution of UA in male and female was shown respectively in **Fig. 1**. The clinical characteristics and biochemistry data of patients by gender-specific tertiles of UA were

represented in **Table 1**. Patients with higher UA were more likely to be younger and obese. The prevalence of CVD was highest but diabetes was lowest in high tertile group. Systolic and diastolic blood pressure, serum albumin, urea nitrogen, creatinine, phosphate, and parathyroid hormone levels increased, but corrected calcium, hemoglobin and total Kt/V decreased in the middle/high tertiles. Serum CRP, triglycerides, total cholesterol, HDL and LDL cholesterol, total Ccr and RRF levels were not significantly different between groups ($P > 0.05$).

The association between UA and outcome

The associations between UA and outcomes were analyzed. First, UA was examined as a continuous variable. Each 1 mg/dL of increase in UA was associated with higher all-cause mortality with 1.05(1.00~1.10) of HR($P = 0.05$) and higher CV mortality with 1.12 (1.05~1.20) of HR($P = 0.001$) after adjusting for age, gender and center size **(Tables 2 and 3)**. We further divided patients into subgroups, i.e.age≥65 years and <65years, with and without CVD, DM and non-DM respectively. For CV mortality rather than all-cause mortality, the prognostic value of UA was significant in low-risk groups such as patients with age<65 years, without CVD or DM at baseline rather than in their counterpars respectively **(Figs. 2 and 3)**. Next, UA was examined as categorical variable by gender-specific tertiles and quartiles (data not shown for the latter). The highest gender-specific tertile of UA predicted higher all-cause mortality with 1.23(1.00~1.52) of HR($P = 0.04$) and higher CV mortality with 1.69 (1.21~2.38) of HR($P = 0.002$) after adjusting for age, gender and center size compared to low tertile of UA. However, the associations of UA and CVD/all-cause mortality weakened after further adjusted for uremia-related factors including serum albumin, hemoglobin, phosphate, and CRP, and disappeared with additional adjustement for traditional CV factors such as CVD history, DM, body mass index, and LDL cholestrol **(Table 2 and 3)**.

Table 1. Clinical characteristics and biochemistry data of patients by gender-specific tertiles of UA.

Variables	Tertile 1 M: 2.09~5.79 mg/dL FM: 1.74~5.37 mg/dL	Tertile 2 M: 5.80~7.38 mg/dL FM: 5.38~6.65 mg/dL	Tertile 3 M: 7.39~16.7 mg/dL FM: 6.66~8.08 mg/dL	P values[&]
N	731	731	731	—
Age, yrs	61.9±15.1***	57.7±15.4$^{\Delta\Delta\Delta}$	54.7±15.3$^{\#\#\#}$	<0.001
Male (%)	49.2	49	49.2	0.99
BMI, Kg/m^2	22.4±3.5***	23.3±3.6	23.1±3.7$^{\#\#\#}$	<0.001
Diabetes (%)	40.2	40.6$^{\Delta\Delta}$	32.8$^{\#\#}$	0.003
CVD history (%)	34.8**	42.7	46.6$^{\#\#\#}$	<0.001
Systolic blood pressure, mmHg	133.5±22.5**	137.8±18.9	138.7±16.5$^{\#\#\#}$	<0.001
Diastolic blood pressure, mmHg	78.4±12.9**	80.5±12.9	82.1±11.2$^{\#\#}$	<0.001
Triglycerides, mmol/L	1.84±1.28	1.94±1.29	1.87±1.08	0.23
Total cholesterol, mmol/L	4.92±1.27	4.97±1.28	4.82±1.23	0.08
HDL cholesterol, mmol/L	1.16±0.38	1.13±0.35	1.14±0.37	0.2
LDL cholesterol, mmol/L	2.71±0.89	2.71±0.96	2.69±0.93	0.97
Albumin, g/L	33.9±5.4***	35.6±5.1$^{\Delta\Delta}$	36.5±5.2$^{\#\#\#}$	<0.001
Hemoglogin, g/dL	103.6±19.5	104.2±18.6	101.7±19.8	0.04
UA, mg/dL	4.5±0.8***	6.3±0.5$^{\Delta\Delta\Delta}$	8.4±1.4$^{\#\#\#}$	<0.001
Urea nitrogen, mmol/L	17.7±6.3***	21.0±6.3$^{\Delta\Delta\Delta}$	23.1±7.1$^{\#\#\#}$	<0.001
Creatinine, umol/L	621.8±242.8***	695.0±246.9$^{\Delta\Delta\Delta}$	728.9±274.5$^{\#\#\#}$	<0.001
Corrected calcium, mmol/L	2.29±0.25	2.29±0.25$^{\Delta\Delta\Delta}$	2.25±0.24$^{\#\#\#}$	<0.001
Parathyroid hormone, pg/ml	157.8 (74.5, 318.9)	163.5(75.9, 314.8)$^{\Delta}$	196.8(91.8, 345.7)$^{\#}$	0.02
Phosphate, mmol/L	1.4±0.4***	1.6±0.4$^{\Delta\Delta\Delta}$	1.7±0.5$^{\#\#\#}$	<0.001
CRP, mg/L	3.1(1.2, 6.9)	2.6(1.0, 7.8)	2.8(1.0, 7.5)	0.32
Total Kt/V	2.19±0.65***	2.01±0.60	1.95±0.63$^{\#\#\#}$	<0.001
Total Ccr, L/w/1.73m2	76.2±30.9	73.5±33.6	73.3±30.3	0.23
RRF, ml/min	3.1(1.4, 5.2)	3.2(1.6, 5.2)	3.7(1.8, 5.8)	0.16

Abbreviations: M, male; FM, female; UA, uric acid; BMI, body mass index; CVD, cardiovascular disease; CRP, C-reactive protein; Ccr, creatinie clearance; RRF, residual renal function.
[&]P for comparisons among tertiles.
*P<0.05, **P<0.01, ***P<0.001 for Tertile 1 vs Tertile 2.
$^{\Delta}$P<0.05, $^{\Delta\Delta}$P<0.01, $^{\Delta\Delta\Delta}$P<0.001 for Tertile 2 vs Tertile 3.
$^{\#}$P<0.05, $^{\#\#}$P<0.01, $^{\#\#\#}$P<0.01 for Tertile 1 vs Tertile 3.

Discussion

In contrast to previous studies on HD patients showing a negative or 'J-shaped' relationship between UA and mortality [16–19], the present PD study did ont indicate similar trends between UA and CV or all-cause mortality. One may suspect that it is due to that the mean UA values in this cohort is quite different. This hypothesis is easily denied since the mean UA values(6.4 mg/dL) for our participants were very close to those reported in HD patients [16–19,23]. It was also hypothesized that the inverse association of UA and outcome previously reported is confounded by nutrition status as indicated from DOPPS data [19]. From our data, although serum UA was also closely associated with higher body mass index, serum albumin, creatinine, phosphorous and better residual renal function, we could not observe a similar trend to HD patients.

The inconsistent trend of UA and outcomes was more likely to be explained by its dual effects on CV outcomes. Excess UA is closely related to components of metabolic syndrome, endothelial dysfunction, inflammation, oxidative stress and activated renin-angiotensin-aldosterone system in general population and patients with CKD [16,24–29]. On the other hand, both in vitro and in vivo studies have shown UA to be a powerful free radical scavenger in humand and could be expected to offer a number of benefits within the cardiovascular system [30,31].Therefore, the final trend for the association of UA and outcomes for a specific population might depend on the balance between the protective and toxic effects of UA. In addition, hyperuricaemia is significantly associated with the rate of decline of RRF [32], and RRF play a critical role in predicting CV events and all-cause death in PD population [33], which might partly contribute to the weakly negative associations of hyperuricaemia and outcomes for our PD patients.

Another interesting finding from our data is that the prognostic value of UA in CV mortality only existed in relatively low-risk patients including ones younger than 65 years, without CVD or DM at the start of PD therapy. This phenomenon has been indicated in previous data. For example, UA levels at either

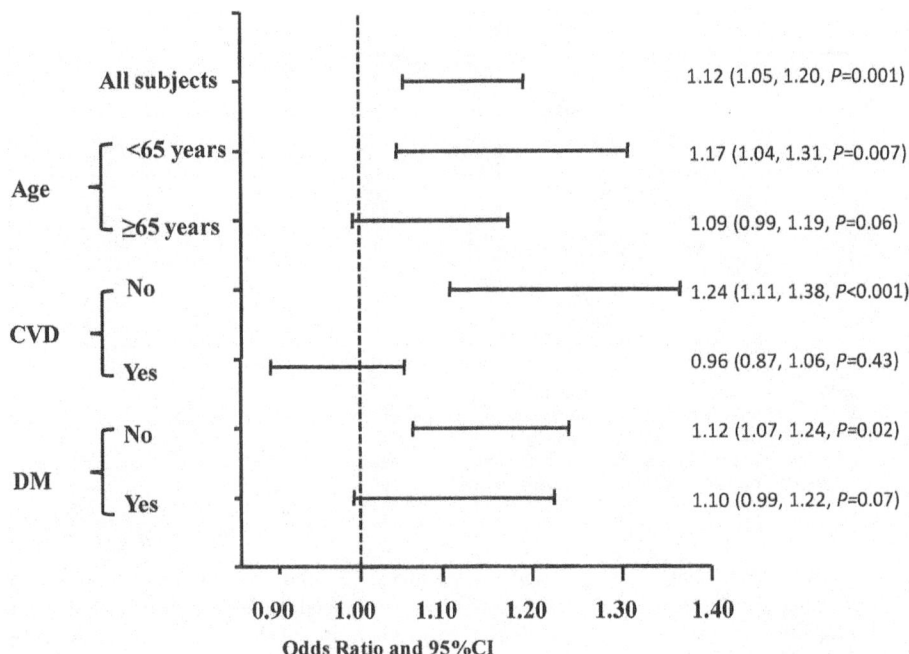

Figure 2. Risk of CVD mortality in all subjects and subgroups. Subgroups were divided by age ≥65 years or <65 years, with or without CVD or DM at baseline. All models are adjusted for age, gender and center size. Abbreviations: UA, uric acid; CDV, cardiovascular disease; DM, diabetes.

extremes predicted higher risk for cardiovascular mortality in general population, which was stronger in subgroups without DM, hypertension, coronary heart disease, stroke, heart failure and CKD [34]. The association between UA and renal function decline was more obvious in subgroups without hypertension and DM from a Chinese population [35]. Inverse associations of serum UA and morbidity of acute ischemic stroke were observed only in non-DM hemodialysis patients [36]. The potential cause for this

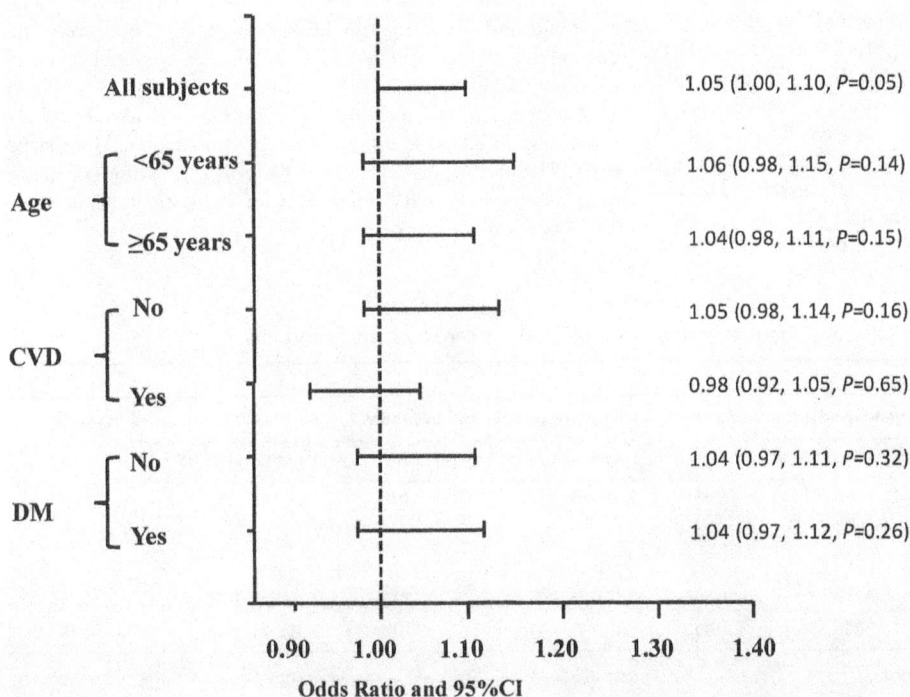

Figure 3. Risk of all-cause mortality in all subjects and subgroups. Subgroups were divided by age ≥65 years or <65 years, with or without CVD or DM at baseline. All models are adjusted for age, gender and center size. Abbreviations: UA, uric acid; CDV, cardiovascular disease; DM, diabetes.

Table 2. The prognostic values of UA as continuous or categorical variable for all-cause mortality.

Subjects	Age, gender-adjusted in Model 1		Multivariate-adjusted in Model 2		Multivariate-adjusted in Model 3	
	Hazard ratio (95% CI)	P	Hazard ratio (95% CI)	P	Hazard ratio (95% CI)	P
UA (per 1 mg/dL increase)	1.05(1.00~1.10)	0.05	1.05(0.98~1.12)	0.15	1.05(0.96~1.14)	0.34
Gender-specific tertiles of UA						
Tertile 1	Reference		Reference		Reference	
Tertile 2	1.09(0.89~1.33)	0.41	1.26 (0.97~1.65)	0.09	1.23 (0.90~1.70)	0.19
Tertile 3	1.23 (1.00~1.52)	0.04	1.30 (0.98~1.75)	0.07	1.21 (0.85~1.73)	0.3

Abbreviation: UA, uric acid; CI, confidence interval.
Model 1: age,center size-adjusted, gender-adjusted only UA as continuous variable.
Model 2: age,residual renal function, serum albumin, hemoglobin,phosphate, C-reactive protein and center size-adjusted, gender-adjusted only UA as continuous variable.
Model 3: age, residual renal function, serum albumin, hemoglobin,phosphate, C-reactive protein, the histroy of cardiovascular disease,diabetes, body mass index, mean arterial pressure, LDL cholestrol and center size-adjusted, gender-adjusted only UA as continuous variable.

phenomena is not clear but it might be relevant to concomitant confounders for CV mortality muting the association of UA and outcome in high-risk subjects. This finding also call us to pay more attention to low-risk subjects with elevated UA value.

Our data further indicated that the association of UA and CV/all-cause mortality was not independent, but rather related to concomitant uremia-related and traditional CV risk factors for PD population. This finding is in accordance with previous data from general population [37–40] and patients with CKD [41,42], showing that independent role of UA weakened or abolished after controlling for some traditional or non-traditional factors. Recently, Chen et al also showed that the association between UA and acute ischemic stroke was confounded by demographic characteristics and malnutrition-microinflammation syndrome in Chinese HD patients [36]. Therefore, whether hyperuricemia represents a marker or a cause for CV events and mortality is still not clear for CKD population [43,44]. Interventional studies should focus on this area to demonstrate if CKD patients would benefit from interventions lowering the elevated UA value.

Our large-scale multi-center cohort study gave us a valuable chance to observe the weak association of UA and CV/all-cause mortality in PD population for the first time. All participants were enrolled from 'core' PD centers of medical school affiliated hospital, which ensure the integrity and accuracy of clinical data

for statistical adjustments. Second, multiple measurements of baseline laboratory were averaged, leading to more reliable data. Only 3.1% of participants missing UA values is also a merit. By contrast, most studies only have one single-point measurement [13,15–17,19,36] or relatively higher percentage of missing values [19].

This study also has several of limitations. First of all, for observational studies where associations do not prove causality, residual confounding cannot entirely be excluded. As a retrospective study, the quality of data collection must have been affected by many uncontrolled factors. There was even no information about the diuretics and/or allopurinol treatment. Smoking habits, alcohol consumption and other non-traditional CV factors were not entirely examined. Howerver, if confounding occurred, it would result in underestimation of the association but not change our main findings at all. In addition, we should be aware of the possibilities of ascertainment bias (totally 3.1% eligible patients were not included).

In conclusion, we suggested that high UA is weakly associated with CV and all-cause mortality for PD population. More large-scale PD cohort studies are needed to verify our findings. Whether high UA levels should be modified for PD patients as done for CKD patients is to be determined.

Table 3. The prognostic values of UA as continuous or categorical variable for cardiovascular mortality.

Subjects	Age, gender-adjusted in Model 1		Multivariate-adjusted in Model 2		Multivariate-adjusted in Model 3	
	Hazard ratio (95% CI)	P	Hazard ratio (95% CI)	P	Hazard ratio (95% CI)	P
UA (per 1 mg/dL increase)	1.12(1.05, 1.20)	0.001	1.05(0.95, 1.17)	0.35	1.04(0.89, 1.20)	0.65
Gender-specific tertiles of UA						
Tertile 1	Reference		Reference		Reference	
Tertile 2	1.56(1.13, 2.15)	0.007	1.48(0.96, 2.29)	0.08	1.29(0.75, 2.23)	0.35
Tertile 3	1.69(1.21, 2.38)	0.002	1.50(0.93, 2.41)	0.09	1.35(0.74, 2.46)	0.33

Abbreviation: UA, uric acid; CI, confidence interval.
Model 1: Age, center size-adjusted, gender-adjusted only UA as continuous variable.
Model 2: Age, residual renal function, serum albumin, hemoglobin,phosphate, C-reactive protein and center size-adjusted, gender-adjusted only UA as continuous variable.
Model 3: Age, residual renal function, serum albumin, hemoglobin,phosphate, C-reactive protein, the history of cardiovascular disease, diabetes, body mass index, mean arterial pressure, LDL cholestrol and center size-adjusted, gender-adjusted only UA as continuous variable.

Acknowledgments

The authors express their appreciation to the patients, doctors, and nursing staff of the peritoneal dialysis center of Peking University First Hospital, Division of Nephrology of Peking University Third Hospital, Division of Nephrology of Huashan Hospital, Fudan University, Division of Nephrology of the second affiliated hospital of Harbin Medical University, Division of Nephrology of Peking University People's Hospital, Division of Nephrology of the first affiliated hospital of Zhejiang University School of Medicine, Division of Nephrology of General Hospital of NingXia Medical University, for their participation in this study.

Author Contributions

Conceived and designed the experiments: JD HYW. Performed the experiments: JD QFH TYZ YPR JHC HPZ MHC RX YW CMH RZ XHZ MW NT. Analyzed the data: JD RX. Contributed reagents/materials/analysis tools: JD RX. Wrote the paper: JD.

References

1. Sarnak MJ, Levey AS, Schoolwerth AC, Coresh J, Culleton B, et al. (2003) Kidney disease as a risk factor for development of cardiovascular disease: a statement from the American Heart Association Councils on Kidney in Cardiovascular Disease, High Blood Pressure Research, Clinical Cardiology, and Epidemiology and Prevention. Hypertension 42: 1050–1065.
2. Elsayed EF, Tighiouart H, Griffith J, Kurth T, Levey AS, et al. (2007) Cardiovascular disease and subsequent kidney disease. Arch Intern Med 167: 1130–1136.
3. USRDS Annual Data Report. Available: http://www.usrds.org/2011/view/v2_04.asp. Accessed 2013 Jun 3.
4. Muntner P, He J, Astor BC, Folsom AR, Coresh J (2005) Traditional and nontraditional risk factors predict coronary heart disease in chronic kidney disease: results from the atherosclerosis risk in communities study. J Am Soc Nephrol 16: 529–538.
5. Stenvinkel P, Carrero JJ, Axelsson J, Lindholm B, Heimburger O, et al. (2008) Emerging biomarkers for evaluating cardiovascular risk in the chronic kidney disease patient: how do new pieces fit into the uremic puzzle? Clin J Am Soc Nephrol 3: 505–521.
6. Navaneethan SD, Nigwekar SU, Perkovic V, Johnson DW, Craig JC, et al. (2009) HMG CoA reductase inhibitors (statins) for dialysis patients. Cochrane Database Syst Rev: CD004289.
7. Pan Y, Guo LL, Cai LL, Zhu XJ, Shu JL, et al. (2012) Homocysteine-lowering therapy does not lead to reduction in cardiovascular outcomes in chronic kidney disease patients: a meta-analysis of randomised, controlled trials. Br J Nutr 108: 400–407.
8. Jun M, Venkataraman V, Razavian M, Cooper B, Zoungas S, et al. (2012) Antioxidants for chronic kidney disease. Cochrane Database Syst Rev 10: CD008176.
9. Palmer SC, Nistor I, Craig JC, Pellegrini F, Messa P, et al. (2013) Cinacalcet in patients with chronic kidney disease: a cumulative meta-analysis of randomized controlled trials. PLoS Med 10: e1001436.
10. Johnson RJ, Kang DH, Feig D, Kivlighn S, Kanellis J, et al. (2003) Is there a pathogenetic role for uric acid in hypertension and cardiovascular and renal disease? Hypertension 41: 1183–1190.
11. Jonasson T, Ohlin AK, Gottsater A, Hultberg B, Ohlin H (2005) Plasma homocysteine and markers for oxidative stress and inflammation in patients with coronary artery disease–a prospective randomized study of vitamin supplementation. Clin Chem Lab Med 43: 628–634.
12. Niskanen LK, Laaksonen DE, Nyyssonen K, Alfthan G, Lakka HM, et al. (2004) Uric acid level as a risk factor for cardiovascular and all-cause mortality in middle-aged men: a prospective cohort study. Arch Intern Med 164: 1546–1551.
13. Madero M, Sarnak MJ, Wang X, Greene T, Beck GJ, et al. (2009) Uric acid and long-term outcomes in CKD. Am J Kidney Dis 53: 796–803.
14. Chen J, Mohler ER 3rd, Xie D, Shlipak MG, Townsend RR, et al. (2012) Risk factors for peripheral arterial disease among patients with chronic kidney disease. Am J Cardiol 110: 136–141.
15. Kanbay M, Yilmaz MI, Sonmez A, Solak Y, Saglam M, et al. (2012) Serum uric acid independently predicts cardiovascular events in advanced nephropathy. Am J Nephrol 36: 324–331.
16. Suliman ME, Johnson RJ, Garcia-Lopez E, Qureshi AR, Molinaei H, et al. (2006) J-shaped mortality relationship for uric acid in CKD. Am J Kidney Dis 48: 761–771.
17. Lee SM, Lee AL, Winters TJ, Tam E, Jaleel M, et al. (2009) Low serum uric acid level is a risk factor for death in incident hemodialysis patients. Am J Nephrol 29: 79–85.
18. Hsu SP, Pai MF, Peng YS, Chiang CK, Ho TI, et al. (2004) Serum uric acid levels show a 'J-shaped' association with all-cause mortality in haemodialysis patients. Nephrol Dial Trandplant 19: 457–462.
19. Latif W, Karaboyas A, Tong L, Winchester JF, Arrington CJ, et al. (2011) Uric acid levels and all-cause and cardiovascular mortality in the hemodialysis population. Clin J Am Soc Nephrol 6: 2470–2477.
20. Xu R, Han QF, Zhu TY, Ren YP, Chen JH, et al. (2012) Impact of individual and environmental socioeconomic status on peritoneal dialysis outcomes: a retrospective multicenter cohort study. PLoS One 7: e50766.
21. Smith SC Jr, Jackson R, Pearson TA, Fuster V, Yusuf S, et al. (2004) Principles for national and regional guidelines on cardiovascular disease prevention: a scientific statement from the World Heart and Stroke Forum. Circulation 109: 3112–3121.
22. Chobanian AV, Bakris GL, Black HR, Cushman WC, Green LA, et al. (2003) The Seventh Report of the Joint National Committee on Prevention, Detection, Evaluation, and Treatment of High Blood Pressure: the JNC 7 report. JAMA 289: 2560–2572.
23. Garg JP, Chasan-Taber S, Blair A, Plone M, Bommer J, et al. (2005) Effects of sevelamer and calcium-based phosphate binders on uric acid concentrations in patients undergoing hemodialysis: a randomized clinical trial. Arthritis Rheum 52: 290–295.
24. Alexander RW (1994) Inflammation and coronary artery disease. N Engl J Med 331: 468–469.
25. Iuliano L (2001) The oxidant stress hypothesis of atherogenesis. Lipids 36 Suppl: S41–44.
26. Caravaca F, Martin MV, Barroso S, Cancho B, Arrobas M, et al. (2005) [Serum uric acid and C-reactive protein levels in patients with chronic kidney disease]. Nefrologia 25: 645–654.
27. Khosla UM, Zharikov S, Finch JL, Nakagawa T, Roncal C, et al. (2005) Hyperuricemia induces endothelial dysfunction. Kidney Int 67: 1739–1742.
28. Kanbay M, Yilmaz MI, Sonmez A, Turgut F, Saglam M, et al. (2011) Serum uric acid level and endothelial dysfunction in patients with nondiabetic chronic kidney disease. Am J Nephrol 33: 298–304.
29. Melendez-Ramirez G, Perez-Mendez O, Lopez-Osorio C, Kuri-Alfaro J, Espinola-Zavaleta N (2012) Effect of the treatment with allopurinol on the endothelial function in patients with hyperuricemia. Endocr Res 37: 1–6.
30. Nieto FJ, Iribarren C, Gross MD, Comstock GW, Cutler RG (2000) Uric acid and serum antioxidant capacity: a reaction to atherosclerosis? Atherosclerosis 148: 131–139.
31. Suzuki T (2007) Nitrosation of uric acid induced by nitric oxide under aerobic conditions. Nitric Oxide 16: 266–273.
32. Park JT, Kim DK, Chang TI, Kim HW, Chang JH, et al. (2009) Uric acid is associated with the rate of residual renal function decline in peritoneal dialysis patients. Nephrol Dial Trandplant 24: 3520–3525.
33. Wang AY (2007) The "heart" of peritoneal dialysis. Perit Dial Int 27 Suppl 2: S228–232.
34. Kuo CF, See LC, Yu KH, Chou IJ, Chiou MJ, et al. (2013) Significance of serum uric acid levels on the risk of all-cause and cardiovascular mortality. Rheumatology (Oxford) 52: 127–134.
35. Zhang L, Wang F, Wang X, Liu L, Wang H (2012) The association between plasma uric acid and renal function decline in a Chinese population-based cohort. Nephrol Dial Trandplant 27: 1836–1839.
36. Chen Y, Ding X, Teng J, Zou J, Zhong Y, et al. (2011) Serum uric acid is inversely related to acute ischemic stroke morbidity in hemodialysis patients. Am J Nephrol 33: 97–104.
37. Culleton BF, Larson MG, Kannel WB, Levy D (1999) Serum uric acid and risk for cardiovascular disease and death: the Framingham Heart Study. Ann Intern Med 131: 7–13.
38. Moriarity JT, Folsom AR, Iribarren C, Nieto FJ, Rosamond WD (2000) Serum uric acid and risk of coronary heart disease: Atherosclerosis Risk in Communities (ARIC) Study. Ann Epidemiol 10: 136–143.
39. Wen CP, David Cheng TY, Chan HT, Tsai MK, Chung WS, et al. (2010) Is high serum uric acid a risk marker or a target for treatment? Examination of its independent effect in a large cohort with low cardiovascular risk. Am J Kidney Dis 56: 273–288.
40. Wannamethee SG, Shaper AG, Whincup PH (1997) Serum urate and the risk of major coronary heart disease events. Heart 78: 147–153.
41. Navaneethan SD, Beddhu S (2009) Associations of serum uric acid with cardiovascular events and mortality in moderate chronic kidney disease. Nephrol Dial Trandplant 24: 1260–1266.
42. Liu WC, Hung CC, Chen SC, Yeh SM, Lin MY, et al. (2012) Association of hyperuricemia with renal outcomes, cardiovascular disease, and mortality. Clin J Am Soc Nephrol 7: 541–548.
43. Tangri N, Weiner DE (2010) Uric acid, CKD, and cardiovascular disease: confounders, culprits, and circles. Am J Kidney Dis 56: 247–250.
44. Badve SV, Brown F, Hawley CM, Johnson DW, Kanellis J, et al. (2011) Challenges of conducting a trial of uric-acid-lowering therapy in CKD. Nat Rev Nephrol 7: 295–300.

High-Sensitivity C-Reactive Protein Predicts Mortality and Technique Failure in Peritoneal Dialysis Patients

Shou-Hsuan Liu[1], Yi-Jung Li[1,2], Hsin-Hsu Wu[1,2], Cheng-Chia Lee[1], Chan-Yu Lin[1], Cheng-Hao Weng[1,2], Yung-Chang Chen[1], Ming-Yang Chang[1], Hsiang-Hao Hsu[1], Ji-Tseng Fang[1], Cheng-Chieh Hung[1], Chih-Wei Yang[1], Ya-Chung Tian[1]*

1 Kidney Research Center, Department of Nephrology, Lin-Kou Chang Gung Memorial Hospital and Department of Medicine, Chang Gung University, Tao Yuan, Taiwan, 2 Graduate Institute of Clinical Medical Sciences, Chang Gung University, Tao Yuan, Taiwan

Abstract

Introduction: An elevated level of serum C-reactive protein (CRP) is widely considered an indicator of an underlying inflammatory disease and a long-term prognostic predictor for dialysis patients. This cross-sectional cohort study was designed to assess the correlation between the level of high-sensitivity CRP (HS-CRP) and the outcome of peritoneal dialysis (PD) patients.

Methods: A total of 402 patients were stratified into 3 tertiles (lower, middle, upper) according to serum HS-CRP level and and followed up from October 2009 to September 2011. During follow-up, cardiovascular events, infection episodes, technique failure, and mortality rate were recorded.

Results: During the 24-month follow-up, 119 of 402 patients (29.6%) dropped out from PD, including 28 patients (7.0%) who died, 81 patients (20.1%) who switched to hemodialysis, and 10 patients (2.5%) who underwent kidney transplantation. The results of Kaplan–Meier analysis and log-rank test demonstrated a significant difference in the cumulative patient survival rate across the 3 tertiles (the lowest rate in upper tertile). On multivariate Cox regression analysis, only higher HS-CRP level, older age, the presence of diabetes mellitus (DM), lower serum albumin level, and the occurrence of cardiovascular events during follow-up were identified as independent predictors of mortality. Every 1 mg/L increase in HS-CRP level was independently predictive of a 1.4% increase in mortality. Multivariate Cox regression analysis also showed that higher HS-CRP level, the presence of DM, lower hemoglobin level, lower serum albumin level, higher dialysate/plasma creatinine ratio, and the occurrence of infective episodes and cardiovascular events during follow-up were independent predictors of technique failure.

Conclusions: The present study shows the importance of HS-CRP in the prediction of 2-year mortality and technique survival in PD patients independent of age, diabetes, hypoalbuminemia, and the occurrence of cardiovascular events.

Editor: Leighton R. James, University of Florida, United States of America

Funding: The authors have no support or funding to report.

Competing Interests: The authors have declared that no competing interests exist.

* E-mail: dryctian@adm.cgmh.org.tw

Introduction

An elevated level of serum C-reactive protein (CRP), an acute-phase reactant, has been found to predict the clinical outcome of various cardiovascular diseases such as myocardial infarction and stroke in the general population and in patients with chronic kidney disease and those undergoing dialysis [1,2]. Some studies reported that CRP itself is pro-inflammatory as it has the ability to bind damaged cells and activate complements [3,4]. A high CRP level is widely considered an indicator of an underlying inflammatory disease or a high oxidative stress condition, and a long-term prognostic predictor for patients undergoing dialysis [5–7]. A high-sensitivity CRP (HS-CRP) test is more sensitive than conventional CRP detection tests and can detect levels of CRP within the reference range [8].

Many studies have recognized uremic milieu as a state of chronic inflammation [9–12]. Even after dialysis, patients remain in an inflammatory status because the serum level of pro-inflammatory cytokines such as interleukin-1 (IL-1), IL-6, and tumor necrosis factor-α are elevated in dialysis patients [13–17]. It has been reported that up to 30–50% of peritoneal dialysis (PD) patients have increased CRP levels [7,18,19]. Although several studies have reported that the elevation of CRP is a useful predictor of the occurrence of cardiovascular events and mortality [7,13,20,21], some demonstrate that CRP is not significantly associated with all-cause mortality [19,22,23]. It has been reported that the characteristics of membrane transporter status and residual renal function affect the serum CRP level [24,25]. Therefore, this discrepancy may be attributed to the sample size, analyzed parameters, and study period.

Table 1. Demographic and laboratory characteristics of the PD patients stratified according to serum HS-CRP levels.

	Total	Lower tertile	Middle tertile	Upper tertile	
	(n = 402)	(n = 134)	(n = 134)	(n = 134)	
HS-CRP (mg/L)	9.57±16.35	0.90±0.43	3.90±1.69	23.90±22.09	P
		(<1.77)	(1.77–7.51)	(>7.51)	
Male	148 (36.8%)	43 (32.1%)	53 (39.6%)	52 (38.8%)	0.38
Age (years)	48.6±14.6	44.3±15.3	49.1±13.0	52.4±14.3	<0.001
Body mass index (kg/m^2)	22.4±3.6	21.1±2.9	22.8±3.6	23.4±3.9	<0.001
Diabetes mellitus	71 (17.7%)	11 (8.2%)	23 (17.2%)	37 (27.6%)	<0.001
PD duration (months)	73.6±41.0	66.9±35.7	76.1±40.4	77.8±45.8	0.07
Residual urine	254 (63.2%)	103 (76.9%)	80 (59.7%)	71 (53.0%)	<0.001
WBC count (1000/μL)	7.655±2.523	6.400±1.959	7.679±2.058	8.866±2.840	<0.001
Hemoglobin (g/dL)	10.06±1.56	10.24±1.56	10.18±1.45	9.66±1.61	<0.001
Platelet count (1000/μL)	257.81±82.63	247.65±79.33	258.69±77.09	266.92±90.35	0.17
AST (U/L)	20.1±11.9	20.3±12.6	19.4±9.3	20.6±13.4	0.73
ALT (U/L)	20.2±18.4	20.3±20.5	19.9±12.2	20.5±21.2	0.9
Total bilirubin (mg/dL)	0.30±0.12	0.28±0.13	0.36±0.12	0.25±0.08	0.20
Albumin (g/dL)	3.96±0.46	4.07±0.38	3.98±0.43	3.85±0.55	<0.001
Total cholesterol (mg/dL)	202.3±49.0	205.6±44.6	203.2±49.5	198.3±52.5	0.48
HDL (mg/dL)	47.4±15.1	55.2±16.0	45.0±13.4	40.9±11.5	<0.001
LDL (mg/dL)	119.7±40.8	121.6±40.6	119.2±41.4	117.9±40.8	0.82
Triglyceride (mg/dL)	190.3±129.3	149.3±79.4	195.4±132.8	224.6±152.5	<0.001
Total patients					
Fasting sugar (mg/dL)	114.7±53.4	103.5±43.7	110.6±40.3	129.9±68.6	<0.001
HbA1c %	5.66±1.03	5.43±0.85	5.61±0.89	5.96±1.23	<0.001
Diabetic patients					
Fasting sugar (mg/dL)	187.4±90.1	194.9±114.9	172.9±61.6	193.8±97.4	0.67
HbA1c %	7.31±1.50	7.81±1.34	7.02±1.36	7.33±1.61	0.40
Non-diabetic patients					
Fasting sugar (mg/dL)	98.8±17.8	94.9±10.2	98.1±16.7	104.5±24.3	<0.001
HbA1c %	5.33±0.38	5.22±0.36	5.35±0.42	5.42±0.33	<0.001
Creatinine (mg/dL)	11.32±3.01	11.73±3.23	11.40±2.83	10.82±2.89	0.046
Uric acid (mg/dL)	6.81±1.32	6.76±1.25	6.73±1.24	6.95±1.45	0.35
Calcium (mg/dL)	10.01±1.00	9.96±1.00	10.12±0.98	9.95±0.99	0.30
Phosphorus (mg/dL)	4.94±1.32	5.09±1.28	4.90±1.27	4.83±1.42	0.26
iPTH (pg/mL)	329.0±388.8	332.8±391.3	285.8±318.3	367.2±443.4	0.25
Transferrin saturation	0.272±0.127	0.295±0.118	0.276±0.134	0.244±0.122	0.01
Ferritin (μg/L)	329.1±510.9	261.9±435.2	371.9±667.9	352.6±382.4	0.20

Note:

Continuous variables given as mean ± standard deviation, and categorical variables, as number (percentage).

Abbreviations: HS-CRP, high-sensitivity C-reactive protein; PD, peritoneal dialysis; WBC, white blood cell; AST, aspartate transaminase; ALT, alanine transaminase; HDL, high-density lipoprotein; LDL, low-density lipoprotein; HbA1c, glycated hemoglobin; iPTH, intact parathyroid hormone.

In addition to predicting mortality, an elevated CRP level has been shown to be linked to technique failure. Nevertheless, only a few studies have assessed the impact of baseline serum CRP level on technique failure, and the association between baseline serum CRP level and subsequent technique failure is still inconclusive. Some studies demonstrated that serum CRP level was independently associated with technique failure [26], whereas others found that serum CRP level was not a predictor for technique failure [27,28]. Therefore, it would be interesting to know whether serum CRP level is correlated with technique failure in PD patients.

Both residual renal function and peritoneal clearance have been reported to be inversely associated with serum CRP level [24,25], whereas some studies demonstrate that serum CRP is not influenced by peritoneal solute transport rate and residual renal function [22,29]. As these 2 factors have also been shown to be predictive markers for mortality and technique failure in PD patients and are associated with CRP, it would be crucial to elucidate whether HS-CRP can predict the clinical outcome in PD patients independently of residual renal function and peritoneal clearance.

Table 2. Peritoneal membrane characteristics of the PD patients stratified according to HS-CRP levels.

	Total	Lower tertile	Middle tertile	Upper tertile	
	(n = 402)	(n = 134)	(n = 134)	(n = 134)	
HS-CRP (mg/L)	9.57±16.35	0.90±0.43	3.90±1.69	23.90±22.09	P
		(<1.77)	(1.77–7.51)	(>7.51)	
Dialysate/plasma creatinine	0.64±0.12	0.62±0.12	0.65±0.10	0.66±0.13	0.01
Peritoneal equilibration test					<0.001
High	28 (7.0%)	5 (3.7%)	6 (4.5%)	17 (12.7%)	
High average	152 (37.8%)	41 (30.6%)	63 (47.0%)	48 (35.8%)	
Low average	179 (44.5%)	66 (49.3%)	55 (41.0%)	58 (43.3%)	
Low	43 (10.7%)	22 (16.4%)	10 (7.5%)	11 (8.2%)	
Weekly CCr (normalized)	59.6±13.9	58.8±13.8	60.3±14.9	59.7±13.1	0.70
Weekly CCr (total)	54.1±14.5	52.0±14.6	55.5±14.9	54.7±13.9	0.12
Weekly CCr (PD)	45.1±12.1	41.0±12.0	47.1±10.6	47.3±12.6	<0.001
Weekly CCr (renal)	8.9±15.2	11.0±13.9	8.2±16.8	7.4±14.6	0.12

Note:
Continuous variables given as mean ± standard deviation, and categorical variables, as number (percentage).
Abbreviations: PD, peritoneal dialysis; HS-CRP, high-sensitivity C-reactive protein; CCr, creatinine clearance.

The aim of this cross-sectional cohort study was to investigate whether serum HS-CRP level was independently associated with mortality and technique failure in PD patients.

Materials and Methods

This cross-sectional cohort study complied with the guidelines of the Declaration of Helsinki and approved by the Medical Ethics Committee of Chang Gung Memorial Hospital, a tertiary referral center located in the northern part of Taiwan. Since this study involved retrospective review of existing data, the Institutional Review Board approval was obtained, but without specific informed consent from patients. In addition, all individual information was securely protected (by delinking identifying information from main data set) and available to investigators only. Furthermore, all the data were analyzed anonymously. The Institutional Review Board of Chang Gung Memorial Hospital has approved this study and no informed consent was requested by the Committee. Finally, all primary data were collected according to strengthening the reporting of observational studies in epidemiology guidelines.

Study Population and Follow-up

This cohort observational study was conducted in the PD unit of Linkou Chang-Gung Memorial Hospital from October 2009 to September 2011 to determine the impact of HS-CRP on the patients' outcome. All the data were obtained from the record of the routine examination. Among 445 patients, 43 patients were excluded owing to recent episodes of peritonitis, active infection, chronic liver disease, autoimmune disease, malignant diseases, or acute myocardial infarction within 3 months. The remaining 402

Table 3. Clinical outcomes in the PD patients stratified according to HS-CRP levels.

	Total	Lower tertile	Middle tertile	Upper tertile	
	(n = 402)	(n = 134)	(n = 134)	(n = 134)	
HS-CRP (mg/L)	9.57±16.35	0.90±0.43	3.90±1.69	23.90±22.09	P
		(<1.77)	(1.77–7.51)	(>7.51)	
Outcomes					
Death	28 (7.0%)	0 (0.0%)	4 (3.0%)	24 (17.9%)	<0.001
Transfer to HD	81 (20.1%)	25 (18.7%)	25 (18.7%)	31 (23.1%)	0.575
Transplantation	10 (2.5%)	3 (2.2%)	4 (3.0%)	3 (2.2%)	0.903
Technique survival	283 (70.4%)	106 (79.1%)	101 (75.4%)	76 (56.7%)	<0.001
Infection episodes	192 (47.8%)	55 (41.0%)	66 (49.3%)	71 (53.0%)	0.14
Cardiovascular events	72 (17.9%)	17 (12.7%)	21 (15.7%)	34 (25.4%)	0.02

Note:
Continuous variables given as mean ± standard deviation, and categorical variables, as number (percentage).
Abbreviations: PD, peritoneal dialysis; HS-CRP, high-sensitivity C-reactive protein; HD, hemodialysis.

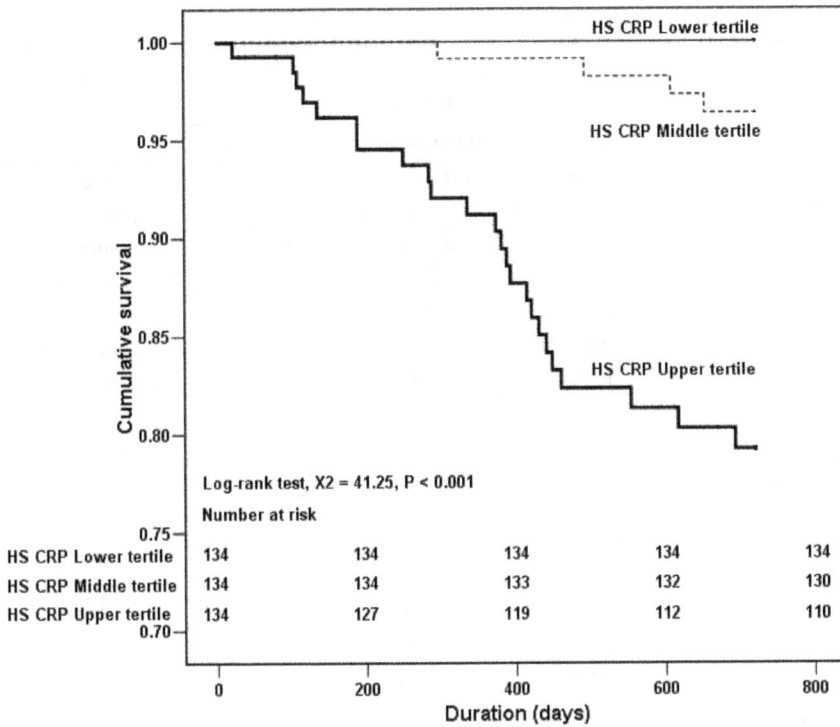

Figure 1. Kaplan–Meier survival curves based on serum HS-CRP levels among PD patients in the 2-year follow-up.

patients were enrolled in this study. All patients had been undergoing PD for >3 months and were observed during a period of 24 months. Patients were categorized into 3 tertiles according to the baseline HS-CRP level in October 2009.

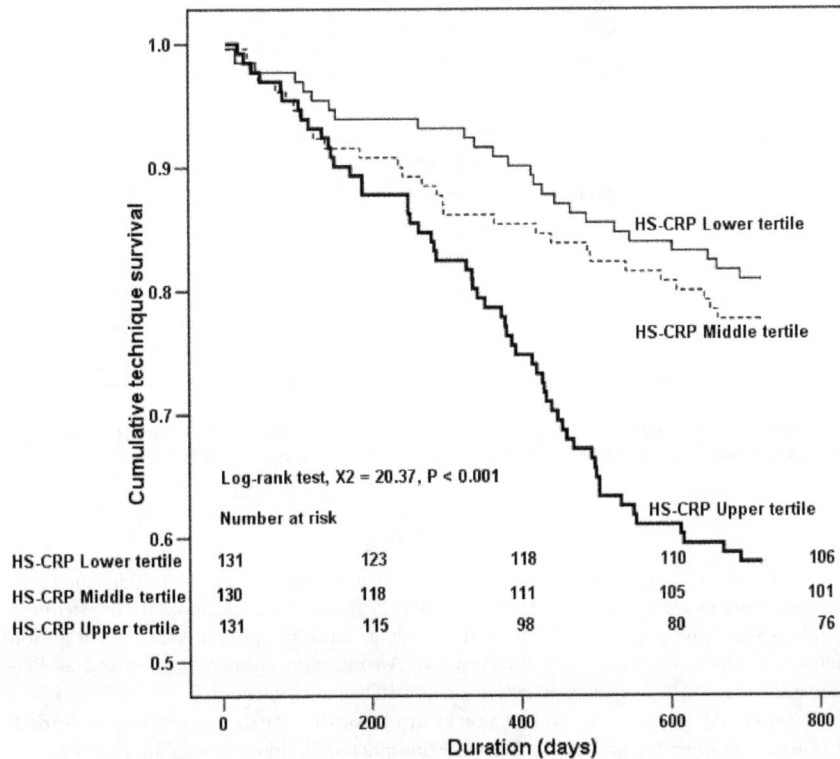

Figure 2. Kaplan–Meier technique survival (transplantation censored) curves based on serum HS-CRP levels among PD patients in the 2-year follow-up.

Table 4. Relative risk of mortality in univariate Cox regression analysis.

		Univariate analysis	
	RR	HR (95% CI)	P
HS-CRP (mg/L)	1.025	1.014–1.035	<0.001
Male	1.692	0.719–3.981	0.23
Age	1.067	1.036–1.098	<0.001
Body mass index (kg/m^2)	1.051	0.954–1.158	0.32
Diabetes mellitus	5.979	2.846–12.560	<0.001
PD duration (months)	0.993	0.982–1.004	0.20
Residual urine	0.700	0.331–1.480	0.35
White blood cell count (1000/µL)	1.158	1.046–1.281	0.01
Hemoglobin (g/dL)	0.859	0.684–1.079	0.19
Platelet count (1000/µL)	1.000	0.996–1.005	0.9
AST (U/L)	1.018	0.996–1.041	0.12
ALT (U/L)	1.003	0.983–1.023	0.80
Total bilirubin (mg/dL)	0.168	0.000–231.652	0.67
Albumin (g/dL)	0.194	0.110–0.341	<0.001
Total cholesterol (mg/dL)	0.996	0.988–1.004	0.31
HDL (mg/dL)	1.002	0.964–1.042	0.9
LDL (mg/dL)	0.991	0.974–1.008	0.28
Triglyceride (mg/dL)	1.001	0.999–1.004	0.34
Sugar (mg/dL)	1.008	1.004–1.012	<0.001
HbA1c %	1.532	1.232–1.905	<0.001
Creatinine (mg/dL)	0.730	0.620–0.858	<0.001
Uric acid (mg/dL)	0.746	0.541–1.028	0.07
Calcium (mg/dL)	0.653	0.476–0.896	0.01
Phosphorus (mg/dL)	0.674	0.488–0.931	0.02
iPTH (pg/mL)	0.999	0.998–1.000	0.11
Transferrin saturation	3.398	0.259–44.651	0.35
Ferritin (µg/L)	1.000	1.000–1.001	0.19
Dialysate/plasma creatinine	19.269	0.942–394.309	0.06
Peritoneal equilibration test (%)	1.612	0.995–2.613	0.05
Weekly CCr (normalized)	0.996	0.969–1.024	0.77
Weekly CCr (total)	0.992	0.966–1.018	0.54
Weekly CCr (PD)	1.003	0.973–1.034	0.85
Weekly CCr (renal)	0.990	0.961–1.019	0.49
Infection episodes	2.434	1.122–5.279	0.02
Cardiovascular events	5.979	2.847–12.557	<0.001

Note:
Abbreviations: RR, relative risk; HR, hazard ratio; CI, confidence interval; HS-CRP, high-sensitivity C-reactive protein; PD, peritoneal dialysis; AST, aspartate transaminase; ALT, alanine transaminase; HDL, high-density lipoprotein; LDL, low-density lipoprotein; HbA1c, glycated hemoglobin; iPTH, intact parathyroid hormone; CCr, creatinine clearance.

Baseline demographic and clinical data, including age, sex, body mass index (BMI), presence of diabetes, duration of PD at the entry of this study, residual renal function, hemogram, and biochemical parameters, were recorded. PD membrane characteristics, including the dialysate/plasma creatinine ratio (D/P$_{Cr}$) and peritoneal equilibrium test (PET) results, were assessed. All of these data were obtained during routine clinical practice. During the 24-month follow-up, cardiovascular events, infection episodes, technique failure, and mortality rate were recorded. A cardiovas-

cular event was defined as acute myocardial infarction, intervention of coronary artery disease with angioplasty or stenting, cerebral vascular accident, and peripheral vascular occlusion requiring intervention. An infection episode was defined as PD-related infection or non-PD-related infection.

No patient was lost to follow-up. Patient deaths were recorded, and those patients who underwent kidney transplantation or were transferred to hemodialysis were censored when they received alterative renal replacement therapy.

Table 5. Relative risk of mortality in multivariate Cox regression analysis.

	RR	Multivariate analysis HR (95% CI)	P
HS-CRP (mg/L)	1.014	1.003–1.026	0.02
Age	1.042	1.011–1.074	0.01
Diabetes mellitus	3.381	1.578–7.243	0.002
Albumin (g/dL)	0.289	0.156–0.535	<0.001
Cardiovascular events	2.839	1.309–6.160	0.008

Note:
Abbreviations: RR, relative risk; HR, hazard ratio; CI, confidence interval; HS-CRP, high-sensitivity C-reactive protein.

Laboratory Parameters

Blood specimens were collected within a few days of clinical examination during stable PD routine examination to minimize the effect of any acute event. Blood was drawn immediately, centrifuged, and then stored at $-70°C$ until used in assays. Serum HS-CRP was analyzed by using immunonephelometry (Nanopia CRP; Daiichi, Tokyo, Japan). Serum intact parathyroid hormone (iPTH) was determined by using a chemiluminometric immunoassay (ADVIA Centaur iPTH; Siemens Medical Solutions Diagnostics, New York, NY, USA) with a reference range of 7–53 pg/mL. All other biochemical parameters were obtained with standard laboratory procedures by using an automatic analyzer.

Peritoneal Dialysis Membrane Characteristics

The adequacy of dialysis was determined by measuring the total weekly creatinine clearance (CCr), which was normalized to 1.73 m^2 of the body surface area. Residual renal CCr was calculated as an average of the 24-h urine urea and CCr. Dialysate creatinine concentration was corrected for interference by glucose. The dialysate/plasma creatinine ratio (D/P_{Cr}) was calculated from the concentrations of creatinine in the 24-h dialysate and the plasma.

Statistical Analysis

Continuous variables are expressed as means and standard deviations, and categorical variables as numbers and percentages in brackets. All data were tested for normality of distribution and equality of standard deviations before analysis. For comparisons between patient groups, one-way ANOVA was used for quantitative variables, whereas chi-square or Fisher's exact test was used for categorical variables. P values were calculated, and the null hypothesis was rejected if the P value was <0.05. The independent links between HS-CRP and variables were analyzed further with simple and stepwise backward multiple linear regression analyses, adjusting for other factors linked with HS-CRP. Mortality was examined by using Kaplan–Meier analysis. Differences in the survival curves among the 3 groups were evaluated by using the log-rank test. An initial univariate Cox regression analysis was performed to compare the frequency of possible risk factors associated with mortality. To control for possible confounding factors, a multivariate Cox regression analysis (stepwise backward approach) was performed to analyze the significant factors (P< 0.05) on the univariate analysis that met the assumptions of a proportional hazard model. The criterion for significance was a 95% confidence interval to reject the null hypothesis (P<0.05). All analyses were performed by using SPSS 12.0 for Windows (SPSS Inc., Chicago, IL, USA).

Results

Baseline Patient Characteristics of Demography and Biochemistry

Of the 402 patients in this cohort observational study, 148 (36.8%) were men and 254 (63.2%) were women. Their mean age was 48.6±14.6 years. The mean duration of PD was 73.6±41.0 months. Table 1 shows the baseline characteristics and laboratory parameters of these 402 patients stratified into 3 tertiles according to the serum HS-CRP level. The mean HS-CRP value in the study patients was 9.57 mg/L. The mean HS-CRP values were 0.90 mg/L (0–1.77 mg/L) in the lower tertile (T1), 3.90 mg/L (1.77–7.51 mg/L) in the middle tertile (T2), and 23.90 mg/L (7.51–45.85 mg/L) in the upper tertile (T3). Among the 3 tertiles, there was no significant difference in sex and PD duration. There was a significant increase (P<0.001) in the mean age across HS-CRP tertiles: 44.3 years in T1, 49.1 years in T2, and 52.4 years in T3. The percentages of patients with diabetes were significantly increased: 8.2% in T1, 17.2% in T2, and 27.6% in T3. A significant increase in the BMI values was also found across the 3 tertiles. Up to 76.9% of patients in T1 had residual renal function, whereas 59.7% of patients in T2 and 53.0% of patients in T3 had residual renal function (P<0.001). The white blood cell count was significantly increased and the hemoglobin level was reduced, whereas the platelet count was not different across these groups. Liver biochemistry test showed no difference in serum aspartate transaminase, alanine transaminase, and total bilirubin levels across the HS-CRP tertiles. The serum albumin level was in inverse proportion to the HS-CRP level, with the lowest level in T3. The examination of lipid profiles revealed a significant decrease in high-density lipoprotein (HDL) levels and an increase in triglyceride levels across the 3 tertiles of increasing HS-CRP, whereas total cholesterol and low-density lipoprotein (LDL) levels were not different across these tertiles. Fasting blood sugar and glycated hemoglobin (HbA1c) levels were examined in every patient, and the results showed a significant increase in these 2 parameters across the 3 tertiles of increasing HS-CRP. Surprisingly, further analysis revealed that in patients without diabetes, fasting blood sugar and HbA1c levels were increased across the 3 tertiles of increasing HS-CRP, whereas in patients with diabetes, blood sugar and HbA1c levels varied and were not different across the HS-CRP tertiles. Compared with patients in the other tertiles, the serum creatinine level was lowest in the patients in T3. Serum uric acid, calcium, phosphorus, and iPTH levels were not significantly different across the HS-CRP tertiles. Transferrin saturation was significantly decreased across the 3 tertiles of increasing HS-CRP. There was a trend toward the higher ferritin

Table 6. Relative risk of technique failure in univariate Cox regression analysis.

		Univariate analysis	
	RR	HR (95% CI)	P
HS-CRP (mg/L)	1.016	1.009–1.023	<0.001
Male	0.364	0.814–1.750	0.36
Age	1.020	1.006–1.034	0.01
Body mass index (kg/m²)	1.028	0.976–1.082	0.30
Diabetes mellitus	2.902	1.946–4.330	<0.001
PD duration (months)	0.995	0.990–1.001	0.08
Residual urine	0.656	0.449–0.958	0.03
White blood cell count (1000/μL)	1.077	1.011–1.147	0.02
Hemoglobin (g/dL)	0.831	0.742–0.931	0.001
Platelet count (1000/μL)	1.001	0.999–1.003	0.23
AST (U/L)	1.008	0.993–1.022	0.30
ALT (U/L)	1.004	0.995–1.013	0.42
Total bilirubin (mg/dL)	0.139	0.000–178.189	0.59
Albumin (g/dL)	0.326	0.233–0.455	<0.001
Total cholesterol (mg/dL)	0.996	0.992–1.000	0.06
HDL (mg/dL)	1.002	0.981–1.024	0.86
LDL (mg/dL)	0.994	0.986–1.003	0.20
Triglyceride (mg/dL)	1.002	0.999–1.003	0.23
Sugar (mg/dL)	1.006	1.004–1.008	<0.001
HbA1c %	1.360	1.193–1.550	<0.001
Creatinine (mg/dL)	0.901	0.839–0.967	0.004
Uric acid (mg/dL)	0.953	0.816–1.113	0.54
Calcium (mg/dL)	0.830	0.691–0.997	0.05
Phosphorus (mg/dL)	0.797	0.681–0.933	0.01
iPTH (pg/mL)	1.000	0.999–1.000	0.21
Transferrin saturation	0.416	0.078–2.207	0.30
Ferritin (μg/L)	1.000	1.000–1.000	0.56
Dialysate/plasma creatinine	19.105	4.168–87.571	<0.001
Peritoneal equilibration test (%)	1.579	1.237–2.014	<0.001
Weekly CCr (normalized)	1.000	0.987–1.014	0.9
Weekly CCr (total)	1.000	0.988–1.013	0.9
Weekly CCr (PD)	1.017	1.001–1.033	0.04
Weekly CCr (renal)	0.988	0.973–1.004	0.13
Infection episodes	5.153	3.225–8.232	<0.001
Cardiovascular events	2.886	1.921–4.275	<0.001

Note:
Abbreviations: RR, relative risk; HR, hazard ratio; CI, confidence interval; HS-CRP, high-sensitivity C-reactive protein; PD, peritoneal dialysis; AST, aspartate transaminase; ALT, alanine transaminase; HDL, high-density lipoprotein; LDL, low-density lipoprotein; HbA1c, glycated hemoglobin; iPTH, intact parathyroid hormone; CCr, creatinine clearance.

level in the upper tertiles, although it did not reach statistical significance.

Baseline Peritoneal Membrane Characteristics

Table 2 outlines the peritoneal membrane characteristics of the PD patients. Among the 3 tertiles of increasing HS-CRP, the value of D/P_{Cr} was significantly increased. According to the results of PET, the peritoneal transport status in the 3 tertiles was significantly different, as 12.7% of patients in T3 were high transporters and 8.2% of patients were low transporters, whereas 3.7% of patients in T1 were high transporters and 16.4% of patients were low transporters. There was no significant difference for the weekly CCr (total) in the 3 tertiles, whereas the weekly CCr (PD) in T1 was significantly lower than that in the other 2 tertiles (P<0.001). There was also a trend toward a lower value of weekly CCr (renal) in T3.

Table 7. Relative risk of technique failure in multivariate Cox regression analysis.

		Multivariate analysis	
	RR	HR (95% CI)	P
HS-CRP (mg/L)	1.009	1.001–1.017	0.03
Diabetes mellitus	2.170	1.424–3.306	<0.001
Hemoglobin (g/dL)	0.877	0.774–0.994	0.04
Albumin (g/dL)	0.631	0.418–0.953	0.03
Dialysate/plasma creatinine	6.133	1.152–32.656	0.03
Infection episodes	4.775	2.931–7.778	<0.001
Cardiovascular events	1.896	1.228–2.927	0.004

Note:
Abbreviations: RR, relative risk; HR, hazard ratio; CI, confidence interval; HS-CRP, high-sensitivity C-reactive protein.

Patient Survival, Technique Survival, Cardiovascular Events, and Infection Episodes during the 24-month Follow-up

During the 24-month follow-up, 119 of 402 patients (29.6%) dropped out from PD, including 28 patients who died (7.0%), 81 patients (20.1%) who switched to hemodialysis, and 10 patients (2.5%) who underwent kidney transplantation (Table 3). There were significant differences in the mortality and technique failure in the three tertiles, whereas there was no significant difference in the number of patients transferring to HD and receiving transplantation among three groups (Table 3).

The results of the Kaplan–Meier analysis and log-rank test also demonstrated that there was significant difference in the cumulative patient survival rate between T3 vs T1 (P<0.001) and T3 vs T2 (P<0.001) (Fig. 1). Nevertheless, despite a trend towards a higher patient survival rate in T1 than that in T2, the difference did not reach statistically significant. In addition, the Kaplan–Meier analysis and log-rank test also revealed that the cumulative technique survival rate in T3 was significantly lower than T1 and T2 (T3 vs. T1, P<0.001; T3 vs. T2, P<0.001) (Fig. 2), whereas the comparison of the cumulative technique survival rate between T1 and T2 was not statistically different.

During the 24-month follow-up, there was no difference in the episodes of PD-related and non-PD-related infection across the 3 tertiles. Because serum CRP level has been identified as a cardiovascular factor, we examined the predictive value of serum HS-CRP level for subsequent cardiovascular events during the 24-month follow-up. More patients (25.4%) in T3 had cardiovascular events during the follow-up period than patients in T2 (15.7%) and T1 (12.7%) (P = 0.018). These results suggest that patients in the high HS-CRP tertiles are at risk of developing cardiovascular events in the following 24 months.

HS-CRP Level is an Independent Predictor of Mortality and Technique Failure

To further assess the independent predictors of mortality, Cox regression analysis was used. The results of univariate Cox regression analysis revealed that higher HS-CRP level, older age, the presence of DM, higher white blood cell count, lower serum albumin level, higher plasma sugar level and HbA1c value, lower serum creatinine level, lower calcium and phosphorus levels, and the occurrence of infection episodes and cardiovascular events during the 24-month follow-up were risk factors for mortality (Table 4). On multivariate Cox regression analysis, only higher HS-CRP level, older age, the presence of DM, lower serum albumin level, and the occurrence of cardiovascular events during follow-up were identified as independent predictors of mortality (Table 5). Every 1 mg/L increase in HS-CRP level was independently predictive of a 1.4% increase in mortality.

To identify the risk factors for technique failure (death or transfer to hemodialysis), univariate and multivariate Cox regression analyses were applied. The results of univariate Cox regression analysis demonstrated that higher HS-CRP level, older age, the presence of DM, the existence of residual urine, higher white blood cell count, lower hemoglobin level, lower serum albumin level, higher plasma sugar level and HbA1c value, lower serum creatinine level, lower serum phosphorus levels, higher dialysate/plasma creatinine ratio, peritoneal equilibration test, higher weekly CCr (PD), and the occurrence of infection episodes and cardiovascular events during follow-up were significant risk factors for technique failure (Table 6). Multivariate Cox regression analysis showed that higher HS-CRP level, the presence of DM, lower hemoglobin level, lower serum albumin level, higher dialysate/plasma creatinine ratio, and the occurrence of infection episodes and cardiovascular events during follow-up were independent predictors of technique failure (Table 7).

Discussion

This study is a cross-sectional cohort study that enrolled 402 patients to assess the impact of serum HS-CRP levels on mortality and technique survival in PD patients. The major causes of death and technique failure in PD patient is attributed to cardiovascular disease, infection, and loss of dialysis adequacy, all of which are associated with inflammation. Our results demonstrate that HS-CRP as an inflammatory marker predicts mortality and technique survival, supporting the hypothesis that inflammation has an adverse effect on the clinical outcome. Our study demonstrates that 42% of PD patients had serum HS-CRP levels more than 5 mg/L, slightly higher than those reported in Chinese PD patients (36%) [7]. In this study, the patients in the high HS-CRP tertile have a higher mortality rate and a lower technique survival rate during the 24-month follow-up. Relatively small number of patient deaths may contribute to insignificant difference in mortality and technique survival rate between T1 (none of patients) vs T2 (4 patients). In accordance, the results of multivariate logistical regression analysis also showed that HS-CRP is an independent predictor of both mortality and technique failure.

During the past decade, CRP has emerged as a powerful predictor of mortality in dialysis patients [10,30–34]. Our study also verifies the importance of HS-CRP in predicting the subsequent survival of PD patients. CRP is the most used inflammatory marker. It has been associated with the nutrition status and its markers, including serum albumin level [35,36]. In accordance, our study also showed that serum albumin level was significantly reduced across the 3 tertiles of increasing HS-CRP. Serum albumin level is an important predictor of all-cause mortality in both PD and hemodialysis patients [37,38]. As frequently there is a reciprocal interaction between serum albumin and CRP levels, some studies have shown that on multivariate Cox regression analysis, serum CRP level instead of serum albumin level remains significant in predicting mortality [39]. In contrast, our study showed that both serum HS-CRP and albumin levels were independent risk factors for mortality and technique failure. This discrepancy may be attributed to the low percentage (17.7%) of patients with diabetes in our study, as serum albumin level has been reported to be lower in diabetic PD patients and may become a confounding factor in studies recruiting a high population of diabetic patients. CRP has been shown to be strongly associated with diabetes in recent years [40,41]. Oh et al. reported that diabetic PD patients had a higher serum HS-CRP level, suggesting an interrelation between diabetes and HS-CRP. Our study demonstrates that on multivariate Cox regression analysis, serum HS-CRP, albumin level, and diabetes all remain independent factors for predicting mortality and technique failure in PD patients.

Both peritoneal clearance and residual renal function are major determinants of survival in PD patients [42–44]. In addition, these 2 factors have been shown to be linked with serum CRP level. Some studies reported that a reduction of residual renal function and peritoneal clearance led to an elevated serum CRP level [24,25,45–47], whereas other studies did not find this correlation [19,22,29,48]. There is therefore a controversy about whether CRP predicts the clinical outcome of PD patients independent of peritoneal clearance and residual renal function. Our study demonstrated that peritoneal clearance was decreased across the 3 tertiles of increasing HS-CRP, whereas there was no significant difference in the CCr of residual renal function across the 3 tertiles. On multivariate logistic regression analysis, serum HS-CRP level instead of peritoneal clearance and residual renal function was a negative predictive marker for both mortality and technique failure. The CANUSA study showed that there was a 12% decrease in the relative risk (RR) of death (RR, 0.88; 95% confidence interval [CI], 0.83 to 0.94) for each 5 L/wk per 1.73 m2 increment in glomerular filtration rate [49]. Compared with the patients in the CANUSA study, our patients had less residual renal function (37.7 L/wk in CANUSA study vs. 8.9 L/wk in our study). Thus, our study might underestimate the contribution of residual renal function to mortality and technique failure.

Technique failure in PD patients is frequently caused by peritonitis or high peritoneal membrane solute transport [42,43,48,50,51]. Our data showed that the patients in the high HS-CRP tertile had a higher value of D/P_{Cr} and a larger proportion of high transporters than those in the other tertiles. In addition, despite having no role in predicting mortality, a high D/P_{Cr} value is indeed a high risk factor for technique failure. Furthermore, high HS-CRP level predicted subsequent technique failure independent of D/P_{Cr}. Being a high transporter has been shown to be a significant risk factor for PD failure in a large-scale

study [48], and associated with a trend to higher technique failure in a meta-analysis report [43]. In addition, Fine et al. have demonstrated that being a high transporter predicts an increase in serum CRP level [45]. Whether the association between a high transporter status and serum HS-CRP level is a causal relation or an epiphenomenon remains elusive.

Cardiovascular events are the most common cause of death in dialysis patients [52,53]. It may be related to uremic toxins, volume status, vascular calcification, anemia, hypoalbuminemia, and chronic inflammation [52,54,55]. An elevated CRP level has been reported to be an independent predictor of myocardial infarction and cardiovascular mortality in PD patients [7,15,19,20]. Our study further demonstrated that although the incidence of cardiovascular events was significantly increased across the increasing HS-CRP tertiles, both HS-CRP and cardiovascular events were independent predictive markers for all-cause mortality on multivariate Cox regression analysis.

Our study also verified some well-established factors associated with HS-CRP (Table 1), including age, DM, BMI, existence of residual urine, white blood cell count, hemoglobin, albumin, HDL, triglycerides, fasting sugar, HbA1c level, and transferrin saturation. Among these factors, it is of interest that fasting sugar and HbA1c levels were significantly increased across the 3 tertiles in non-diabetic patients, whereas it lost statistical significance in diabetic patients. In addition to blood sugar control, chronic inflammation and oxidant stress have been found to be elevated in diabetic dialysis patients. Our finding may suggest that other factors, such as oxidative stress and chronic inflammation, in diabetic PD patients may surpass the influence of blood sugar control on serum HS-CRP level, whereas blood sugar level is still associated with the elevated serum HS-CRP level in nondiabetic PD patients. Nevertheless, except HS-CRP, age, DM, and hypoalbuminemia, all of these factors, including fasting sugar and HbA1c level, failed to predict mortality and technique failure on multivariate logistical regression analysis.

This study has several limitations. First, this study was restricted to a single-center observation. Second, this study is cross-sectional and includes prevalent patients. As HS-CRP is associated with high mortality in PD patients, this study enrolled only prevalent patients and may have underestimated the impact of HS-CRP on mortality owing to censoring bias. Nevertheless, the large number of PD patients and the extensive analysis of possible parameters that can affect clinical outcome in this study reduce these limitations.

In conclusion, the present study shows the importance of HS-CRP in predicting the 2-year mortality and technique survival in PD patients independent of age, diabetes, hypoalbuminemia, and the occurrence of cardiovascular events.

Acknowledgments

The authors thank all the members of the PD unit, Chang Gung Memorial Hospital, Linkou, for their invaluable help.

Author Contributions

Conceived and designed the experiments: SHL YCT. Performed the experiments: SHL YCT. Analyzed the data: SHL YCT. Contributed reagents/materials/analysis tools: YJL HHW CCL CYL CHW YCC MYC HHH JTF CCH CWY. Wrote the paper: SHL YCT.

References

1. Yeun JY, Levine RA, Mantadilok V, Kaysen GA (2000) C-Reactive protein predicts all-cause and cardiovascular mortality in hemodialysis patients. Am J Kidney Dis 35: 469–476.

2. Ridker PM, Cushman M, Stampfer MJ, Tracy RP, Hennekens CH (1997) Inflammation, aspirin, and the risk of cardiovascular disease in apparently healthy men. N Engl J Med 336: 973–979.

3. Volanakis JE, Narkates AJ (1981) Interaction of C-reactive protein with artificial phosphatidylcholine bilayers and complement. J Immunol 126: 1820–1825.

4. Torzewski J, Torzewski M, Bowyer DE, Frohlich M, Koenig W, et al. (1998) C-reactive protein frequently colocalizes with the terminal complement complex in the intima of early atherosclerotic lesions of human coronary arteries. Arterioscler Thromb Vasc Biol 18: 1386–1392.

5. Windgassen EB, Funtowicz L, Lunsford TN, Harris LA, Mulvagh SL (2011) C-reactive protein and high-sensitivity C-reactive protein: an update for clinicians. Postgrad Med 123: 114–119.

6. Chen HY, Chiu YL, Hsu SP, Pai MF, Lai CF, et al. (2010) Elevated C-reactive protein level in hemodialysis patients with moderate/severe uremic pruritus: a potential mediator of high overall mortality. QJM 103: 837–846.

7. Wang AY, Woo J, Lam CW, Wang M, Sea MM, et al. (2003) Is a single time point C-reactive protein predictive of outcome in peritoneal dialysis patients? J Am Soc Nephrol 14: 1871–1879.

8. Corrado E, Novo S (2007) [High sensitivity of C-reactive protein in primary prevention]. G Ital Cardiol (Rome) 8: 327–334.

9. Panichi V, Migliori M, De Pietro S, Taccola D, Bianchi AM, et al. (2000) C-reactive protein as a marker of chronic inflammation in uremic patients. Blood Purif 18: 183–190.

10. Meuwese CL, Stenvinkel P, Dekker FW, Carrero JJ (2011) Monitoring of inflammation in patients on dialysis: forewarned is forearmed. Nat Rev Nephrol 7: 166–176.

11. Filiopoulos V, Vlassopoulos D (2009) Inflammatory syndrome in chronic kidney disease: pathogenesis and influence on outcomes. Inflamm Allergy Drug Targets 8: 369–382.

12. Wanner C, Drechsler C, Krane V (2009) C-reactive protein and uremia. Semin Dial 22: 438–441.

13. Choi HY, Lee JE, Han SH, Yoo TH, Kim BS, et al. (2010) Association of inflammation and protein-energy wasting with endothelial dysfunction in peritoneal dialysis patients. Nephrol Dial Transplant 25: 1266–1271.

14. Honda H, Qureshi AR, Heimburger O, Barany P, Wang K, et al. (2006) Serum albumin, C-reactive protein, interleukin 6, and fetuin a as predictors of malnutrition, cardiovascular disease, and mortality in patients with ESRD. Am J Kidney Dis 47: 139–148.

15. Wang AY, Lam CW, Chan IH, Wang M, Lui SF, et al. (2009) Long-term mortality and cardiovascular risk stratification of peritoneal dialysis patients using a combination of inflammation and calcification markers. Nephrol Dial Transplant 24: 3826–3833.

16. Filiopoulos V, Hadjiyannakos D, Takouli L, Metaxaki P, Sideris V, et al. (2009) Inflammation and oxidative stress in end-stage renal disease patients treated with hemodialysis or peritoneal dialysis. Int J Artif Organs 32: 872–882.

17. Stenvinkel P, Ketteler M, Johnson RJ, Lindholm B, Pecoits-Filho R, et al. (2005) IL-10, IL-6, and TNF-alpha: central factors in the altered cytokine network of uremia–the good, the bad, and the ugly. Kidney Int 67: 1216–1233.

18. Yeun JY, Kaysen GA (1997) Acute phase proteins and peritoneal dialysate albumin loss are the main determinants of serum albumin in peritoneal dialysis patients. Am J Kidney Dis 30: 923–927.

19. Herzig KA, Purdie DM, Chang W, Brown AM, Hawley CM, et al. (2001) Is C-reactive protein a useful predictor of outcome in peritoneal dialysis patients? J Am Soc Nephrol 12: 814–821.

20. Ducloux D, Bresson-Vautrin C, Kribs M, Abdelfatah A, Chalopin JM (2002) C-reactive protein and cardiovascular disease in peritoneal dialysis patients. Kidney Int 62: 1417–1422.

21. Avram MM, Fein PA, Paluch MM, Schloth T, Chattopadhyay J (2005) Association between C-reactive protein and clinical outcomes in peritoneal dialysis patients. Adv Perit Dial 21: 154–158.

22. Oh KH, Moon JY, Oh J, Kim SG, Hwang YH, et al. (2008) Baseline peritoneal solute transport rate is not associated with markers of systemic inflammation or comorbidity in incident Korean peritoneal dialysis patients. Nephrol Dial Transplant 23: 2356–2364.

23. Cho JH, Hur IK, Kim CD, Park SH, Ryu HM, et al. (2010) Impact of systemic and local peritoneal inflammation on peritoneal solute transport rate in new peritoneal dialysis patients: a 1-year prospective study. Nephrol Dial Transplant 25: 1964–1973.

24. Perez-Flores I, Coronel F, Cigarran S, Herrero JA, Calvo N (2007) Relationship between residual renal function, inflammation, and anemia in peritoneal dialysis. Adv Perit Dial 23: 140–143.

25. Chung SH, Heimburger O, Stenvinkel P, Bergstrom J, Lindholm B (2001) Association between inflammation and changes in residual renal function and peritoneal transport rate during the first year of dialysis. Nephrol Dial Transplant 16: 2240–2245.

26. Zalunardo NY, Rose CL, Ma IW, Altmann P (2007) Higher serum C-reactive protein predicts short and long-term outcomes in peritoneal dialysis-associated peritonitis. Kidney Int 71: 687–692.

27. Westhuyzen J, Mills K, Healy H (2005) Predicting clinical outcomes in peritoneal dialysis patients using small solute modeling. Ann Clin Lab Sci 35: 46–53.

28. Noh H, Lee SW, Kang SW, Shin SK, Choi KH, et al. (1998) Serum C-reactive protein: a predictor of mortality in continuous ambulatory peritoneal dialysis patients. Perit Dial Int 18: 387–394.

29. Wang T, Heimburger O, Cheng HH, Bergstrom J, Lindholm B (1999) Does a high peritoneal transport rate reflect a state of chronic inflammation? Perit Dial Int 19: 17–22.

30. Kaysen GA (2009) Biochemistry and biomarkers of inflamed patients: why look, what to assess. Clin J Am Soc Nephrol 4 Suppl 1: S56–63.

31. Pecoits-Filho R, Stenvinkel P, Wang AY, Heimburger O, Lindholm B (2004) Chronic inflammation in peritoneal dialysis: the search for the holy grail? Perit Dial Int 24: 327–339.

32. Wanner C, Metzger T (2002) C-reactive protein a marker for all-cause and cardiovascular mortality in haemodialysis patients. Nephrol Dial Transplant 17 Suppl 8: 29–32; discussion 39–40.

33. Stenvinkel P, Lindholm B (2005) C-reactive protein in end-stage renal disease: are there reasons to measure it? Blood Purif 23: 72–78.

34. Lacson E, Jr., Levin NW (2004) C-reactive protein and end-stage renal disease. Semin Dial 17: 438–448.

35. Don BR, Kaysen GA (2000) Assessment of inflammation and nutrition in patients with end-stage renal disease. J Nephrol 13: 249–259.

36. Kaysen GA, Dubin JA, Muller HG, Rosales LM, Levin NW (2000) The acute-phase response varies with time and predicts serum albumin levels in hemodialysis patients. The HEMO Study Group. Kidney Int 58: 346–352.

37. Jones CH, Newstead CG, Wills EJ, Davison AM (1997) Serum albumin and survival in CAPD patients: the implications of concentration trends over time. Nephrol Dial Transplant 12: 554–558.

38. Owen WF, Jr., Lew NL, Liu Y, Lowrie EG, Lazarus JM (1993) The urea reduction ratio and serum albumin concentration as predictors of mortality in patients undergoing hemodialysis. N Engl J Med 329: 1001–1006.

39. Kang SH, Cho KH, Park JW, Yoon KW, Do JY (2012) Risk factors for mortality in stable peritoneal dialysis patients. Ren Fail 34: 149–154.

40. Kaul K, Hodgkinson A, Tarr JM, Kohner EM, Chibber R (2010) Is inflammation a common retinal-renal-nerve pathogenic link in diabetes? Curr Diabetes Rev 6: 294–303.

41. Calle MC, Fernandez ML (2012) Inflammation and type 2 diabetes. Diabetes Metab.

42. Churchill DN, Thorpe KE, Nolph KD, Keshaviah PR, Oreopoulos DG, et al. (1998) Increased peritoneal membrane transport is associated with decreased patient and technique survival for continuous peritoneal dialysis patients. The Canada-USA (CANUSA) Peritoneal Dialysis Study Group. J Am Soc Nephrol 9: 1285–1292.

43. Brimble KS, Walker M, Margetts PJ, Kundhal KK, Rabbat CG (2006) Meta-analysis: peritoneal membrane transport, mortality, and technique failure in peritoneal dialysis. J Am Soc Nephrol 17: 2591–2598.

44. Liao CT, Chen YM, Shiao CC, Hu FC, Huang JW, et al. (2009) Rate of decline of residual renal function is associated with all-cause mortality and technique failure in patients on long-term peritoneal dialysis. Nephrol Dial Transplant 24: 2909–2914.

45. Fine A (2002) Relevance of C-reactive protein levels in peritoneal dialysis patients. Kidney Int 61: 615–620.

46. Chung SH, Heimburger O, Stenvinkel P, Qureshi AR, Lindholm B (2003) Association between residual renal function, inflammation and patient survival in new peritoneal dialysis patients. Nephrol Dial Transplant 18: 590–597.

47. Ates K, Ates A, Ekmekci Y, Nergizoglu G (2005) The time course of serum C-reactive protein is more predictive of mortality than its baseline level in peritoneal dialysis patients. Perit Dial Int 25: 256–268.

48. Rumpsfeld M, McDonald SP, Johnson DW (2006) Higher peritoneal transport status is associated with higher mortality and technique failure in the Australian and New Zealand peritoneal dialysis patient populations. J Am Soc Nephrol 17: 271–278.

49. Bargman JM, Thorpe KE, Churchill DN (2001) Relative contribution of residual renal function and peritoneal clearance to adequacy of dialysis: a reanalysis of the CANUSA study. J Am Soc Nephrol 12: 2158–2162.

50. Mujais S, Story K (2006) Peritoneal dialysis in the US: evaluation of outcomes in contemporary cohorts. Kidney Int Suppl: S21–26.

51. Kavanagh D, Prescott GJ, Mactier RA (2004) Peritoneal dialysis-associated peritonitis in Scotland (1999–2002). Nephrol Dial Transplant 19: 2584–2591.

52. Krediet RT, Balafa O (2010) Cardiovascular risk in the peritoneal dialysis patient. Nat Rev Nephrol 6: 451–460.

53. Li PK, Chow KM (2005) The clinical and epidemiological aspects of vascular mortality in chronic peritoneal dialysis patients. Perit Dial Int 25 Suppl 3: S80–83.

54. Johnson DW, Craven AM, Isbel NM (2007) Modification of cardiovascular risk in hemodialysis patients: an evidence-based review. Hemodial Int 11: 1–14.

55. Nolan CR (2005) Strategies for improving long-term survival in patients with ESRD. J Am Soc Nephrol 16 Suppl 2: S120–127.

Glycosylated Hemoglobin and Albumin-Corrected Fructosamine are Good Indicators for Glycemic Control in Peritoneal Dialysis Patients

Szu-Ying Lee[1*◗], Yin-Cheng Chen[2◗], I-Chieh Tsai[2], Chung-Jen Yen[3], Shu-Neng Chueh[4], Hsueh-Fang Chuang[5], Hon-Yen Wu[3,6], Chih-Kang Chiang[7], Hui-Teng Cheng[8], Kuan-Yu Hung[3], Jenq-Wen Huang[3]

1 Department of Internal Medicine, National Taiwan University Hospital, Yun-Lin Branch, Yunlin County, Taiwan, 2 Department of Internal Medicine, Department of Health, Taipei Hospital, Taiwan, 3 Department of Internal Medicine, National Taiwan University Hospital and College of Medicine, Taipei, Taiwan, 4 Department of Nursing, National Taiwan University Hospital and College of Medicine, Taipei, Taiwan, 5 Department of Nursing, National Taiwan University Hospital, Bei-Hu Branch, Taipei, Taiwan, 6 Department of Internal Medicine, Far Eastern Memorial Hospital, New Taipei City, Taiwan, 7 Department of Integrated Diagnostics and Therapeutics, National Taiwan University Hospital and College of Medicine, Taipei, Taiwan, 8 Department of Internal Medicine, National Taiwan University Hospital, Hsin-Chu Branch, Hsinchu City, Taiwan

Abstract

Purpose: Diabetes mellitus (DM) is the most common cause of end-stage renal disease and is an important risk factor for morbidity and mortality after dialysis. However, glycemic control among such patients is difficult to assess. The present study examined glycemic control parameters and observed glucose variation after refilling different kinds of fresh dialysate in peritoneal dialysis (PD) patients.

Methods: A total of 25 DM PD patients were recruited, and continuous glucose monitoring system (CGMS) was applied to measure interstitial fluid (ISF) glucose levels at 5-min intervals for 3 days. Patients filled out diet and PD fluid exchange diaries. The records measured with CGMS were analyzed and correlated with other glycemic control parameters such as fructosamine, albumin-corrected fructosamine (AlbF), glycosylated hemoglobin (HbA1c), and glycated albumin levels.

Results: There were significant correlations between mean ISF glucose and fructosamine ($r = 0.45$, $P < 0.05$), AlbF ($r = 0.54$, $P < 0.01$), and HbA1c ($r = 0.51$, $P < 0.01$). The ISF glucose levels in glucose-containing dialysate increased from approximately 7–8 mg/dL within 1 hour of exchange in contrast to icodextrin dialysate which kept ISF glucose levels unchanged.

Conclusion: HbA1c and AlbF significantly correlated with the mean ISF glucose levels, indicating that they are reliable indices of glycemic control in DM PD patients. Icodextrin dialysate seems to have a favorable glycemic control effect when compared to the other glucose-containing dialysates.

Editor: Emmanuel A. Burdmann, University of Sao Paulo Medical School, Brazil

Funding: This work was supported by a grant from the Department of Health, Taipei Hospital. The funders had no role in study design, data collection and analysis, decision to publish, or preparation of the manuscript.

Competing Interests: The authors have declared that no competing interests exist.

* E-mail: 007378@ntuh.gov.tw

◗ These authors contributed equally to this work.

Introduction

Peritoneal dialysis (PD) is a renal replacement therapy that uses high glucose content to create an osmotic gradient between PD fluid and plasma to achieve ultrafiltration. We previously conducted study to show that higher PD glucose levels had adverse effects on patient survival [1–3]. The other effects of glucose absorption via the peritoneum will contribute to hyperglycemia, dyslipidemia, and other metabolic abnormalities in PD patients. However, appropriate glycemic control parameters that can accurately monitor glucose control among PD patients remain to be established. In addition, the real-time glycemic effects of different dialysate are difficult to demonstrate with conventional glucometer or repeated phlebotomy.

Traditionally, glycosylated hemoglobin (HbA1c) has been used to monitor glycemic control in diabetes mellitus (DM) patients. However, HbA1c in chronic kidney disease (CKD) can be influenced by anemia [4] and uremia [5–10]. Therefore, HbA1c may not be an ideal measure of blood glucose control in DM CKD patients. Several alternative indices of glycemic control have been reported in literature; these include fructosamine [11], albumin-corrected fructosamine (AlbF) [12], and glycated albumin (GA) levels [13]. All have been reported to accurately reflect glycemic control better than HbA1c levels in CKD patients [14]. However, these studies used only casual fasting blood glucose as the gold standard for comparison with the abovementioned glycemic control parameters.

The continuous glucose-monitoring system (CGMS), which measures interstitial fluid (ISF) glucose levels at 5-min intervals over a couple days, can provide continuous and detailed records of glucose levels of subjects [15]. The CGMS has been validated as a reliable and accurate measurement of blood glucose levels in nonuremic DM patients [16], and it has been recently applied for the assessment of glycemic control in DM hemodialysis (HD) [17] and PD [18] patients.

In this study, we applied the CGMS method to PD patients to test the accuracy of fasting glucose, HbA1c, fructosamine, AlbF, and GA as glycemic control parameters. We found that both HbA1c and AlbF were good indicators of glycemic control in PD patients. In addition, the glycemic effects of variable dialysate were also demonstrated by CGMS.

Materials and Methods

Patient Data Collection

From June 2010 to October 2011, DM patients aged more than 20 years who underwent maintenance PD for more than 3 months were enrolled in our study. We excluded patients who had undergone a prior renal transplant, and those who had been newly identified DM after PD. We also excluded patients who could not operate a capillary glucometer. All these patients fitted the DM diagnostic criteria of the American Diabetes Association [19]. In brief, patients with an HbA1c $\geq 6.5\%$, fasting plasma glucose level ≥ 126 mg/dL, or 2-h plasma glucose ≥ 200 mg/dL during an oral glucose-tolerance test at diagnosis and who had received stable anti-diabetic treatment for minimum 6 months were diagnosed with diabetes. Information collected from these participants included demographic data, and data on height, weight, PD modality, glucose concentration of dialysate, and the medication for DM. Peritoneal membrane transport characteristics were defined based on the results of the most recent peritoneal equilibration test (PET) [20]. Residual renal function was measured by calculating the renal Kt/V with a 24-h urine collection. PD adequacy was measured as the sum of peritoneal Kt/V and renal Kt/V. A fasting blood sample was obtained before implanting the CGMS device whichever dialysate in the peritoneal cavity. The blood was centrifuged immediately at 4°C with 3000 rpm. It was then stored at –80°C until measurement.

We collected the information of the monthly doses of erythrocyte stimulating agents (ESA) three months before CGMS. Potency of darbepoetin alfa (NESP, Taiyo Pharmaceutical Industry, Japan) and methoxy polyethylene glycol- epoetin beta (Mircera, Roche Diagnostics GmbH, Germany) were converted to international unit (IU) with a ratio of 1 µg = 200 IU as epoetin beta (Recormon, Roche Diagnostics GmbH, Germany) [21,22].

Ethical Considerations

This study was approved by the ethic committees of National Taiwan University Hospital and Taipei Hospital, Department of Health. The approval numbers were NTUH-REC No. 200912044R and THIRB-10-08, respectively. Patients provided written informed consent before participating in the study.

CGMS Data Collection

Over the past decade, several CGMS have been developed [23], and these equipments measure variations in the glucose levels continuously over a couple days as a Holter system [15]. This demonstrates the true pattern of glucose levels other than the spot levels of fasting or postprandial glycemic levels. Analysis of the CGMS data provides more information about the efficacy of anti-diabetic agents or insulin regimen [24].

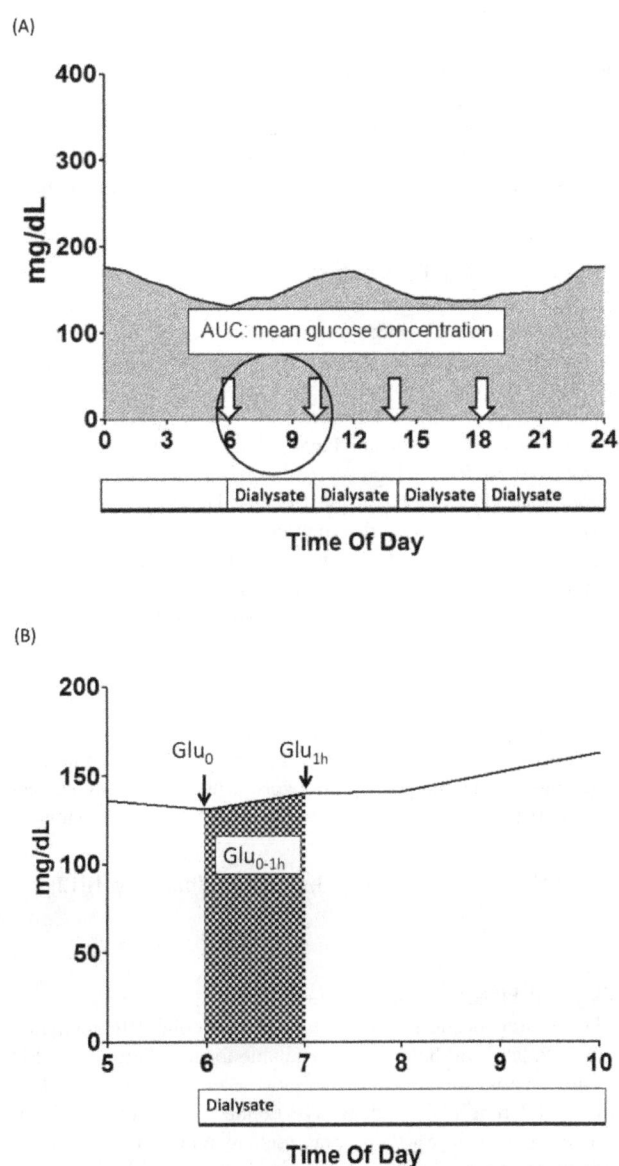

Figure 1. The symbols used to represent the glucose level change by continuous glucose monitoring system.

After adequate informed consent, enrolled patients were implanted with a "Medtronic MiniMed" CGMS (Medtronic MiniMed, CA). Through a needle-type glucose sensor inserted subcutaneously into the abdominal wall, CGMS could be used to record ISF glucose levels, which represent the blood glucose levels. The monitor recorded ISF levels every 10 s and then stored a smoothed average over 5 min. The range of ISF detection was 40–400 mg/dL. Glucose oxidase reaction was applied to measure glucose concentration; this serves as a suitable monitor for patients using icodextrin solution [15].

During CGMS implantation, patients were asked to measure capillary glucose 4 times a day and record the time and content of any oral intake. The time of PD fluid exchange and glucose concentration of dialysate were also recorded. After 3 days of continuous measurement, patients returned to the hospital to remove the device; at that time, the results were downloaded and patients submitted their diet and PD fluid exchange diaries.

Mean glucose level within the first hour of exchanging dialysate (Glu$_{0-1\,h}$) was calculated by measuring the area under the curve (AUC) in this period. Data from patients who had food intake within 1 hr before or after refilling PD fluid were excluded to avoid any interference of diet. Three-day AUC of ISF glucose levels was also calculated to represent the mean 3-day glycemic levels and compare with other glycemic control parameters.

Glycemic Control Parameters

Samples drawn preceding CGMS insertion were checked for levels of the following: fasting glucose, HbA1c, insulin, fructosamine, and GA. HbA1c was analyzed on a cation exchange column chromatograph using an automated high-pressure liquid chromatography instrument (HLC-723 G7, Tosoh Corporation, Tokyo, Japan). This HbA1c assay would be elevated to falsely high by carbamylated hemoglobin [25]. Commercial kits of Cobas Mira (Roche Diagnostics, Mannheim, Germany) were used to determinate fructosamine level which had the ability to reduce nitroblue tetrazolium in alkaline medium. The rate of formation of formazane was directly proportional to the fructosamine concentration and was measured photometrically at 552 nm. We determined GA by commercial kits (Exocell Inc. Philadelphia, PA) with monoclonal antibodies that specifically recognized the glycated lysine residue in GA which was also ketoamine formed by a non-enzymatic oxidation of glucose. These measurements were conducted according to manufacturers' protocols. The method of correction of fructosamine by albumin was described as following:

$$AlbF = fructosamine(mmol/l)/serum\,albumin(g/l)\,[12]$$

Dialysate Effects on Glycemia in PD

Different concentrations of glucose-based dialysate including 1.36%, 2.25% and 3.86% were available for ultrafiltration in PD therapy. Thus, we analyzed the short-term glycemic variations among different PD solutions. We defined 4 parameters. First, baseline glucose levels (Glu$_0$) was used to represent the glucose level at the time of refilling fresh dialysate, and this signified a baseline glucose level. Second, Glu$_{1\,h}$ – Glu$_0$, difference between the glucose level at 1 hr (Glu$_{1\,h}$) after PD fluid exchange and base line Glu$_0$, represented the magnitude of change in ISF glucose concentration within the first hour. Third, Glu$_{0-1\,h}$ calculated from the AUC within the first hour after refilling fresh dialysate represented the average ISF glucose concentration in this period as the above mentioned. Fourth, Glu$_{0-1\,h}$ – Glu$_0$, difference between mean ISF glucose in first hour Glu$_{0-1\,h}$ and the baseline Glu$_0$ level, represented the mean glycemic effects of PD fluid within the first hour (Figure 1).

Statistical Analysis

All variables are reported as mean ± SD or median (25%, 75%) where appropriate for continuous variables and as frequencies or percentages for categorical variables. Student's t-test or non-parametric t-test was used for analysis between groups, wherever appropriate. Differences in frequency were tested using Chi-square analysis. Relationships between variables were tested with Pearson correlation. P values <0.05 were considered significant. All statistical analyses were conducted using SPSS 13.0 for Windows (SPSS Inc., IL, USA).

Results

Clinical Characteristics and Glycemic Parameters

A total of 25 DM patients were recruited in this study. The demographic data and clinical characteristics of these patients are shown in Table 1. Forty-eight percent of study participants were women, and the mean age of the participants was 59±13 years. They had body mass index of 24.7±3.4 kg/m^2 with mean PD vintage of 18±14 months. Their glycemic control parameters were shown in Table 2. Mean values for serum fasting glucose, HbA1c, fructosamine, AlbF, and %GA were 187±82 mg/dL, 8.1±1.4%, 368±64 μmol/L, 972±203 μ mol/g, and 1.72±1.56%, respectively. The mean ISF glucose level calculated from 3-day AUC of glucose levels measured by CGMS was 215±53 mg/dL. Our patients were relatively more obese, and their glycemic controls were poor. The mean doses of ESA at the month of CGMS and one, two and three months prior to CGMS were 14880±6508 IU, 12320±8035 IU, 11840±6780 IU, and 15920±6041 IU, respectively. There was no difference among these groups ($P=0.138$ with non-parametric t-test). The doses of ESA had not changed before the preceding 3 months of the study.

Glycemic Control Parameters Correlate the Glucose Levels Measured by CGMS

To test whether glycemic control parameters could predict chronic glucose control in PD patients, we analyzed the relationships between the data measured by CGMS and other clinically used glycemic control parameters (Figure 2). 3-day mean AUC of glucose levels were significantly correlated with fructosa-

Table 1. Demographic data and clinical characteristics of the enrolled diabetic peritoneal dialysis patients.

	Mean±SD
Sex (man/woman)	13/12
Age	59±13
Body mass index (Kg/m^2)	24.7±3.4
Dialysis modality (CAPD/APD)	16/9
PD vintage (months)	18±14
D4/D0 glucose	0.40±0.07
4 hr D/P creatinine	0.67±0.10
Peritoneal Kt/V	1.78±0.36
Renal Kt/V	0.17±0.22
Total Kt/V	1.95±0.38
nPCR (gm/Kg/day)	0.88±0.19
UN(mg/dL)	55.3±15.2
Creatinine (mg/dL)	10.8±3.2
Albumin (gm/dL)	3.8±0.8
Hb (g/dL)	10.2±1.8
Cholesterol (mg/dL)	212±55
Triglyceride (mg/dL)	157±194
LDL(mg/dL)	99±39
HDL(mg/dL)	44±10
CRP(mg/dL)	0.77±0.87

Continuous ambulatory peritoneal dialysis (CAPD).
Automated peritoneal dialysis (APD).
Normalized protein catabolic rate (nPCR).

Table 2. Glycemic control parameters among the recruited peritoneal dialysis patients.

	Mean±SD
Fasting glucose (mg/dL)	187±82
HbA1c (%)	8.1±1.4
Fructosamine (umol/L)	368±64
Albumin-corrected fructosamine(umol/g)	972±203
Glycated albumin %	1.72±1.56
3-day mean glucose AUC by CGMS (mg/dL)	215±53
Insulin (μU/mL)	13.95±6.23

AUC: area under curve.
Continuous glucose monitoring system (CGMS).
Diet/antidiabetic agent (ADA)/ADA+insulin/insulin (n): 3/4/6/12.

mine (r = 0.45, $P<0.05$), AlbF (r = 0.54, $P<0.01$), and HbA1c (r = 0.51, $P<0.01$). However, there was no correlation between mean AUC and single serum fasting glucose (r = 0.36, $P = 0.08$) or %GA (r = –0.26, $P = 0.26$). These results suggested that HbA1c and AlbF could represent chronic glucose control accurately in PD patients.

Glycemic Change within the First Hour of Dialysate Exchange

Next, we assessed short-term change in glucose levels during PD fluid exchange. There were 16 continuous ambulatory peritoneal dialysis (CAPD) patients enrolled in our study. ISF glucose variations within 1 h of refilling fresh dialysate were further analyzed, and these variations were shown in Fig. 3A. Since the Glu_0 for each dialysate were not identical, the changes in ISF glucose concentrations within the first hour ($Glu_{1\ h}$ – Glu_0) of exchanging fresh dialysate were studied (Fig. 3B). The levels of change were similar between the 1.36% and 2.25% glucose dialysate. However, there were prominent increments in ISF glucose levels after exchanging 3.86% glucose dialysate. Icodextrin dialysate administration had no effect or even lowered the ISF glucose levels.

There was a trend towards increased ISF glucose concentration as the dialysate glucose increased (Table 3). Since CGMS had serial glucose measurement, mean ISF glucose level within 1 h ($Glu_{0–1\ h}$) and the mean increment of glucose levels within 1 h ($Glu_{0–1\ h}$ – Glu_0) could be calculated with these data. $Glu_{0–1\ h}$ was highest after 3.86% glucose indwelling, but the sample number was only 3. $Glu_{0–1\ h}$ – Glu_0 was similar for 1.36% and 2.25% glucose dialysate use, and icodextrin had the lowest increment of ISF glucose levels (Table 3).

The above results suggested that baseline Glu_0 was higher when patients used high glucose concentration dialysate. The Pearson correlation was used to clarify this relationship, and a reverse correlation between Glu_0 and ($Glu_{1\ h}$ – Glu_0) (r = –0.22, $P<0.01$) or ($Glu_{0–1\ h}$ – Glu_0) (r = –0.16, $P = 0.05$) was found. When the extent of changes in glucose concentration were further analyzed, ($Glu_{1\ h}$ – Glu_0)/Glu_0 and ($Glu_{0–1\ h}$ – Glu_0)/Glu_0 were significantly inversely correlated with baseline glucose levels (r = –0.37, $P<0.01$ and r = –0.25, $P<0.01$, respectively, Figure 4).

Peritoneal Membrane Transport Characeristics and Glycemic Control Parameters

Since dialysate dextrose concentration was correlated with peritoneal membrane transport function, we examined the correlation between PET and glycemic control parameters. 4 hrD/P creatinine was correlated with HbA1c (r = 0.41, $P<0.05$), fructosamine (r = 0.41, $P<0.05$), AlbF (r = 0.56, $P<0.01$), and mean AUC of CGMS (r = 0.53, $P<0.01$).

We also examined PET on the changes in glucose levels within the first hour of dialysate exchange. 4 hrD/P creatinine was correlated with (Glu_0) (r = 0.57, $P<0.05$) or ($Glu_{0–1\ h}$) (r = 0.62, $P<0.01$) and D4/D0 glucose was inversely correlated with ($Glu_{1\ h}$-Glu_0) (r = –0.51, $P<0.05$) or ($Glu_{0–1\ h}$-Glu_0) (r = –0.48, $P<0.05$).

Effects of Dialysate on HbA1c

Since HbA1c was positively correlated with the mean ISF glucose when using CGMS, we divided the participants into 2 groups according to median HbA1c levels. One group had HbA1c levels <8% (n = 12), and the other group had HbA1c levels ≥8% (n = 13). We analyzed the effect of dialysates on glucose levels of the 2 groups. Mean glucose concentration within the first hour ($Glu_{0–1\ h}$) of PD fluid exchange was found to be higher in the high HbA1c group with marginal significance ($P = 0.05$, Table 4). However, there was no difference in absolute value or extent of glucose increment, $Glu_{1\ h}$ – Glu_0 or $Glu_{0–1\ h}$ – Glu_0, between these 2 groups (Table 4).

Discussion

In this study, HbA1c and AlbF levels were found to be reliable indices of glycemic control in DM patients receiving PD since these levels were significantly correlated with the mean ISF glucose levels when CGMS was used as a standard of chronic glycemic control. In addition, CGMS demonstrated that icodextrin dialysate had more favorable glycemic effect than other glucose-based dialysates.

Traditional criteria for DM diagnosis are based on spot values of blood glucose levels. However, one study found that spot values were not associated with chronic glycemic control, and there was no association of spot values with DM complications [26]. HbA1c levels, which reflect chronic blood glucose concentration, are a better index of overall glycemic control and provide risk assessment for long-term complications [27]. However, HbA1c levels can be lower along with reduced red cell survival by uremic toxin as well as increased turnover by erythropoietic agents [4]. On the other hand, they become higher under high carbonyl stress in uremia milieu [5–10]. Therefore, it is still not known whether HbA1C can accurately assess glycemic control in CKD patients.

Using the CGMS, we found that HbA1c, AlbF, and fructosamine were good markers of glycemic control in DM PD patients; this was especially true for HbA1c and AlbF. These 2 parameters represented the mean glucose levels better than others, and this finding was inconsistent with other studies that reported that HbA1c levels, as compared to GA%, underestimated glycemic control in dialysis patients [13,14,28]. However, in those studies, either random serum glucose concentration or the mean of monthly fasting serum glucose concentrations were used as the standard of comparison. In our study, on the other hand, single fasting glucose level was correlated with mean ISF glucose level with only marginal significance (Figure 2). It is, therefore, not appropriate to use single fasting sugar level as a standard to monitor glycemic control in DM PD patients.

For PD patients, protein loss from effluent about 5 to 15 g daily with little variation [29]. However, both glycated and non-

(A)

(B)

(C)

(D)

(E)

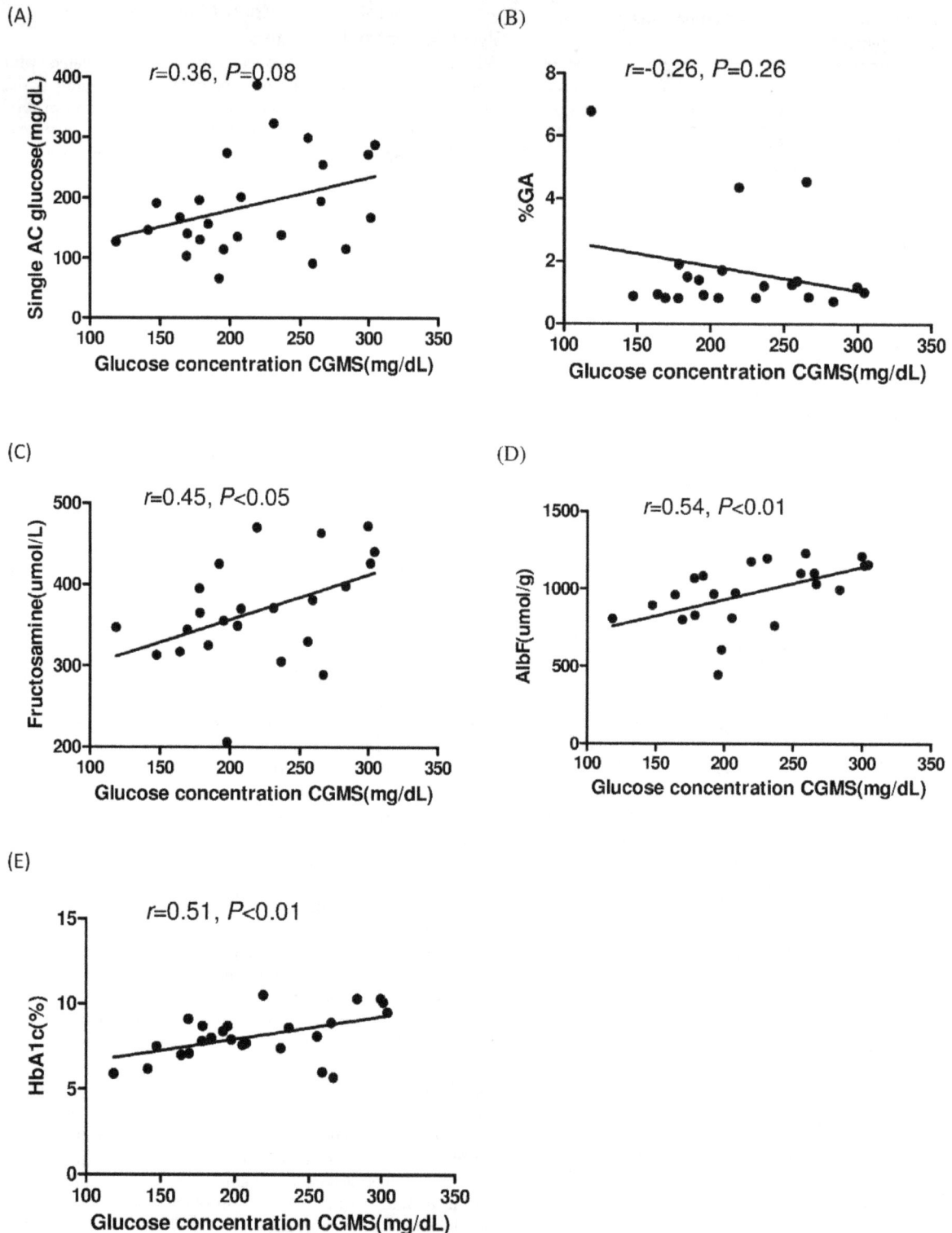

Figure 2. Correlation between ISF glucose and glycemic control parameters. Correlation between 3-day mean interstitial fluid glucose levels measured with continuous glucose monitoring system and levels of single-fasting serum glucose (A), glycated albumin percent (B), fructosamine (C), albumin-corrected fructosamine (D), and glycosylated hemoglobin (E).

glycated protein will exist in effluent with similar ratio as in blood. Therefore, AlbF and GA% will not be affected by the extent of protein loss. This result might explain that the AlbF might be more accurate than fructosamine alone to represent glycemic control.

For GA, an inappropriate glycemic index in this study, molecular weight is higher than that of fructosamine (179 daltons) and the measurement methods for fructosamine and GA are quite different. We are not sure whether the result is related to the

(A)

(B)

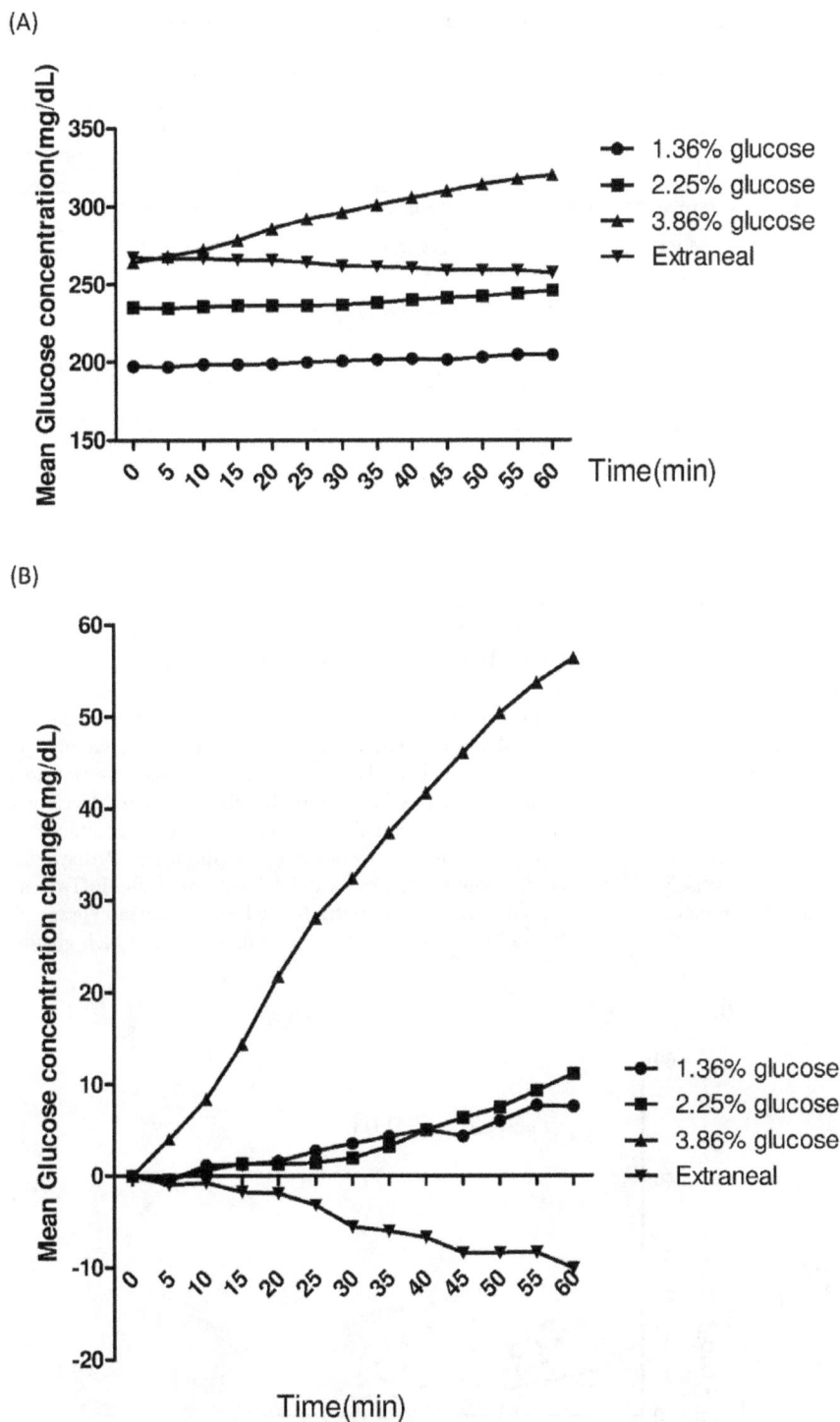

Figure 3. Glucemic change within the first hour of dialysate exchange. The time course of interstitial fluid (ISF) glucose levels (A), and the change of ISF glucose levels (B) within the first hour of refilling fresh dialysate among different kinds of dialysates, including 1.36%, 2.25%, 3.86% glucose dialysate, and Extraneal.

methodology we applied. A number of previous studies showed that icodextrin reduced the burden of glucose overexposure and facilitated glycemic control in DM patients [30,31]. Our results further confirmed that glucose levels increased approximately 4–5% at first hour after exchanging conventional glucose-based dialysate. CGMS could clearly demonstrated that icodextrin

dialysate had no effect or even lowered ISF glucose levels. This result reinforced the advantages of icodextrin-based dialysate use in DM patients.

The reverse relationship between Glu_0 and glucose changes $(Glu_{1\ h} - Glu_0)/Glu_0$ and $(Glu_{0-1\ h} - Glu_0)/Glu_0$ indicated that higher baseline glucose levels reflected smaller changes of ISF

Table 3. The change in interstitial fluid glucose concentration within the first hour of peritoneal dialysis fluid exchange among different kinds of dialysates.

	1.36% glucose	2.25% glucose	3.86% glucose	Extraneal
n	**53**	**77**	**3**	**22**
	Median(25%, 75%)	**Median(25%, 75%)**	**Median(25%, 75%)**	**Median(25%, 75%)**
Glu_0*	192(145, 252)	236(166, 302)	254(201, 337)	264(174, 374)
Glu_{1h}– Glu_0	8(−8, 25)	7(−6, 31)	60(−45, 64)	−7(−34, 14)
Glu_{0-1h} *	191(153, 261)	228(171, 310)	291(233, 359)	249(166, 361)
Glu_{0-1h} – Glu_0*	2(−6, 12)	1(−7, 14)	32(22, 37)	−4(−22, 13)
$(Glu_{1h}$– $Glu_0)/Glu_0$(%)	5(−5, 17)	4(−3, 13)	25(−13,30)	−3(−11, 8)
$(Glu_{0-1h}$ – $Glu_0)/Glu_0$(%)*	1(−3, 8)	0(−3, 7)	15(7, 16)	−2(−9, 6)

*$P<0.05$ with non-parametric t-test.
Glu_{1h}– Glu_0: Glucose increment at 1 h.
Glu_{0-1h}: Mean glucose level within 1 h of fresh dialysate exchange.
Glu_{0-1h} – Glu_0: Mean increment of glucose levels within 1 h.

glucose levels after PD fluid exchange (Figure 4). These results could explain the similar magnitude of increment in glucemic levels for 1.36% and 2.25% glucose dialysate since the Glu_0 levels in the 2.25% dialysate were higher than those of the 1.36% dialysate (Table 3).

Poor sugar control forced diabetic PD patients to higher glucose dialysate to maintain ultrafiltration with subsequent peritoneum damage and higher peritoneal transporting capacity. Therefore, 4 hrD/P creatinine was correlated with HbA1c, fructosamine, AlbF, and mean AUC of CGMS. The lower D4/D0 glucose indicated the higher glucose absorption and was inversely correlated with the increment of glucose levels after refilling dialysate.

Finally, for the patients with HbA1c <8% and ≥8%, Glu_{0-1h} appeared to be higher in the HbA1c ≥8% group with marginal significance. However, there was no difference in $(Glu_{0-1h} – Glu_0)$ or $(Glu_{0-1h} – Glu_0)/Glu_0$ between these 2 groups. Baseline glucose levels (Glu_0) might play a major role in Glu_{0-1h} levels, and the glucose load from dialysate had a fixed extent of increment of glucose in each patient (Table 4). Reduced Glu_0 may be more important in the reduction of HbA1c. Higher glucose levels will need more high glucose dialysate usage to facilitate ultratfiltration and might also contribute to elevating the Glu_0 levels. Perhaps, the vicious cycle could be broken with icodextrin dialysate. In Taiwan, the insurance regulation restricts icodextrin dialysate usage in HbA1C more than 7% or using more than a half of high glucose

(A)

(B)

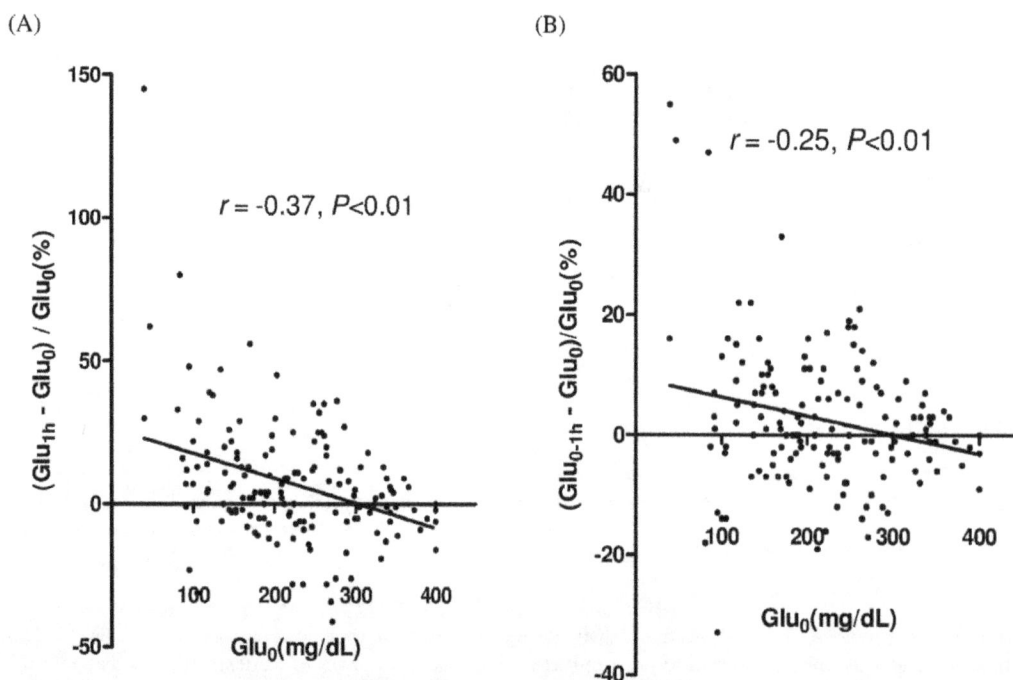

Figure 4. Glucemic change within the first hour of dialysate exchange. Within the first hour of peritoneal dialysis (PD) fluid exchange, correlation between Glu0 and (Glu1 h − Glu0)/Glu0 (A) and (Glu0–1 h − Glu0)/Glu0 (B).

Table 4. Comparison of ISF glucose concentration change within the first hour of PD fluid exchange between patients with HbA1c levels <8% and ≥8%.

	HbA1c <8(n = 12)	HbA1c ≥ 8(n = 13)	
Dialysis modality (CAPD/APD)	9/3	7/6	
The first hour after PD fluid exchange in CAPD patients			
Glu_0 (mg/dL)	191(153, 258)	249(183, 294)	$P = 0.086$
$Glu_{0-1 h}$ (mg/dL)	198(159, 264)	273(182, 299)	$P = 0.050$
$Glu_{1 h} - Glu_0$ (mg/dL)	11(1, 18)	15(7, 22)	$P = 0.414$
$Glu_{0-1 h} - Glu_0$ (mg/dL)	4(−2, 8)	6(−1, 12)	$P = 0.221$
$(Glu_{1 h} - Glu_0)/Glu_0$ (%)	8(1, 15)	5(3, 16)	$P = 0.806$
$(Glu_{0-1 h} - Glu_0)/Glu_0$ (%)	3(−95, 70)	2(−18, 10)	$P = 0.514$
Single fasting glucose	179(136, 242)	156(115, 280)	$P = 0.644$
Mean ISF glucose*	188(155, 225)	236(188, 291)	$P = 0.039$

*$P < 0.05$ with non-parametric t-test.
Interstitial fluid (ISF).

(≥2.25%) dialysate use. So the baseline Glu_0 was higher in the data collected for the icodextrin. On the other hand, use of icodextrin dilysate to achieve adequate ultrafiltration can avoid the further elevation in glucose levels by using high glucose dialysate.

There are limitations in this study. First, we enrolled 25 patients, but only 16 patients received CAPD. For those patients who received automated PD with a cycler, dialysate glucose concentration could not accurately define if the PD fluid containing mixed different glucose concentration dialysate. Second, we conducted only a cross-sectional study and lack of a prospective follow-up. Third, CGMS can only record 3-day glucose levels; it remains unclear whether these data can represent 3 weeks for fructosamine or even 3 months for HbA1 levels. However, 3-day serial measurement by CGMS is more accurate than spot blood glucose levels. Finally, there was no uniform prescription for each patient, so we can't have the same sample numbers of different dialysates in the same patients, however, this will be an universal limitation in the PD dialysate study.

In conclusion, serial measurement of 3-day glucose levels by using CGMS demonstrated that HbA1c and AlbF are appropriate indices of glycemic control in DM patients receiving PD. Higher baseline glucose levels indicate higher glucose concentration dialysate usage with a vicious cycle. Icodextrin-based dialysate which provides a more favorable glycemic control effect.might play a role to brake the cycle.

Acknowledgments

The authors thank the staff of Second Core Lab, Department of Medical Research, National Taiwan University Hospital for technical support.

Author Contributions

Conceived and designed the experiments: JWH. Performed the experiments: SYL YCC. Analyzed the data: ICT CJY CKC HTC. Contributed reagents/materials/analysis tools: SNC HFC HYW JWH. Wrote the paper: KYH SYL YCC.

References

1. Wu HY, Hung KY, Huang TM, Hu FC, Peng YS, et al. (2012) Safety issues of long-term glucose load in patients on peritoneal dialysis–a 7-year cohort study. PLoS One 7: e30337.

2. Wu HY, Hung KY, Huang JW, Chen YM, Tsai TJ, et al. (2008) Initial glucose load predicts technique survival in patients on chronic peritoneal dialysis. Am J Nephrol 28: 765–771.

3. Wu HY, Hung KY, Hu FC, Chen YM, Chu TS, et al. (2010) Risk factors for high dialysate glucose use in PD patients–a retrospective 5-year cohort study. Perit Dial Int 30: 448–455.

4. Ly J, Marticorena R, Donnelly S (2004) Red blood cell survival in chronic renal failure. Am J Kidney Dis 44: 715–719.

5. Goldstein DE, Little RR, Lorenz RA, Malone JI, Nathan D, et al. (1995) Tests of glycemia in diabetes. Diabetes Care 18: 896–909.

6. Panzer S, Kronik G, Lechner K, Bettelheim P, Neumann E, et al. (1982) Glycosylated hemoglobins (GHb): an index of red cell survival. Blood 59: 1348–1350.

7. Smith WG, Holden M, Benton M, Brown CB (1989) Glycosylated and carbamylated haemoglobin in uraemia. Nephrol Dial Transplant 4: 96–100.

8. Tzamaloukas AH (1996) Interpreting glycosylated hemoglobin in diabetic patients on peritoneal dialysis. Adv Perit Dial 12: 171–175.

9. Joy MS, Cefalu WT, Hogan SL, Nachman PH (2002) Long-term glycemic control measurements in diabetic patients receiving hemodialysis. Am J Kidney Dis 39: 297–307.

10. Nakao T, Matsumoto H, Okada T, Han M, Hidaka H, et al. (1998) Influence of erythropoietin treatment on hemoglobin A1c levels in patients with chronic renal failure on hemodialysis. Intern Med 37: 826–830.

11. Coronel F, Macia M, Cidoncha A, Sanchez A, Tornero F, et al. (1991) Fructosamine levels in CAPD: its value as glycemic index. Adv Perit Dial 7: 253–256.

12. Mittman N, Desiraju B, Fazil I, Kapupara H, Chattopadhyay J, et al. (2010) Serum fructosamine versus glycosylated hemoglobin as an index of glycemic control, hospitalization, and infection in diabetic hemodialysis patients. Kidney Int Suppl: S41–45.

13. Freedman BI, Shenoy RN, Planer JA, Clay KD, Shihabi ZK, et al. (2010) Comparison of glycated albumin and hemoglobin A1c concentrations in diabetic subjects on peritoneal and hemodialysis. Perit Dial Int 30: 72–79.

14. Peacock TP, Shihabi ZK, Bleyer AJ, Dolbare EL, Byers JR, et al. (2008) Comparison of glycated albumin and hemoglobin A(1c) levels in diabetic subjects on hemodialysis. Kidney Int 73: 1062–1068.

15. Gross TM, Bode BW, Einhorn D, Kayne DM, Reed JH, et al. (2000) Performance evaluation of the MiniMed continuous glucose monitoring system during patient home use. Diabetes Technol Ther 2: 49–56.

16. McGahan L (2002) Continuous glucose monitoring in the management of diabetes mellitus. Issues Emerg Health Technol: 1–4.

17. Riveline JP, Teynie J, Belmouaz S, Franc S, Dardari D, et al. (2009) Glycaemic control in type 2 diabetic patients on chronic haemodialysis: use of a continuous glucose monitoring system. Nephrol Dial Transplant 24: 2866–2871.

18. Marshall J, Jennings P, Scott A, Fluck RJ, McIntyre CW (2003) Glycemic control in diabetic CAPD patients assessed by continuous glucose monitoring system (CGMS). Kidney Int 64: 1480–1486.

19. (2010) Executive summary: Standards of medical care in diabetes–2010. Diabetes Care 33 Suppl 1: S4–10.

20. Hung KY, Huang JW, Tsai TJ, Chen WY (2000) Natural changes in peritoneal equilibration test results in continuous ambulatory peritoneal dialysis patients: a retrospective, seven year cohort survey. Artif Organs 24: 261–264.

21. Bock HA, Hirt-Minkowski P, Brunisholz M, Keusch G, Rey S, et al. (2008) Darbepoetin alpha in lower-than-equimolar doses maintains haemoglobin levels in stable haemodialysis patients converting from epoetin alpha/beta. Nephrol Dial Transplant 23: 301–308.

22. Sulowicz W, Locatelli F, Ryckelynck JP, Balla J, Csiky B, et al. (2007) Once-monthly subcutaneous C.E.R.A. maintains stable hemoglobin control in patients with chronic kidney disease on dialysis and converted directly from epoetin one to three times weekly. Clin J Am Soc Nephrol 2: 637–646.

23. Reach G (2008) Continuous glucose monitoring and diabetes health outcomes: a critical appraisal. Diabetes Technol Ther 10: 69–80.

24. Reach G, Choleau C (2008) Continuous glucose monitoring: physiological and technological challenges. Curr Diabetes Rev 4: 175–180.

25. Weykamp CW, Miedema K, de Haan T, Doelman CJ (1999) Carbamylated hemoglobin interference in glycohemoglobin assays. Clin Chem 45: 438–440.

26. Wong TY, Liew G, Tapp R, Schmidt MI, Wang JJ, et al. (2008) Relation between fasting glucose and retinopathy for diagnosis of diabetes: three population-based cross-sectional studies (vol 371, pg 736, 2008). Lancet 371: 1838–1838.

27. Gillett MJ (2009) International Expert Committee report on the role of the A1c assay in the diagnosis of diabetes: Diabetes Care 2009; 32(7): 1327–1334. Clin Biochem Rev 30: 197–200.

28. Inaba M, Okuno S, Kumeda Y, Yamada S, Imanishi Y, et al. (2007) Glycated albumin is a better glycemic indicator than glycated hemoglobin values in hemodialysis patients with diabetes: Effect of anemia and erythropoietin injection. Journal of the American Society of Nephrology 18: 896–903.

29. Blumenkrantz MJ, Gahl GM, Kopple JD, Kamdar AV, Jones MR, et al. (1981) Protein losses during peritoneal dialysis. Kidney Int 19: 593–602.

30. Paniagua R, Ventura MD, Avila-Diaz M, Cisneros A, Vicente-Martinez M, et al. (2009) Icodextrin improves metabolic and fluid management in high and high-average transport diabetic patients. Perit Dial Int 29: 422–432.

31. Babazono T, Nakamoto H, Kasai K, Kuriyama S, Sugimoto T, et al. (2007) Effects of icodextrin on glycemic and lipid profiles in diabetic patients undergoing peritoneal dialysis. Am J Nephrol 27: 409–415.

Histological and Clinical Findings in Patients with Post-Transplantation and Classical Encapsulating Peritoneal Sclerosis

Joerg Latus[1⑨], Sayed M. Habib[2⑨], Daniel Kitterer[1], Mario R. Korte[3], Christoph Ulmer[4], Peter Fritz[5], Simon Davies[6], Mark Lambie[7], M. Dominik Alscher[1], Michiel G. H. Betjes[2¶], Stephan Segerer[8¶], Niko Braun[1*¶] on behalf of the European EPS study group[‡]

1 Department of Internal Medicine, Division of Nephrology, Robert-Bosch-Hospital, Stuttgart, Germany, 2 Department of Internal Medicine, Division of Nephrology and Transplantation, Erasmus Medical Center, Rotterdam, The Netherlands, 3 Department of Internal Medicine, Division of Nephrology, Albert Schweitzer Hospital, Dordrecht, The Netherlands, 4 Department of General, Visceral and Trauma Surgery, Robert-Bosch-Hospital, Stuttgart, Germany, 5 Department of Diagnostic Medicine, Division of Pathology, Robert-Bosch Hospital, Stuttgart, Germany, 6 Institute for Science and Technology in Medicine, Keele University, Keele, United Kingdom, 7 Department of Nephrology, University Hospital of North Staffordshire, Stoke-on-Trent, United Kingdom, 8 Division of Nephrology, University Hospital, Zurich, Switzerland

Abstract

Background: Encapsulating peritoneal sclerosis (EPS) commonly presents after peritoneal dialysis has been stopped, either post-transplantation (PT-EPS) or after switching to hemodialysis (classical EPS, cEPS). The aim of the present study was to investigate whether PT-EPS and cEPS differ in morphology and clinical course.

Methods: In this European multicenter study we included fifty-six EPS patients, retrospectively paired-matched for peritoneal dialysis (PD) duration. Twenty-eight patients developed EPS after renal transplantation, whereas the other twenty-eight patients were classical EPS patients. Demographic data, PD details, and course of disease were documented. Peritoneal biopsies of all patients were investigated using histological criteria.

Results: Eighteen patients from the Netherlands and thirty-eight patients from Germany were included. Time on PD was 78(64–95) in the PT-EPS and 72(50–89) months in the cEPS group (p>0.05). There were no significant differences between the morphological findings of cEPS and PT-EPS. Podoplanin positive cells were a prominent feature in both groups, but with a similar distribution of the podoplanin patterns. Time between cessation of PD to the clinical diagnosis of EPS was significantly shorter in the PT-EPS group as compared to cEPS (4(2–9) months versus 23(7–24) months, p<0.001). Peritonitis rate was significantly higher in cEPS.

Conclusions: In peritoneal biopsies PT-EPS and cEPS are not distinguishable by histomorphology and immunohistochemistry, which argues against different entities. The critical phase for PT-EPS is during the first year after transplantation and therefore earlier after PD cessation then in cEPS.

Editor: Lucienne Chatenoud, Université Paris Descartes, France

Funding: These authors have no support or funding to report.

Competing Interests: The EPS-study group is supported by Baxter. Baxter did not fund this study. There are no patents, products in development or marketed products to declare. This does not alter the authors' adherence to all the PLoS ONE policies on sharing data and materials.

* Email: Niko.braun@rbk.de

⑨ These authors contributed equally to this work.

¶ These authors are joint senior authors on this work.

‡ Membership of the European EPS study group is provided in the Acknowledgments.

Introduction

Prolonged time on peritoneal dialysis (PD) could be complicated by encapsulating peritoneal sclerosis (EPS), a rare but severe complication [1–6]. Nowadays, three diagnostic hallmarks are used, i.e. clinical symptoms, radiologic findings and macroscopical/histological criteria [7–9]. In 2000, the International Society for Peritoneal Dialysis (ISPD) defined EPS by clinical signs of abdominal pain, bowel obstruction or weight loss in late stages of the disease [10]. Vlijm et al. [11] and Tarzi et al. [12] published computed tomography (CT)-based scores to diagnose EPS by radiological findings. Several working groups studied histological findings in EPS. However, diagnostic criteria are not well defined [13–15]. Recently, we established a scoring system based on morphological and immunohistochemical features [8]. This study was performed to distinguish simple sclerosis from EPS, more than 20 histological findings were studied and described.

Several risk factors for development of EPS have been reported. The risk of EPS increases with longer time on PD. Additionally younger age, glucose load, peritonitis rate, and cessation of PD are factors illustrated in some studies [5,16,17]. EPS may occur when patients are on dialysis (classical EPS, cEPS) or after undergoing a kidney transplantation (post-transplantation EPS, PT-EPS). The prevalence of PT-EPS has been reported to be between 1 and 3%. This presentation of EPS seems to occur shortly after kidney transplantation in former PD patients [18–21].

The pathophysiology of EPS is still unknown. The widely discussed second-hit theory assumes that the peritoneal membrane is "preconditioned" by the prolonged use of dialysis fluids resulting in a repair process with inflammation and fibrosis, so called simple fibrosis [21–23]. When the second-hit occurs, for example an inflammatory stimulus like bacterial peritonitis, or discontinuation of PD, EPS can develop [24]. There are several hypotheses how transplantation might act as a "second-hit". These include discontinuation of peritoneal lavage of proinflammatory factors, direct apposition of damaged peritoneal membrane or, after successful kidney transplantation, concomitant use of profibrotic calcineurin inhibitors (CNIs) [7,20,21,25]. Previously, Khanna et al. showed that both, Ciclosporine and Tacrolimus can enhance TGB-ß expression and subsequent fibrosis [26].

From a clinical point of view, both cEPS and PT-EPS are similar with regard to clinical presentation and radiological findings. However, post-transplantation EPS seems to be associated with less systemic inflammation at time of presentation and a better outcome [19,21]. The purpose of the current analysis was to determine whether the morphological features of patients presenting with PT-EPS are different to cEPS, thus suggesting a different clinical entity. The clinical course following cessation of PD is also compared. For this purpose we combined peritoneal biopsies from two countries of an European consortium [7].

Materials and Methods

Study population

In the present study, 56 peritoneal biopsies were studied. All biopsies (n = 9) of PT-EPS cases in the biobank of the Dutch EPS registry and Rotterdam PA database (Netherlands) were selected and for each PT-EPS biopsy, one biopsy of a cEPS case was selected resulting in a total number of 18 biopsies [3]. Likewise, a total number of 38 biopsies (including 19 PT-EPS biopsies and 19 cEPS biopsies) were selected from the biobank of the Robert Bosch Hospital in Stuttgart (Germany).

In total, 28 biopsies from patients with PT-EPS were included in the present study. PT-EPS was defined as EPS in former PD patients undergoing a kidney transplantation, after which they developed EPS while having a functioning renal allograft. All 28 biopsies of cEPS patients were paired-matched for PD duration. After cessation of PD, none of the patients performed peritoneal lavage. Classical EPS was defined as EPS in patients who had been or were treated with PD without undergoing prior kidney transplantation.

For the diagnosis of EPS we used clinical criteria stated by Nakamoto et al. [27], radiological criteria by Vlijm et al. [11] and histological criteria by Braun and Honda et al [13,28].

Data collection included demographic data, PD details at start of dialysis. The study protocol was approved by the medical ethics committee of Erasmus Medical Center and by the local ethics committee in Germany (#322/2009BO1, Eberhard-Karls University Tuebingen, Germany). All patients gave written informed consent before participating in the study.

Peritoneal biopsies and analysis

Biopsies from the visceral peritoneum were formalin-fixed in 4% buffered formalin and paraffin-embedded following routine protocols [29]. All peritoneal biopsies were taken from patients at the time of catheter removal or during abdominal surgery (e.g. enterolysis, peritonectomy and enterolysis (PEEL)) following the protocol published by Williams et al. [30] in the time period from February 2002 to December 2012. Staining for podoplanin with the monoclonal antibody D2-40 has been used in several previous studies demonstrating the expression and pattern in EPS [8,28,31]. A monoclonal mouse antihuman podoplanin antibody (D2-40, DAKO, Baar, Switzerland) was used on all biopsies [8,32]. A negative control specimen was created by omitting the primary antibody. Podoplanin was evaluated as either vascular or podoplanin avascular (0, 1, 2, 3). Furthermore, the histological description and pattern(s) of podoplanin-positive cells in peritoneal biopsies were investigated. The biopsies were separated into four groups ("low" podoplanin pattern, "organized" pattern, "diffuse" pattern and "mixed" pattern with features of both "organized" and "diffuse" patterns) [31].

From each slide hematoxylin and eosin staining was done for morphological analysis as previously described [8]: fibrosis: absent, 1–10%/low-power field (LPF), 11–50%/LPF, >51%/LPF (0, 1, 2, 3). Fibroblast-like cells (FLC): absent, 1/5 high-power fields (HPFs), 2–4/5 HPFs, >5/5 HPFs (0, 1, 2, 3); exudation: absent, 1 small area in 1 MPF, 1 area <50%/MPF, 1 area >50%/medium-power field (MPF) (0, 1, 2, 3); cellularity was evaluated as 0(1–2 nuclei/HPF), 1(3–5 nuclei/HPF) 2(6–20 nuclei/HPF) and 3(>20 nuclei/HPF); vessel density: absent, 1–5/HPF, 6–10/HPF, >10/HPF in the submesothelial cell layer (0, 1, 2, 3), acute inflammation (neutrophiles): absent, 1/HPF, 2–5/HPF, >5/HPF (0, 1, 2, 3); chronic inflammation (round cells): absent, 1–5/HPF, 6–20/HPF, >20/HPF (0, 1, 2, 3); hemorrhage: absent extravasal erythrocytes, 1 area <10%/5 LPF, 2+3 area/5 LPF or 1 area 11–30%/LPF, 4+5 area/5 LPF or 1 area >30%/LPF (0, 1, 2, 3); fibrin deposits: absent eosinophilic area, 1 area <5%/5 MPF, 1 area 6–20%/5 MPF, 1 area >20%/5 MPF (0, 1, 2, 3); presence of vasculopathy: thickening of vessel walls and/or inflammation of the vessel wall (0, 1); mesothelial denudation: no visible mesothelium (0, 1); presence of acellular areas (0, 1); presence of brown, probably iron deposits (0, 1); presence of blue, probably calcium deposits (0, 1), and osseous metaplasia (0, 1). FLC were defined as elongated cells, separated from vessel lumen with vesicular nucleus and one to three nucleoli. Acute inflammatory reaction was defined by the presence of neutrophilic granulocytes. Chronic inflammatory reaction was defined by the presence of round cells without taking into consideration further subclasses such as lymphocytes, plasma cells, monocytes and histiocytes. Furthermore thickness of the sub mesothelial cell (SMC) zone was measured as was descripted previously [30,33,34]. $HPF = 0.26 \text{ mm}^2$, $MPF = 0.91 \text{ mm}^2$, $LPF = 3.2 \text{ mm}^2$. Two experienced observer (one pathologist and one nephrologist) blinded to the specimen's diagnosis evaluated each section.

Statistical analysis

Continuous data are expressed as mean ± standard deviation (SD). Variables were classified as either binary (present or absent) or ordinal. The ordinal variables were discriminated as absent, low grade, moderate grade and high grade. We compared a four level classification system with a two level classification system. Each parameter was analyzed for its inter-observer variability. Comparisons between different disease groups were made using analysis of variances (ANOVA) and the

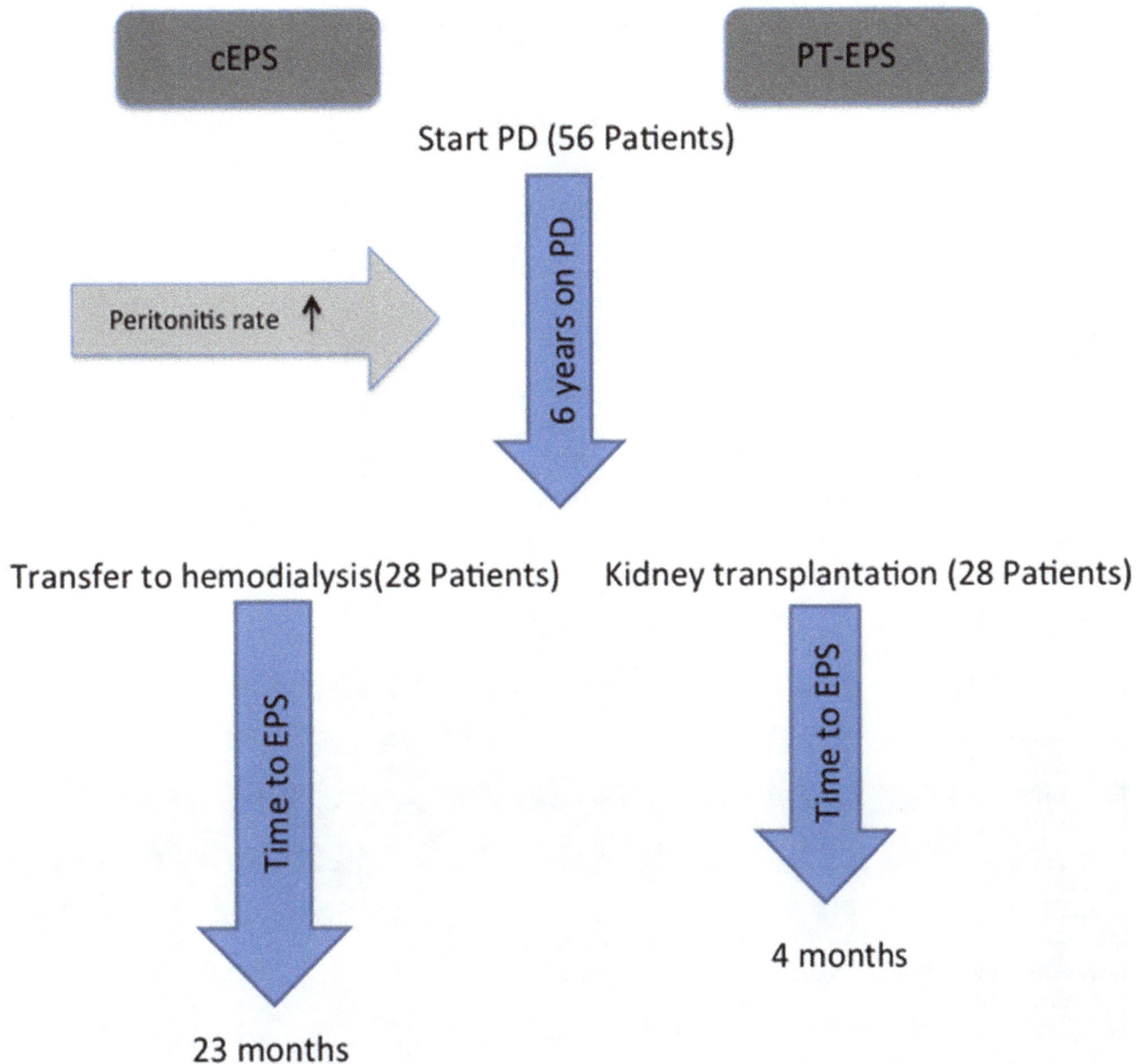

Figure 1. Schematic course of the studied patients. Fifty-six patients started PD. After a mean of approximately six years, twenty-eight patients were transferred to HD, whereas the other twenty-eight patients received a functioning renal allograft. Peritonitis rate was higher and the use of Icodextrin more common in the cEPS compared to the PT-EPS group. Time between transfer to hemodialysis and development of EPS was significantly longer, compared to time between transplantation and development of EPS (23(7–24) months vs. 4(2–9) months, p<0.001; cEPS classical EPS, PT-EPS post-transplantation EPS).

Fisher-test. Statistical results with a p-value≤0.05 were considered as statistically significant.

Results

The baseline clinical characteristics of the study population are shown in table 1. A total of 56 EPS patients were included (28 PT-EPS and 28 cEPS patients, Figure 1). Eighteen patients from the Netherlands and thirty-eight patients from Germany were included. Time on PD was 78(64–95) months in the PT-EPS and 72(50–89) months in the cEPS group without a significant difference between the groups, indicating successful

matching. In both groups, there were more female than male (p>0.05). Patients with cEPS demonstrated a significant higher rate of peritonitis episodes (most common organisms were *Staphylococcus aureus* followed by *coagulase negative Staphylococci* in both groups) and a more frequent use of Icodextrin (table 1).

The time between cessation of PD and diagnosis of EPS was significantly longer in cEPS compared to time after transplantation in PT-EPS group (23(7–24) months vs. 4(2–9) months, p< 0.001) (table 1 and figure 1). Time from onset of symptoms associated with EPS to requirement of surgery was 8(5–11) months in the PT-EPS and 5(4–8) months in the cEPS group

Table 1. Clinical data of PT-EPS and cEPS patients; PD, peritoneal dialysis; EPS, encapsulating peritoneal sclerosis; PET, peritoneal equilibrium test, PDF, peritoneal dialysis fluid, *p<0.05, **p<0.001, #median and interquartile range.

Variable	Post-transplantation EPS	Classical EPS
N	28	28
Age (years)#	52 (46–58)	55 (52–63)
Female/Male	17/11	21/7
CT diagnostic	28	28
Peritoneal thickening	13	12
Bowel dilatation	15	16
Calcification	7	9
Ascites	19	14
Clinical features		
Bowel obstruction		
Nausea and vomiting	23	22
Loss of appetite	18	15
Abdominal pain	28	26
Diarrhea	9	10
Inflammation		
Fever	10	7
PD details		
PD-duration at time of EPS diagnosis in months#	78 (64–95)	72 (50–89)
PET (switch to HD/NTx)	21	22
Low/low average	7	5
High average/high	14	17
Composition of PDF		
Neutral pH	6	10
Acidic pH	11	11
Both	8	3
N.D.	3	4
Icodextrin*	13/24	22/25
Peritonitis*	45 in 1990 months 1:44.2	103 in 1913 months 1:18.6
No peritonitis episodes	8/28	3/28
1–4 peritonitis episodes	19/28	17/28
>4 peritonitis episodes	1/28	8/28
Reason for cessation PD		
Peritonitis		10
Ultrafiltration failure		13
Technical failure		5
Age at time of NTx#	39 (32–47)	
Transfer to HD or NTx to diagnosis EPS (months)**#	4 (2–9)	23 (7–24)
Treatment after transplantation		
Tacrolimus	13	
Ciclosporin	9	
Both	6	
Follow-up		
Follow-up time (months)#	29 (22–74) months	31 (20–63) months
Alive/Dead	19/9	14/14

(p = 0.7). Other parameters including outcome were not significantly different between the groups. All patients in the PT-EPS group were treated with CNIs as part of the transplant immunosuppressive protocol. Six out of twenty-eight patients in the PT-EPS group were exposed to both, Ciclosporin and Tacrolimus.

PT-EPS

cEPS

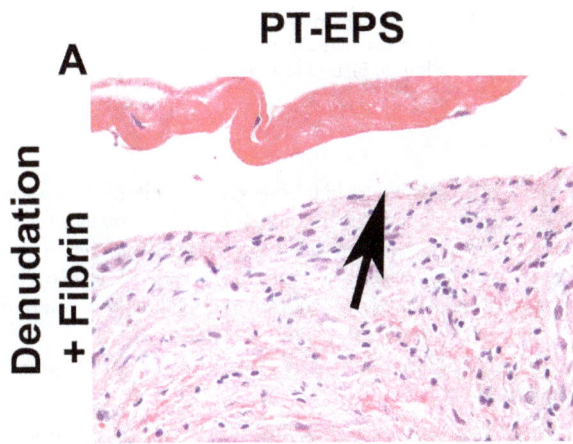

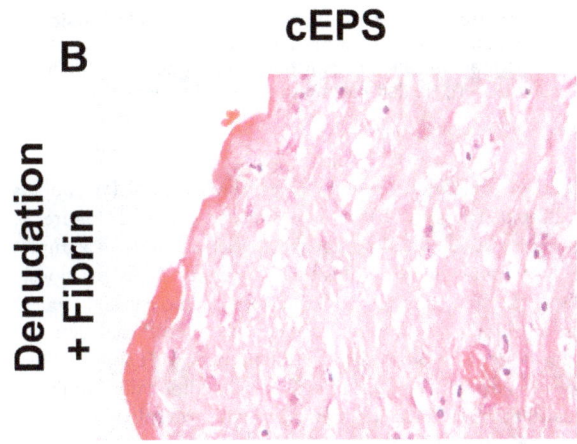

Denudation + Fibrin

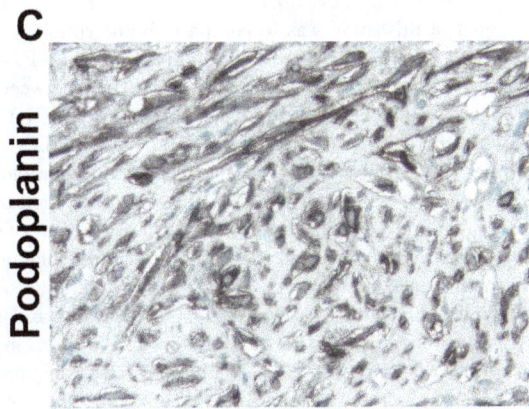

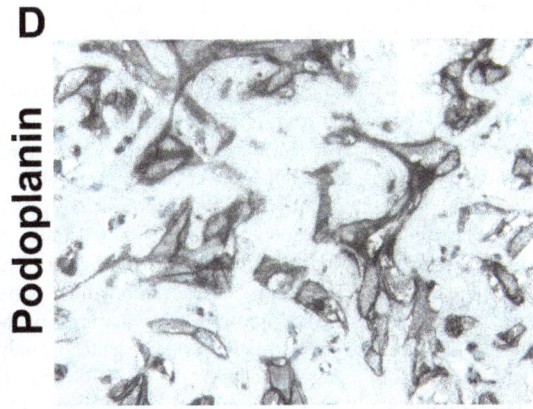

Podoplanin

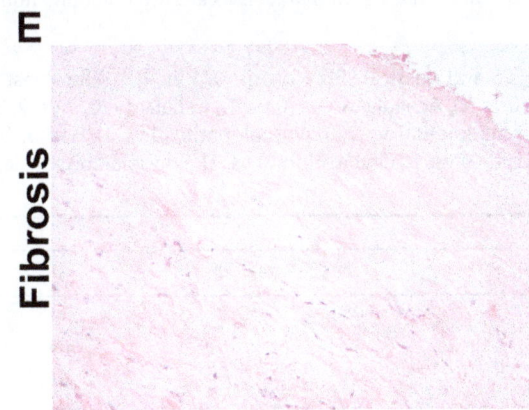

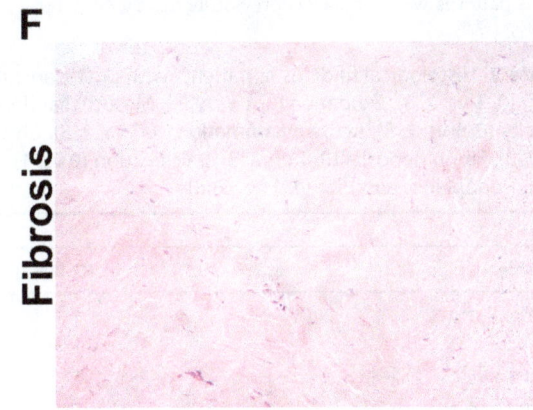

Fibrosis

Acellular areas

Figure 2. Morphologogical evaluation of peritoneal biopsies in PT-EPS and cEPS. Peritoneal biopsies were either stained with PAS (A, B, E–H) or by immunohistochemistry with a monoclonal antibody against podoplanin (D2-40, C, D, original magnifications X 400 in A–D, G, H, X200 in E, F). The morphological evaluation demonstrated similar degrees of denodation and fibrin deposition (A, B), podoplanin positive cells (C, D), fibrosis (E, F) and acellular ares (G, H). (left column post transplant EPS; PT-EPS, right column classical EPS, cEPS).

A detailed evaluation of the biopsies from 28 PT-EPS patients and of 28 patients with cEPS was performed (Table 2, Figure 2). Two observer blinded to the diagnosis studied the slides. Examples of the 17 parameters were illustrated in figure 2. As previously described the majority of EPS biopsies demonstrated severe fibrosis, accumulation of fibroblast like cells, mesothelial denudation, fibrin deposits and chronic inflammation (Table 2). The degree of fibrosis was measured and additionally analyzed semiquantitatively. Measurement of fibrosis revealed a fibrosis zone of 1369 μm [IQR 946–2551] in cEPS and 1690 μm [IQR 1356–2598] in PT-EPS (p = 0.17). Furthermore, podoplanin positive cells and podoplanin positive lymphatic vessels were prominent features (Figure 2).

Based on the morphological evaluation the biopsies with PT-EPS could not be separated from cEPS (Figure 2). There was no significant difference in any of the scored parameters (Table 2). The prominent staining for podoplanin in EPS biopsies was seen to be identical in both country sources, reproducing previous findings. The scores for podoplanin were not significantly different. The peritoneal biopsies were separated into four groups: "low" podoplanin pattern, "organized" podoplanin pattern, "diffuse" pattern and "mixed" pattern with features of both "organized" and "diffuse" patterns). Using this detailed analysis, no differences could be detected between the PT-EPS and cEPS group (all p>0.05) (table 3). Importantly, the percentages of the various patterns were similar as previously described [31].

To avoid a systematic bias between the peritoneal biopsies from different sources (i.e. the Netherlands and Germany), the results were compared between the biopsies from different countries. There was no statistically significant difference between the peritoneal biopsies from the German patient cohort compared to the patients from the Netherlands (table 4).

Discussion

Previous studies suggest, that the clinical course of cEPS differs from patients who develop EPS after transplantation. Therefore, the goal of this study was to compare the morphology of a high number of peritoneal biopsies from patients with PT-EPS and cEPS to detect possible histological differences between the two groups. We matched the groups according to "time on PD", the most relevant risk factor for the development of EPS. A separation of the two groups on morphological grounds would provide evidence that these reflect two different pathological entities. Inflammation, angiogenesis and fibrosis are the main features of EPS, resulting in exudations of fibrin and chronic inflammation of the peritoneal membrane [35]. This leads to adhesions, development of a fibrous cocoon covering the intestines and results in symptoms of bowel obstruction [10,36]. The biopsies included in our study demonstrated the typical (but non-specific) morphological features described for EPS. We could not confirm the hypothesis that PT-EPS and cEPS are two different entities, as the

Table 2. Histological findings in patients with post-transplantation EPS and classical EPS; Fibrosis (0, 1 vs. 2, 3), Fibroblast-like-cells (FLC) (0, 1 vs. 2, 3), Exudation (0, 1 vs. 2, 3), Mesothelial denudation (0 vs. 1), Acellular areas (0 vs. 1), Cellularity (0, 1 vs. 2, 3), Vessel density (0, 1 vs. 2, 3), Acute inflammation (0, 1 vs. 2, 3), Chronic inflammation (0, 1 vs. 2, 3), Vasculopathy (0 vs. 1), Hemorrhage (0, 1 vs. 2, 3), Fibrin deposits (0, 1 vs. 2, 3), Calcification (0 vs. 1), Iron deposits (0 vs. 1), Ossification (0 vs. 1), Podoplanin vascular (0, 1 vs. 2, 3), Podoplanin avscular (0, 1 vs. 2, 3).

Variable	PT-EPS (n = 28)	cEPS (n = 28)	p
Fibrosis	1/27	2/26	1
FLC	14/14	10/18	0.4
Exudation	12/16	14/14	0.8
Mesothelial denudation	0/28	0/28	1
Acellular areas	16/12	21/7	0.3
Cellularity	12/16	8/20	0.4
Vessel density	9/19	5/23	0.4
Acute inflammation	24/4	23/5	0.3
Chronic inflammation	16/12	13/15	1
Vasculopathy	5/23	6/22	1
Hemorrhage	17/11	15/13	0.8
Fibrin deposits	11/17	10/18	1
Calcification	25/3	26/2	1
Iron deposits	11/17	10/18	1
Ossification	0/0	0/0	1
Podoplanin vascular	16/12	17/11	1
Podoplanin avascular	11/17	10/18	1

Table 3. Podoplanin patterns [31] in post-transplantation and classical EPS patients; Organized pattern (0 vs. 1), Diffuse pattern (0 vs. 1), Low pattern (0 vs. 1), Mixed pattern (0 vs. 1).

Variable	Post-transplantation EPS (n = 28)	Classical EPS (n = 28)	p
Organized pattern	10	8	0.8
Diffuse pattern	7	6	1
Low pattern	1	5	0.2
Mixed pattern	4	4	1

histological evaluation could not separate biopsies from the groups. Although, we applied all ever published histological features in EPS, we found no significant differences between the two groups [8]. Immunohistochemstry with podoplanin, including an extensive pattern analysis revealed no difference between the groups. Recently, Kinashi et al. showed that peritoneal tissue from patients with ultrafiltration failure (UFF) contained more lymphatic vessels than tissue from patients without UFF [37]. Podoplanin was found to be a good marker for lymphatic endothelial cells, but is expressed by peritoneal mesothelial and fibroblast-like-cells (FLC) too [8,38]. In our patient cohort, approximately fifty-percent of the patients in both groups showed a strong expression of podoplanin, but no difference in the expression pattern. Hence, podoplanin seems to play an role in the pathogenesis of EPS, but does not differentiate between cEPS and PT-EPS.

The incidence of EPS increases with time on PD (other factors like peritonitis rate, male gender, younger age, smoking and glucose exposure are under debate) [5,16,32,39–44]. The group of

patients with cEPS demonstrated a higher-rate of peritonitis, and the use of icodextrin was more common, whereas the time to diagnosis after cessation of PD was longer in the cEPS group. The shorter time to clinically symptomatic EPS in patients after kidney transplantation has previously been described [21,45]. Interestingly, there were no differences regarding morphological findings, and particularly no differences in the severity of fibrosis, using both, semi-quantitative and quantitative analysis. This could argue that factors in the PT-EPS group resulted in a faster progression of the disease. It is likely that the time to the clinical manifestation is based on the ratio of pro fibrotic factors (e.g. time on PD, surgery, peritonitis, calcineurin-inhibitors) and factors which might inhibit the disease process (e.g. steroids, rinsing the abdominal cavity). The combination of pro-fibrotic factors after transplantation might result in a faster disease process, although the major players in the pathogenesis have not been defined [21].

It has been recently shown in a rat model of peritoneal exposure to dialysis fluid that additional administration of Ciclosporin leads to EPS like abnormalities [46]. The calcineurin-inhibitors

Table 4. Histological findings in patients with EPS (post-transplantation EPS and classical EPS) in the study population of the Netherlands and Germany; Fibrosis (0, 1 vs. 2, 3), Fibroblast-like-cells (FLC) (0, 1 vs. 2, 3), Exudation (0, 1 vs. 2, 3), Mesothelial denudation (0 vs. 1), Acellular areas (0 vs. 1), Cellularity (0, 1 vs. 2, 3), Vessel density (0, 1 vs. 2, 3), Acute inflammation (0, 1 vs. 2, 3), Chronic inflammation (0, 1 vs. 2, 3), Vasculopathy (0 vs. 1), Hemorrhage (0, 1 vs. 2, 3), Fibrin deposits (0, 1 vs. 2, 3), Calcification (0 vs. 1), Iron deposits (0 vs. 1), Ossification (0 vs. 1), Podoplanin vascular (0, 1 vs. 2, 3), Podoplanin avscular (0, 1 vs. 2, 3).

Variable	Netherlands (n = 18)	Germany (n = 38)	p
Fibrosis	2/16	1/37	0.2
FLC	10/8	14/24	0.3
Exudation	8/10	18/20	1
Mesothelial denudation	0/18	0/38	0.3
Acellular areas	13/5	24/14	0.6
Cellularity	6/12	14/24	1
Vessel density	3/15	11/38	0.5
Acute inflammation	14/4	33/5	0.4
Chronic inflammation	11/7	18/20	0.4
Vasculopathy	5/13	6/32	0.3
Hemorrhage	12/6	20/18	0.8
Fibrin deposits	9/9	12/26	0.2
Calcification	18/0	33/5	0.2
Iron deposits	4/14	17/21	0.1
Ossification	0/0	0/0	1
Podoplanin vascular	13/5	20/18	0.2
Podoplanin avascular	9/9	12/26	0.2

(Ciclopsorin and Tacrolimus) can lead to enhanced expression of transforming growth factor-β (TGF-β), demonstrated in a preconditioned peritoneal membrane, which already demonstrated up-regulation of TGF-β. This results in increasing fibrosis and neoangiogenesis of the peritoneal membrane [21,26,47]. Due to the lack of biopsies at the time of transfer to either dialysis or transplantation we cannot prove the differences in progression. It is less likely that PT-EPS patients would have had more severe membrane injury at the time of modality transfer compared to the cEPS group who likely had complications leading to technique failure as evidenced by their higher rate of peritonitis episodes and greater need of Icodextrin, suggesting either UFF or less residual renal function. This raises an important question: could the morphological evaluation at the time of transfer to a different form of renal replacement therapy add value to an overall risk assessment (including time on treatment, peritonitis history and ultrafiltration failure) in predicting the development of EPS? This requires a high number of patients with biopsies at transfer when removing the PD catheter, and we will try to answer this question within the European patient cohort in the future.

An alternative explanation for the differences between the time to manifestation would be that patients after transplantation might be seen more often in the transplant clinics and/or symptoms might rather be ignored in patients on hemodialysis, as had been reported by patients [48]. In 9 interviews of patients with EPS the patients described a loss of trust in the doctors as symptoms while being on dialysis were not taken seriously [48].

If patients after transplantation would be detected earlier in the diseases course due to more frequent doctor visits, it would be expected that the histological finding would be less extensive in patients with PT-EPS. Particularly, the fibrosis scores should be less severe, but no differences could be detected and time from onset of symptoms associated with EPS to requirement of surgery was not different between both groups. Therefore this argument is less convincing than a faster disease process.

The limitations of the study design of course leaves unanswered questions and room for future studies. The available data from these two referral centers provided in the registers were limited. We could not provide more sophisticated information about membrane function (e.g. osmotic conductance or glucose exposure during PD) [49]. We were unable to fully comply with suggested standards for reporting clinical features of EPS as the data was collected prospectively, before the standards were suggested [50]. Survival was not significantly different between the groups, even so there was a trend towards a better outcome in the PT-EPS group (p = 0.3). This does not contradict previous reports, which demonstrated a better outcome of PT-EPS, as the study was not powered to find such a difference [19,45]. The younger age of PT-EPS patients and the better overall condition of patients with a functioning kidney allograft would be likely explanations for a better outcome [19].

In conclusion, this analysis did not support the hypothesis that EPS following transplantation is a different clinico-pathological entity, despite differences in the time taken between stopping PD and diagnosis and possible differences in known risk factors such membrane failure.

Acknowledgments

The study was supported by Baxter.

European EPS study group: Andreas Vychytil, Division of Nephrology and Dialysis, Department of Medicine III, Medical University of Vienna, Vienna, Austria; Eric Goffin, Université catholique de Louvain, Brussels, Belgium; Guido Garosi, Azienda Ospedaliera Universitaria Senese, Siena, Italy; Rafael Selgas, Department of Nephrology, Hospital Universitario La Paz, IdiPAZ, Madrid, Spain; Alferso C. Abrahams University Medical Center Utrecht,Utrecht, Netherlands; Bengt Lindholm, Divisions of Renal Medicine and Baxter Novum, Department of Clinical Science, Intervention and Technology, Karolinska University Hospital K56, Karolinska Institutet, 14186, Stockholm, Sweden; Paul Brenchley, Manchester Institute of Nephrology and Transplantation, Central Manchester University Hospital NHS Trust, Oxford Road, Manchester M13 9WL, UK; Angela Summers, Manchester Royal Infirmary, Manchester, UK.

Author Contributions

Conceived and designed the experiments: JL SS MB DK NB MDA PF. Performed the experiments: JL SS MB DK NB MDA PF CU SMH. Analyzed the data: JL SS MB DK NB MDA PF CU MK SD ML SMH. Contributed reagents/materials/analysis tools: JL SS MB DK NB MDA PF CU MK SD ML SMH. Wrote the paper: JL SS MB DK NB MDA PF CU MK SD ML SMH.

References

1. Maruyama Y, Nakayama M (2008) Encapsulating peritoneal sclerosis in Japan. Perit Dial Int 28 Suppl 3: S201–204.

2. Latus J, Ulmer C, Fritz P, Rettenmaier B, Biegger D, et al. (2013) Encapsulating peritoneal sclerosis: a rare, serious but potentially curable complication of peritoneal dialysis-experience of a referral centre in Germany. Nephrol Dial Transplant 28: 1021–1030.

3. Korte MR, Boeschoten EW, Betjes MG (2009) The Dutch EPS Registry: increasing the knowledge of encapsulating peritoneal sclerosis. Neth J Med 67: 359–362.

4. Habib SM, Betjes MG, Fieren MW, Boeschoten EW, Abrahams AC, et al. (2011) Management of encapsulating peritoneal sclerosis: a guideline on optimal and uniform treatment. Neth J Med 69: 500–507.

5. Brown MC, Simpson K, Kerssens JJ, Mactier RA (2009) Encapsulating peritoneal sclerosis in the new millennium: a national cohort study. Clin J Am Soc Nephrol 4: 1222–1229.

6. Sampimon DE, Korte MR, Barreto DL, Vlijm A, de Waart R, et al. (2010) Early diagnostic markers for encapsulating peritoneal sclerosis: a case-control study. Perit Dial Int 30: 163–169.

7. Summers AM, Abrahams AC, Alscher MD, Betjes M, Boeschoten EW, et al. (2011) A collaborative approach to understanding EPS: the European perspective. Biomarkers of EPS: can we go "back to the future"? Perit Dial Int 31: 245–248.

8. Braun N, Fritz P, Ulmer C, Latus J, Kimmel M, et al. (2012) Histological criteria for encapsulating peritoneal sclerosis - a standardized approach. PLoS One 7: e48647.

9. Latus J, Ulmer C, Fritz P, Rettenmaier B, Biegger D, et al. (2013) Phenotypes of encapsulating peritoneal sclerosis–macroscopic appearance, histologic findings, and outcome. Perit Dial Int 33: 495–502.

10. Kawaguchi Y, Kawanishi H, Mujais S, Topley N, Oreopoulos DG (2000) Encapsulating peritoneal sclerosis: definition, etiology, diagnosis, and treatment. International Society for Peritoneal Dialysis Ad Hoc Committee on Ultrafiltration Management in Peritoneal Dialysis. Perit Dial Int 20 Suppl 4: S43–55.

11. Vlijm A, Stoker J, Bipat S, Spijkerboer AM, Phoa SS, et al. (2009) Computed tomographic findings characteristic for encapsulating peritoneal sclerosis: a case-control study. Perit Dial Int 29: 517–522.

12. Tarzi RM, Lim A, Moser S, Ahmad S, George A, et al. (2008) Assessing the validity of an abdominal CT scoring system in the diagnosis of encapsulating peritoneal sclerosis. Clin J Am Soc Nephrol 3: 1702–1710.

13. Honda K, Nitta K, Horita S, Tsukada M, Itabashi M, et al. (2003) Histologic criteria for diagnosing encapsulating peritoneal sclerosis in continuous ambulatory peritoneal dialysis patients. Adv Perit Dial 19: 169–175.

14. Garosi G, Di Paolo N, Sacchi G, Gaggiotti E (2005) Sclerosing peritonitis: a nosological entity. Perit Dial Int 25 Suppl 3: S110–112.

15. Sherif AM, Yoshida H, Maruyama Y, Yamamoto H, Yokoyama K, et al. (2008) Comparison between the pathology of encapsulating sclerosis and simple sclerosis of the peritoneal membrane in chronic peritoneal dialysis. Ther Apher Dial 12: 33–41.

16. Johnson DW, Cho Y, Livingston BE, Hawley CM, McDonald SP, et al. (2010) Encapsulating peritoneal sclerosis: incidence, predictors, and outcomes. Kidney Int 77: 904–912.

17. Oules R, Challah S, Brunner FP (1988) Case-control study to determine the cause of sclerosing peritoneal disease. Nephrol Dial Transplant 3: 66–69.

18. Fontana I, Bertocchi M, Santori G, Ferrari G, Barabani C, et al. (2012) Encapsulating peritoneal sclerosis after kidney transplantation: a single-center experience from 1982 to 2010. Transplant Proc 44: 1918–1921.

19. Habib SM, Korte MR, Betjes MG (2013) Lower mortality and inflammation from post-transplantation encapsulating peritoneal sclerosis compared to the classical form. Am J Nephrol 37: 223–230.

20. Fieren MW, Betjes MG, Korte MR, Boer WH (2007) Posttransplant encapsulating peritoneal sclerosis: a worrying new trend? Perit Dial Int 27: 619–624.

21. Korte MR, Habib SM, Lingsma H, Weimar W, Betjes MG (2011) Posttransplantation encapsulating peritoneal sclerosis contributes significantly to mortality after kidney transplantation. Am J Transplant 11: 599–605.

22. Saito A (2005) Peritoneal dialysis in Japan: the issue of encapsulating peritoneal sclerosis and future challenges. Perit Dial Int 25 Suppl 4: S77–82.

23. Kawanishi H, Kawaguchi Y, Fukui H, Hara S, Imada A, et al. (2004) Encapsulating peritoneal sclerosis in Japan: a prospective, controlled, multicenter study. Am J Kidney Dis 44: 729–737.

24. Honda K, Oda H (2005) Pathology of encapsulating peritoneal sclerosis. Perit Dial Int 25 Suppl 4: S19–29.

25. Korte MR, Yo M, Betjes MG, Fieren MW, van Saase JC, et al. (2007) Increasing incidence of severe encapsulating peritoneal sclerosis after kidney transplantation. Nephrol Dial Transplant 22: 2412–2414.

26. Khanna A, Plummer M, Bromberek C, Bresnahan B, Hariharan S (2002) Expression of TGF-beta and fibrogenic genes in transplant recipients with tacrolimus and cyclosporine nephrotoxicity. Kidney Int 62: 2257–2263.

27. Nakamoto H (2005) Encapsulating peritoneal sclerosis–a clinician's approach to diagnosis and medical treatment. Perit Dial Int 25 Suppl 4: S30–38.

28. Braun N, Alscher DM, Fritz P, Edenhofer I, Kimmel M, et al. (2011) Podoplanin-positive cells are a hallmark of encapsulating peritoneal sclerosis. Nephrol Dial Transplant 26: 1033–1041.

29. Braun N, Reimold F, Biegger D, Fritz P, Kimmel M, et al. (2009) Fibrogenic growth factors in encapsulating peritoneal sclerosis. Nephron Clin Pract 113: c88–95.

30. Williams JD, Craig KJ, Topley N, Von Ruhland C, Fallon M, et al. (2002) Morphologic changes in the peritoneal membrane of patients with renal disease. J Am Soc Nephrol 13: 470–479.

31. Braun N, Alscher MD, Fritz P, Latus J, Edenhofer I, et al. (2012) The spectrum of podoplanin expression in encapsulating peritoneal sclerosis. PLoS One 7: e53382.

32. Braun N, Alscher DM, Fritz P, Edenhofer I, Kimmel M, et al. (2010) Podoplanin-positive cells are a hallmark of encapsulating peritoneal sclerosis. Nephrol Dial Transplant.

33. Shimaoka T, Hamada C, Kaneko K, Io H, Sekiguchi Y, et al. (2010) Quantitative evaluation and assessment of peritoneal morphologic changes in peritoneal dialysis patients. Nephrol Dial Transplant 25: 3379–3385.

34. Honda K, Hamada C, Nakayama M, Miyazaki M, Sherif AM, et al. (2008) Impact of uremia, diabetes, and peritoneal dialysis itself on the pathogenesis of peritoneal sclerosis: a quantitative study of peritoneal membrane morphology. Clin J Am Soc Nephrol 3: 720–728.

35. Bozkurt D, Sipahi S, Cetin P, Hur E, Ozdemir O, et al. (2009) Does immunosuppressive treatment ameliorate morphology changes in encapsulating peritoneal sclerosis? Perit Dial Int 29 Suppl 2: S206–210.

36. Alscher DM, Braun N, Biegger D, Fritz P (2007) Peritoneal mast cells in peritoneal dialysis patients, particularly in encapsulating peritoneal sclerosis patients. Am J Kidney Dis 49: 452–461.

37. Kinashi H, Ito Y, Mizuno M, Suzuki Y, Terabayashi T, et al. (2013) TGF-beta1 promotes lymphangiogenesis during peritoneal fibrosis. J Am Soc Nephrol 24: 1627–1642.

38. Kalof AN, Cooper K (2009) D2-40 immunohistochemistry-so far! Adv Anat Pathol 16: 62–64.

39. Guest S (2009) Hypothesis: gender and encapsulating peritoneal sclerosis. Perit Dial Int 29: 489–491.

40. Korte MR, Sampimon DE, Lingsma HF, Fieren MW, Looman CW, et al. (2011) Risk factors associated with encapsulating peritoneal sclerosis in Dutch EPS study. Perit Dial Int 31: 269–278.

41. Martikainen TA, Teppo AM, Gronhagen-Riska C, Ekstrand AV (2005) Glucose-free dialysis solutions: inductors of inflammation or preservers of peritoneal membrane? Perit Dial Int 25: 453–460.

42. Posthuma N, Verbrugh HA, Donker AJ, van Dorp W, Dekker HA, et al. (2000) Peritoneal kinetics and mesothelial markers in CCPD using icodextrin for daytime dwell for two years. Perit Dial Int 20: 174–180.

43. Brown EA, Van Biesen W, Finkelstein FO, Hurst H, Johnson DW, et al. (2009) Length of time on peritoneal dialysis and encapsulating peritoneal sclerosis: position paper for ISPD. Perit Dial Int 29: 595–600.

44. Kawanishi H, Moriishi M (2005) Epidemiology of encapsulating peritoneal sclerosis in Japan. Perit Dial Int 25 Suppl 4: S14–18.

45. Balasubramaniam G, Brown EA, Davenport A, Cairns H, Cooper B, et al. (2009) The Pan-Thames EPS study: treatment and outcomes of encapsulating peritoneal sclerosis. Nephrol Dial Transplant 24: 3209–3215.

46. van Westrhenen R, Aten J, Hajji N, de Boer OJ, Kunne C, et al. (2007) Cyclosporin A induces peritoneal fibrosis and angiogenesis during chronic peritoneal exposure to a glucose-based, lactate-buffered dialysis solution in the rat. Blood Purif 25: 466–472.

47. Margetts PJ, Bonniaud P, Liu L, Hoff CM, Holmes CJ, et al. (2005) Transient overexpression of TGF-{beta}1 induces epithelial mesenchymal transition in the rodent peritoneum. J Am Soc Nephrol 16: 425–436.

48. Hurst H, Summers AM, Beaver K, Caress AL (2014) Living with Encapsulating Peritoneal Sclerosis (Eps): The Patient's Perspective. Perit Dial Int.

49. Lambie ML, John B, Mushahar L, Huckvale C, Davies SJ (2010) The peritoneal osmotic conductance is low well before the diagnosis of encapsulating peritoneal sclerosis is made. Kidney Int 78: 611–618.

50. Lambie M, Braun N, Davies SJ (2013) Towards standardized reporting in studies of encapsulating peritoneal sclerosis. Perit Dial Int 33: 482–486.

Serum Potassium Levels and its Variability in Incident Peritoneal Dialysis Patients: Associations with Mortality

Qingdong Xu, Fenghua Xu, Li Fan, Liping Xiong, Huiyan Li, Shirong Cao, Xiaoyan Lin, Zhihua Zheng, Xueqing Yu, Haiping Mao*

Department of Nephrology, The First Affiliated Hospital, Sun Yat-sen University, Key Laboratory of Nephrology, Ministry of Health of China, Guangzhou, China

Abstract

Background: Abnormal serum potassium is associated with an increased risk of mortality in dialysis patients. However, the impacts of serum potassium levels on short- and long-term mortality and association of potassium variability with death in peritoneal dialysis (PD) patients are uncertain.

Methods: We examined mortality-predictability of serum potassium at baseline and its variability in PD patients treated in our center January 2006 through December 2010 with follow-up through December 2012. The hazard ratios (HRs) were used to assess the relationship between baseline potassium levels and short-term (≤ 1 year) as well as long-term (>1 year) survival. Variability of serum potassium was defined as the coefficient of variation of serum potassium (CVSP) during the first year of PD.

Results: A total of 886 incident PD patients were enrolled, with 248 patients (27.9%) presented hypokalemia (serum potassium <3.5 mEq/L). During a median follow-up of 31 months (range: 0.5–81.0 months), adjusted all-cause mortality hazard ratio (HR) and 95% confidence interval (CI) for baseline serum potassium of <3.0, 3.0 to <3.5, 3.5 to <4.0, 4.5 to <5.0, and ≥ 5.0 mEq/L, compared with 4.0 to <4.5 (reference), were 1.79 (1.02–3.14), 1.15 (0.72–1.86), 1.31 (0.82–2.08), 1.33 (0.71–2.48), 1.28 (0.53–3.10), respectively. The increased risk of lower potassium with mortality was evident during the first year of follow-up, but vanished thereafter. Adjusted all-cause mortality HR for CVSP increments of 7.5% to $<12.0\%$; 12.0% to $<16.7\%$ and $\geq 16.7\%$, compared with $<7.5\%$ (reference), were 1.35 (0.67–2.71), 2.00 (1.05–3.83) and 2.18 (1.18–4.05), respectively. Similar association was found between serum potassium levels and its variability and cardiovascular mortality.

Conclusions: A lower serum potassium level was associated with all-cause and cardiovascular mortality during the first year of follow-up in incident PD patients. In addition, higher variability of serum potassium levels conferred an increased risk of death in this population.

Editor: Emmanuel A. Burdmann, University of Sao Paulo Medical School, Brazil

Funding: This work was supported by grants from the National Key Technology Research and Development Program of the Ministry of Science and Technology of China (No. 2011BAI10B05), the National Science Fund for Distinguished Young Scholars of China (No. 30925019), 5010 Clinical Program of Sun Yat-sen University (No. 2007007) and the Guangzhou Committee of Science and Technology of China (No. 2010U1-E00831). The funders had no role in study design, data collection and analysis, decision to publish, or preparation of the manuscript.

Competing Interests: The authors have declared that no competing interests exist.

* E-mail: haipingmao@126.com

Introduction

Disorder of potassium homeostasis may contribute to a higher risk of death in patients on dialysis. In patients with chronic kidney disease or those under hemodialysis (HD), a link between serum potassium levels and mortality is evident, with mortality risk significantly greater at potassium <4.0 mEq/L [1,2]. Unlike HD patients, hypokalemia (serum potassium <3.5 mEq/L) is common in peritoneal dialysis (PD) patients, at a frequency ranging from 10 to 36% [3,4,5]. The reasons for this wide range of prevalence of hypokalemia are unknown, but may depend on studying different populations, time point of baseline serum potassium levels, and study period.

It has been well documented that low potassium levels are associated with general and sudden death among patients with cardiovascular disease [6,7]. Among Chinese continuous ambulatory peritoneal dialysis (CAPD) patients, Szeto *et al.* has demonstrated that hypokalemia at baseline is an independent prognostic indicator of survival [8]. Recently, a large study from the United States showed that a time-averaged, but not baseline, serum potassium <3.5 mEq/L was associated with a higher adjusted risk for all-cause and cardiovascular mortality in a cohorts of prevalent PD patients [9]. Low potassium may affect myocardial resting membrane potential, repolarization and conduction velocity, suggesting that it causes negative short-term effects on mortality and becomes weaker following correction over longer period of time. However, the time discrepancy of serum potassium on mortality has not been evaluated in prior studies. Moreover, stability of potassium levels, rather than those absolute values of baseline, may be more closely relevant to mortality [10]. To the best of our knowledge, there is a lack of study that determines the

Table 1. Baseline characteristics of PD patients according to categories of serum potassium.

Variables	Baseline levels of serum potassium (mEq/L)						P-value
	<3.0	3.0 to <3.5	3.5 to <4.0	4.0 to <4.5	4.5 to <5.0	≥5.0	
No. of patients (%)	(n = 66, 7.4%)	(n = 182, 20.5%)	(n = 284, 32.1%)	(n = 220, 24.8%)	(n = 96, 10.8%)	(n = 38, 4.3%)	–
Age (years)	54.1±17.3	50.7±16.5	47.7±15.0	47.1±14.7	47.0±14.5	46.0±12.7	0.005*
Female (%)	35 (53.0%)	85 (46.7%)	120 (42.3%)	92 (41.8%)	35 (36.5%)	13 (34.2%)	0.34
BMI (kg/m^2)	20.2±2.9	21.4±2.7	21.7±3.2	22.2±3.1	22.6±3.5	22.7±3.4	<0.001*
Etiology of ESRD							0.1
CGN (%)	32 (48.5%)	88 (48.4%)	164 (57.7%)	128 (58.7%)	51 (53.1%)	19 (50.0%)	
DN (%)	15 (22.7%)	46 (25.3%)	50 (17.6%)	52 (23.9%)	25 (26.0%)	11 (28.9%)	
HN (%)	9 (13.6%)	11 (6.0%)	28 (9.9%)	12 (5.5%)	4 (4.2%)	0 (0%)	
Others (%)	10 (15.2%)	37 (20.3%)	42 (14.8%)	26 (11.9%)	16 (16.7%)	8 (21.1%)	
Diabetes (%)	17 (25.8%)	47 (25.8%)	56 (19.7%)	55 (25.0%)	25 (26.0%)	12 (31.6%)	0.38
Charlson Comorbidity Index	4.26±1.87	3.95±2.02	3.49±1.73	3.54±1.88	3.50±2.08	3.32±1.54	0.006*
Use of ACEI/ARB at study initiation (%)	43 (65.2%)	120 (65.9%)	188 (66.2%)	134 (60.9%)	68 (70.8%)	26 (68.4%)	0.35
SBP (mmHg)	142.1±19.8	140.8±15.9	141.2±17.8	140.7±17.3	140.7±15.9	141.2±18.8	0.99
DBP (mmHg)	84.2±14.4	85.4±12.0	84.7±12.9	85.1±13.4	86.1±12.4	86.5±10.7	0.89
Potassium (mEq/L)	2.66±0.25	3.25±0.13	3.69±0.13	4.20±0.15	4.72±0.15	5.51±0.35	<0.001*
Hemoglobin (g/dL)	10.9±2.1	10.8±2.0	11.0±1.9	11.2±2.1	11.3±2.0	10.6±2.0	0.1
Albumin (g/dL)	3.63±0.53	3.69±0.54	3.80±0.49	3.87±0.43	3.91±0.41	3.85±0.52	<0.001*
Hs-CRP (mg/L)	2.32 (0.55, 8.00)	1.97 (0.66, 8.36)	2.04 (0.63, 6.83)	1.69 (0.58, 6.21)	1.51 (0.52, 4.55)	1.16 (0.49, 5.14)	0.39
FBG (mg/dL)	97.1±37.0	104.8±49.0	95.7±37.3	98.2±41.8	97.1±35.0	81.2±22.0	0.13
rGFR (ml/min/1.73 m^2)	3.01 (1.08, 4.29)	2.26 (1.13, 3.92)	2.62 (0.99, 4.68)	2.37 (1.13, 3.62)	2.58 (1.27, 4.17)	3.13 (0.78, 4.76)	0.84
Total Kt/V$_{urea}$	2.23±0.61	2.40±0.68	2.29±0.59	2.27±0.62	2.20±0.55	2.50±0.91	0.3
WCCr (L/w/1.73 m^2)	83.6±29.4	85.4±33.0	83.0±25.9	80.5±25.3	84.8±32.7	96.8±34.7	0.15
Net UF (ml/day)	420 (188, 630)	445 (220, 660)	420 (200, 678)	470 (220, 685)	460 (145, 675)	565 (328, 775)	0.52
Urine output (ml/day)	600 (373, 1000)	630 (400, 803)	620 (400, 878)	620 (370, 870)	690 (390, 978)	500 (230, 880)	0.56
D/P Cr	0.73±0.13	0.70±0.12	0.71±0.11	0.70±0.11	0.71±0.12	0.72±0.11	0.8
PDV/BSA (L/m^2/day)	4.77±0.64	4.73±0.68	4.71±0.52	4.55±0.63	4.46±0.72	4.49±0.75	<0.001*
Estimated peritoneal glucose exposure (g/day)	130.2±27.5	132.2±25.2	133.2±23.1	128.4±24.8	130.0±26.7	131.7±34.2	0.01*

Values expressed as mean ± SD, number (percent), or median (interquartile range). Conversion factors for units: albumin and hemoglobin in g/dL to g/L, × 10; FBG in mg/dL to mmol/L, × 0.05551. No conversion necessary for serum potassium in mEq/L and mmol/L. Abbreviations and definitions: BMI, body mass index; ESRD, end-stage renal disease; CGN, chronic glomerulonephritis; DN, diabetic nephropathy; HN, hypertensive nephrosclerosis; ACEI, angiotensin-converting enzyme inhibitors; ARB, angiotensin II receptor blockades; SBP, systolic blood pressure; DBP, diastolic blood pressure; hs-CRP, high-sensitivity C-reactive protein; FBG, fast blood glucose; rGFR, residual glomerular filtration rate; WCCr, total weekly creatinine clearance; Net UF, net ultrafiltration; D/P Cr, dialysate-to-plasma ratio of creatinine; PDV/BSA, peritoneal dialysis volume per unit of body surface area.

serum potassium variability with respect to mortality in PD patients.

In this study, we assessed the associations of baseline serum potassium levels with both short- and long-term mortality and evaluated the relationship between serum potassium variability and mortality in incident PD patients.

Methods

Ethics Statement

This study was approved by the First Affiliated Hospital of Sun Yet-sen University Institutional Review Boards. All participants provided their written informed consent before inclusion.

Patients

A total of 1149 incident CAPD patients with 18 years or older and being treated with PD more than 3 months at our centre from

January 1, 2006 to December 31, 2010 were studied. All patients were treated with Dianeal solution which does not contain potassium (Baxter China Ltd., Guangzhou, China). We excluded 67 patients because of lack of available baseline potassium and 196 patients with PD-related peritonitis or other acute infection, severe gastrointestinal disease, prescription of diuretics, or concomitant potassium supplementation during the month before the study. 886 patients were enrolled in the final analysis.

Patients were categorized according to baseline serum potassium levels (<3.0, 3.0 to <3.5, 3.5 to <4.0, 4.0 to <4.5, 4.5 to <5.0, and ≥5.0 mEq/L) to examine the association between serum potassium and mortality. Because relatively few patients (17, 1.9%) presented hyperkalemia (serum potassium ≥5.5 mEq/L), we grouped patients with serum potassium ≥5.0 mEq/L into one category for analysis.

To investigate the relation of serum potassium variability and mortality, patients surviving more than one year with at least three

Table 2. Variables correlation with baseline levels of serum potassium.

Variables	r	P-value
Age	−0.11	0.001*
Gender	−0.08	0.02*
BMI	0.18	<0.001*
Charlson Comorbidity Index	−0.1	0.004*
Diabetes	−0.01	0.74
Use of ACEI/ARB	−0.02	0.58
SBP (mmHg)	−0.02	0.56
DBP (mmHg)	0.03	0.36
Hemoglobin (g/dL)	0.04	0.24
Albumin (g/dL)	0.16	<0.001*
Hs-CRP (mg/L)	−0.08	0.02*
FBG (mg/dL)	−0.07	0.03*
rGFR (ml/min/1.73 m^2)	0.02	0.51
Total Kt/V$_{urea}$	−0.02	0.73
WCCr (L/w/1.73 m^2)	0.02	0.61
Net UF (ml/day)	−0.01	0.8
Urine output (ml/day)	0.05	0.17
D/P Cr	0.01	0.73
PDV/BSA (L/m^2/day)	−0.15	<0.001*
Estimated peritoneal glucose exposure (g/day)	−0.02	0.63

Abbreviations and definitions as listed in Table 1.

Table 3. Multivariate analysis of clinical measures associated with levels of serum potassium.

Variables	Standard Error	Standardized β	t	P-value
Age (years)	0.002	−0.084	−1.607	0.108
Gender	0.046	−0.008	−0.221	0.825
BMI (kg/m^2)	0.007	0.158	4.453	<0.001*
Charlson Comorbidity Index	0.019	0.033	0.608	0.543
Albumin (g/dL)	0.005	0.117	3.377	0.001*
Hs-CRP (mg/L)	0.005	−0.061	−1.808	0.071
FBG (mg/dL)	0.001	−0.05	−1.343	0.18
PDV/BSA (L/m^2/day)	0.038	−0.091	−2.536	0.011*

Abbreviations and definitions as listed in Table 1.

Daily exchange volume of peritoneal dialysate was defined as peritoneal dialysis volume per unit of body surface area (PDV/BSA). The number, volume and concentration of glucose exchanges were recorded based on the PD regimen during the first 3 months of PD treatment, and the estimated peritoneal glucose exposure was calculated by the product of the volume and the glucose concentration of each exchange [15]. All biochemical and hematological tests were measured in the biochemical laboratory of the First Affiliated Hospital of Sun Yat-sen University.

Detection and Management of Hypokalemia and Hyperkalemia

All patients were follow-up every 3 months with serum potassium measured at each visit, and additional measurement would be determined according to patients' condition. Hypoka-

check-ups for serum potassium were selected. We excluded 96 patients who commenced PD for less than one year due to following reasons: death (n = 53), transfer to HD (n = 10), renal transplantation (n = 32), and loss to follow-up (n = 1). We also excluded another 99 patients who had less than three times measurement of serum potassium levels because they lived far away from our PD center. Thus, 691 of 886 patients were included in this analysis. Serum potassium variability was expressed as the within-patient standard deviation (SDSP) and the coefficient of variation of serum potassium (CVSP). CVSP was calculated as the ratio of SDSP and the within-patient mean of serum potassium. Patients were split into four categories according quartiles (Q) of CVSP: Q1: <7.5%; Q2:7.5 to <12.0%; Q3:12.0 to <16.7%; Q4: ≥16.7%.

Demographic and Clinical Data

All data were obtained at the time of PD initiation, including demographic details, etiology of end-stage renal disease (ESRD), presence of diabetes, and comorbidity score. Comorbidity was measured using the modified Charlson Comorbidity Index (CCI) [11].

Baseline biochemical data, a standard peritoneal equilibration test (PET) and Kt/V was evaluated in the first 3 months of PD therapy, as previous described [12]. Urine and ultrafiltration volumes during Kt/V test [13], peritoneal transport status (D/P Cr), and adequacy of dialysis [total Kt/V$_{urea}$ and total weekly creatinine clearance (WCCr)] were measured using PD Adequest software (Baxter Healthcare Corporation, Chicago, 1L, USA). Residual glomerular filtration rate (rGFR) was calculated as the average of 24-hour urinary urea and creatinine clearance [14].

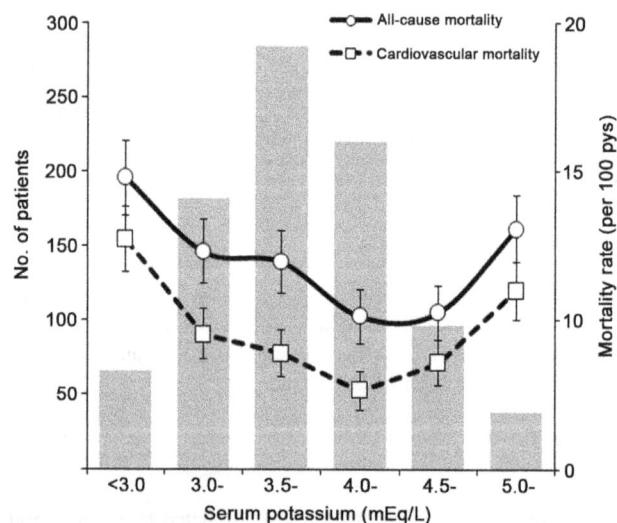

Figure 1. Distribution of baseline serum potassium levels and corresponding mortality rates. Gender- and age- standardized all-cause and cardiovascular mortality rates (per 100 patient-years) with 95% confidence intervals according to serum potassium categories at baseline.

Table 4. Rates and hazard ratios for all-cause and cardiovascular mortality according to categories of serum potassium.

	Baseline levels of serum potassium (mEq/L)					
	<3.0	3.0 to <3.5	3.5 to <4.0	4.0 to <4.5	4.5 to <5.0	≥5.0
No. of patients	66	182	284	220	96	38
All-cause mortality						
No. of deaths	25	43	49	30	15	6
[a]Rate (per 100 pys)	9.77 (8.52–11.01)	7.29 (6.21–8.36)	6.94 (5.89–7.99)	5.12 (4.22–6.03)	5.25 (4.34–6.16)	8.06 (6.95–9.19)
Unadjusted HR	2.51 (1.48–4.28)	1.70 (1.06–2.70)	1.34 (0.85–2.11)	1.0 (Reference)	1.16 (0.62–2.15)	1.17 (0.49–2.82)
[b]Adjusted HR	1.79 (1.02–3.14)	1.15 (0.72–1.86)	1.31 (0.82–2.08)	1.0 (Reference)	1.33 (0.71–2.48)	1.28 (0.53–3.10)
Cardiovascular mortality						
No. of deaths	19	25	26	16	10	5
[a]Rate (per 100 pys)	7.71 (6.60–8.81)	4.52 (3.67–5.36)	2.63 (1.99–3.28)	3.88 (3.09–4.66)	3.57 (2.82–4.32)	6.0 (5.04–6.98)
Unadjusted HR	3.61 (1.85–7.02)	1.87 (1.00–3.50)	1.34 (0.72–2.49)	1.0 (Reference)	1.47 (0.67–3.25)	1.83 (0.67–5.01)
[b]Adjusted HR	2.35 (1.16–4.75)	1.25 (0.66–2.37)	1.24 (0.65–2.33)	1.0 (Reference)	1.71 (0.77–3.79)	1.85 (0.67–5.11)

Abbreviations: pys, patient-years; HR, hazard ratio, and other abbreviations and definitions as listed in Table 1.
[a]Age- and gender-standardized Mortality rate.
[b]Adjusted for age, gender, BMI, diabetic status, CCI, hemoglobin, serum albumin, hs-CRP, and PDV/BSA.

lemia (serum potassium <3.5 mEq/L) or hyperkalemia was informed to the clinics urgently for immediate recheck or treatment. In brief, patients with a potassium level of 3.0–3.5 mEq/L were commonly prescribed oral potassium supplementation and educated on a high potassium diet. Intravenous potassium was required in patients with a potassium level of

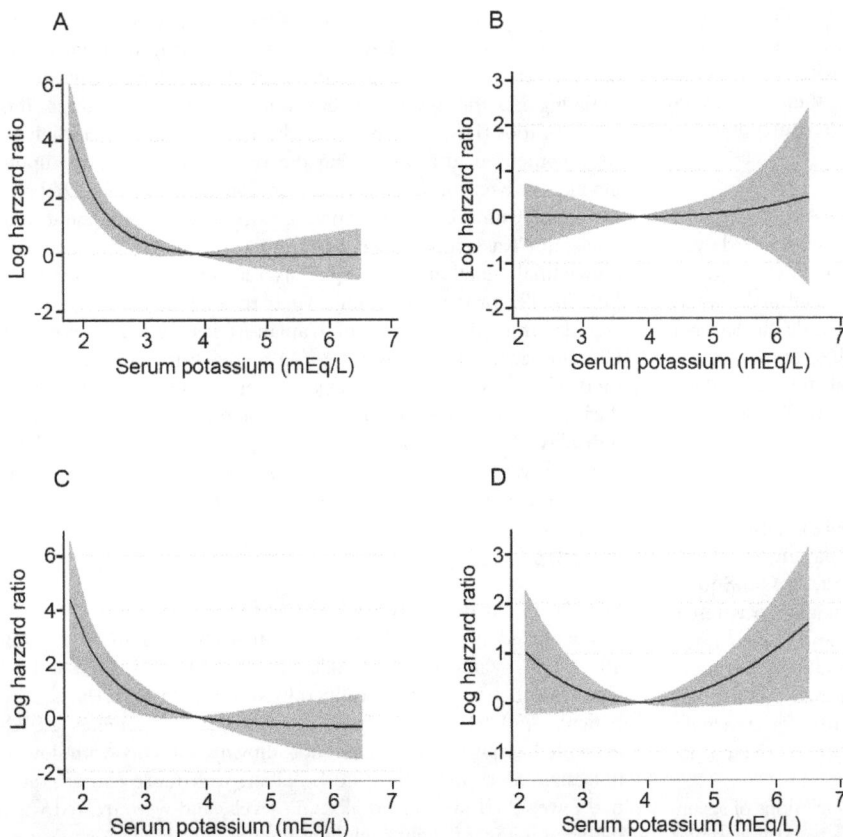

Figure 2. Fractional polynomial graphs depicting the relationship between serum potassium and mortality risk. The relation between serum potassium and all-cause (A, B) and cardiovascular mortality (C, D) in term of short- and long-term mortality rates was expressed by the log-HR ratio. Baseline serum potassium levels were modeled as a continuous variable, and the model was adjusted for age, gender, BMI, diabetic status, CCI, hemoglobin, serum albumin, hs-CRP, and PDV/BSA. Shaded areas indicate the 95% confidence interval.

Table 5. Association of serum potassium levels and all-cause and cardiovascular mortality by follow-up time.

	Baseline levels of serum potassium (mEq/L)					
	<3.0	3.0 to <3.5	3.5 to <4.0	4.0 to <4.5	4.5 to <5.0	≥5.0
All-cause mortality						
No. of deaths (≤1 years)	10	18	15	5	4	1
[a]Adjusted HR	4.34 (1.44–13.1)	2.80 (1.03–7.65)	2.10 (0.75–5.88)	1.0 (Reference)	1.81 (0.48–6.89)	1.16 (0.14–10.1)
No. of deaths (>1 years)	15	25	34	25	11	5
[a]Adjusted HR	1.31 (0.66–2.60)	0.81 (0.46–1.44)	1.16 (0.69–1.97)	1.0 (Reference)	1.24 (0.60–2.55)	1.38(0.52–3.67)
Cardiovascular mortality						
No. of deaths (≤1 years)	7	12	9	2	2	0
[a]Adjusted HR	7.17 (1.44–35.8)	4.61 (1.01–20.9)	3.12 (0.66–14.7)	1.0 (Reference)	2.45 (0.34–17.7)	–[b]
No. of deaths (>1 years)	12	13	17	14	8	5
[a]Adjusted HR	1.70 (0.74–3.92)	0.76 (0.35–1.64)	0.97 (0.47–2.01)	1.0 (Reference)	1.53 (0.63–3.74)	2.29 (0.80–6.53)

Abbreviations: HR, hazard ratio, and other abbreviations and definitions as listed in Table 1.
[a]Adjusted for age, gender, BMI, diabetic status, CCI, hemoglobin, serum albumin, hs-CRP, and PDV/BSA.
[b]Number of events in this category is too low to obtain an effect estimate.

<2.5 mEq/L. To avoid bacterial contamination of the dialysis solution, we did not add potassium chloride to solution. For patients with a potassium level ≥5.5 mEq/L, high potassium diet and hyperkalemia generating drugs (angiotensin converting enzyme inhibitors, angiotension receptor antagonists, and potassium-sparing diuretics) would be stopped immediately. Furosemide was prescribed to the patients with urine output >500 ml/day. Intermittent peritoneal dialysis (IPD) or HD was used remove extra potassium in anuric patients or patients with potassium of >6.0 mEq/L. Serum potassium levels were then monitored closely and maintained in the normal range (serum potassium concentration of 3.5 to <5.5 mEq/L).

Outcomes

Our primary outcomes were all-cause mortality and cardiovascular mortality. Cardiovascular mortality was defined as death from acute heart failure, myocardial infarction, fatal arrhythmia, stroke, peripheral artery disease [16,17], or sudden death. Survival was defined as the time from enrollment to death or administrative censoring (i.e. transfer to hemodialysis, renal transplantation, transfer to other dialysis centers, loss to follow-up, or end of the study period) at December 31, 2012.

Statistical Analyses

Results are expressed as mean ± standard deviation (SD) unless otherwise specified. Comparisons between parameters were performed using ANOVA, Kruskal-Wallis H test, or Chi-Square test, as appropriate. The bivariate correlation analysis was tested to assess the associations of demographic and biochemical characteristics with baseline levels of serum potassium. Spearman's correlation coefficients were used for non-normally distributed variables and Pearson's correlation coefficients for normally distributed variables. Significant parameters were selected for further multivariable linear regression analysis.

Survival analyses were performed to assess associations of serum potassium levels with all-cause mortality and cardiovascular mortality, with the category of serum potassium 4.0 to <4.5 mEq/L as the reference group. The following models were performed sequentially to estimate mortality rates (per 100 patient-years, pys) during follow-up period according to baseline serum potassium categories: (1) unadjusted; (2) the Cox models were constructed by adjusted for age, gender, body mass index (BMI), diabetic status, CCI, hemoglobin, serum albumin level, high-sensitivity C-reactive protein (hs-CRP), and PDV/BSA, because these parameters were related to serum potassium levels and/or significantly associated with mortality in univariate Cox proportional hazard regression analyses. Conditional Cox regression analysis [18] was carried out to determine the time-stratified effects of baseline serum potassium on mortality. Short-term survival was defined as 1-year patient survival and long-term survival as initiating PD therapy more than one year. In this analysis, the hazard ratios (HRs) for mortality during the first year of dialysis were compared to those during the year after, conditional upon having survived the first year. In addition, to avoid the problems associated with arbitrary selection of categories, the baseline serum potassium was modeled as a continuous predictor by fractional polynomial function to examine its relationship with outcomes [19,20]. The prognostic significance of serum potassium variability was determined by means of Kaplan-Meier survival curve and Cox proportional hazards regression model. Survival analysis was modeled considering the behavior of serum potassium variability during the first year of follow-up as a predictor of subsequent mortality. All statistical analyses were performed using the SPSS software, version 13.0 (SPSS Inc., Chicago, IL, USA). A P-value <0.05 was considered statistically significant.

Results

Baseline Characteristics of Study Cohort

We included 886 incident PD patients with a mean age of 48.5±15.4 years, 42.9% female. Table 1 showed the baseline characteristics of patients stratified by serum potassium levels. 248 patients (27.9%) suffered from hypokalemia, 17 patients (1.9%) presented hyperkalemia (data not shown). Patients with lower potassium were more likely to be older, with more comorbidity, had lower BMI and serum albumin levels, and were treated with higher amount of daily exchange volume and glucose exposure, when compared to patients with normal serum potassium. When patients were further stratified into three groups according to daily urine output at baseline (>500 ml, 100–500 ml, and <100 ml), we found that mean urine output was 673±423 ml/day with 63.2% of the patients having a urine output >500 ml/day and

Table 6. Patient baseline characteristics by serum potassium variability during the first year of PD treatment.

Variables	Categories of serum potassium variability (CVSP)				P-value
	Q1 (n = 170)	Q2 (n = 176)	Q3 (n = 173)	Q4 (n = 172)	
Within-patient mean of serum potassium (mEq/L)	3.93±0.49	3.93±0.59	3.93±0.57	3.87±0.61	0.62
SDSP (mEq/L)	0.19±0.07	0.38±0.08	0.55±0.09	0.85±0.25	<0.001*
CVSP (%)	4.94±1.75	9.62±1.30	14.1±1.3	22.1±5.8	<0.001*
Age (years)	45.9±13.3	46.9±15.6	48.1±15.3	52.3±15.8	<0.001*
Female (%)	67 (39.4%)	77 (43.8%)	76 (43.9%)	86 (50.0%)	0.27
BMI (kg/m²)	22.1±2.9	22.1±3.3	22.3±3.5	21.3±3.1	0.02*
Etiology of ESRD					0.55
CGN (%)	98 (57.6%)	94 (53.4%)	93 (53.8%)	81 (47.1%)	
DN (%)	34 (20.0%)	35 (19.9%)	39 (22.5%)	50 (29.1%)	
HN (%)	14 (8.2%)	16 (9.1%)	12 (6.9%)	11 (6.4%)	
Others (%)	24 (14.1%)	31 (17.6%)	29 (16.8%)	30 (17.4%)	
Diabetes (%)	36 (21.2%)	39 (22.2%)	41 (23.7%)	53 (30.8%)	0.15
Charlson Comorbidity Index	3.34±1.72	3.55±1.83	3.55±1.79	4.19±2.10	<0.001*
Use of ACEI/ARB at study initiation (%)	108 (63.5%)	119 (67.6%)	114 (65.9%)	110 (64.0%)	0.85
SBP (mmHg)	140.9±17.3	142.0±18.0	138.6±15.3	142.0±17.4	0.21
DBP (mmHg)	85.9±12.4	85.2±14.6	85.2±10.6	85.7±12.2	0.93
Hemoglobin (g/dL)	11.1±1.9	11.2±1.8	11.2±1.9	11.2±2.0	0.83
Albumin (g/dL)	3.91±0.46	3.85±0.43	3.86±0.45	3.75±0.46	0.009*
Hs-CRP (mg/L)	1.64 (0.64, 6.52)	2.04 (0.69, 6.46)	2.45 (0.52, 8.22)	1.93 (0.61, 6.20)	0.74
FBG (mg/dL)	95.5±35.8	95.6±37.8	96.7±42.0	104.3±45.8	0.14
rGFR (ml/min/1.73 m²)	2.36 (0.98, 4.41)	2.09 (0.94, 3.68)	2.64 (1.13, 4.37)	2.58 (1.19, 4.54)	0.29
Total Kt/V$_{urea}$	2.32±0.72	2.27±0.60	2.22±0.54	2.26±0.60	0.73
WCCr (L/w/1.73 m²)	81.5±27.9	81.4±24.6	82.8±29.7	86.4±31.4	0.53
Net UF (ml/day)	400 (200, 650)	450 (200, 648)	460 (165, 670)	570 (210, 750)	0.16
Urine output (ml/day)	670 (378, 900)	605 (393, 930)	620 (385, 880)	580 (323, 795)	0.36
D/P Cr	0.70±0.12	0.72±0.12	0.71±0.11	0.71±0.11	0.55
PDV/BSA (L/m²/day)	4.62±0.57	4.63±0.57	4.58±0.63	4.71±0.70	0.27
Estimated peritoneal glucose exposure (g/day)	131.2±24.2	131.7±25.7	130.9±23.3	131.7±29.4	0.98

Note: Values expressed as mean ± SD, number (percent), or median (interquartile range). Conversion factors for units: albumin and hemoglobin in g/dL to g/L, × 10; FBG in mg/dL to mmol/L, × 0.05551. No conversion necessary for serum potassium in mEq/L and mmol/L.
Abbreviations: CVSP, coefficient variation of serum potassium; SDSP, standard deviation of serum potassium; and other abbreviations as listed in Table 1.

7.3% of anuric (<100 ml/day) patients. However, neither potassium levels nor hypokalemia prevalence at baseline, and potassium variability was statically different across the groups (data not shown).

Univariate analysis revealed that baseline serum potassium level was positively correlated with BMI and serum albumin and negatively correlated with age, comorbidity score, hs-CRP, fast blood glucose, and PDV/BSA (Table 2). On multivariate analysis, serum potassium level remained positively associated with BMI ($\beta = 0.158$; P<0.001) and serum albumin ($\beta = 0.117$; P = 0.001) and negatively associated with PDV/BSA ($\beta = -0.091$; P = 0.011) (Table 3).

Serum Potassium Levels and Mortality

During a median follow-up of 31 months (range: 0.5–81.0 months), 168 patients (19.0%) died. 101 (60.1%) of which were attributed to cardiovascular causes: 72 deaths were cardiac, 27 deaths were due to cerebrovascular disease, and 2 deaths were due to peripheral vascular accident (including one patient with a pulmonary embolism and another with a ruptured abdominal aortic aneurysm). Of all deaths, 53 died within one year, including 32 cardiovascular and 21 non-cardiovascular deaths. As shown in Figure 1 and Table 4, the relationship between baseline serum potassium and all-cause and cardiovascular mortality was U-shaped, with lowest mortality rates observed in patients with potassium levels of 4.0 to 4.5 mEq/L (5.12 and 3.88 death/100 pys, respectively) and highest in that of potassium <3.0 mEq/L. (9.77 and 7.71 death/100 pys, respectively). Both all-cause and cardiovascular mortality rates were higher for potassium levels of ≥5.0 mEq/L (8.06 and 6.0 death/100 pys, respectively), compared with those with levels between 4.0 and 4.5 mEq/L. In unadjusted model, serum potassium levels <3.0 and 3.0 to <3.5 mEq/L were associated with increased risk of all-cause and cardiovascular mortality. After adjustments, the risk of all-cause and cardiovascular death was only significant in those with potassium of <3.0 mEq/L [HR, 1.79 (1.02–3.14) and 2.35 (1.16–4.75), respectively]. In contrast, patients with potassium levels of

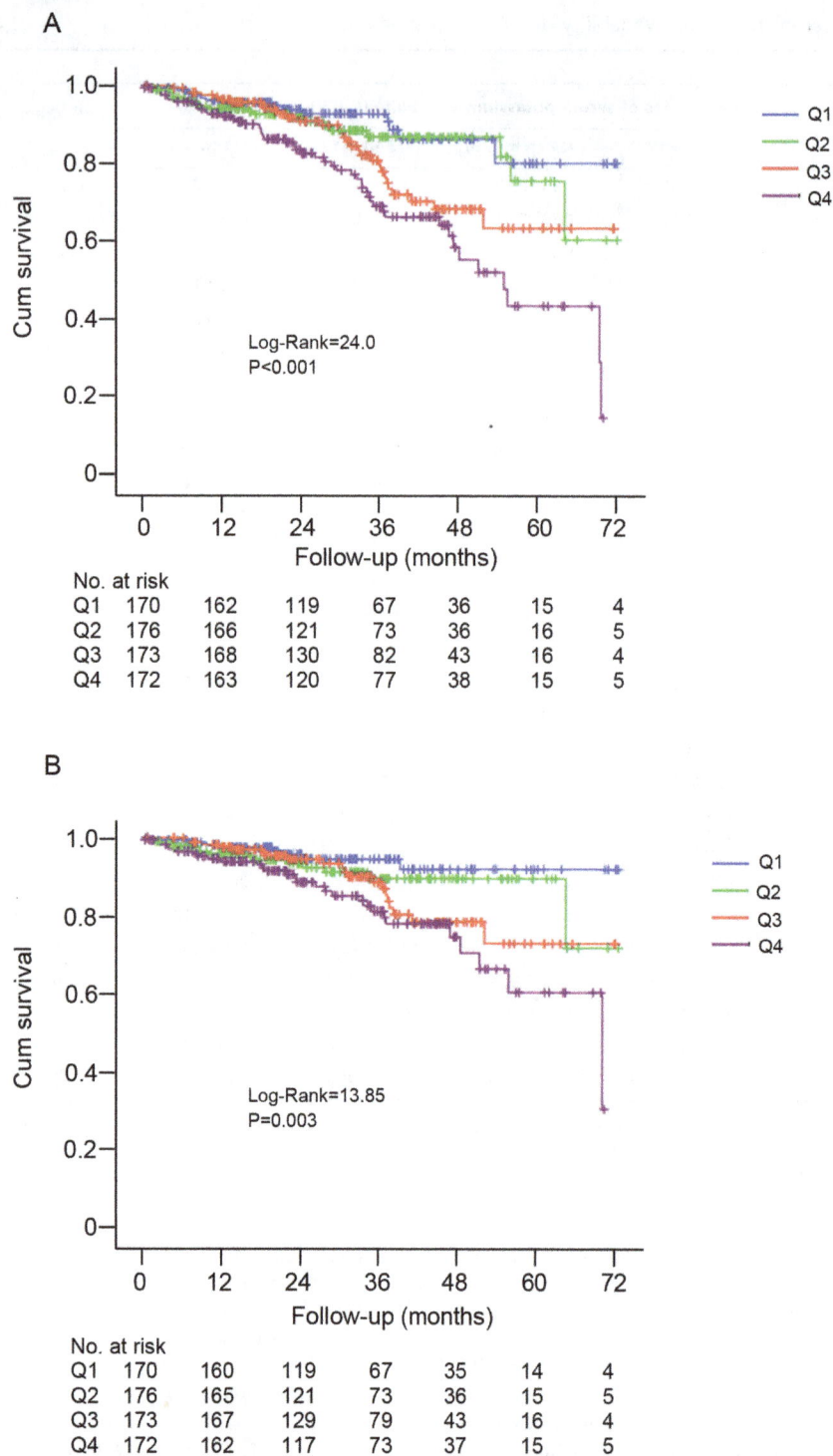

Figure 3. Kaplan-Meier survival curves for mortality according to serum potassium variability. (A) all-cause mortality; (B) cardiovascular mortality. Patients were split into four categories according quartiles (Q) of coefficient of variation of serum potassium (CVSP): Q1: <7.5%; Q2:7.5 to <12.0%; Q3:12.0 to <16.7%; Q4: ≥16.7%. The P values refer to the significance of the log-rank test across quartiles.

≥5.0 mEq/L showed an increased tendency of mortality, although not statistically significant.

In conditional Cox analysis, compared with the reference group (4.0 to <4.5 mEq/L), patients with potassium levels of 3.0 to <3.5 mEq/L had a greater than twice-fold increased risk of all-cause death within the first year of follow-up (adjusted HR, 2.80;

95% CI, 1.03–7.65), and much higher at that of <3.0 mEq/L (adjusted HR, 4.34; 95% CI, 1.44–13.1). Moreover, the corresponding adjusted HRs for cardiovascular mortality were 4.61 (95% CI, 1.01–20.9) and 7.17 (95% CI, 1.44–35.8) for serum potassium levels of 3.0–3.5 mEq/L and <3.0 mEq/L, respectively. The increased risk of lower potassium with mortality was

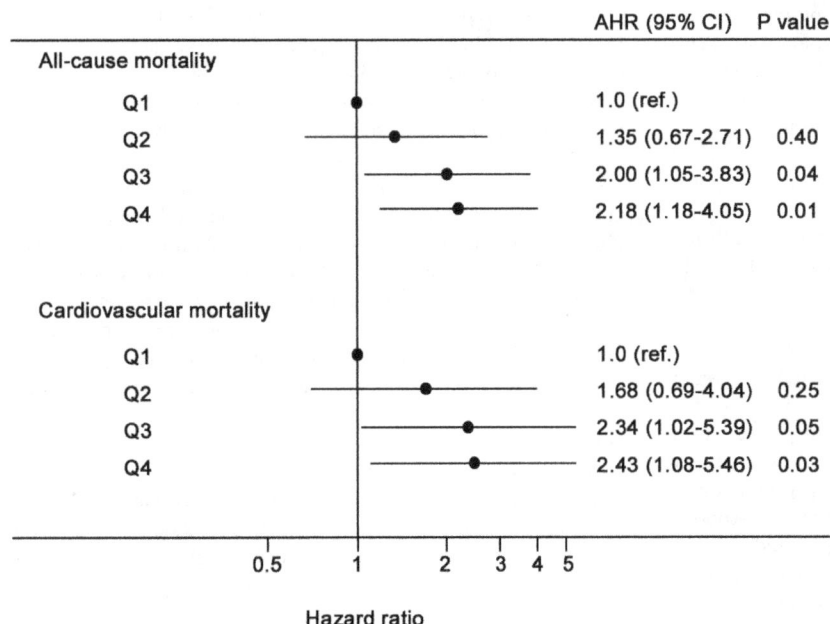

Figure 4. Hazard ratio for all-cause and cardiovascular mortality according to serum potassium variability. Adjustments included age at initiation of PD, gender, BMI, diabetes status, CCI, hemoglobin, serum albumin, hs-CRP, PDV/BSA, and within-patient mean of serum potassium. Q1: (CVSP) <7.5%; Q2: (CVSP) 7.5 to <12.0%; Q3: (CVSP) 12.0 to <16.7%; Q4: (CVSP) ≥16.7%.

evident only during the first year of follow-up. And this relationship was no longer pronounced in the subsequent years of observation (Table 5), indicating the predictive value of hypokalemia for short-term mortality among incident PD patients.

When baseline serum potassium was modeled as a continuous predictor, as shown in Figure 2, both the short-term all-cause (A) and cardiovascular mortality (C) risk was lowest for serum potassium values of approximately 4 mEq/L and increased steadily with lower serum potassium. However, association of baseline serum potassium levels and long-term mortality became less pronounced (B, D).

Serum Potassium Variability and Mortality

We further investigated the risk of all-cause mortality according to the quartiles of serum potassium variability (expressed as CVSP). When comparing baseline clinical characteristics between included and excluded patients (99 patients with fewer than 3 serum potassium levels measurements plus 96 patients with less than one year on PD therapy), we found that excluded patients had lower BMI, hemoglobin, serum albumin and serum potassium, while no significant difference between two groups with respect to other variables. As shown in Table 6, the baseline characteristics of included patients across quartiles of CVSP were highly comparable with the exception of age, BMI, comorbidity score, and serum albumin. Patients in the highest quartile of CVSP (≥16.7%) were more likely to be older and had more comorbidity and lower BMI and serum albumin levels (P<0.05 for all).

Figure 3 displayed the Kaplan–Meier survival curves for all-cause (A) and cardiovascular (B) mortality across quartiles of CVSP (Q1, Q2, Q3, and Q4), indicating that patients with higher serum potassium variability (Q3 and Q4) had significantly poorer all-cause (P<0.001) and cardiovascular mortality (P=0.003), compared to those with relatively stable potassium levels (Q1).

The relative risks of mortality in relation to serum potassium variability showed in Figure 4, with the Q1 group as a reference.

All-cause mortality risk in the Q3 group was higher and appeared to increase steadily in the Q4 group, with adjusted hazard ratios of 2.00 (1.05–3.83) and 2.18 (1.18–4.05), respectively, independently of the within-patient mean of serum potassium. However, the Q2 group was not associated with a higher risk for all-cause death. Similar results were observed with regard to cardiovascular mortality, with adjusted hazard ratios 2.34 (1.02–5.39) and 2.43 (1.08–5.46) for the Q3 and Q4 groups, respectively.

Discussion

In the present study, we demonstrated that 27.9% of incident PD patients presented hypokalemia. There was a U-shaped association of baseline serum potassium levels and all-cause and cardiovascular mortality, with the highest mortality rate observed for potassium levels <3.0 mEq/L. After adjustment for confounders, the relationship between hypokalemia and mortality risk was evident only during the first year, but not thereafter. Furthermore, higher serum potassium variability conferred an increased mortality risk, which was independent of the average serum potassium levels.

The risk factors for hypokalemia in PD patients are complex, many factors are involved. Associations of chronic inflammation and malnutrition with potassium levels have been described previously [8,21,22,23]. Indeed, we found that patients with a lower potassium levels were older and had more comorbidities, lower albumin and BMI. Given that peritoneal dialysate is potassium-free, ongoing losses of potassium into dialysate may contribute to hypokalemia in some patients. Our results were in accordance with previous studies [24,25], revealing that an elevated dialysis dose was independently related to decreased serum potassium levels. In addition, potassium redistribution into the intracellular compartment, stimulated by insulin release due to continuous peritoneal glucose infusion was thought to be another important risk factor for hypokalemia [23]. However, we were unable to demonstrate a relationship between serum potassium and daily glucose exposure. Because we did not measure the absolute amount of peritoneal glucose absorption, and the effects of cellular uptake on potassium levels couldn't be excluded. Moreover, in line with previous studies [8,26], we did not found any association between serum potassium levels and urine volume or residual renal function, suggesting that the removal of potassium from urinary might be insufficient to develop hypokalemia in our study population.

A relation of serum potassium levels with the risk of death has been reported by Szeto et al. [8], indicating a higher risk for all-cause mortality in PD patients with baseline serum potassium <3.5 mEq/L. In the most recent and robust evidence from a large, contemporary cohort of dialysis population showed a clear U-shaped relationship between time-averaged serum potassium levels and all-cause and cardiovascular mortality in prevalent PD patients, and the lowest mortality was observed in patients with serum potassium of 4.0–4.5 mEq/L, while increased mortality for serum potassium <4.0 mEq/L and ≥5.5 mEq/L [9]. Our results were somewhat consistent with previous study that a U-shaped association of baseline serum potassium and age - and gender-standardized all-cause and cardiovascular mortality rates in incident PD patients, with the highest mortality rate observed for potassium levels <3.0 mEq/L. However, our study showed that patients with potassium levels ≥5.0 mEq/L had an increased tendency of mortality rate, though without statistically significance, probably due to the small number of PD patients in this category (4.3% of the total patients).

Abnormal serum potassium levels most prominently affect the cardiovascular system and have been implicated in many aspects of cardiovascular disease including atrial fibrillation, stroke, heart attack, hypertension, and sudden cardiac death [27]. Therefore, any abnormalities in serum potassium are usually corrected as soon as possible in our clinical practices. To our knowledge, this is the first study to examine the relationship between time discrepancy of serum potassium levels and mortality in PD patients. We found that the association between hypokalemia and mortality risk was evident only within the first year, but vanished in the subsequent years. This relationship remained significant after adjustment for confounders. Our data revealed the importance of early correction of abnormal serum potassium in this population. Consistently, we demonstrated that patients with lower or higher serum potassium levels had increased rates of cardiovascular mortality. Another potential explanation is malnutrition, one of the confounders, termed as a "short-term killer" [28,29], because hypokalemia was closely associated with malnutrition and severe coexisting comorbid conditions, which might be responsible for the poor short-term outcome.

It has been reported that the variability of heart rate [30], blood pressure [31], hemoglobin [32], as well as variability of serum calcium and phosphorus [33] are closely associated with clinical outcomes. Additionally, highest risk of death was found on the days following the longest interval without dialysis [34]. Rapid reduction of potassium after HD may be one of vital contributors, since the excessive variability in serum potassium levels can enhance the risk for cardiac arrhythmia and sudden death. However, the relationship between distribution of serum potassium variability and mortality risk has not been investigated in PD patients. We found that patients with a relative stable serum potassium levels during one year's observation appeared to have a pronouncedly better survival. An excessive fluctuation in serum potassium was associated with significantly increased mortality, which was independent of the within-patient average serum potassium levels.

Nonetheless, our study has several limitations. First, an observational study cannot prove causality. Second, there is a potential selection bias when we evaluated the association between serum potassium variability and mortality. Because we enrolled patients who had received PD for more than one year with at least three check-ups of serum potassium, patients with relatively lower or higher serum potassium levels might died within the first year of therapy. Thus, these data may underestimate the negative roles of serum potassium variability in mortality. Third, relatively few patients presented abnormally high serum potassium levels. Hence, a small number of patients with hyperkalemia may result in the lack of significant association with mortality. Finally, factors affecting serum potassium levels, such as dietary intake, loss via dialysate and urine, were not examined in the present study.

In conclusion, our study demonstrates for the first time that association between hypokalemia at baseline and mortality risk is evident only during the first year of follow-up period. In addition, the higher serum potassium variability may contribute substantially to both all-cause and cardiovascular mortality risk in this population. Our findings emphasize the importance of early achieving the optimal and stable serum potassium levels in patients initiating PD therapy.

Author Contributions

Conceived and designed the experiments: HPM XQY ZHZ QDX. Performed the experiments: QDX FHX LPX HYL SRC XYL. Analyzed the data: QDX FHX LF. Contributed reagents/materials/analysis tools: XQY HPM. Wrote the paper: QDX HPM.

References

1. Korgaonkar S, Tilea A, Gillespie BW, Kiser M, Eisele G, et al. (2010) Serum potassium and outcomes in CKD: insights from the RRI-CKD cohort study. Clin J Am Soc Nephrol 5: 762–769.
2. Kovesdy CP, Regidor DL, Mehrotra R, Jing J, McAllister CJ, et al. (2007) Serum and dialysate potassium concentrations and survival in hemodialysis patients. Clin J Am Soc Nephrol 2: 999–1007.
3. Oreopoulos DG, Khanna R, Williams P, Vas SI (1982) Continuous ambulatory peritoneal dialysis - 1981. Nephron 30: 293–303.
4. Rostand SG (1983) Profound hypokalemia in continuous ambulatory peritoneal dialysis. Arch Intern Med 143: 377–378.
5. Khan AN, Bernardini J, Johnston JR, Piraino B (1996) Hypokalemia in peritoneal dialysis patients. Perit Dial Int 16: 652.
6. Go AS, Chertow GM, Fan D, McCulloch CE, Hsu CY (2004) Chronic kidney disease and the risks of death, cardiovascular events, and hospitalization. N Engl J Med 351: 1296–1305.
7. Harrison TR, Pilcher C, Ewing G (1930) STUDIES IN CONGESTIVE HEART FAILURE: IV. The Potassium Content of Skeletal and Cardiac Muscle. J Clin Invest 8: 325–335.
8. Szeto CC, Chow KM, Kwan BC, Leung CB, Chung KY, et al. (2005) Hypokalemia in Chinese peritoneal dialysis patients: prevalence and prognostic implication. Am J Kidney Dis 46: 128–135.
9. Torlen K, Kalantar-Zadeh K, Molnar MZ, Vashistha T, Mehrotra R (2012) Serum potassium and cause-specific mortality in a large peritoneal dialysis cohort. Clin J Am Soc Nephrol 7: 1272–1284.
10. Kwan BC, Szeto CC (2012) Dialysis: Hypokalaemia and cardiac risk in peritoneal dialysis patients. Nat Rev Nephrol 8: 501–503.
11. Beddhu S, Zeidel ML, Saul M, Seddon P, Samore MH, et al. (2002) The effects of comorbid conditions on the outcomes of patients undergoing peritoneal dialysis. Am J Med 112: 696–701.
12. Rocco MV, Jordan JR, Burkart JM (1994) Determination of peritoneal transport characteristics with 24-hour dialysate collections: dialysis adequacy and transport test. J Am Soc Nephrol 5: 1333–1338.
13. Konings CJ, Kooman JP, Schonck M, Struijk DG, Gladziwa U, et al. (2003) Fluid status in CAPD patients is related to peritoneal transport and residual renal function: evidence from a longitudinal study. Nephrol Dial Transplant 18: 797–803.

14. van Olden RW, Krediet RT, Struijk DG, Arisz L (1996) Measurement of residual renal function in patients treated with continuous ambulatory peritoneal dialysis. J Am Soc Nephrol 7: 745–750.
15. Davies SJ, Phillips L, Naish PF, Russell GI (2001) Peritoneal glucose exposure and changes in membrane solute transport with time on peritoneal dialysis. J Am Soc Nephrol 12: 1046–1051.
16. Wang AY, Wang M, Woo J, Lam CW, Li PK, et al. (2003) Cardiac valve calcification as an important predictor for all-cause mortality and cardiovascular mortality in long-term peritoneal dialysis patients: a prospective study. J Am Soc Nephrol 14: 159–168.
17. Chertow GM, Block GA, Correa-Rotter R, Drueke TB, Floege J, et al. (2012) Effect of cinacalcet on cardiovascular disease in patients undergoing dialysis. N Engl J Med 367: 2482–2494.
18. Dekker FW, de Mutsert R, van Dijk PC, Zoccali C, Jager KJ (2008) Survival analysis: time-dependent effects and time-varying risk factors. Kidney Int 74: 994–997.
19. McDonald SP, Collins JF, Johnson DW (2003) Obesity is associated with worse peritoneal dialysis outcomes in the Australia and New Zealand patient populations. J Am Soc Nephrol 14: 2894–2901.
20. Royston P (2000) A strategy for modelling the effect of a continuous covariate in medicine and epidemiology. Statistics in medicine 19: 1831–1847.
21. Chuang YW, Shu KH, Yu TM, Cheng CH, Chen CH (2009) Hypokalaemia: an independent risk factor of Enterobacteriaceae peritonitis in CAPD patients. Nephrol Dial Transplant 24: 1603–1608.
22. Jung JY, Chang JH, Lee HH, Chung W, Kim S (2009) De novo hypokalemia in incident peritoneal dialysis patients: a 1-year observational study. Electrolyte Blood Press 7: 73–78.
23. Tziviskou E, Musso C, Bellizzi V, Khandelwal M, Wang T, et al. (2003) Prevalence and pathogenesis of hypokalemia in patients on chronic peritoneal dialysis: one center's experience and review of the literature. Int Urol Nephrol 35: 429–434.
24. Gao H, Lew SQ, Bosch JP (1999) Biochemical parameters, nutritional status and efficiency of dialysis in CAPD and CCPD patients. Am J Nephrol 19: 7–12.
25. Newman LN, Weiss MF, Berger J, Priester A, Negrea LA, et al. (2000) The law of unintended consequences in action: increase in incidence of hypokalemia with improved adequacy of dialysis. Adv Perit Dial 16: 134–137.
26. Li PK, Chow KM, Wong TY, Leung CB, Szeto CC (2003) Effects of an angiotensin-converting enzyme inhibitor on residual renal function in patients receiving peritoneal dialysis. A randomized, controlled study. Ann Intern Med 139: 105–112.
27. Sica DA, Struthers AD, Cushman WC, Wood M, Banas JS Jr, et al. (2002) Importance of potassium in cardiovascular disease. J Clin Hypertens (Greenwich) 4: 198–206.
28. Fleischmann EH, Bower JD, Salahudeen AK (2001) Risk factor paradox in hemodialysis: better nutrition as a partial explanation. ASAIO J 47: 74–81.
29. Kalantar-Zadeh K, Block G, Humphreys MH, Kopple JD (2003) Reverse epidemiology of cardiovascular risk factors in maintenance dialysis patients. Kidney Int 63: 793–808.
30. Chan CT (2008) Heart rate variability in patients with end-stage renal disease: an emerging predictive tool for sudden cardiac death? Nephrol Dial Transplant 23: 3061–3062.
31. Di Iorio B, Pota A, Sirico ML, Torraca S, Di Micco L, et al. (2012) Blood pressure variability and outcomes in chronic kidney disease. Nephrol Dial Transplant 27: 4404–4410.
32. Kainz A, Mayer B, Kramar R, Oberbauer R (2010) Association of ESA hypo-responsiveness and haemoglobin variability with mortality in haemodialysis patients. Nephrol Dial Transplant 25: 3701–3706.
33. Kalantar-Zadeh K, Kuwae N, Regidor DL, Kovesdy CP, Kilpatrick RD, et al. (2006) Survival predictability of time-varying indicators of bone disease in maintenance hemodialysis patients. Kidney Int 70: 771–780.
34. Bleyer AJ, Russell GB, Satko SG (1999) Sudden and cardiac death rates in hemodialysis patients. Kidney Int 55: 1553–1559.

Permissions

All chapters in this book were first published in PLOS ONE, by The Public Library of Science; hereby published with permission under the Creative Commons Attribution License or equivalent. Every chapter published in this book has been scrutinized by our experts. Their significance has been extensively debated. The topics covered herein carry significant findings which will fuel the growth of the discipline. They may even be implemented as practical applications or may be referred to as a beginning point for another development.

The contributors of this book come from diverse backgrounds, making this book a truly international effort. This book will bring forth new frontiers with its revolutionizing research information and detailed analysis of the nascent developments around the world.

We would like to thank all the contributing authors for lending their expertise to make the book truly unique. They have played a crucial role in the development of this book. Without their invaluable contributions this book wouldn't have been possible. They have made vital efforts to compile up to date information on the varied aspects of this subject to make this book a valuable addition to the collection of many professionals and students.

This book was conceptualized with the vision of imparting up-to-date information and advanced data in this field. To ensure the same, a matchless editorial board was set up. Every individual on the board went through rigorous rounds of assessment to prove their worth. After which they invested a large part of their time researching and compiling the most relevant data for our readers.

The editorial board has been involved in producing this book since its inception. They have spent rigorous hours researching and exploring the diverse topics which have resulted in the successful publishing of this book. They have passed on their knowledge of decades through this book. To expedite this challenging task, the publisher supported the team at every step. A small team of assistant editors was also appointed to further simplify the editing procedure and attain best results for the readers.

Apart from the editorial board, the designing team has also invested a significant amount of their time in understanding the subject and creating the most relevant covers. They scrutinized every image to scout for the most suitable representation of the subject and create an appropriate cover for the book.

The publishing team has been an ardent support to the editorial, designing and production team. Their endless efforts to recruit the best for this project, has resulted in the accomplishment of this book. They are a veteran in the field of academics and their pool of knowledge is as vast as their experience in printing. Their expertise and guidance has proved useful at every step. Their uncompromising quality standards have made this book an exceptional effort. Their encouragement from time to time has been an inspiration for everyone.

The publisher and the editorial board hope that this book will prove to be a valuable piece of knowledge for researchers, students, practitioners and scholars across the globe.

List of Contributors

Wim Van Biesen
University Hospital Ghent, Ghent, Belgium

John D. Williams
University Hospital of Wales College of Medicine, Cardiff, United Kingdom

Adrian C. Covic
University "Gr T Popa" and University Hospital "C I Pharon", Iasi, Romania

Stanley Fan
The Royal London Hospital, London, United Kingdom

Kathleen Claes
University Hospital Leuven, Leuven, Belgium

Monika Lichodziejewska-Niemierko
Dialysis Center NephroCare, Gdansk University, Gdansk, Poland

Christian Verger
University Hospital René Dubos, Pontoise, France

Jurg Steiger
University Hospital Basel, Basel, Switzerland

Volker Schoder, Peter Wabel, Adelheid Gauly, Rainer Himmele
Fresenius Medical Care Deutschland GmbH, Bad Homburg, Germany

Shirong Cao, Huiyang Li, Liping Xiong, Yi Zhou, Jinjin Fan, Xueqing Yu, Haiping Mao
Department of Nephrology, The First Affiliated Hospital, Sun Yat-sen University, Key Laboratory of Nephrology, Ministry of Health, Guangzhou, China

Shu Li
Department of Nephrology, The First Affiliated Hospital, Sun Yat-sen University, Key Laboratory of Nephrology, Ministry of Health, Guangzhou, China
Department of Rheumatology, The Second Xiangya Hospital, Central South University, Changsha, Hunan, China

Valentín Ceña
Unidad Asociada Neurodeath, Departamento de Ciencias Médicas, CSIC-Universidad de Castilla-La Mancha, Albacete, Spain
CIBERNED, Instituto de Salud Carlos III, Madrid, Spain

Juan Pérez-Martínez, Jesús Masiá, Agustín Ortega
Department of Nephrology, Complejo Hospitalario Universitario, Albacete, Spain

Francisco C. Pérez-Martínez, Blanca Carrión
Department of Research and Development, NanoDrugs, S.L., Parque Científico y Tecnoló gico, Albacete, Spain

Esther Simarro
Department of Clinical Chemistry, Complejo Hospitalario Universitario, Albacete, Spain

Syong H. Nam-Cha
Department of Pathology, Complejo Hospitalario Universitario, Albacete, Spain

Carolina Caballo, Marta Palomo, Ana M. Galán, Patricia Molina, Gines Escolar, Maribel Diaz-Ricart
Hemotherapy-Hemostasis Department, Centre de Diagnòstic Biomèdic, Institut d'Investigacions Biom èdiques August Pi i Sunyer, Hospital Clinic, Universitat de Barcelona, Barcelona, Spain

Aleix Cases, Manel Vera
Nephrology Department, Institut d'Investigacions Biomèdiques August Pi i Sunyer, Hospital Clinic, Universitat de Barcelona, Barcelona, Spain

Xavier Bosch
Cardiology Department, Institut d'Investigacions Biomèdiques August Pi i Sunyer, Hospital Clinic, Universitat de Barcelona, Barcelona, Spain

Qunying Guo, Chunyan Yi, Jianying Li, Xiaofeng Wu, Xiao Yang, Xueqing Yu
Department of Nephrology, The First Affiliated Hospital, Sun Yat-sen University, Guangzhou, Guangdong, China

Dong Eun Yoo, Jung Tak Park, Hyung Jung Oh, Seung Jun Kim, Mi Jung Lee, Dong Ho Shin, Seung Hyeok Han, Tae-Hyun Yoo, Kyu Hun Choi, Shin-Wook Kang
Department of Internal Medicine, College of Medicine, Brain Korea 21 for Medical Science, Severance Biomedical Science Institute, Yonsei University, Seoul, Korea

Jenq-Wen Huang, Chung-Jen Yen, Kuan-Yu Hung
Department of Internal Medicine, National Taiwan University College of Medicine and Hospital, Taipei, Taiwan

Chih-Kang Chiang
Department of Internal Medicine, National Taiwan University College of Medicine and Hospital, Taipei, Taiwan
Department of Integrated Diagnostics and Therapeutics, National Taiwan University College of Medicine and Hospital, Taipei, Taiwan

Hon-Yen Wu
Department of Internal Medicine, National Taiwan University College of Medicine and Hospital, Taipei, Taiwan
Department of Internal Medicine, Far Eastern Memorial Hospital, New Taipei City, Taiwan

Chun-Chun Pan, Tsai-Wei Hung
Department of Nursing, National Taiwan University College of Medicine and Hospital, Taipei, Taiwan

Yu-Chung Lien
Department of Internal Medicine, Buddhist Tzu Chi General Hospital, Taipei Branch, New Taipei City, Taiwan

Chi-Ting Su
Department of Internal Medicine, National Taiwan University College of Medicine and Hospital, Yun-Lin Branch, Yun-Lin County, Taiwan

Hui-Teng Cheng
Department of Internal Medicine, National Taiwan University College of Medicine and Hospital, Hsin-Chu Branch, Hsin Chu City, Taiwan

Rong Xu, Jie Dong, Hai-Yan Wang
Renal Division, Department of Medicine, Peking University First Hospital, Institute of Nephrology, Peking University, Key Laboratory of Renal Disease, Ministry of Health, Key Laboratory of Renal Disease, Ministry of Education, Beijing, China

Qing-Feng Han, Yue Wang
Department of Nephrology, Peking University Third Hospital, Beijing, China

Tong-Ying Zhu, Chuan-Ming Hao
Department of Nephrology, Huashan Hospital of Fudan University, Shanghai, China

Ye-Ping Ren, Rui Zhang
Department of Nephrology, Second Affiliated Hospital of Harbin Medical University, Heilongjiang, China

Jiang-Hua Chen, Xiao-Hui Zhang
Kidney Disease Center, The First Affiliated Hospital, College of Medicine, Zhejiang University, Hangzhou, China

Mei Wang, Hui-Ping Zhao
Department of Nephrology, Peking University People's Hospital, Beijing, China

Meng- Hua Chen, Na Tian
Department of Nephrology, General Hospital of Ningxia Medical University, Ningxia, China

Tae Ik Chang, Ea Wha Kang, Yong Kyu Lee, Sug Kyun Shin
Department of Internal Medicine, NHIC Medical Center, Ilsan Hospital, Goyangshi, Gyeonggi–do, Republic of Korea

Valèria C. Ferreira, Carlos F. M. A. Rodrigues
Nefroclínica de Uberlândia, Minas Gerais, Brazil

Sebastião R. Ferreira-Filho, Gilberto R. Machado
Nefroclínica de Uberlândia, Minas Gerais, Brazil
Federal University of Uberlândia, Minas Gerais, Brazil

Thyago Proenca de Moraes, Marcia Olandoski, Roberto Pecoits-Filho
Center for Health and Biological Sciences, Pontifícia Universidade Católica do Paraná, Curitiba, Brazil

Josè C. Divino-Filho
Baxter Healthcare, Division of Baxter Novum and Renal Medicine, CLINTEC, Karolinska Institute, Stockholm, Sweden

Christopher McIntyre
Faculty of Medicine & Health Sciences, University of Nottingham, Nottingham, United Kingdom

Ruchir Chavada, Sebastiaan van Hal
Department of Microbiology and Infectious Diseases, Sydney South West Pathology Service, Liverpool Hospital, Liverpool, Australia

Jen Kok, Sharon C-A. Chen
Centre for Infectious Diseases and Microbiology Laboratory Services, Institute of Clinical Pathology and Medical Research, Westmead Hospital, Westmead, Australia

Sander M. Hagen, Jeffrey A. Lafranca, Jan N. M. IJzermans, Frank J. M. F. Dor
Department of Surgery, Erasmus MC, University Medical Center, Rotterdam, The Netherlands

Ewout W. Steyerberg
Department of Public Health, Erasmus MC, University Medical Center, Rotterdam, The Netherlands

Chin-Chung Shu
Department of Traumatology, National Taiwan University Hospital, Taipei City, Taiwan
College of Internal Medicine, National Taiwan University, Taipei City, Taiwan

Vin-Cent Wu, Jann-Yuan Wang, Jann-Tay Wang
College of Internal Medicine, National Taiwan University, Taipei City, Taiwan
Department of Internal Medicine, National Taiwan University Hospital, Taipei City, Taiwan

Sung-Ching Pan
Department of Internal Medicine, National Taiwan University Hospital, Taipei City, Taiwan

Feng-Jung Yang
Department of Internal Medicine, National Taiwan University Hospital, Yun- Lin Branch, Yun-Lin County, Taiwan

Tai-Shuan Lai
Department of Internal Medicine, National Taiwan University Hospital, Bei-Hu Branch, Taipei City, Taiwan

Li-Na Lee
Department of Laboratory Medicine, National Taiwan University Hospital, Taipei City, Taiwan

Yu-Sen Peng
Department of Internal Medicine, Far Eastern Memorial Hospital, New Taipei City, Taiwan
Department of Internal Medicine, National Taiwan University Hospital, Taipei, Taiwan

Hon-Yen Wu
Department of Internal Medicine, Far Eastern Memorial Hospital, New Taipei City, Taiwan
Department of Internal Medicine, National Taiwan University Hospital, Taipei, Taiwan
Department of Internal Medicine, Yun-Lin Branch, National Taiwan University Hospital, Yun-Lin, Taiwan

Tzong-Shinn Chu, Tun-Jun Tsai, Kwan-Dun Wu, Jenq-Wen Huang, Shuei-Liong Lin
Department of Internal Medicine, National Taiwan University Hospital, Taipei, Taiwan

Kuan-Yu Hung
Department of Internal Medicine, National Taiwan University Hospital, Taipei, Taiwan
Center of Quality Management, National Taiwan University Hospital, Taipei, Taiwan

Yung-Ming Chen, Tao-Min Huang
Department of Internal Medicine, National Taiwan University Hospital, Taipei, Taiwan
Department of Internal Medicine, Yun-Lin Branch, National Taiwan University Hospital, Yun-Lin, Taiwan

Fu-Chang Hu
National Center of Excellence for General Clinical Trial and Research, National Taiwan University Hospital, Taipei, Taiwan
International Harvard Statistical Consulting Company, Taipei, Taiwan

Niko Braun, Joerg Latus, Martin Kimmel
Department of Internal Medicine, Division of General Internal Medicine and Nephrology, Robert-Bosch-Hospital, Stuttgart, Germany

M. Dominik Alscher
Department of Internal Medicine, Division of General Internal Medicine and Nephrology, Robert-Bosch-Hospital, Stuttgart, Germany
Institute of Digital Medicine, Stuttgart, Germany

Fabian Reimold
Department of Internal Medicine, Division of General Internal Medicine and Nephrology, Robert-Bosch-Hospital, Stuttgart, Germany
Division of Nephrology, Beth Israel Deaconess Medical Center, Department of Medicine, Harvard Medical School, Boston, United States of America

Peter Fritz
Institute of Digital Medicine, Stuttgart, Germany
Department of Diagnostic Medicine, Division of Pathology, Robert-Bosch-Hospital, Stuttgart, Germany

Rudolf P. Wüthrich
Division of Nephrology, University Hospital, Zurich, Switzerland

Ilka Edenhofer, Stephan Segerer
Division of Nephrology, University Hospital, Zurich, Switzerland
Institute of Anatomy, University of Zurich, Zurich, Switzerland

Maja Lindenmeyer, Clemens D. Cohen
Division of Nephrology, University Hospital, Zurich, Switzerland
Institute of Physiology, University of Zurich, Zurich, Switzerland

Seth L. Alper
Division of Nephrology, Beth Israel Deaconess Medical Center, Department of Medicine, Harvard Medical School, Boston, United States of America

Dagmar Biegger
Margarete Fischer-Bosch Institute of Clinical Pharmacology, University of Tuebingen, Stuttgart, Germany

Jacqueline C. T. Caramori, Alessandro L. Mondelli, Pasqual Barretti
Departamento de Clínica Médica, Faculdade de Medicina, UNESP - Universidade Estadual Paulista, Botucatu, São Paulo, Brazil

Taíse M. C. Moraes, Carlos H. Camargo, Augusto C. Montelli
Departamento de Clínica Médica, Faculdade de Medicina, UNESP - Universidade Estadual Paulista, Botucatu, São Paulo, Brazil
Departamento de Microbiologia e Imunologia, Instituto de Biociências, UNESP - Universidade Estadual Paulista, Botucatu, São Paulo, Brazil

Maria de Lourdes R. S. da Cunha
Departamento de Microbiologia e Imunologia, Instituto de Biociências, UNESP - Universidade Estadual Paulista, Botucatu, São Paulo, Brazil

Fabian R. Reimold
Renal Division, Beth Israel Deaconess Medical Center, Harvard Medical School, Boston, Massachusetts, United States of America
Department of Medicine, Harvard Medical School, Boston, Massachusetts, United States of America
Department of General Internal Medicine and Nephrology, Robert-Bosch Hospital, Stuttgart, Germany

S. Ananth Karumanchi, Seth L. Alper
Renal Division, Beth Israel Deaconess Medical Center, Harvard Medical School, Boston, Massachusetts, United States of America
Department of Medicine, Harvard Medical School, Boston, Massachusetts, United States of America
Center for Vascular Biology Research, Beth Israel Deaconess Medical Center and Harvard Medical School, Boston, Massachusetts, United States of America

Isaac E. Stillman
Renal Division, Beth Israel Deaconess Medical Center, Harvard Medical School, Boston, Massachusetts, United States of America
Department of Pathology, Beth Israel Deaconess Medical Center and Harvard Medical School, Boston, Massachusetts, United States of America

Hakan R. Toka
Renal Division, Beth Israel Deaconess Medical Center, Harvard Medical School, Boston, Massachusetts, United States of America
Division of Nephrology and Department of Medicine, Brigham and Women's Hospital and Harvard Medical School, Boston, Massachusetts, United States of America

Manoj K. Bhasin
Department of Medicine, Harvard Medical School, Boston, Massachusetts, United States of America
Division of Interdisciplinary Medicine and Biotechnology and Department of Medicine, Beth Israel Deaconess Medical Center and Harvard Medical School, Boston, Massachusetts, United States of America

Niko Braun, Joerg Latus, M. Dominik Alscher
Department of General Internal Medicine and Nephrology, Robert-Bosch Hospital, Stuttgart, Germany
Institute of Digital Medicine, Stuttgart, Germany

Zsuzsanna K. Zsengellér
Department of Pathology, Beth Israel Deaconess Medical Center and Harvard Medical School, Boston, Massachusetts, United States of America

Peter Fritz
Division of Pathology, Department of Diagnostic Medicine, Robert-Bosch Hospital, Stuttgart, Germany

Dagmar Biegger
Division of Pathology, Department of Diagnostic Medicine, Robert-Bosch Hospital, Stuttgart, Germany, Margarete Fischer-Bosch Institute of Clinical Pharmacology, Stuttgart, Germany

Stephan Segerer
Division of Nephrology, University Hospital Zurich, Zurich, Switzerland

Zhi-Kai Yang, Jie Dong, Hai-Yan Wang
Renal Division, Department of Medicine, Peking University First Hospital, Institute of Nephrology, Peking University, Key Laboratory of Renal Disease, Ministry of Health, Key Laboratory of Renal Disease, Ministry of Education, Beijing, China

Qing-Feng Han, Yue Wang
Department of Nephrology, Peking University Third Hospital, Beijing, China

Tong-Ying Zhu, Chuan- Ming Hao
Department of Nephrology, Huashan Hospital of Fudan University, Shanghai, China

Rui Zhang, Ye-Ping Ren
Department of Nephrology, Second Affiliated Hospital of Harbin Medical University, Heilongjiang, China

Jiang-Hua Chen, Xiao-Hui Zhang
Kidney Disease Center, The First Affiliated Hospital, College of Medicine, Zhejiang University, Hangzhou, China

Hui-Ping Zhao, Mei Wang
Department of Nephrology, Peking University People's Hospital, Beijing, China

Meng-Hua Chen, Na Tian
Department of Nephrology, General Hospital of Ningxia Medical University, Ningxia, China

Feng He, Xianfeng Wu, Xi Xia, Fenfen Peng, Fengxian Huang, Xueqing Yu
Department of Nephrology, The First Affiliated Hospital, Sun Yat-sen University, Guangzhou, China

Jie Dong, Rong Xu, Hai-Yan Wang
Renal Division, Department of Medicine, Peking University First Hospital; Institute of Nephrology, Peking University; Key Laboratory of Renal Disease, Ministry of Health; Key Laboratory of Renal Disease, Ministry of Education; Beijing, China

Qing-Feng Han, Yue Wang
Department of Nephrology, Peking University Third Hospital, Beijing, China

Tong-Ying Zhu, Chuan-Ming Hao
Department of Nephrology, Huashan Hospital of Fudan University, Shanghai, China

Ye-Ping Ren, Rui Zhang
Department of Nephrology, Second Affiliated Hospital of Harbin Medical University, Heilongjiang, China

Jiang-Hua Chen, Xiao-Hui Zhang
Kidney Disease Center, The First Affiliated Hospital, College of Medicine, Zhejiang University, Hangzhou, China

Hui-Ping Zhao, Mei Wang
Department of Nephrology, Peking University People's Hospital, Beijing, China

Meng-Hua Chen, Na Tian
Department of Nephrology, General Hospital of Ningxia Medical University, Ningxia, China

Cheng-Chia Lee, Chan-Yu Lin, Yung-Chang Chen, Ming-Yang Chang, Hsiang-Hao Hsu, Ji-Tseng Fang, Cheng-Chieh Hung, Chih- Wei Yang, Ya-Chung Tian, Shou-Hsuan Liu
Kidney Research Center, Department of Nephrology, Lin-Kou Chang Gung Memorial Hospital and Department of Medicine, Chang Gung University, Tao Yuan, Taiwan

Yi-Jung Li, Hsin-Hsu Wu, Cheng-Hao Weng
Kidney Research Center, Department of Nephrology, Lin-Kou Chang Gung Memorial Hospital and Department of Medicine, Chang Gung University, Tao Yuan, Taiwan
Graduate Institute of Clinical Medical Sciences, Chang Gung University, Tao Yuan, Taiwan

Szu-Ying Lee
Department of Internal Medicine, National Taiwan University Hospital, Yun-Lin Branch, Yunlin County, Taiwan

Yin-Cheng Chen, I-Chieh Tsai
Department of Internal Medicine, Department of Health, Taipei Hospital, Taiwan

Chung-Jen Yen, Kuan-Yu Hung, Jenq-Wen Huang
Department of Internal Medicine, National Taiwan University Hospital and College of Medicine, Taipei, Taiwan

Hon-Yen Wu
Department of Internal Medicine, National Taiwan University Hospital and College of Medicine, Taipei, Taiwan
Department of Internal Medicine, Far Eastern Memorial Hospital, New Taipei City, Taiwan,

Shu-Neng Chueh
Department of Nursing, National Taiwan University Hospital and College of Medicine, Taipei, Taiwan

Hsueh-Fang Chuang
Department of Nursing, National Taiwan University Hospital, Bei-Hu Branch, Taipei, Taiwan

Chih-Kang Chiang
Department of Integrated Diagnostics and Therapeutics, National Taiwan University Hospital and College of Medicine, Taipei, Taiwan

Hui-Teng Cheng
Department of Internal Medicine, National Taiwan University Hospital, Hsin-Chu Branch, Hsinchu City, Taiwan

Joerg Latus, Daniel Kitterer, M. Dominik Alscher, Niko Braun
Department of Internal Medicine, Division of Nephrology, Robert-Bosch-Hospital, Stuttgart, Germany

Sayed M. Habib, Michiel G. H. Betjes
Department of Internal Medicine, Division of Nephrology and Transplantation, Erasmus Medical Center, Rotterdam, The Netherlands

Mario R. Korte
Department of Internal Medicine, Division of Nephrology, Albert Schweitzer Hospital, Dordrecht, The Netherlands

Christoph Ulmer
Department of General, Visceral and Trauma Surgery, Robert-Bosch-Hospital, Stuttgart, Germany

Peter Fritz
Department of Diagnostic Medicine, Division of Pathology, Robert-Bosch Hospital, Stuttgart, Germany

Simon Davies
Institute for Science and Technology in Medicine, Keele University, Keele, United Kingdom

Mark Lambie
Department of Nephrology, University Hospital of North Staffordshire, Stoke-on-Trent, United Kingdom

Stephan Segerer
Division of Nephrology, University Hospital, Zurich, Switzerland

Qingdong Xu, Fenghua Xu, Li Fan, Liping Xiong, Huiyan Li, Shirong Cao, Xiaoyan Lin, Zhihua Zheng, Xueqing Yu, Haiping Mao
Department of Nephrology, The First Affiliated Hospital, Sun Yat-sen University, Key Laboratory of Nephrology, Ministry of Health of China, Guangzhou, China

Index

A

Albumin, 1, 3-4, 6-7, 11, 19, 33, 41-43, 45-48, 50, 52-53, 55, 57, 59-63, 65-70, 72-79, 82, 102-106, 113, 141, 146, 148-150, 162-164, 166, 172-178, 180-182, 197-201, 203

Albumin-corrected Fructosamine, 178, 181-182

All-cause Mortality, 51, 54-55, 57, 64, 88, 149, 154-155, 158-159, 161-168, 176-177, 196, 199-200, 202-203, 205

Antifungal Agent, 86-87, 89

Autoimmune Disease, 103-105, 170

B

Bacterial Peritonitis, 86-90, 131, 134, 188

Blood Urea Nitrogen, 52, 60-61, 63, 74, 110, 112-113, 134

Body Mass Index (BMI), 45, 52, 59-60, 67, 74, 81-82, 108, 148-149, 162, 172, 200

C

C-reactive Protein, 11, 26, 42, 52, 73-75, 77, 90, 116-117, 119-120, 146, 155-157, 159, 162, 164, 166-170, 172-177, 197, 200

Cardiac Dysfunction, 1, 41

Cardiac Event Rate, 41, 44, 48-49

Cardiovascular Disease, 32, 35, 37-40, 42, 44-45, 48, 51-54, 58, 66-69, 72-73, 75-78, 80, 83, 85, 133, 148, 150, 153-157, 160, 162, 164-167, 175-177, 196, 204-205

Chronic Dialysis, 22-24, 28-29, 113

Chronic Kidney Disease (CKD), 20, 32, 59, 80, 161, 178

Chronic Peritoneal Dialysis, 8, 26-27, 30, 49, 100, 114, 131-132, 136, 153, 177, 185, 194, 205

Coagulase-negative Staphylococcus (CONS), 125

Continuous Ambulatory Peritoneal Dialysis (CAPD), 11, 103, 145, 154, 180-181, 196

D

Diabetes Mellitus, 11, 44, 51, 57-58, 60, 62-63, 66-67, 75, 83-84, 88-89, 104-106, 108, 110-113, 125, 129, 148-150, 154-157, 159-160, 162, 168-169, 172-175, 178, 185

Diabetic Nephropathy, 51-52, 55-57, 69, 144, 149, 154-159, 163, 197

Diabetic Patients, 31, 38, 46-47, 51, 55, 57-58, 129, 154, 169, 176, 185-186

Diastolic Blood Pressure, 3, 54, 155-157, 162-164, 197

E

Edema, 7, 11, 41, 43, 45-46, 48, 60, 80-85

Encapsulating Peritoneal Sclerosis (EPS), 115, 132, 187, 195

End-stage Renal Disease (ESRD), 32, 51, 73, 91, 108, 154, 161, 198

End-stage Renal Failure, 22, 26, 50

Endothelial Activation and Damage, 32-38

Euvolemia, 1, 7-8

F

Fibronectin 1, 132, 134, 139, 142-143

Fluconazole, 86-87, 89-90

Fluid Overload, 1-4, 7-8, 41-43, 46, 48-49, 80, 85

Fluid Status, 1-2, 4, 7-8, 39, 41-42, 45, 47-50, 80, 85, 204

Fungal Peritonitis, 19, 86-90

G

Glucose Concentration, 19, 38, 42-43, 45, 47, 49, 108-113, 179-181, 184-185, 198

Glycemic Control, 7, 51-53, 55-58, 178-183, 185

Glycosylated Hemoglobin, 58, 178, 182, 185

H

Hemoglobin, 3-4, 11, 33, 43, 52-54, 58, 65-70, 81, 103, 110-111, 134, 141, 148-150, 155-157, 162-163, 166, 168-169, 172-176, 178, 180, 182, 185-186, 197-201, 203-204

Human Immunodeficiency Virus, 103

Hyperlipidemia, 32, 37, 146, 161-162

Hypertension, 6-9, 31-33, 41-42, 48-50, 52, 71, 73, 75, 80-81, 84-85, 88, 116-117, 122-123, 134, 144, 155-158, 161-162, 165, 167, 204

Hypervolemia, 1, 8, 80

Hypoalbuminemia, 73, 75-78, 84, 103, 106, 168, 176

I

Incident Peritoneal Dialysis, 71, 78-80, 153, 196, 205

Initial-episode Peritonitis, 147, 149, 152

K

Kidney Transplantation, 48, 145, 155, 168, 172, 175, 188, 193-195

L

Latent Tuberculosis Infection (ltbi), 102, 105

Lean Body Mass, 59-64, 74-77, 113, 142

Liver Cirrhosis, 103, 109

Long-term Glucose Load, 108, 111, 114, 185

Lymphatic Endothelial Cells, 115, 118, 124, 193

M

Mortality Rate, 60, 86, 89, 102, 154, 168, 172, 175, 199, 203-204

Myocardial Infarction, 31, 44-45, 67-69, 74, 148, 155, 162-163, 168, 170, 172, 176, 200

Myofibroblasts, 115, 117, 119, 121, 123, 143

N

Nfkb, 32-34, 36-39, 139
Nuclear Protein, 10, 13, 20

O

Osmotic Agent, 22, 37
Oxacillin Resistance, 125, 128, 131

P

Pd Catheter Insertion, 91, 93-94, 96-98
Peripheral Arterial Disease, 67-69, 78, 148, 155, 162-163, 167
Peritoneal Biopsies, 115, 117-120, 122, 124, 187-188, 192
Peritoneal Dialysis (PD), 1, 10, 22, 35-36, 51, 59, 65, 73, 80, 86, 91, 102, 108, 115, 125, 132-133, 147, 155, 161, 168, 178, 184, 187, 196
Peritoneal Equilibration Test, 8, 19, 26, 28-29, 60, 74, 78, 109-110, 113-114, 170, 172, 174-175, 179, 186, 198
Peritoneal Fibrosis, 22, 27, 31, 121, 132-133, 136, 141, 143-146, 195
Peritoneal Inflammation, 10, 12, 14-15, 78, 146, 177
Peritoneal Membrane, 3, 7, 9-10, 22, 24, 26, 28-31, 73, 78, 84, 115, 145-146, 170, 174, 176-177, 179, 181, 188, 192, 194-195
Peritoneal Mesothelial Cell Line, 10-11, 19
Peritoneal Protein Clearance, 73-78
Peritoneal Solute Transport Rate, 73, 169, 177
Peritoneal Tissue, 122, 132-133, 141, 143-144, 193
Peritonitis, 10-17, 19-21, 38, 52, 59-60, 62, 65, 67-72, 86-91, 93-94, 96, 99-101, 110, 116-117, 119, 121-131, 134, 141, 145, 147-149, 152-153, 170, 176-177, 187-190, 197, 205
Pneumonia, 52, 154-160

Pneumonia-related Mortality, 154-155, 157-159
Podoplanin Expression, 115, 117, 119-120, 122, 124, 195
Primary Renal Disease, 19, 52, 56, 67, 122, 148, 162-163
Protein Catabolic Rate, 52-53, 59-61, 63, 74-77, 180
Protein-energy Wasting, 41-42, 48-50, 59, 64, 78, 177
Pulse Pressure, 3, 73-75, 77, 79

R

Renal Replacement Therapy, 59, 71, 80, 85, 88, 114, 132, 152, 172, 178, 194
Renin Angiotensin Aldosterone System (RAAS), 133
Renin-angiotensin-aldosterone System, 22, 31
Residual Renal Function, 2, 7-8, 33, 38, 42-45, 48-50, 53-54, 59-64, 66-69, 74, 83-85, 91, 100, 103, 108, 114, 131, 136, 148, 150, 162, 164, 172-173, 179, 194, 204-205

S

S. Aureus Peritonitis, 125-131
Staphylococcus Aureus, 125, 127, 129, 131, 189
Systemic Arterial Hypertension (SAH), 80
Systolic Blood Pressure, 1, 3-7, 41-42, 45-49, 156-157, 164, 197

T

Thrombospondin 1, 132, 134, 139, 142-143
Tunnel Infection, 93, 96

U

Ultrafiltration, 1-4, 6-7, 9, 12, 15, 22, 26, 29-30, 42-43, 45, 48-50, 68-69, 81, 85, 108, 110, 113, 133, 178, 180, 184-185, 190, 193-194, 197-198
Uremia, 32-35, 38, 40, 116, 141, 144, 160-163, 166, 177-178, 181, 195
Uric Acid, 52, 161, 163-167, 169, 172-174